The Kidney
and Body Fluids in
Health and Disease

The Kidney and Body Fluids in Health and Disease

Edited by
SAULO KLAHR, M.D.

Washington University School of Medicine
St. Louis, Missouri

SPRINGER SCIENCE+BUSINESS MEDIA, LLC

Library of Congress Cataloging in Publication Data

Main entry under title:

The Kidney and body fluids in health and disease.

Includes bibliographies and index.
1. Kidneys—Diseases. 2. Body fluid disorders. 3. Kidneys. I. Klahr, Saulo.
[DNLM: 1. Body fluids. 2. Kidney—Physiology. 3. Kidney dis-
eases—Physiopathology. 4. Water–electrolyte balance. 5. Water–electrolyte im-
balance—Physiopathology. WJ 300 K455]
RC903.K45 1983   616.6'1   82-15128
ISBN 978-1-4613-3526-9   ISBN 978-1-4613-3524-5   (eBook)
DOI 10.1007/978-1-4613-3524-5

© 1983 Springer Science+Business Media New York
Originally published by Plenum Publishing Corporation in 1983
Softcover reprint of the hardcover 1st edition 1983

This book is dedicated to the memory of

Dr. Carl V. Moore

Chairman, Department of Internal Medicine
Washington University School of Medicine
St. Louis, Missouri
1955–1972

Contributors

Elsa Bello-Reuss, M.D., Assistant Professor of Medicine, Departments of Medicine, and Physiology and Biophysics, Washington University School of Medicine and The Jewish Hospital of St. Louis, St. Louis, Missouri 63110

John Buerkert, M.D., Associate Professor of Medicine, Department of Medicine, Washington University School of Medicine and The Jewish Hospital of St. Louis, St. Louis, Missouri 63110

Barbara R. Cole, M.D., Associate Professor of Pediatrics, Department of Pediatrics, Washington University School of Medicine, St. Louis, Missouri 63110

James A. Delmez, M.D., Assistant Professor of Medicine, Department of Medicine, Washington University School of Medicine, St. Louis, Missouri 63110

Jeffrey Freitag, M.D., Chief Medical Resident, Department of Medicine, Washington University School of Medicine, St. Louis, Missouri 63110. *Present address:* Saginaw General Hospital, Saginaw, Michigan 48602

Herschel R. Harter, M.D., Associate Professor of Medicine, Department of Medicine, Washington University School of Medicine, St. Louis, Missouri 63110

Phillip Hoffsten, M.D., Assistant Professor of Medicine, Department of Medicine, Washington University School of Medicine, St. Louis, Missouri 63110. *Present address:* Medical Associates Clinic, Pierre, South Dakota 57501

Keith Hruska, M.D., Associate Professor of Medicine, Department of Medicine, Washington University School of Medicine and The Jewish Hospital of St. Louis, St. Louis, Missouri 63110

Saulo Klahr, M.D., Professor of Medicine, Department of Medicine, Washington University School of Medicine, St. Louis, Missouri 63110

Kevin Martin, M.D., Assistant Professor of Medicine, Department of Medicine, Washington University School of Medicine, St. Louis, Missouri 63110

Aubrey R. Morrison, M.D., Assistant Professor of Medicine and Pharmacology, Departments of Medicine and Pharmacology, Washington University School of Medicine, St. Louis, Missouri 63110

Luis Reuss, M.D., Professor of Physiology and Biophysics, Department of Physiology and Biophysics, Washington University School of Medicine, St. Louis, Missouri 63110

Alan M. Robson, M.D., Professor of Pediatrics, Department of Pediatrics, Washington University School of Medicine, St. Louis, Missouri 63110

Hector J. Rodriguez, M.D., Ph.D., Assistant Professor of Medicine, Department of Medicine, Washington University School of Medicine, St. Louis, Missouri 63110. *Present address:* 9400 Brighton Way, Beverly Hills, California 90210

Eduardo Slatopolsky, M.D., Professor of Medicine, Department of Medicine, Washington University School of Medicine, St. Louis, Missouri 63110

Andres J. Valdes, M.D., Clinical Assistant Professor of Pathology and Associate Pathologist and Director of Clinical Immunology, Department of Pathology, Washington University School of Medicine and St. John's Mercy Medical Center, St. Louis, Missouri 63110

Preface

This volume was designed as a text for medical students, house officers, and even clinicians. It deals with the most common problems in nephrology, providing new insight into how to improve clinical skills. A comprehensive overview of renal physiology and electrolyte disorders lays the groundwork for a clear presentation of the pathophysiological principles that underlie these disorders and a step-by-step presentation of the mechanisms behind the signs and symptoms of kidney failure.

The origins of this book can be traced to the teaching of a Renal Pathophysiology course at the Washington University School of Medicine, beginning in the mid-1960s. When changes in the medical school curriculum took place in the early 1970s, an effort was made to synthesize the minimum core curriculum for sophomore medical students, and the distillation of "essential material" to be covered in the area of renal pathophysiology led to the development of the first edition of a renal syllabus. This syllabus has been used in our department since 1974, and, following some of the recommendations and critiques of students and faculty, it has been entirely reworked many times to improve its effectiveness and value.

This book is a direct extension of that syllabus, integrated with contributions from faculty members in our Renal Division, and expanded to include a section on therapy in most chapters. It is our hope that this format will serve the needs of not only sophomore and senior medical students, but also house officers, nephrology fellows, and clinicians.

The book is divided into seven sections. Section I describes the basic concepts of fluid, electrolyte, and renal physiology and comprises three chapters entitled "Introduction to the Physiology of Body Fluids," "Homeostatic and Excretory Functions of the Kidney," and "Nonexcretory Functions of the Kidney." The second section discusses the pathophysiology of fluid and electrolyte disorders, including the regulation of volume sodium metabolism, the development of edema and edema-forming states, the pathophysiological basis for alterations in water balance, the pathophysiology of potassium metabolism, the pathophysiology of acid–base metabolism, and the pathophysiology of calcium, magnesium, and phosphorus metabolism. Section III comprises a single chapter devoted to the pathophysiology of hypertension. Section IV, "Pathophysiology of Proteinuric Renal Disease," is divided into two chapters, "Proteinuria and the Nephrotic Syndrome" and "Pathology and Pathophysiology of Proteinuric Glomerular Disease." Section V, "Renal Failure," contains chapters on the pathophysiology of acute renal failure, the pathophysiology of chronic renal failure, and the pathophysiological principles underlying the treatment of patients with renal failure. Section VI contains a single chapter, "Pathophysiology of Nephrolithiasis," and Section VII discusses renal pharmacology.

Every attempt has been made to make the chapters uniform. No attempt has been made to be comprehensive and exhaustive, but we believe that most of the fundamental developments in each field have been included. All the authors of this book are or have been affiliated with the Washington University School of Medicine; most of them have been long-standing members of the Division of Pediatric or Renal Medicine at Washington University, a fact that greatly facilitated the writing and editing of this book. We hope that our readers will find this volume useful, and look forward to their constructive criticism for use in future editions.

Saulo Klahr, M.D.

Contents

2. Homeostatic and Excretory Functions of the Kidney

Elsa Bello-Reuss and Luis Reuss

3. Nonexcretory Functions of the Kidney

Saulo Klahr

II. Pathophysiology of Fluid and Electrolyte Disorders

4. Pathophysiology of Volume Regulation and Sodium Metabolism

Elsa Bello-Reuss

5. Edema and Edema-Forming States
Alan M. Robson

6. The Pathophysiologic Bases for Alterations in Water Balance
John Buerkert

7. Pathophysiology of Potassium Metabolism
Hector J. Rodriguez and Saulo Klahr

8. Pathophysiology of Acid–Base Metabolism

Keith Hruska

9. Pathophysiology of Calcium, Magnesium, and Phosphorus Metabolism

Eduardo Slatopolsky

III. Pathophysiology of Hypertension

10. Pathophysiology of Hypertension
Herschel R. Harter

IV. Pathophysiology of Proteinuric Renal Disease

11. Proteinuria and the Nephrotic Syndrome
Alan M. Robson

12. Pathology and Pathophysiology of Proteinuric Glomerular Disease

Barbara R. Cole and Andres J. Valdes

V. Renal Failure

13. Pathophysiology of Acute Renal Failure

Kevin Martin

14. Pathophysiology of Chronic Renal Failure

Phillip Hoffsten and Saulo Klahr

15. Pathophysiological Principles in the Treatment of Patients with Renal Failure

James A. Delmez

VI. Pathophysiology of Nephrolithiasis

16. Pathophysiology of Nephrolithiasis

Jeffrey Freitag and Keith Hruska

VII. Renal Pharmacology

17. Renal Pharmacology

Aubrey R. Morrison

I

Basic Concepts of Fluid, Electrolyte, and Renal Physiology

In multicellular higher organisms the cells are bathed by an extracellular fluid *(ECF) or internal medium whose volume and composition are finely regulated within a narrow range. Normal cell function and life itself depend on the maintenance of the volume and composition of the ECF.*

The ECF is distributed in two compartments: intravascular (plasma) and interstitial. These compartments and the intracellular fluid (ICF) are in dynamic equilibrium, but are also independent of one another because of the different properties of the membranes (barriers) between them. Plasma volume is important for circulation and therefore for assuring adequate rates of both supply of nutrients to all cells and removal of potentially toxic products of cell function. The composition of the extracellular fluid influences directly the function of some cells. For instance, changes of extracellular potassium concentration have important effects on cell membrane potentials, and therefore alter the function of excitable cells, and can also exert effects on the composition of the intracellular fluid. For example, if the osmolality of the extracellular fluid falls, because of a reduction of total concentration of solute particles, a net water flux ensues toward the cell interior, with the end result of dilution of the intracellular fluid and alteration of a number of cell functions.

Homeostasis of water and electrolytes results from a number of complicated negative feedback mechanisms which include the participation of the central nervous system, the endocrine system, and the kidney.

This section is divided into three chapters: Chapter 1 deals with the physiology of body fluids (distribution, composition and general mechanisms of regulation of both), Chapter 2 discusses the homeostatic and excretory functions of the kidney, and Chapter 3 the nonexcretory functions of the kidney.

Introduction to the Physiology of Body Fluids

LUIS REUSS and ELSA BELLO-REUSS

I. HOMEOSTASIS OF WATER AND ELECTROLYTES: AN OVERVIEW

Life of complicated pluricellular organisms depends upon the preservation of a very narrow range of volume and composition of body fluids. Water, inorganic substances, and organic molecules are taken up from the external medium and distributed in one or more body fluid compartments. Some of them are eventually utilized for energy production, growth, and repair. Others, such as water and electrolytes, provide the environment in which the physical and chemical processes characteristic of cell, tissue, and organ function take place.

Epithelial tissues, such as the lining of the gastrointestinal tract and the renal tubule, function as both limiting barriers and pathways for transport between body and external world. Their function is oriented to maintain constant the volume and composition of body fluids by adjusting the rates of uptake and excretion of a number of substances and by preventing

LUIS REUSS • Department of Physiology and Biophysics, Washington University School of Medicine, St. Louis, Missouri 63110.   ELSA BELLO-REUSS • Departments of Medicine, and Physiology and Biophysics, Washington University School of Medicine and The Jewish Hospital of St. Louis, St. Louis, Missouri 63110.

accumulation of materials produced by cell metabolism which can eventually be toxic. The concept of *homeostasis*, introduced by Claude Bernard, refers to this condition, or dynamic equilibrium between inflow and outflow, in which volume and composition of body fluids remain constant. This equilibrium is attained by negative feedback mechanisms which include the participation of the central nervous system, the endocrine system, and transport organs such as the intestine and the kidney.

As a first approximation, body fluids are distributed in two major compartments: *intracellular* and *extracellular*. The barrier separating them is the *cell membrane* or plasmalemma. The extracellular fluid is distributed in two subcompartments: *intravascular* (plasma) and *extravascular* (interstitial fluid and lymph), anatomically separated by the *capillary endothelium*. These two subcompartments are in dynamic equilibrium, similar to the equilibrium between ECF and ICF. The properties and function of the barriers—cell membranes and capillary endothelium—are essential in the maintenance of normal exchanges between these compartments.

In the first two chapters of this book water and electrolyte metabolism will be reviewed from a physiologic point of view.

Chapter 1 deals with the problems of volume, distribution, and composition of body fluids. The specific mechanisms of regulation of water and electrolyte balance are treated later in the text. An Appendix has been added at the end of the chapter in which membrane transport processes relevant to the subject matter of Chapter 1 are treated in some detail. The material covered in this Appendix includes the different mechanisms of transport and the effects of concentration differences across biological membranes, i.e., Gibbs–Donnan equilibrium and membrane electrical potentials. The treatment is elementary, with a minimum of equations. The reader is advised to review this section and decide whether its detailed study is necessary.

Chapters 2 and 3 are reviews of renal physiology, from the point of view of homeostatic and excretory functions (Chapter 2) and from the point of view of metabolic and endocrine functions (Chapter 3). Again, these chapters are introductory to the study of renal pathophysiology and are intended to refresh and stress essential notions to be used in the later chapters, devoted to abnormal processes.

II. BODY WATER: VOLUME AND DISTRIBUTION

Water, the most abundant molecular component of living matter, is a very appropriate solvent for many ions and nonelectrolytes present both inside and outside cells. Water allows fast diffusion of most solutes and, because of its high dielectric constant, reduces the field between ions of opposite charge, thereby increasing their mobility. The high heat capacity, heat conductivity, and heat of evaporation of water make it very important for body temperature regulation.

Water makes up 40%–80% of total body weight in humans. The main variable affecting this percentage is the amount of fat (adipose tissue contains little water), which varies with age, sex, and nutritional status. Typical total body water values for males are 75% at birth, 60% from one year of age to middle age, and about 50% after middle age. Values for females are about 5% lower from puberty to old age, because of a relatively higher fat content. Obesity reduces and leanness increases these percentages at any age, in either sex.

Water is distributed in several compartments. The measurement of the volume of these compartments is accomplished by the use of the *indicator-dilution technique*. A substance known or presumed to distribute in one or several compartments is administered and its concentration in serum is measured until equilibrium is reached. At this time, the volume of distribution of the substance can be determined from the following equation:

$$V_d = \frac{C_a V_a - C_e V_e}{C_d}$$

where V_d is the volume of distribution, $C_a V_a$ is the administered amount (concentration $\times$ volume), $C_e V_e$ is the excreted amount (usually by the kidneys), and C_d is the final, steady state serum concentration.

Examples of indicators are deuterium oxide (total body water), inulin (extracellular fluid), and red cells tagged with ^{51}Cr (intravascular volume). Compartments not directly measurable can be calculated from substraction of the above ones.

On the basis of both anatomic and kinetic considerations, Edelman and Leibman proposed the distribution scheme shown in Figure 1A.

The main compartments are as follows:

1. *Intracellular fluid (ICF)*, bounded by the cell membranes, contained in cells of soft tissues, equivalent to 55% of body water.
2. *Extracellular fluid (ECF)*, separated from the external medium by epithelia, and from the ICF by the cell membranes. Its volume is about 27.5% of body water. The ECF is subdivided into an intravascular compartment (plasma, contained inside the endothelial membranes) and an interstitial-lymph compartment in contact with most cells. They represent 7.5% and 20% of total body water, respectively.

Although also extracellular, the following two compartments are better considered separately.

3. *Slowly exchanging water compartments*, which include dense connective tissue, cartilage, and bone. Their sum corresponds to about 15% of total body water.
4. *Transcellular fluids*, whose composition is influenced by transepithelial transport, and in most cases are not really inside the body. They can be, however, a reservoir for the extracellular space, and are, ob-

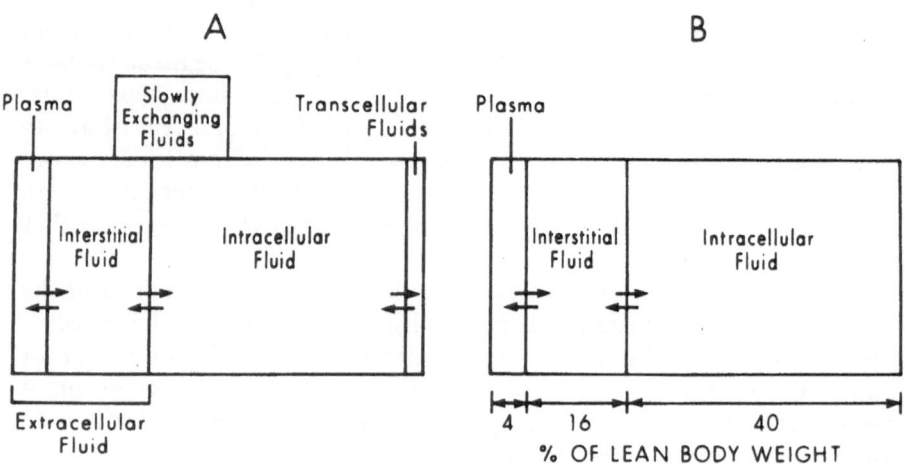

Figure 1. Body fluid compartments. Diagram (A) shows the distribution described by Edelman and Leibman. Diagram (B) is a simplified scheme applicable to clinical situations. Volumes of the main compartments are given as percents of lean body weight.

viously, a part of body weight. Under normal conditions, the only two transcellular fluids of quantitative importance are the gastrointestinal contents and the intratubular fluid and urine present in the kidneys and lower urinary tract. Transcellular fluids, which also include cerebrospinal and ocular fluids, normally amount to 2.5% of total body water.

Edelman's distribution can be simplified, for practical purposes (mainly clinical considerations), to the diagram shown in Figure 1B, where the ICF is two thirds and the ECF is one third of total body water. One fourth of the ECF is plasma and three fourths are interstitial fluid and lymph. The barriers are the cell membranes (between ICF and ECF) and the vascular endothelium (between plasma and interstitial fluid). Skin and other epithelia provide the barrier between the body and the external medium, with or without an interposed transcellular fluid.

III. IONIC COMPOSITION OF BODY FLUIDS

Concentrations of ions in body fluids are best expressed in millimoles or milliequivalents per kilogram H_2O (molal concentration) because these units indicate real concentrations in the solvent, and therefore reflect the chemical activity of the solute. Because of practical considerations, however, concentrations are usually measured per liter of solution (molar concentration). Under normal conditions the difference between molal and molar concentration is negligible, but if a large fraction of the solution is made up by solids (e.g., proteins, lipids) ion concentrations can be significantly underestimated. In such a case, the molal concentration of Na (mEq/kg H_2O) will be far larger than its molar concentration (mEq/liter plasma).

A. Ionic Composition of the Main Two Subcompartments of the Extracellular Fluid

The average normal electrolyte concentrations in the ECF are shown in Table I. The main common characteristics of plasma and interstitial fluid are as follows: (1) The main cation is Na^+, which, together with the accompanying anions, accounts for most of the osmolality of both fluids. (2) The concentrations of K^+, Ca^{2+}, and Mg^{2+} are small, although extremely important: consider the influence of $[K^+]_{out}$ on the electrical potential of most cells, and the effect of $[Ca^{2+}]_{out}$ on neuromuscular excitability. (3) Cl^- and HCO_3^- are the principal anions. Besides its osmotic role, HCO_3^- is the anion of the main extracellular buffer. Among anions present at lower concentrations, phosphate plays an important role in renal excretion of acid.

The most important composition differences between plasma and interstitial fluid are the following: (1) the higher protein concentration in plasma (proteins permeate slowly the vascular endothelium); (2) ionic asymmetries resulting from the Gibbs–Donnan equilibrium (see Appendix) caused by the protein concentration difference across the vascular wall, reflected in Na, Cl, and HCO_3 concentration differences between the two compartments; and (3) lower interstitial concentrations of divalent cations, because of partial binding to plasma proteins.

Table I. Average Normal Electrolyte Concentrations in Extracellular Fluid

Electrolyte	Concentration (mEq/liter)	
	Plasma[a]	Interstitial fluid[b]
Cations		
Na^+	142	145
K^+	4	4
Ca^{2+}	5	
Mg^{2+}	2	
Anions		
Cl^-	103	114
HCO_3^-	26	31
Phosphate	1	
Sulfate	1	
Proteins	16	
Organic acids	6	

[a] Plasma osmolality, 289 mOsm/kg; plasma pH, 7.40.
[b] Values of divalent and polyvalent ions in interstitial fluid are uncertain.

Table II. Electrolyte Concentrations in
Intracellular Fluid

Electrolyte	Concentration (mEq/liter)
Cations	
K^+	155
Mg^{2+}	26
Na^+	10
Ca^{2+}	3
Anions	
Cl^-	3
HCO_3^-	10
Organic phosphate	95
Sulfate	20
Proteins	55

B. Ionic Composition of the Intracellular Fluid

Electrolyte concentrations in the ICF are difficult to measure accurately because of the problems involved in obtaining large samples uncontaminated by ECF. In any event, rather large differences exist among different cells types, e.g., the high Cl concentration of red cells, which is an exception to the rule of low Cl concentration in the ICF. In addition, the ICF is not a homogeneous fluid, as is the ECF. Different subcellular compartments have diverse ionic compositions. An average representative analysis of human ICF, with emphasis on skeletal muscle, is shown in Table II.

The prominent features, as compared to the composition of the ECF, are that K^+ is the principal cation, having an osmotic role similar to the one of Na^+ in the ECF, that Mg^{2+} is far more concentrated than in the ECF, that Cl^- and HCO_3^- concentrations are very low (the main intracellular anions are proteins and organic phosphate ions), and that large fractions of intracellular divalent cations are bound. The large differences in ionic composition of ECF and ICF, combined with the selective permeability of the cell membranes to some ions, result in an electrical potential difference across the cell membrane. In most cases, the cell is 50–90 millivolts (mV) negative to the ECF.

C. Osmolality of Body Fluids

Osmolality and osmolarity are expressions of the total concentration of solute per kilogram of water (osmolality) or per liter of solution (osmolarity). The osmotic effect of a solute is independent of its charge and only related to the concentration of particles. *Osmole* is a unit of amount of solute, equivalent to 1 mole if the solute is not dissociated. The common unit is the *milliosmole* (mOsm). It follows that 1 mmole of urea is equivalent to 1 mOsm, whereas 1 mmole of NaCl is equivalent to 2 mOsm.

The largest portions of both ECF and ICF osmolality are contributed by the electrolytes present in these compartments: sodium salts in the ECF and potassium salts in the ICF. Since the membranes of most cells are highly permeable to water, the osmolality of the ICF is equal to that of the ECF. Addition of solute or water, or removal of solute or water from either side of a water-permeable membrane, results in rapid water flow through the membrane, until a new osmotic equilibrium is reached.

IV. BALANCE OF WATER AND ELECTROLYTES

A. Concept of Balance

Normally, the volume and composition of body fluids remain essentially constant, i.e., the gains of ions and water are equal to the losses and hence the net balance is zero. Under normal conditions water or ion balance can be different from zero only transiently. Physiological feedback mechanisms tend to bring back the two parameters to the steady state condition. Disregarding the positive water and electrolyte balance which is part of the growth process, persistent deviations from zero balance are abnormal.

B. Pathways of Gains and Losses

There are two normal sources of water gain: (1) water intake (as such, in fluids, or as a constituent of solid food) and (2) metabolic water production (water being produced by catabolism of carbohydrates, proteins, and lipids). Per unit weight, lipids yield more water than carbohydrates and proteins.

Water losses can be classified as (1) insensible (evaporation through respiratory tract and skin) or (2) sensible (urine, feces).

Rough estimates of the magnitude of water gains and losses in a healthy adult, in a balanced diet and in moderate weather, are presented in Figure 2.

The electrolytes and other solutes present in body fluids are, as water, normally maintained in a zero-balance condition.

The gains of electrolytes are usually dependent only on the intake. Normally, virtually all of the losses are by means of urinary and fecal excretion. Approximate gains and losses of cations in normal adults, in an average diet, are shown in Figure 3. Urinary excretion of both Na and K is more than 90% of the total losses, whereas in the case of Ca and Mg fecal losses, which are due in part to incomplete gastrointestinal absorption of these cations, constitute the largest fraction of total excretion.

In general, monovalent anion balances are closely related to monovalent cation balances. Under physiologic conditions, Cl^- balance follows Na^+ balance. However, in certain pathologic situations in which HCO_3^- balance is perturbed, the close relationship between Na^+ and Cl^- can be lost.

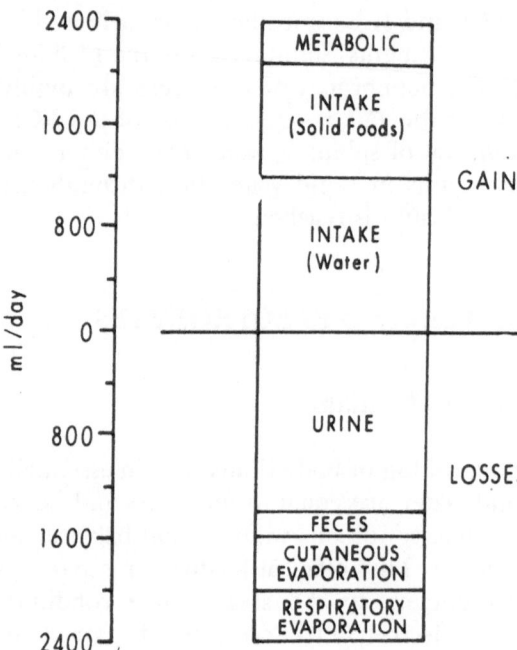

Figure 2. Water balance under normal conditions, in a benign climate. Water gains consist of intake (fluids and water contained in solid foods) and metabolic (oxidative) production. Water losses are sensible (urine and feces) and insensible (cutaneous and respiratory evaporation). Water evaporation depends on ambient temperature and humidity.

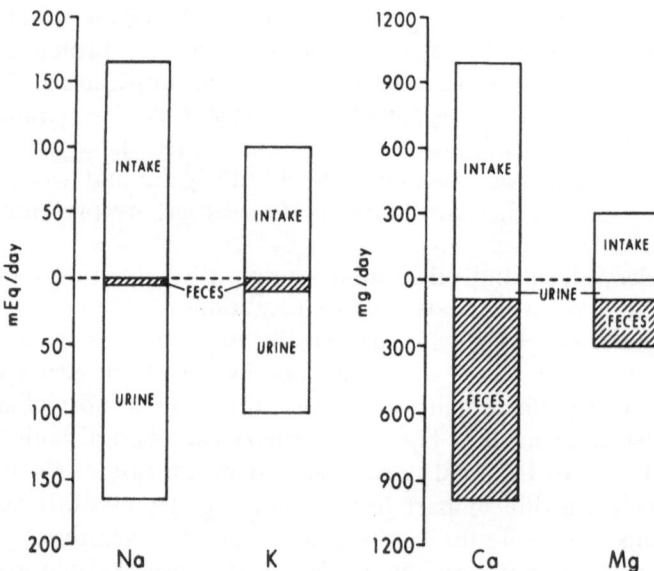

Figure 3. Cation balance under normal conditions in an average Western World diet. The main pathway for losses of Na and K is the urine, whereas the main pathway for losses of Ca and Mg is the feces.

It must be stressed that this description of balances of water and electrolytes is a simplified view that holds only under strictly physiologic conditions in a benign environment. The relative importances of different pathways for gains or losses can be drastically altered by changes in the environmental conditions or by disease. In pathologic and therapeutic conditions, other pathways of gains and losses of water and electrolytes have to be considered in addition to those illustrated in Figures 2 and 3. Abnormal pathways for gains include tube feeding, intravenous administration, and dialysis; abnormal pathways for losses include sweating, vomiting, diarrhea, drainage, fistulas, fluid suction from gastrointestinal tract, and dialysis.

C. Overview of the Mechanisms of Regulation of Salt and Water Balance

Although detailed discussions of the control mechanisms of water and electrolyte balance are presented in several other chapters of this book, an introduction to these mechanisms is appropriate here.

1. Control of Salt Balance

Sodium salts are the principal osmotic component of the extracellular fluid. The amount of sodium in the extracellular fluid determines not only the ECF volume but total body water as well. The cell membranes are in general highly permeable to water. Therefore, changes of osmotic pressure secondary to alterations in the extracellular amount of sodium salts cause changes not only in water intake but also in net water fluxes between extracellular and intracellular compartments, and the osmolalities of the two spaces are kept equal. The end result of these processes is a direct relationship between ECF volume and total ECF sodium mass: the volume of the ECF depends on the amount of ECF sodium salts. Quite correctly, the mechanisms of regulation of sodium balance are usually referred to as the *mechanisms of ECF volume regulation.*

The end point of the physiologic control of sodium balance is to keep the amount in the ECF constant. In principle, this can be achieved by regulation of the intake, the excretion, or both.

It is uncertain whether sodium intake is regulated in man under normal conditions. It is known, however, that in pathophysiologic states, such as adrenal insufficiency, a preference for high salt foods develops.

The *main mechanism* of regulation of Na balance is the control of Na excretion. Although sodium is excreted also in feces, the principal pathway for excretion is the urine. This fraction is regulated physiologically by feedback mechanisms signaled by ECF volume changes. Primary changes in Na balance result in alterations of ECF volume in the same direction. These, in turn, are sensed by specific receptors, which change their activity and hence modify renal Na excretion. Several kinds of receptors are thought to participate in these responses: intra- and extravascular baroreceptors, distension or flow receptors, and chemoreceptors.

Sodium excretion by the kidneys is regulated by changes in the filtered load and the rate of tubular reabsorption. The filtered load of sodium is equal to the product of plasma Na concentration and the rate of glomerular filtration (GFR). GFR is physiologically regulated by sympathetic activity, which controls the degree of renal vasoconstriction. With negative salt balance, the fall in arterial pressure results in an increase of sympathetic activity and in a reduction of both GFR and filtered load of Na. GFR is referred to as the *first factor* in the control of Na balance. The *second factor* is the adrenocortical hormone aldosterone, whose secretion is controlled principally by the renin–angiotensin system. Negative sodium balance causes increases of plasma renin and angiotensin, stimulation of aldosterone secretion, and increased Na reabsorption by the distal and collecting segments of the renal tubule.

A number of factors other than GFR and aldosterone are known or presumed to modify renal sodium excretion. They are collectively referred to as the *third factor*, and include (1) hydrostatic and colloid-osmotic pressure differences across the tubule wall, (2) a possible natriuretic hormone, (3) changes in the distribution of renal blood flow, and (4) direct effects of catecholamines on tubule transport. The importance of these mechanisms is uncertain at present.

2. Control of Water Balance

As ECF volume is ultimately the parameter regulated by the mechanisms of control of sodium balance, ECF osmolality is the parameter regulated by the mechanisms of control of water balance. In contrast with the regulation of sodium balance, water balance is controlled by both changes of intake and excretion. Intake depends on the sensation of thirst, and water excretion in the urine depends on the action of antidiuretic hormone (ADH) on the collecting segments of the renal tubule. The principal stimulus of both thirst and ADH secretion is an increase in ECF osmolality, sensed by osmoreceptors in the hypothalamus. Secondary stimuli include decreases of extracellular fluid volume (sensed by baroreceptors), pain and stress, and pharmacologic agents.

3. Interrelations between the Control Mechanisms of Salt and Water Balance

Although for didactic reasons the control mechanisms of salt and water balance are separated, they are frequently interrelated.

(1) Alterations of water balance secondary to primary alterations of salt balance: Isoosmotic losses of salt and water do not change ECF osmolality,

but the volume reduction stimulates thirst and ADH secretion, resulting in a tendency to positive water balance and a reduction in body fluid osmolality. Angiotensin II, which increases in plasma in response to decreases of ECF volume, may be the stimulus of thirst and ADH secretion in this condition.

(2)   Alterations in sodium balance secondary to primary alterations of water balance: Large positive or negative water balances can alter significantly ECF volume, and hence cause secondary alterations of sodium balance even if ECF sodium content is initially normal. These alterations are mediated by changes in GFR, aldosterone secretion, and other factors.

V. BARRIERS FOR WATER AND ION DISTRIBUTION

To understand the bases of the mechanisms by which water and/or electrolyte balance or distribution can be altered we need to identify and characterize the barriers separating the compartments shown in Figure 1B.

Exchanges of water and solute can take place at three barriers: the cell membranes (exchanges between ECF and ICF), the capillary walls (exchanges between plasma and interstitial-lymph compartment), and transporting epithelia (exchanges between ECF and external medium). We will now study these barriers and the mechanisms of transport across them. Some general principles of transport across membranes are presented in the Appendix.

A. Properties of the Cell Membrane as Related to Water and Electrolyte Metabolism

1. Water

With the exception of some epithelial cells, the cell membrane has a relatively high water permeability. In the absence of osmotic or hydrostatic pressure differences, water molecules move in both directions by simple diffusion, with no net flux. If there are osmotic or hydrostatic pressure differences, net fluxes of water take place. This flux appears to occur, at least in part, through small pores in the membrane. In practice, net movements of water through the cell membrane occur because of osmotic pressure differences, or, in other words, because there is a difference in total solute concentration between ICF and ECF. Significant hydrostatic pressure differences across the cell membrane are unlikely. However, it is known that cells swollen by exposure to a hypoosmotic medium extrude some fluid after an initial gain of volume. Some investigators think that the mechanism of this volume regulation could be an increase of hydrostatic pressure in a restricted intracellular compartment, which results in fluid filtration across the cell membrane.

Addition of different solutes to the ECF will not result necessarily in identical changes in the effective osmotic pressure of this fluid, even if the final concentrations of added substances, in number of particles, are the same. As explained in the Appendix, the effective osmotic pressure depends on the reflection coefficient of the solute. Therefore, solutes that penetrate the cell membrane (low reflection coefficient) will have a smaller osmotic effect than less permeant solutes (high reflection coefficient). For example, in the presence of insulin glucose is taken up by the cells. Therefore, the administration of isoosmotic glucose solutions is eventually equivalent to the administration of water. Obviously, this is not the case if an isoosmotic NaCl solution is administered, since NaCl will be effectively excluded from the intracellular compartment.

Because of the high water permeability of the cell membrane, changes in osmolality in the ECF (or ICF) result in swift net fluxes of water in the direction of the osmotic pressure difference, and a new steady state situation is achieved at which the osmotic pressures of the two compartments are equal again. The osmotic gradient is very short lived.

2. Electrolytes

Although permeable to most physiologically significant ions (K^+, Na^+, Cl^-), the cell membrane maintains steep concentration gradients because of the operation of ionic pumps, particularly the Na^+ pump (Na–K-activated ATPase) which extrudes actively Na^+ and takes up K^+. Cl^- in most cells is distributed passively according to the membrane potential. Cell membranes also transport other ions in an uphill fashion. Two examples are H^+ and Ca^{2+}. H^+ extrusion is well known to occur in epithelia such as the gastric mucosa and the renal tubule, but it has been demonstrated also in other tissues, such as muscle and nerve cells. Ca^{2+} is kept at a very low concentration in the cytoplasm by two mechanisms: "sequestration," which appears to take place mostly in mitochondria, and extrusion, which seems to be of two kinds: secondary active transport linked to Na entry (downhill) and a Ca^{2+} pump (Ca^{2+}-activated ATPase). These mechanisms result in a low intracellular ionized calcium concentration. Increases in this concentration trigger specific cell functions such as muscle contraction and secretion.

The energy metabolism of the cells and the proper operation of the ionic pumps are essential to maintain the ion concentration gradients across the cell membranes, and these, in turn, are essential for life. A good example is the distribution of K^+ across the cell membrane, and the ominous results of a net K^+ efflux to the ECF. To maintain the K^+ distribution it is necessary to have a normal operation of the Na^+ pump, a normal supply of metabolic energy, and a normal acid–base status, because H^+ fluxes through the cells membrane influence K^+ distribution. Defects in any of these can result in a net K^+ efflux from the cells, which can exert profound effects on cell function (see Chapter 7).

B. Properties of the Capillary Endothelium as Related to Water and Electrolyte Metabolism

The barrier separating plasma from interstitial fluid is the capillary endothelium. This membrane is highly permeable to water and crystalloids (i.e., solutes of lower molecular weight), but has a low permeability for colloids (proteins, lipoproteins). The difference in concentration of nondiffusible anions across the capillary wall results in changes in the concentration of diffusible ions, a condition known as *Gibbs–Donnan equilibrium*. The steady state situation is characterized by a lower concentration of diffusible anions and a higher concentration of diffusible cations in the side containing the impermeant anion, as compared to the other side. A more detailed analysis of Gibbs–Donnan equilibrium can be found in the Appendix. In addition, since divalent cations such as calcium are partly bound to plasma proteins, their total concentration in the interstitial fluid is lower than in plasma.

Exchanges between plasma and interstitial fluid occur by diffusion and by bulk flow. For definitions and descriptions of these processes, see the Appendix. Diffusion is favored by the high permeability of the capillary for most low-molecular-weight substances. Bulk flow, in which water and solutes move together, greatly increases the turnover rate of the intercellular fluid required to provide oxygen and remove catabolic products. Bulk flow can occur in both directions (plasma toward interstitium, or vice versa) according to the differences of hydrostatic and colloid-osmotic (oncotic) pressure (Landis and Pappenheimer; Starling):

$$J_v = L_p \left(\Delta P - \Delta \pi_{onc} \right)$$

where J_v is the net fluid flow through the wall, L_p is the hydraulic permeability coefficient, and ΔP and $\Delta \pi_{onc}$ are the transmural hydrostatic and colloid osmotic pressure differences, respectively. A positive J_v indicates flow toward the interstitial fluid.

At the *arteriolar end* of the capillary (where $\Delta P > \Delta \pi$) filtration will occur, while at the venous end (where ΔP has dropped and $\Delta \pi$ has increased, because of the filtration of protein-free fluid) the gradient reverses and reabsorption takes place. Alternatively, it is possible that, according to the degree of contraction of precapillary sphincters, a whole capillary vessel can function as a filtration element (high ΔP) or as a reabsorption element (low ΔP). Interstitial fluid filtered at the capillaries returns to the intravascular compartment not only by reabsorption across the capillary wall, but also through the lymphatic system.

Alterations in ΔP or $\Delta \pi_{onc}$ across the capillary wall can result in large changes of the distribution of fluid between the two subcompartments of the ECF. Two illustrative examples are the increase of ΔP secondary to cardiac failure, which tends to increase filtration, and the reduction of $\Delta \pi_{onc}$ (e.g., protein malnutrition, or abnormal protein losses), which also causes an increase of net filtration. In both conditions, edema (fluid accumulation in the interstitium) will result.

C. Properties of Epithelia as Related to Water and Electrolyte Metabolism

1. General Considerations

Transporting epithelia are differentiated tissues in which cells are closely apposed to each other, as flat sheets or tubules. Epithelia exhibit morphologic and functional polarity: the membrane facing the lumen (or external side) is different in its transport properties from the membrane facing the ECF. This polarity allows transepithelial net transport to take place even when the fluids bathing both sides of the tissue have identical composition.

Net transepithelial transport is ultimately accounted for by active mechanisms, i.e., by utilization of metabolic energy in translocating substances through the cell membranes. In many cases only a few substances are transported actively. Coupling mechanisms allow downhill or secondary active transport of other species (see Appendix).

The epithelial cells are held together at their apical ends by specialized discrete contacts of the cell membranes that form the limiting junctions or tight junctions (a misnomer—sometimes they are leaky). In the remainder of their height, the cells are separated by usually convoluted lateral intercellular spaces. Since it has been observed that the width of these spaces varies directly with the rate of transepithelial transport, it is thought that fluid is transported from the cell into the spaces across the lateral portion of the basolateral membrane, in addition to transport across its basal portion. Additional circumstantial evidence for this interpretation is provided by the demonstration that the sodium pump, believed to be responsible for salt transport by epithelia, is located in the basolateral membrane of several absorbing epithelial tissues.

The capillary bed toward which transport occurs is usually very rich and close to the epithelial cells. In the case of the kidney, blood flow is about 25% of cardiac output, i.e., one of the highest of the body per unit tissue weight. This enormous flow rate makes plasma a practically infinite sink or source of water or solutes transported in either direction.

2. Mechanisms of Transepithelial NaCl Transport

Salt and fluid transport across epithelia are widely believed to involve Na transport as a primary event. A coherent mechanism of epithelial sodium transport was proposed by Ussing and co-workers, and is usually referred to as the *two-membrane hypothesis*. This hypothesis, originally stated to explain Na^+ transport by the frog skin *in vitro*, was later extended to other epithelia. It is thought that Na^+ is transported passively across the outer membrane of the cell, into a cytoplasmic pool, and then from this pool, across the inner membrane, to the extracellular fluid of the animal. The mechanism of transport across the inner barrier is presumed to be active, by the operation of the Na^+ pump. The net effects of the pump are to decrease Na^+ and to

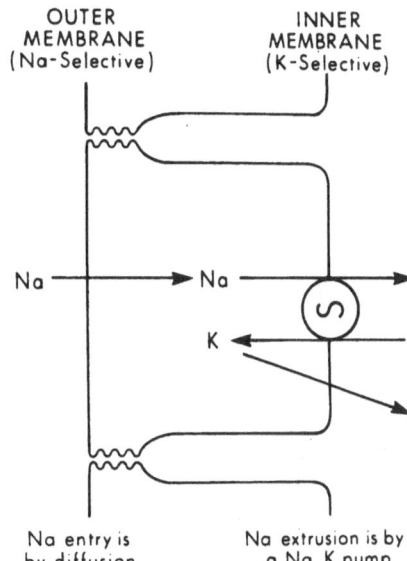

OUTER
MEMBRANE
(Na-Selective)

INNER
MEMBRANE
(K-Selective)

Na → Na →

K ←

Na entry is
by diffusion

Na extrusion is by
a Na, K pump

Figure 4. Two-membrane hypothesis of the mechanism of sodium transport in tight epithelia, as proposed by Koefoed-Johnsen and Ussing. The active element is a Na,K pump at the inner membrane, which transports Na from cell to ECF. The electrochemical gradient across the outer (luminal) membrane favors downhill Na entry. The outer membrane is Na permeable, whereas the inner membrane is K permeable.

increase K^+ concentration in the cells. The reduction in intracellular Na^+ concentration results, in turn, in a favorable gradient for downhill Na^+ entry across the outer membrane, which has a high Na permeability and a low K permeability. The inner membrane is, on the contrary, selectively permeable to K^+. Under steady state conditions, then, Na^+ transport occurs in the following way: entry at the apical membrane (downhill, because of the low Na^+ intracellular concentration), mixing in the intracellular pool, and active extrusion at the basolateral membrane. Na^+ extrusion at this barrier is coupled to K^+ uptake, by the operation of the Na pump. The coupling ratio (Na flux:K flux) can be, in principle, one (neutral pump) or greater (electrogenic pump). K^+ leaves the cells by diffusion through the basolateral membrane, and therefore the intracellular K^+ concentration is maintained constant (Figure 4).

This model, with suitable modifications, accounts for most of the features of sodium transport in *tight epithelia* (frog skin, urinary bladder of most vertebrates, distal and collecting segments of the nephron, large intestine). All of these epithelia develop a relatively high transepithelial electrical potential difference when incubated with the same physiologic salt solution on both sides and have relatively low overall permeability to ions. In many tight epithelia sodium is thought to be the sole ion actively transported. Chloride transport is believed to be passive, driven by the lumen-negative electrical potential difference generated by active Na^+ transport.

The two-membrane hypothesis does not account for the mechanism of Na^+ transport in all epithelia, as shown initially by Diamond in the gallbladder. Gallbladder epithelium transports Na^+ but does not develop a sizable transepithelial electrical potential difference (V_t). A similar situation (i.e., a low or negligible V_t) is observed under transporting conditions in all *leaky*

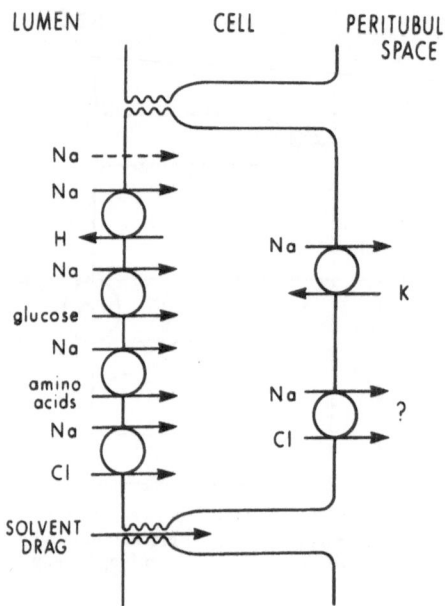

LUMEN   CELL   PERITUBULAR
                                      SPACE

Na

Na

H

Na

glucose

Na

amino
acids

Na

Cl

SOLVENT
DRAG

Na

K

Na

Cl

?

Figure 5. Mechanisms of Na transport in leaky epithelia. This figure summarizes results obtained in renal proximal tubule, small intestine, and gallbladder. Na entry is not only by diffusion (uniport), but also coupled to transport with other species; exchange (antiport) with H^+, or cotransport (symport) with a number of solutes: Cl, glucose, amino acids, and (not shown) lactate and phosphate. Na extrusion from the cells has also been proposed to follow parallel pathways: in addition to a "classical" Na,K pump, a neutral mechanism of NaCl transport is postulated. The high permeability of the limiting junctions suggests that salt transport is partly by solvent drag, bypassing the cells.

epithelia, i.e., tissues such as the renal proximal tubule, the small intestine, and the choroid plexus. The differences between tight and leaky epithelia have not been completely explained. However, two features seem to be present in leaky and not in tight Na^+-transporting epithelia: a high overall permeability to water, ions, and small nonelectrolytes, which appears to be due to a high permeability of the limiting junctions, and a mechanism of Na^+ transport at the luminal membrane that includes carrier-mediated cotransport with other solutes and is not by simple electrodiffusion, as in tight epithelia.

As it will be described in detail in the next chapter, Na^+ transport at the luminal membrane of the proximal tubule, for example, is only in part by diffusion; sizable fractions of Na^+ entry occur by coupling to glucose, amino acids, and probably Cl^-. NaCl-coupled entry, which has been demonstrated in several leaky epithelia, is an electrically neutral process. It has also been proposed that transport of Na^+ across the basolateral membrane in leaky epithelia is not entirely through the Na^+,K^+ pump, but can in part be through a neutral NaCl transport mechanism.

In summary, in tight epithelia Na^+ is thought to be transported in two steps: passive entry at the luminal membrane and active extrusion across the basolateral membrane. Transepithelial Cl^- transport is downhill in most cases, and results from the establishment of a large electrical potential difference which makes the mucosal (or luminal) solution negative. The pathway of Cl^- transport (transcellular, intercellular) has not been clarified. In leaky epithelia, Na^+ enters the cell mostly by carrier-mediated downhill mechanisms (coupled to Cl and/or glucose and amino acids). Na^+ exit at the basolateral membrane is, at least in part, through the Na^+,K^+ pump, but there is also the possibility of a parallel NaCl extrusion mechanism. These features are summarized in Figure 5.

The presence, in the limiting junctions and lateral intercellular spaces of leaky epithelia, of a pathway of high ionic permeability suggests that this intercellular (or shunt) pathway plays a role in the general function of these tissues. For instance, even small electrical potential differences across the tissue can result in large passive fluxes across the shunt pathway: in the case of lumen-negative leaky epithelia, a fraction of Cl^- transport could be passive, driven electrically through the shunt. The trade-off of this advantage is that a backleak of Na^+ transported by the cells would occur through the shunt for the same reason (lumen-negative potential). Another important physiological role of the shunt pathway can be to *permit* solvent drag (see Appendix). If NaCl transport into the lateral intercellular spaces raises locally the osmotic pressure, and if the limiting junctions are water permeable, transcellular salt transport would result in intercellular water transport. The water flow through the limiting junctions would be expected to carry, by solvent drag, small solutes which are highly permeant through the junctions.

In conclusion, transepithelial salt transport appears to occur by basically different mechanisms in different epithelia. The two-membrane hypothesis is consistent with most observations in tight epithelia, while in leaky epithelia other processes have to be considered such as neutral salt uptake and solvent drag. These tend to increase the rate of transport and to make the transported fluid similar to the luminal fluid, and therefore limit the possibility of the establishment of large concentration differences across the epithelium.

Leaky and tight absorbing epithelia have clearly different overall functions: leaky epithelia absorb rather nonselectively large quantities of fluid and cannot generate or maintain large osmotic or ion concentration differences across the wall; tight epithelia absorb very selectively some of the molecular species present in the lumen and are capable of establishing or maintaining large concentration gradients between luminal and extracellular fluid.

3. Mechanisms of Transepithelial Water Transport

Leaky and tight epithelia differ radically in terms of their water permeability. Tight epithelia, under control conditions, are water impermeable. Under the action of antidiuretic hormone (ADH), some of them increase their water permeability (cortical and medullary collecting duct, amphibian skin and urinary bladder). The site of increase of water permeability appears to be the luminal membrane of the cells, which is the main barrier for water permeation in the absence of ADH. Other water-tight epithelia, e.g., the thick ascending segment of the loop of Henle and the mammalian lower urinary tract, do not increase their water permeability in response to ADH. Net water transport across ADH-sensitive tight epithelia is a function of ADH activity and occurs down an osmotic gradient. In the renal medulla, this osmolality gradient is built up by solute accumulation in the interstitial fluid.

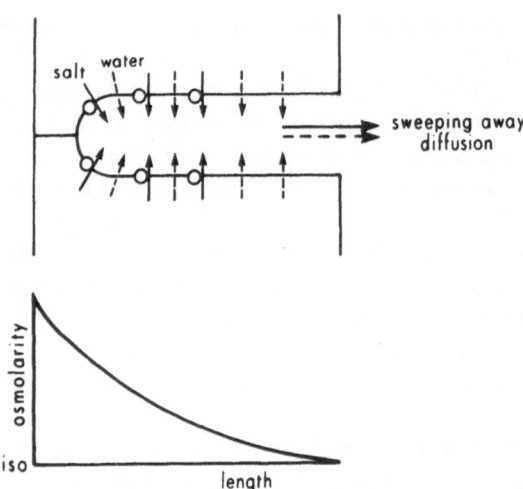

Figure 6. Standing osmotic gradient hypothesis of water transport by epithelia (Diamond and Bossert). Salt transport into the lateral intercellular spaces renders the solution hyperosmotic, resulting in passive water flow from the cells to the spaces. The fluid in the latter becomes progressively less hypertonic as it approaches the basal pole of the cells.

In leaky epithelia, water is transported in isoosmotic proportions with solute transport. About 1 liter of H_2O is transported for every 300 mOsm of solute in the absence of a measurable osmotic gradient (i.e., when luminal and ECF osmolalities do not differ). Since a favorable osmotic gradient is not present in the bulk solutions, it was thought that water transport could result from the presence of a restricted intraepithelial compartment, made hyperosmotic by salt transport, into which water would be dragged, building up hydrostatic pressure and therefore resulting in bulk flow to the ECF. The right location for such a compartment is just beneath the basolateral cell membrane, including the lateral intercellular space. To account for the maintenance of a permanent hyperosmolality, the compartment has to be effectively unstirred, i.e., not mixed with the bulk extracellular solution.

Detailed models along these lines have been proposed by Curran and McIntosh (three-compartment model) and by Diamond and Bossert (standing osmotic gradient hypothesis). The standing osmotic gradient hypothesis is illustrated in Figure 6.

An alternative explanation of isoosmotic fluid transport across the proximal renal tubule has been recently proposed. This is based on the

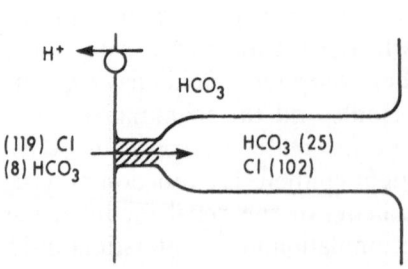

Figure 7. Asymmetric composition of bulk solutions as a mechanism of water transport in leaky epithelia. In the renal proximal tubule, preferential bicarbonate reabsorption results in an increase of luminal Cl concentration equivalent to the decrease of luminal HCO_3 concentration. The total osmolality of the luminal and peritubular fluids are identical, but an effective osmotic pressure difference is caused by the high reflection coefficient of HCO_3, compared to Cl. Therefore, a lumen-to-interspace water flow is produced (arrow). Concentrations in mEq/liter. See text.

experimental observation of *preferential bicarbonate reabsorption* (over Cl^-) as the anion accompanying Na. The result of this process is an increase of luminal Cl^- concentration and a decrease of HCO_3^- concentration, as compared to the concentrations in plasma (and interstitial fluid). Because the tubule is more permeable to Cl^- than to HCO_3^-, the net effect is an increased effective osmolality of the peritubular fluid, even though the total concentrations on both sides are identical. This effective osmotic pressure difference drives water from lumen to blood. Additional effects to the one of HCO_3, in the same direction, are provided by the complete reabsorption of glucose and amino acids (Figure 7).

4. Mechanisms of Transepithelial Transport of Other Substances

In addition to NaCl and water, epithelia transport a variety of other substances, including ions such as H^+, HCO_3^-, phosphate, divalent cations, organic acids and bases, and nonelectrolytes, e.g., sugars, amino acids, lipids, and urea. A detailed discussion of these processes is beyond the scope of this chapter. However, we should stress that transport of some of these substrates is coupled in one of several ways to active transport of other substances. The most obvious example of coupling through a pump is the extrusion of Na^+ and uptake of K^+ by the Na^+ pump. Other coupling mechanisms are the following: electrical (Cl^- transport in tight epithelia), osmotic (passive water transport secondary to salt transport), and carrier-mediated cotransport (Na^+ and Cl^-, or Na^+ and glucose or amino acids in some epithelia). The essential notion involved is that the energy that the cell provides for transport of one species is indirectly used to transport other substances. The obvious convenience of this design, in terms of utilization of metabolic energy, is offset, in part. by the loss of flexibility of the system: if the primary step (Na transport) fails, transport of a large number of substances is compromised.

APPENDIX: MEMBRANE TRANSPORT PROCESSES
Luis Reuss

A. Introduction

Transport through a biological membrane can be of two general types, defined by a comparison of the direction of the net flux of the substance and the direction of the net force present across the membrane: (1) *Uphill transport*, where the net flow of the substance takes place against or in the absence of an external net force. An example is Na transport from the cells to the extracellular fluid, which occurs even though the membrane potential is cell negative and the Na concentration is higher in the ECF than in the ICF. (2) *Downhill transport*, where the net flow of the substance takes place by the presence of an external force or concentration difference. An example is water reabsorption by the collecting duct of the nephron, which occurs from a compartment with high water concentration, the tubule lumen, to a compartment with low water concentration, the medullary interstitium.

Transport through biological membranes has been ascribed to various *mechanistic models*. The main ones are the following:

1. Diffusion. The substance present in the aqueous phase on one side "dissolves" in the membrane, migrates to the other side, and finally moves to the aqueous phase on the opposite side of the membrane. It is better to refer to this mechanism as solubility diffusion. An essential idea here is that the diffusional flows obey the independence principle: the flux of one species is not "coupled" to movements of other species.

2. Permeation through Pores. It is postulated that there are water-filled pores in the membrane that communicate the two external phases. Water and some solutes cross the membrane through these preferential pathways.

3. Carrier-Mediated Transport. Molecules in the membrane have sites that bind on one side the transported particle and move it to the other side by migration through the membrane, rotation, or a change in conformation.

4. Transport by Pumps. Specific molecules in the membrane translocate the substrate uphill; the energy necessary for the translocation is supplied by cell metabolism.

5. Transport by Membrane Vesicles. Membrane material surrounds a small portion of solvent and solute on one side, forming a vesicle. The vesicle separates from the membrane and eventually releases its contents on the opposite side.

There are arguments which indicate that all of these mechanisms may operate in biological membranes. Solubility diffusion is the preferred mode of transport of liposoluble substances. Pores appear to be the main pathway for passive permeation of water and small hydrophilic solutes. Carriers are invoked to explain transport of a variety of substrates such as sugars and amino acids. Finally, vesicle formation accounts for uptake (endocytosis) or release (exocytosis) of large molecules.

We will now turn our attention to the mechanisms of downhill and uphill transport.

B. Downhill Transport

As stated above, downhill transport occurs in the presence of a favorable driving force across the membrane. Three modes of downhill transport can be recognized: diffusion, bulk flow, and facilitated diffusion.

1. Diffusion

Diffusion is the effect of the random thermal movement of particles in solution. If a membrane separates two identical solutions, with no net force acting across the membrane, and if the only mechanism by which a substance

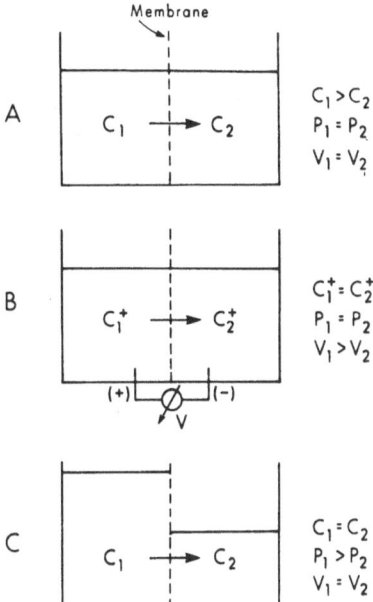

Figure 8. Mechanisms of downhill, diffusional solute transport. C_1 and C_2 are the solute concentrations in two compartments separated by a membrane permeable to the solute. P_1 and P_2 are the hydrostatic pressures exerted on the membranes. V_1 and V_2 are the electrical potentials in the two solutions. In all three cases, the solute net flow is from left to right. The driving forces are (A) concentration difference ($C_1 > C_2$), (B) electrical potential difference ($V_1 > V_2$), and (C) hydrostatic pressure difference ($P_1 > P_2$). See text.

(e.g., a solute) can move through the membrane is by diffusion, the unidirectional fluxes (i.e., the amounts of solute that cross the membrane in one direction per unit time and per unit area) will be equal. Therefore, no net flux will take place. The reason is that, since the two solutions are identical, the number of random collisions of the solute per unit time and per unit area are equal on both surfaces of the membrane.

Diffusion can result in a net flux through a membrane if the number of collisions is greater on one side than on the other. There are three ways in which this can occur: (1) The concentration of solute is higher on one side (and therefore the number of collisions is greater on that side of the membrane). (2) The solute has an electric charge (i.e., it is an ion) and there is an electric field across the membrane. The effect of this superimposed force will be to increase one of the unidirectional fluxes and to decrease the other one, according to the charge of the solute and the orientation of the electric field. For example, if a cell interior is electrically negative to the ECF and a cation is originally present in ICF and ECF at the same concentration, its flux inward will be greater than the flux outward. (3) There is a pressure difference across the membrane which results in a larger flow of both solvent and solute in one direction. The hydrostatic and/or osmotic pressure difference provides the energy required for the net flux. These mechanisms are illustrated in Figure 8. Note that the operation of all of them requires that the structure of the membrane be such that the solute can move through it; the membrane must be permeable to the solute.

Diffusion is a transport mechanism in which the permeating particles (solvent, solute, or both) do not interact between themselves during the translocation; in other words, they obey the independence principle. This can occur, for water and hydrophilic small solutes (ions, urea, other none-lectrolytes), either by a so-called solubility-diffusion mechanism or by permeation through pores. A solubility-diffusion mechanism will result in a net flux through the membrane only if a concentration difference exists between the two aqueous phases or a driving force (electric or mechanic, i.e., pressure) is present across the membrane. The pore hypothesis proposes that water and hydrophilic solutes do not dissolve in the membrane lipids, but move from one side to the other through these water-filled channels. In the absence of a net force that results in a flux of water through the membrane, solute and water fluxes through pores can be treated by the laws of diffusion; one must only consider that the effective area of the membrane available for diffusion is only a fraction of the total membrane surface area. When a pressure gradient is present and water flows through pores, however, both the water and the accompanying solute flow do not obey the simple laws of diffusion.

2. Bulk Flow

When a hydrostatic or an osmotic pressure difference exists across a porous membrane, the resulting flow of fluid through the pores is not diffusional in character: because of frictional intermolecular forces, water molecules "drag" other water molecules and solute molecules. This form of flux is called viscous flow or *bulk flow*. The fact that the solute moves with the water is referred to as *solvent drag*.

Bulk flow, if the solute is impermeant, is described by the following equation:

$$J_v = L_p \left(\Delta p - \Delta \pi \right)$$

where J_v is the volume flow, L_p is a permeability coefficient, the hydraulic conductivity of the membrane, Δp is the hydrostatic pressure difference, and $\Delta \pi$ is the osmotic pressure difference across the membrane.

The *osmotic pressure* of an aqueous solution results from the presence of solute particles, which reduces the concentration (or, better, the chemical activity) of water. If a membrane permeable to water but not to the solute is exposed to aqueous solutions of different concentrations, with no initial hydrostatic pressure difference, water will flow to the high-concentration side until a hydrostatic pressure difference equivalent to the osmotic pressure difference is established (Figure 9).

The net flow from right to left at time = 0 occurs because the activity of water is greater on the right-hand side. At the steady state the water activity on the right is still greater, but a force (dependent on Δp) acts in the opposite direction, increasing the motion of the water particles from left to

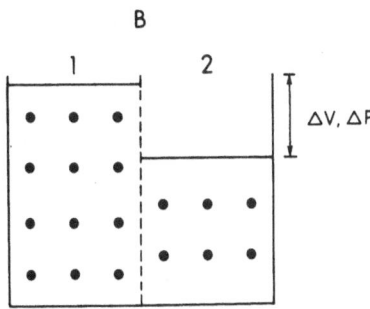

Figure 9. Osmotic pressure. The membrane separating compartments 1 and 2 is permeable to water but not to the solute (circles). At time = 0, diagram (A), the concentration of the solute is greater in side 1, the activity of water is greater in side 2, and therefore water flows from 2 to 1. At equilibrium, diagram (B), the net water flow has caused a volume (and hydrostatic pressure) difference. There is still a water concentration difference favoring flow from 2 to 1, but this is balanced by the hydrostatic pressure difference (Δp), which tends to move water in the opposite direction.

right. Equilibrium occurs when $\Delta \pi = \Delta p$ and J_v ceases. The osmotic pressure is related to the concentration of the solute (C_s) by van't Hoff's law:

$$\pi = RTC_s$$

where R is the gas constant and T the absolute temperature. Note that C_s is concentration of particles. The osmotic pressure of a sodium chloride solution (in which the salt is completely dissociated in Na^+ and Cl^-) is approximately twice the osmotic pressure of a glucose solution of the same molar concentration. For the calculation of osmotic pressures the number of solute particles is expressed in osmoles (abbreviated Osm). One osmole is the equivalent of 1 mole of undissociated solute. Concentrations can be expressed as osmolality (Osm/kg solvent) or osmolarity (Osm/liter solution). The osmolality of body fluids in man is close to 300 mOsm/kg. The hydrostatic pressure equivalent to this osmolality is 25.5 atm (19,300 mm Hg).

If an experiment similar to the one shown in Figure 9 is performed with a membrane permeable to both the solute and the solvent, a net flux of the latter can take place. Let us analyze the situation if the membrane is exposed to identical solutions and a hydrostatic pressure difference is imposed (Figure 10). The pressure difference will result in water flow from left to right. Because of frictional interaction of water and solute molecules in the pores, a net solute flow from left to right will also take place. This flux of both solute and solvent is referred to as bulk flow. The process described is analogous to the common experience of filtration of a solution by gravity: if

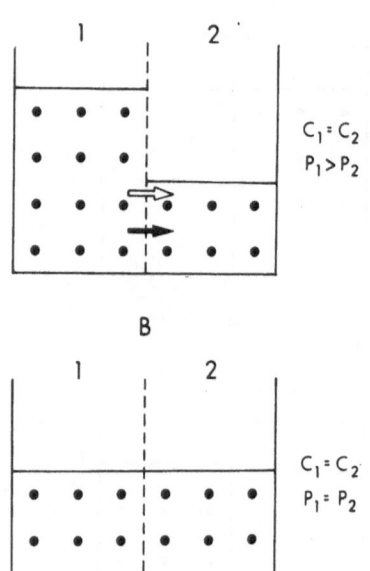

Figure 10. Bulk flow. The membrane is permeable to both water and solute. At time $= 0$, diagram (A), the solute concentrations in the two compartments are equal, but there is a hydrostatic pressure difference, which drives *both* water (open arrow) and solute (solid arrow) to compartment 2. At equilibrium, diagram (B), volume and concentrations are equal.

the filter is permeable to the solute, the solute will move through the filter with the water. The magnitude of the solute flux depends on the magnitude of the volume flux, the solute concentration, and the relative permeabilities of the membrane for water and solute. A simple way of expressing the latter is by the use of Staverman's reflection coefficient of the solute (σ_s). The reflection coefficient of a solute, for a given membrane, is unity when the solute is impermeant (i.e., all the solute particles are "reflected" by the membrane) and zero when the solute is as permeant as water (no solute particles are reflected).

An osmotic pressure difference across a porous membrane will result (as in the case of a hydrostatic pressure difference) in bulk flow, i.e., in net flow of water *and* permeant solutes. As stated before, the solute net flux which results from bulk flow is referred to as solvent drag.

The magnitude of the solute flow (J_s) is given by

$$J_s = J_v \cdot C_s (1 - \sigma_s)(\Delta p - \Delta \pi)$$

where J_v is the volume flow, C_s is the average concentration of the solute in the pores, σ_s is the reflection coefficient, and $\Delta p - \Delta \pi$ is the net driving pressure. Note that if $\sigma_s = 0$ (solute as permeant as water) the solute flow is a maximum for given values of J_v, C_s, and driving pressure; if $\sigma_s = 1$, $1 - \sigma_s = 0$, and J_s is zero.

The notion of reflection coefficient is also useful in understanding the concept of *effective osmotic pressure*. Consider a membrane exposed to pure water on one side and to a solution on the other. If the reflection coefficient of the solute is zero, no net flow will occur, even though there is an absolute osmotic pressure difference between the two solutions. The reason is that since the solute is as permeable as water ($\sigma_s = 0$) the net water flux toward the side containing solution will be equal to the net solute flux toward the side originally containing water. Even though net fluxes of water and solute take place, no net volume flow occurs across the membrane. Therefore, the *effective* osmotic pressure of the solution is zero. If $\sigma_s = 1$, the effective osmotic pressure of the solution equals the total osmotic pressure. Obviously, the effective osmotic pressure depends on σ_s, and thus on the properties of both the solute and the membrane. In general,

$$\pi_{eff} = \sigma_s\, \pi_{total} = \sigma_s\, RT\, C_s$$

This indicates that net flow of water and solute can take place through a membrane exposed to two solutions of identical total osmotic pressure if the reflection coefficients of the solutes differ. This mechanism has been proposed to account for a fraction of fluid reabsorption in the late proximal tubule, as explained on pages 20–21 of this chapter and also in Chapter 2, pages 50–52.

3. Facilitated Diffusion

Some solutes are transported through cell membranes much faster than one would expect from their permeability in lipids, their molecular size, or both. To account for these observations, the hypothesis of *membrane carriers* has been proposed. It is thought that the binding of the substrate (transported molecule) to the carrier (which is a membrane component) results in a better penetration into the membrane than possible for the substrate alone. By migration, rotation, or change in conformation, the carrier–substrate complex changes its position, and the substrate is released on the other side of the membrane. Carrier-mediated transport shows the following features: (1) some degree of specificity with respect to the substrate, (2) saturation kinetics (the number of molecules of the carrier is limited), (3) competitive and noncompetitive inhibition, (4) activation by ions, cofactors, and cosubstrates, (5) genetic and feedback regulation (inducers, hormones, metabolic intermediates of the substrate), and (6) trans-effects (dependence of the transport in one direction on the nature and concentrations of substances present on the other side of the membrane). These properties allow the design of very specific tests to demonstrate and characterize carrier-mediated transport. Among other substances, sugar and amino acids appear to be transported across cell membranes by this mechanism.

C. Uphill Transport

Uphill transport is demonstrated by the observation of net transport of a substance in the absence of or against a net driving force present in the system. In the case of ions, this force is proportional to the electrochemical potential difference across the membrane. In the case of nonelectrolytes, the force is proportional to the chemical potential difference. At constant temperature, the chemical potential difference of a substance across a membrane depends on the concentration difference and the net driving pressure ($\Delta p - \Delta \pi$) across the membrane. The electrochemical potential difference has as a third term the difference in electrical potential. When establishing if a substance is transported uphill, all of these terms have to be considered.

Uphill transport can occur only if there is a force that opposes the one given by the electrochemical potential difference. This force derives from metabolic energy sources (e.g., the hydrolysis of ATP). According to whether this force acts directly or indirectly on the substrate translocation, we distinguish two mechanisms of uphill transport: *primary active transport* and *secondary active transport*.

1. Primary Active Transport

Cellular metabolic energy is directly invested in the translocation of the substrate; the biological unit responsible for the process is a *pump*. A typical example is the Na,K-activated ATPase, i.e., the sodium pump. Uphill movement of Na and K is directly driven by the energy produced by hydrolysis of ATP.

2. Secondary Active Transport

Net movement of substrate is uphill (i.e., it occurs in the absence of or against an electrochemical potential gradient); however, energy is not invested directly in its translocation. A typical example is the absorption of glucose by intestine and renal tubule cells. It has been shown that glucose concentration in the cells, in both cases, becomes greater than that in the lumen (uphill transport) and depends on the luminal presence of Na. Several lines of evidence indicate that the luminal cell membrane contains a carrier that binds both Na and glucose, thereby causing uptake of both. This overall process is downhill, because the electrochemical potential difference which favors Na entry (cell negative, lower [Na] in the cell) is greater than the chemical potential difference that opposes glucose entry. In this case, therefore, the Na pump, responsible for the Na electrochemical gradient in the first place, provides indirectly the energy necessary for uphill glucose transport.

D. Effects of Concentration Differences across Biological Membranes: Gibbs–Donnan Equilibrium and Membrane Potentials

It should be apparent from the preceding discussion that transport across biological membranes can and does result in differences in the compositions of the fluid compartments separated by these membranes. The sodium pump, for instance, is responsible for the maintenance of large differences in Na and K concentrations between ICF and ECF.

1. Gibbs–Donnan Equilibrium

Another mechanism of generation of concentration differences is the impermeability or low permeability of the membrane to solutes originally present on one side only. This situation arises both at the cell membranes, because of the presence of large intracellular anions (proteins, organic phosphates) and across the capillary wall, because of the high plasma protein concentration as compared to the low protein concentration in the interstitial fluid.

Consider a membrane permeable only to K^+ and Cl^-, impermeable to water, separating two compartments which contain solutions of KCl and KP, respectively, at the same concentration. P is a large impermeant anion (Figure 11).

At first, the chemical activity gradients will result in a Cl^- flux from left

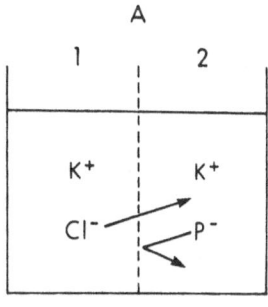

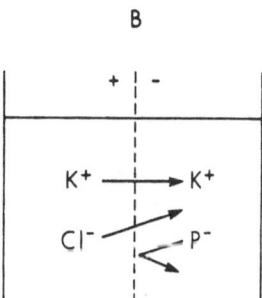

Figure 11. Gibbs–Donnan equilibrium. The membrane separating compartments 1 and 2 is permeable to K^+ and Cl^-, and impermeable to water and the large anion P^-. At time = 0, diagram (A), the salt concentrations (KCl and KP) are equal. The Cl concentration difference results in a net flux from 1 to 2 (P^- cannot cross the membrane). As shown in diagram (B), the Cl^- flux causes a potential difference across the membrane which drive K^+ in the same direction (1 to 2). The net result is, therefore, a KCl flux from 1 to 2. The equilibrium condition is described in the text.

to right. Although the gradient is the same for P^-, no P^- flux will take place because this ion is impermeant. K^+ initially will not tend to move, because its concentrations are equal on both sides. Once Cl^- moves across the membrane, separation of electrical charge takes place (anions are lost from the left-hand side and added to the right-hand side) and therefore an electrical potential difference develops across the membrane. Because of this potential difference, K^+ will now move from left to right. The end result is salt (KCl) net flux in that direction. It should be mentioned that only a minute net flow of charge through biological membranes is required to produce potential differences of the magnitude measured in cells. For all practical purposes, the principle of electroneutrality is obeyed in both compartments.

The KCl flux from left to right will continue until equilibrium is achieved, at which time

$$[K]_r \times [Cl]_r = [K]_l \times [Cl]_l$$

i.e., the products of the concentrations of diffusible anion and cation are equal on both sides.

At equilibrium, by definition, net fluxes of each ion through the membrane are zero. The electrical potential difference, which favors a K^+ flux to the right and a Cl^- flux to the left, is exactly compensated by the concentration differences, which favor fluxes in the opposite directions. Both permeant ions (K^+ and Cl^-) are distributed at equilibrium.

This analysis, albeit didactic, is unrealistic in biological situations (cell membrane, capillary endothelium), because these membranes, in general, have high water permeability, and we have assumed the membrane to be impermeable to water. Since in the situation described the initial total concentrations were the same on both sides, and a net flux of KCl resulted, the total concentration at equilibrium (and therefore the osmotic pressure at this time) is greater on the side containing the impermeant ion. Therefore, to prevent water flow from left to right it would be necessary to exert a hydrostatic pressure Δp on the right-hand side, such that $\Delta p = \Delta \pi$ (i.e., the osmotic pressure difference). This particular osmotic pressure, exerted by large, impermeant molecules, is referred to as *colloid-osmotic* pressure or *oncotic* pressure.

There are two ways in which the presence of a colloid-osmotic pressure difference ($\Delta \pi_{onc}$) across a biological membrane will not result in a net flow of water through such membrane. First, the side with the high π_{onc} has also a higher hydrostatic pressure. This is the situation across the capillary endothelium, where filtration driven by the intracapillary pressure is balanced by reabsorption driven by the higher protein concentration in the blood compartment. Second, an osmotically active substance is present in the compartment opposite to the one containing the oncotic agent and balances the effect of the latter. This substance has to be effectively excluded by the membrane. This mechanism appears to operate in most cells. It was thought for a long time that the cell membrane was impermeable to sodium ions, and that, in consequence, the presence of a higher Na^+ concentration in the ECF would result in an osmotic pressure difference which exactly balanced the oncotic pressure difference across the cell membrane. With the use of radioactive tracers, however, it has been shown that the cell membranes are permeable to Na^+. From this observation, the existence of a mechanism that *actively* extrudes Na^+ from the cell (i.e., the Na^+ pump) was proposed. Sodium, therefore, is excluded from the cells by active transport, not by impermeability of the membrane for this cation. Consistent with this notion, cells swell when the pump is inhibited directly or indirectly (cardiotonic steroids and anoxia, or metabolic poisons, respectively).

The steady state condition described is Donnan and osmotic equilibrium. Its main characteristics, if we look at the side containing the large anion, are lower total concentration of diffusible anions and higher total concentration of diffusible cations.

2. Membrane Potentials

An electrical potential difference across a biological membrane implies separation of charge by the membrane. This can occur by two general mechanisms: electrodiffusion and the presence of electrogenic pumps. The *electrodiffusion mechanism* (diffusion potentials) is explained by the existence of differences in ionic concentrations on both sides of the membranes, associated with different permeabilities of the membrane for the different ions. Consider, for example, a membrane permeable to K^+ but not to Na^+ or Cl^- which separates solutions of NaCl and KCl at identical concentrations. The chemical potential difference will cause a K^+ net flux across the membrane (no other ion can move through it) and therefore an electrical potential difference. *Electrogenic pumps* are ion pumps that transfer charge through the membrane, contributing directly to the membrane potential, and not only because they establish and maintain ion concentration differences. An example is the Na pump, which in most cells appears to transport three Na^+ and two K^+ for each ATP molecule hydrolyzed.

a. Electrodiffusion and Membrane Potentials

In the simplest case of only one permeant ion (for instance, K^+) The potential is given by the Nernst equation

$$\Delta\psi = -\frac{RT}{zF} \ln \frac{C_i}{C_o}$$

where $\Delta\psi$ is the potential difference, R is the gas constant, T is the absolute temperature, z is the valence ($+1$ in the case of K), F is the Faraday ($\sim$96,500 coulombs/equivalent), and C_i and C_o are the K^+ concentrations inside and outside, respectively. In practice, this equation can be simplified by inserting the value of (RT/zF) and changing the natural logarithm to decimal logarithm. For a monovalent cation, at 37°C, $\Delta\psi$ (in mV) is

$$\Delta\psi = -61.8 \log \frac{C_i}{C_o}$$

This is the maximum potential that can result from an ionic concentration difference across a permselective membrane. Note that if $C_i = 10 \times C_o$ the decimal logarithm of the ratio is 1 and $\Delta\psi = -61.8$ mV.

If the membrane is permeable to more than one ion, the electrodiffusional component of the membrane potential is given by the Goldman–Hodgkin–Katz equation (written below for the prevalent monovalent ions, at 37°C):

$$\Delta\psi = -61.8 \log \frac{P_K [K]_i + P_{Na} [Na]_i + P_{Cl} [Cl]_o}{P_K [K]_o + P_{Na} [Na]_o + P_{Cl} [Cl]_i}$$

Note that now the potentials depend not only on the concentration ratios, but also on the permeabilities of the ions. If P_{Na} and P_{Cl} are zero, the Na and Cl terms in numerator and denominator disappear, P_K cancels, and the equation becomes the Nernst equation. In other words, if only one ion is permeant the diffusion potential is the same regardless of the absolute permeability of the membrane for the ion.

The generation of electrodiffusional potentials across membranes is related to both the presence of nondiffusible ions on one side (proteins and large organic phosphates in the cells) and also to the maintenance of large gradients of concentrations across the membranes by the operation of pumps. Most cells have a high K^+ concentration and a low Na^+ concentration, maintained by the Na^+ pump. Excluding the case of excitable tissues during the action potential and some cell membranes of transporting epithelia, cell membranes are far more permeable to K^+ than to Na^+. Therefore, the main determinant of the membrane potential is the K concentration ratio. Cl is usually quite permeant and distributes secondarily to this K diffusion potential; hence the intracellular Cl concentration is low.

b. Electrogenic Pumps and Membrane Potentials

This general picture is somewhat complicated by the existence, in some membranes at least, of electrogenic pumps. As stated before, ion transport through an electrogenic pump results in net tranfer of charge through the membrane. The Na^+ pump is presumably electrogenic, with "coupling ratio" (Na flux : K flux) of 1.5, in most systems so far studied. The contribution of this "pump current" to $\Delta\psi$ depends on the total ionic permeability of the membrane (i.e., on its total conductance), since according to Ohm's law

$$V = i/G$$

where V is potential, i current, and G conductance ($G = 1/R$, where R is the electrical resistance).

For a given pump current, V is inversely proportional to G: in high-conductance (low-resistance) membranes, the contribution of an electrogenic pump to the potential is small. It has been estimated that the contribution of the Na pump to the membrane potential in cells under steady state conditions ranges from a fraction of 1 mV to about 12 mV.

SUGGESTED READINGS

Diamond, J. M.: The epithelial junction: bridge, gate and fence. *Physiologist* 20:10, 1977.

Diamond, J. M., and Bossert, W. H.: Standing-gradient osmotic flow: a mechanism for coupling of water and solute transport in epithelia. *J. Gen. Physiol.* 50:2061–2083, 1967.

Edelman, F. S., Olney, J. M., James, A. H., Brooks, L., and Moore, F. D.: Body composition: studies in the human being by the dilution principle. *Science* 115:447, 1952.

Erlij, D.: Solute transport across isolated epithelia. *Kidney Int.* 9:76, 1976.

Erlij, D., and Martinez-Palomo, A.: Role of tight junctions in epithelial function, in Giebisch, G., Tosteson, D. C., and Ussing, H. H. (eds.): *Membrane Transport in Biology*, Vol. III. Springer-Verlag, Berlin, 1978, p. 27.

Frizzell, R. A., Field, M., and Schultz, S. G.: Sodium-coupled chloride transport by epithelial tissues. *Am. J. Physiol.* 5:F1, 1979.

Hays, R. M.: Dynamics of body water and electrolytes, in Maxwell, M. H., and Kleeman, C. R. (eds.): *Clinical Disorders of Fluid and Electrolyte Metabolism.* McGraw-Hill, New York, 1980, p. 1.

Koefoed-Johnsen, V., and Ussing, H. H.: The nature of the frog skin potential. *Acta Physiol. Scand.* 42:298, 1958.

Landis, E. M., and Pappenheimer, J.R.: Exchange of substances through the capillary walls, in Hamilton, W. F., and Dow, P. (eds.): *Handbook of Physiology*, Section 2, Circulation, Vol. II. American Physiological Society, Washington, D.C., 1963, pp. 961–1034.

Maffly, R. H.: The body fluids: volume, composition and physical chemistry, in Brenner, B. M., and Rector, F. C. (eds.): *The Kidney.* Saunders, Philadelphia, 1981, p. 76.

Reineck, H. J., and Stein, J. H.: Regulation of sodium balance, in Maxwell, M. H., and Kleeman, C. R. (eds.): *Clinical Disorders of Fluid and Electrolyte Metabolism.* McGraw-Hill, New York, 1980, p. 89.

Renkin, E. M., and Curry, F. E.: Transport of water and solutes across capillary endothelium, in Giebisch, G., Tosteson, D. C., and Ussing, H. H. (eds.): *Membrane Transport in Biology*, Vol. IVA. Springer-Verlag, Berlin, 1979, p. 1.

Starling, E. H.: On the absorption of fluids from the connective tissue spaces. *J. Physiol. (London)* 19:312–326, 1896.

Schultz, S. G.: Transport across epithelia: some basic principles. *Kidney Int.* 9:65, 1976.

Schultz, S. G.: *Basic Principles of Membrane Transport.* Cambridge University Press, Cambridge, 1980.

Ussing, H. H., and Leaf, A.: Transport across multimembrane systems, in Giebisch, G., Tosteson, D. C., and Ussing, H. H. (eds.): *Membrane Transport in Biology*, Vol. III. Springer-Verlag, Berlin, 1978, p. 1.

Appendix

Andreoli, T. E., Hoffman, J. F., and Fanestil, D. D. (eds.): *Physiology of Membrane Disorders.* Plenum, New York, 1978.

Hebert, S. H., Schafer, J. A., and Andreoli, T. E.: Principles of membrane transport, in Brenner, B. M., and Rector, F. C. (eds.): *The Kidney.* Saunders, Philadelphia, 1981, p. 116.

Katz, B.: *Nerve, Muscle, and Synapse.* McGraw-Hill, New York, 1966.

Kotyk, A., and Janacek, K.: *Cell Membrane Transport. Principles and Techniques.* Plenum, New York, 1975.

Schafer, J. A.: Membrane transport, in Klahr, S., and Massry, S. (eds.): *Contemporary Nephrology,* Vol. 1. Plenum, New York, 1981, pp. 1–57.

Schultz, S. G.: *Basic Principles of Membrane Transport.* Cambridge University Press, Cambridge, 1980.

2

Homeostatic and Excretory Functions of the Kidney

ELSA BELLO-REUSS and LUIS REUSS

I. INTRODUCTION

A. Renal Homeostatic Function

The kidneys have a central role in the homeostasis of water and electrolytes, i.e., in the maintenance of volume and ionic composition of body fluids. This function is accomplished by appropriate changes in the rate of renal excretion of water and electrolytes, controlled by feedback mechanisms which involve participation of the nervous system, the endocrine system, or both. The homeostatic functions of the kidney include the control of the balance of water, sodium, chloride, potassium, calcium, magnesium, hydrogen ions, and phosphate. The adaptability of the kidney to the requirements of homeostasis is demonstrated by the large changes in urine volume and composition which occur in response to alterations in the diet. There is no fixed normal composition of the urine. Normal homeostatic renal function is defined by the capacity of the organ to vary the volume and composition of the urine over a wide range, according to requirements imposed by intake, extrarenal losses, and other factors.

ELSA BELLO-REUSS • Departments of Medicine, and Physiology and Biophysics, Washington University School of Medicine and The Jewish Hospital of St. Louis, St. Louis, Missouri 63110.   LUIS REUSS • Department of Physiology and Biophysics, Washington University School of Medicine, St. Louis, Missouri 63110.

B. Renal Excretory Function

The urine is the main pathway for elimination from the body of fixed (nonvolatile) metabolic products. Many of these substances serve no biological function and are potentially toxic. Examples are urea (end product of protein metabolism), uric acid (end product of nucleic acid catabolism), creatinine (end product of creatine metabolism), metabolites of hormones, and foreign chemicals and their derivatives.

C. Overview of Glomerular Filtration and Tubular Transport

The kidneys receive 20%–25% of the cardiac output, a fraction disproportionately high when one considers their weight. The renal circulation is characterized by two capillary beds in series: the glomerular capillaries and the peritubular capillaries. This arrangement is intimately related to the functional properties of the organ. The first capillary segment (glomerulus) has a high luminal hydrostatic pressure, as compared to other capillary systems, because it is interposed between two arterioles, i.e., resistive vessels. Therefore, filtration is favored at this level. The second capillary system (peritubular capillaries in the cortex, vasa recta in the medulla) is a high-flow, low-pressure system which acts as sink or reservoir for tubular reabsorption and secretion, respectively.

Renal handling of substances, excluding those produced or utilized by the renal tissue, takes place by glomerular filtration and/or tubular transport. The latter can occur from lumen to blood (reabsorption) or in the opposite direction (secretion). Some substances are both absorbed and secreted by the renal tubule. This results in quite flexible mechanisms of regulation of their excretion.

The fact that the renal tubule consists of several segments in series with widely different transport properties allows for additional functional flexibility. As a first approximation, the tubule can be divided in three functionally distinct segments: (1) The *proximal tubule* is a typical leaky epithelium (see Chapter 1) that transports fluid isoosmotically at a very high rate, modifying only moderately the composition of the filtrate. (2) The *loop of Henle* consists of several segments with different active and passive transport properties. Because of both these transport properties and the hairpin arrangement of the ascending and descending limbs, the loop functions as a countercurrent multiplier, and is responsible for the hyperosmolality of the interstitial fluid in the renal medulla, which eventually drives water reabsorption. (3) The *distal nephron*, consisting of distal and collecting segments, is a tight epithelium. Transport is slower than in the proximal tubule, but the low permeability of the wall permits these segments to establish or maintain large osmotic, electric, and chemical concentration differences. Final regulation of the volume and composition of the urine takes place in the distal nephron.

The function of any segment of the renal tubule depends, in general, on three factors: (1) its intrinsic transport properties, (2) the action of modulating factors, such as physical forces acting across the wall and hormones, and (3) the rate of delivery and composition of the luminal fluid entering the segment. The latter factor is particularly important in the case of the loop of Henle and the distal nephron, which have a much lower reabsorptive capacity than the proximal tubule. Reduction of proximal tubule fluid transport can result in overloading of these segments and large changes in urine volume and composition even if they are structurally and functionally intact.

II. QUANTITATIVE ANALYSIS OF RENAL FUNCTION

A. Clearance

The rate of excretion of a substance (e.g., in mmoles/min), although an important piece of information to evaluate renal function, does not provide insight into the renal mechanism of handling of the substance because filtration, reabsorption, and secretion can occur in a wide variety of combinations to satisfy practically every excretion rate.

The notion of clearance treats the kidney as a black box, and is valid only if the substance under study is not produced, accumulated, or consumed by the organ. In the following discussion, plasma concentrations (Ps) refer to the concentration of ultrafilterable solute.

From the law of conservation of matter, the *rate of extraction of substance x from the blood equals the rate of excretion in the urine*. The amount excreted per unit time can be expressed as $U_x \cdot V$, that is, the product of the urinary concentration (U_x) and the urine flow rate (V), and, analogously, the amount extracted can be expressed as $P_x \cdot C_x$, where P_x is the plasma concentration of substance x, and C_x is the volume of plasma which contains the amount of substance excreted per unit time. Since excretion equals extraction,

$$P_x \cdot C_x = U_x \cdot V$$

and

$$C_x = \frac{U_x \cdot V}{P_x}$$

where C_x is the clearance of the substance x and can be defined as the virtual volume of plasma that has been cleared of the substance per unit time. U_x and P_x have the dimensions of concentrations (in the same units) and C_x and V have the dimensions of volume per unit time, usually ml/min.

Two particular clearances have important physiologic and clinical significance.

Several substances (e.g., the polysaccharide inulin) filter freely and are not transported by the tubule. Therefore, the rate of filtration equals the rate of excretion, or, according to the above equations,

$$P_{inulin} \cdot C_{inulin} = U_{inulin} \cdot V$$

Since the amount filtered per unit time is equal to $P_{inulin} \times$ GFR (glomerular filtration rate) it can be seen that C_{inulin} equals GFR:

$$C_{inulin} = \frac{U_{inulin} \cdot V}{P_{inulin}} = \text{GFR [ml/min]}$$

Therefore, the measurement of the clearance of inulin, or substances with the same properties, allows one to estimate the rate of glomerular filtration.

Other substances (e.g., para-amino hippurate, or PAH) are freely filtered and are also secreted by the tubule. If the plasma concentration is not too high, and transport by the tubule is not saturated, the rate of extraction can be high enough to eliminate essentially all the substance from the blood in a single renal passage. Since the amount of PAH that reaches the kidneys per unit time is almost totally excreted, it is obvious that is was contained in a plasma volume that approximates the total volume of plasma flowing through the kidneys per unit time. Therefore, the clearance of PAH approximates the renal plasma flow (RPF):

$$C_{PAH} = \frac{U_{PAH} \cdot V}{P_{PAH}} \simeq \text{RPF [ml/min]}$$

A small portion of RPF does not perfuse functional renal tissue, but is directly shunted through nonfunctional tissue (renal capsule, renal pelvis, etc). Therefore, it is better to refer to C_{PAH} as an estimation of *effective RPF* (ERPF), meaning plasma flow of functional renal tissue. As stated above, PAH is secreted by a saturable transport system. If the PAH plasma concentration is high enough, saturation of the transport mechanism will occur, a large portion of PAH will not be secreted, and C_{PAH} will be significantly lower than ERPF. In this case, P_{PAH} would have to be determined in arterial blood and in renal venous blood, applying *Fick's principle* to calculate effective renal plasma flow.

Renal blood flow (RBF) can be computed from RPF and the hematocrit (Hct):

$$RBF = \frac{RPF}{1 - Hct}$$

Renal clearances can range from zero (filtration and 100% reabsorption, e.g., glucose) to about 600 ml/min, i.e., ERPF (essentially complete excretion by a combination of filtration and secretion). Inulin clearance (C_{in} = GFR) is about 120 ml/min. If a freely filterable substance has a clearance C_x such that $0 < C_x < C_{in}$, the net effect of tubular transport must be reabsorption. If $C_x = C_{in}$, the substance is not subject to *net* tubular transport (but reabsorption could take place, if secretion occurs at the same rate). If $C_{in} < C_x < C_{PAH}$, the substance must be secreted (or secretion > reabsorption). If $C_x = C_{PAH}$, the substance is excreted, as PAH, by a combination of filtration and secretion.

B. *U/P* Concentration Ratio

In the clearance equation, the U_x/P_x ratio indicates the degree to which x has been concentrated from the filtrate to the final urine. In order to compare the rate of reabsorption of x with the rate of water reabsorption, one can estimate the latter from the *U/P* inulin ratio. Since inulin is not transported by the tubules, U differs from P only because water ("inulin free") is reabsorbed. Rewriting the clearance equation for inulin,

$$\frac{U_{in}}{P_{in}} = \frac{GFR}{V}$$

Or, in other words, the value of $(U/P)_{in}$ is equal to the reciprocal of the fraction of filtered water not reabsorbed by the tubule. Therefore, fractional water reabsorption is

$$\frac{GFR - V}{GFR} = 1 - \frac{P_{in}}{U_{in}}$$

For instance, if $(U/P)_{in} = 2$, fractional water reabsorption is 0.5 (or 50%); if $(U/P)_{in} = 10$, fractional water reabsorption is 0.9 (or 90%).

In many situations the value of *U/P* for other substances is of importance. For example, in patients with oliguria it is necessary to distinguish between the possibilities of (1) a homeostatic response to severe reduction of ECF volume, with normal function, and (2) abnormal tubular function because of ischemic renal damage. In the first case, the mechanisms of sodium retention will operate at a maximum and thus $(U/P)_{Na}$ will be low. If there is renal damage, the capacity of the renal tubules to respond to stimuli for Na reabsorption will be diminished and $(U/P)_{Na}$ will be high.

C. Osmolar Clearance

From urine flow rate and osmolalities of urine and plasma, the renal clearance of *total solute* can be calculated:

$$C_{osm} = \frac{U_{osm} \cdot V}{P_{osm}}$$

According to the definition of clearance, C_{osm} represents the virtual volume of plasma cleared of all solutes per unit time. Comparison of the values of C_{osm} and V can be very useful in understanding the physiology and pathophysiology of concentration and dilution of the urine. If $C_{osm} = V$, according to the equation above $U_{osm} = P_{osm}$. In other words, the net effect of tubular transport has been reabsorption of a fluid isoosmotic to plasma. If the values of C_{osm} and V differ, one must conclude that, in addition to isoosmotic fluid reabsorption, (1) solute (water free) was reabsorbed, in which case $V > C_{osm}$, or (2) water (solute free) was reabsorbed, in which case $C_{osm} > V$.

In case (1) a *free-water clearance* (C_{H_2O}) can be calculated:

$$C_{H_2O} = V - C_{osm}$$

In case (2), essentially the same equation holds, but the sign of C_{H_2O} is negative. In practice, the following formula is employed:

$$T^c_{H_2O} = V - C_{osm}$$

"Free water" is formed, in the absence of antidiuretic hormone, in the diluting segments of the nephron (cortical thick ascending limb of the loop of Henle, distal convoluted tubule, and cortical collecting tubule). Reabsorption of water to increase U_{osm} above P_{osm} takes place in the medullary collecting ducts.

D. Kinetics of Transport by the Renal Tubule: T_m and Gradient-Time Limited Transport

The renal tubule reabsorbs or secretes some substances by saturable transport mechanism. Two examples are glucose reabsorption and PAH secretion. When plasma glucose concentration is progressively increased, therefore increasing the amount filtered per unit time, at a given load glucose appears in the urine, indicating that the reabsorptive mechanism is saturable. The renal tubules can reabsorb glucose until a maximum rate (mmoles/min) is reached. A similar observation can be made for substances subject to tubular secretion. This rate of *maximum tubular transport* is called T_m (tubular transport maximum). At loads equal or larger than the one necessary to produce glycosuria, $T_m = $ (filtered load) − (excreted load). The experimental study of these relationships, by gradual elevation of the plasma concentration of the solute, while measuring simultaneously GFR and plasma concentration and urinary excretion of the solute is usually referred to as a *titration experiment*. A glucose titration of the renal tubules is shown in Figure 1.

Glucose, phosphate, sulfate, amino acids, organic anions, uric acid, and proteins are reabsorbed by T_m-limited processes. The *titration curves*, such as

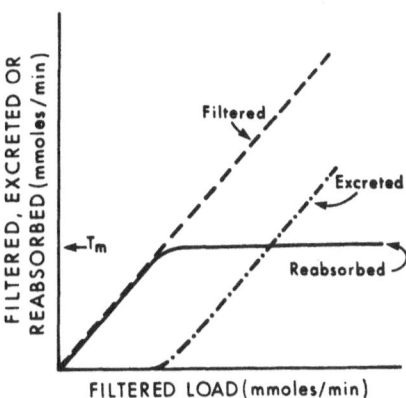

Figure 1. Glucose titration of the renal tubules. The filtered glucose load is increased by increasing plasma glucose concentration. At a certain load, glucose appears in the urine (curve labeled "excreted") indicating that reabsorption has saturated (curve labeled "reabsorbed"). The rate of reabsorption after saturation is the T_m for glucose. Note that the curves exhibit splay. See text. (Figure modified from Pitts, 1974.)

the one illustrated above, are not straight lines, but exhibit "splay," i.e., curvilinear slow rise of the excreted load when excretion starts, and curvilinear flattening of the curve of reabsorbed glucose as the T_m value is approached. Splay is thought to be caused by two mechanisms. First, the affinity of the carrier molecule for the solute is not infinite, and therefore some solute will escape transport when the carrier is still not fully saturated; second, the nephrons are heterogenous, i.e., in some the carrier will be saturated at a lower load than in others.

Substances excreted by T_m-limited secretion are drugs (penicillin, salicylate), and other exogenous substances such as PAH, phenol red, Diodrast (a radiopaque material), and vitamin B_1.

The renal handling of many solutes, however, does not exhibit these simple T_m kinetics. Sodium and potassium, for instance, do not have a definite upper limit for reabsorption or secretion, respectively. When the rate of delivery of Na to the proximal tubule increases, Na reabsorption also increases, without clear saturation within the range in which it can be explored. This kind of tubular transport has been classically called *gradient-time limited transport*.

III. RENAL HEMODYNAMICS

A. Magnitude and Measurement of Renal Blood Flow

Total renal blood flow (RBF) in adult humans is about 1.1 liters/min, or 20%–25% of cardiac output. This is one of the highest organ blood flows per unit weight. For a normal hematocrit of 0.45, total renal plasma flow (RPF) is about 600 ml/min. 20% of RPF is filtered at the glomeruli every minute (GFR – 120 ml/min).

Most of the pressure drop from renal artery to renal vein takes place at the two glomerular arterioles (afferent and efferent), as shown in Figure 2.

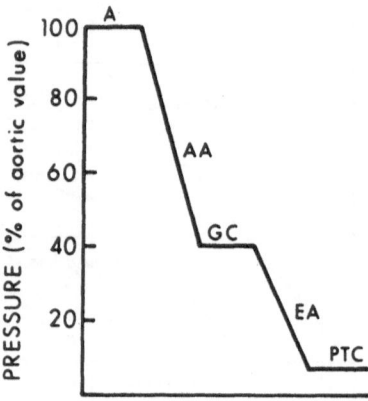

Figure 2. Pressures and resistances in renal circulation. The diagram shows that the resistive vessels of the kidneys are the afferent and efferent arterioles of the glomeruli, as indicated by the large drops in pressure at both sites. Differential constriction of the arterioles can increase or decrease the hydrostatic pressure of the glomerular capillaries. Symbols: A, aorta; AA, afferent arteriole; GC, glomerular capillary; EA, efferent arteriole; PTC, peritubular capillary.

The glomerular arterioles are responsible for the baseline renal vascular resistance (RVR) and therefore for renal blood flow. At constant mean arterial blood pressure, changes in arteriolar resistances (inversely proportional to the fourth power of the radius of the vessel) alter RBF, as they would alter flow in any other tissue.

Total RBF can be measured directly, with an electromagnetic flowmeter attached to the renal artery, or indirectly by means of clearance techniques as discussed in the preceding section.

Estimations of the intrarenal distribution of blood flow are technically difficult. They include procedures such as washout curves of inert gases and systemic injection of particles (labeled microspheres) slightly larger in diameter than the glomerular capillaries: the particles are trapped in the capillary beds in proportion to the total blood flow of the organ, and their distribution in the tissue is proportional to blood flow distribution. Cortical blood flow is about 93% of total RBF. The remaining 7% of RBF is medullary. Only 1/7 of the latter fraction (1% of total RBF) reaches the papillary tissue.

The large blood flow of the kidneys is not an adaptive mechanism to provide large amounts of oxygen. In fact, the arteriovenous O_2 difference is very small (1–2 vol%), and quite constant. The high renal blood flow serves the purpose of providing a high rate of filtration of fluid in the glomeruli. Renal O_2 consumption is directly related to blood flow, or better, to the filtered Na load, and thus to absolute Na reabsorption. Over a wide range of the latter, the ratio of Na reabsorbed to O_2 consumed (T_{Na}/Q_{O_2}) has been observed to remain constant at about 20–30 Eq Na/mole O_2.

B. Autoregulation of Renal Blood Flow

Renal blood flow remains relatively constant as perfusion pressure (i.e., mean pressure in the renal artery) is altered over a rather wide range. It has already been stated that a similar relationship holds for the rate of glomerular filtration. These phenomena are illustrated in Figure 3.

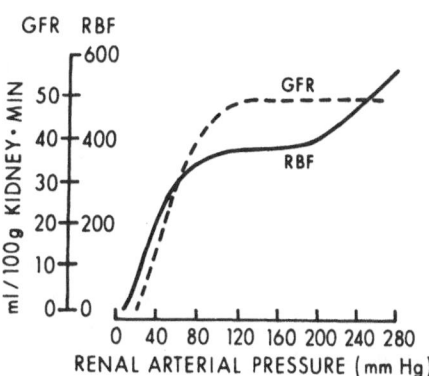

Figure 3. Renal blood flow and glomerular filtration rate autoregulation in the dog kidney. Renal blood flow (RBF) and glomerular filtration rate (GFR) are plotted as function of renal arterial pressure. In the range from about 80 to about 180 mm Hg, RBF and GFR remain almost constant, even though the perfusion pressure increases by more than twofold. (Figure modified from Pitts, 1974.)

The significance of these *autoregulatory mechanisms* is to maintain GFR more or less constant even if arterial pressure changes. This is achieved by changes of RVR in proportion to the changes in perfusion pressure (*P*). Since RBF = *P*/RVR, proportional changes of *P* and RVR in the same direction do not alter RBF. Inasmuch as GFR is also autoregulated, the glomerular capillary hydrostatic pressure (P_{GC}) also remains constant when *P* changes. The change in RVR indicates that one or both arterioles have changed their tone: an elevation of *P* causes arteriolar constriction, whereas a reduction of *P* causes arteriolar dilation. In addition, the fact that GFR, and hence P_{GC}, remain constant indicates that the vascular resistance change is mainly or exclusively preglomerular, i.e., at the afferent arteriole. An increase of *P* by itself, in the absence of effects on arteriolar tone, would

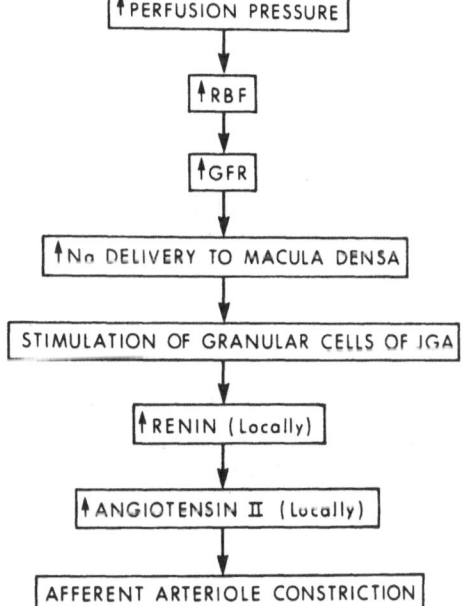

Figure 4. Chemoreceptor (macula densa) hypothesis of renal blood flow autoregulation. The diagram illustrates the operation of the system for primary increases of perfusion pressure. Factors other than Na delivery have been proposed as the stimulus of the chemoreceptor.

tend to increase P_{GC} and therefore GFR. To keep both constant, the increase of RVR has to take place at the afferent arteriole. Thus, when the perfusion pressure increases, the pressure drop across the afferent arteriole rises and P_{GC} does not increase.

Autoregulation is an intrinsic process, which does not require extrarenal neural or hormonal actions. Its precise mechanism has not been clarified.

One possibility, referred to as the *macula densa feedback hypothesis*, is that the rate of Na delivery to the macula densa controls renin production by the granular cells of the juxtaglomerular apparatus (JGA), and that *in situ* renin release leads to local production of angiotensin II. Angiotensin II, in turn, would control the degree of contraction of the afferent arteriole. The operation of this mechanism in case of an initial rise in perfusion pressure is summarized in Figure 4. The overall evidence in favor of this hypothesis is not conclusive.

C. Neurogenic Control of Renal Blood Flow

The kidneys are richly innervated by adrenergic nerve fibers. Under basal physiologic conditions there seems to be no significant renal sympathetic tone, because denervation does not increase RBF, and α- and/or β-adrenergic receptor blockers do not alter RBF. However, increased sympathetic activity produces large reductions of RBF, mediated by increased renal vascular resistance. Both afferent and efferent arterioles contract, producing a smaller proportional drop of GFR than of RBF. Thus, the filtration fraction (FF = GFR/RPF) *rises*, or at least does not fall. During activation of the sympathetic system the decrease of RBF is distributed homogenously in the cortex. Major redistribution of blood flow does not occur.

IV. GLOMERULAR FILTRATION

The net effect of the hydrostatic and colloid-osmotic pressure differences across the glomerular capillary wall is the production of an almost ideal *ultrafiltrate*, that is, a solution which contains water and crystalloids, but not colloids.

A. Mechanism of Glomerular Filtration

The rate of filtration at the glomerulus is controlled by the same forces which act in other capillary beds:

$$GFR = K_f(\Delta P - \Delta \pi) = K_f[(P_{GC} - P_T) - (\pi_{GC} - \pi_T)]$$

Figure 5. Driving forces for glomerular filtration. ΔP ($P_{GC} - P_T$, where P_{GC} is the glomerular capillary hydrostatic pressure and P_T the urinary space hydrostatic pressure) and $\Delta\pi$ (the analogous difference of colloid-osmotic pressures, normally essentially equal to the glomerular colloid-osmotic pressure, π_{GC}) are plotted as a function of length along the capillary. The diagram on the left illustrates a situation of filtration pressure equilibrium ($\Delta P - \Delta\pi = 0$ before the end of the vessel); the diagram on the right illustrates the situation of filtration pressure disequilibrium ($\Delta P > \Delta\pi$ at the end of the capillary). The table at the bottom shows mean values of pressures at afferent and efferent ends of the capillary in the two conditions. Data from Brenner and co-workers (equilibrium) and from Arendhorst and Gottschalk (disequilibrium). P_{UF}, the effective filtration pressure, is $\Delta P - \Delta\pi$, or $P_{GC} - P_T - \pi$. See text.

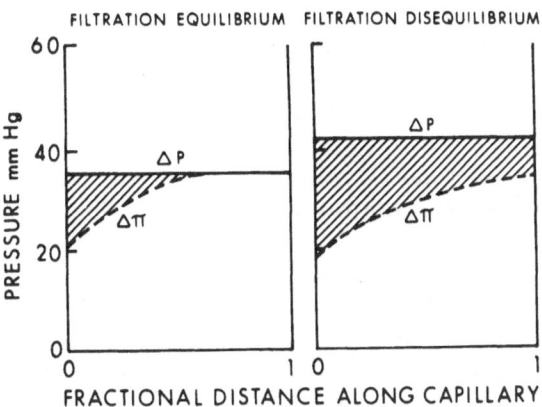

FILTRATION EQUILIBRIUM   FILTRATION DISEQUILIBRIUM

FRACTIONAL DISTANCE ALONG CAPILLARY

Pressures (mm Hg)

	Equilibrium		Disequilibrium	
P_{GC}	45	45	55	55
π_{GC}	20	35	18.5	35
P_T	10	10	13	13
P_{UF}	15	0	23.5	7

where GFR is the rate of glomerular filtration, K_f is the filtration coefficient, which includes hydraulic permeability of the wall (L_p) and total area available for filtration (S), Ps are hydrostatic pressures, and πs are colloid-osmotic pressures. The subscripts GC and T indicate glomerular capillary lumen and tubular space, respectively. Δs stand for differences across the capillary wall. Because of its small value, π_T can usually be neglected. Glomerular ultrafiltration of proteins is normally negligible. Since ΔP favors filtration and $\Delta\pi$ opposes filtration, the driving pressure or effective pressure for ultrafiltration (P_{UF}) can be expressed as

$$P_{UF} = \Delta P - \Delta\pi$$

Recent work in a strain of rats with superficial glomeruli (accessible to puncture) has permitted a direct quantitative analysis of glomerular filtration. Mean results are summarized in Figure 5.

P_{GC} is thought to decrease along the capillary by a very small amount. π_{GC}, however, undergoes a large progressive increase, because filtration of "protein-free plasma" results in an increase of protein concentration in the capillary lumen. The mean effective pressure for ultrafiltration (P_{UF}) is a function of the area between the ΔP and $\Delta\pi$ curves shown in the figure.

P_{GC}, measured directly, was smaller than previously estimated by indirect techniques, and the hydraulic permeability coefficient of the glomerular capillary was estimated to be 10–100 times larger than those of most other capillary beds. In addition, in these rats with superficial glomeruli the rise in glomerular capillary oncotic pressure as a function of length is such that P_{UF} becomes zero before the end of the capillary. In other words, *filtration pressure equilibrium* ($P_{GC} = \pi_{GC} + P_T$) occurs, and filtration ceases. This fact makes glomerular filtration rate highly flow dependent. The reason is that at high flow rates the rise of π_{GC} will be slow, and therefore P_{UF} will not drop to zero as fast. It is not certain, however, that filtration pressure equilibrium is a general phenomenon.

GFR autoregulation is secondary to RBF autoregulation (see above). When perfusion pressure drops, the resistance of the afferent arteriole falls. Thus, RPF drops only moderately, and GFR varies in parallel with RPF, maintaining an essentially constant filtration fraction.

As explained in reference to the mechanism of renal blood flow autoregulation, it has been suggested that the composition of the luminal fluid at the level of the macula densa controls the degree of contraction of the afferent arteriole, and hence renal blood flow and glomerular filtration rate. The relationship between fluid composition and GFR, supported by several experimental observations, is referred to as *glomerulo-tubular feedback*. The proposed role of the juxtaglomerular apparatus in this process is referred to as the macula densa feedback hypothesis (see Section III.B).

B. Measurement of Glomerular Filtration Rate

As discussed before, total kidney GFR can be measured by the clearance of freely filterable substances which are not subject to tubular transport, renal metabolism, or accumulation in the organ. The typical substance for this purpose is *inulin*, a fructose polymer of molecular weight ~5200 and effective molecular radius ~14 Å. Inulin clearance in adult man is about 125 ml/min. It is advisable to relate the value of C_{in} to body surface for standardization purposes.

Creatinine has the advantage, as compared to inulin, of being produced in muscle cells at a relatively constant rate, independent of diet and physical activity. Therefore, an intravenous infusion is not needed. In man, however, creatinine is not only filtered, but is also secreted by the proximal tubule. Exogenous C_{creat} is about 40% greater than C_{in}. At the physiological plasma creatinine concentrations secretion is less, and C_{creat} is higher than C_{in} by about 7%, when true creatinine, and not other chromogens, are measured in plasma and urine. When the total chromogen (Folin picrate) method (the usual clinical laboratory method) is employed, C_{creat} is indistinguishable from C_{in} if GFR is normal. At very low GFR, C_{creat} measured by the total chromogen method rises as compared to C_{in}, because plasma creatinine concentration represents a larger fraction of total plasma chromogens and because the fraction of creatinine excreted by secretion increases. At a GFR of 20 ml/min, C_{creat} is about 50% higher than C_{in} and true GFR.

The clearance of urea was used in the past to estimate GFR. There is no good reason to maintain this practice. On the average, $C_{urea} \sim 0.6$ GFR (because of tubular reabsorption of urea, in addition to filtration). Furthermore, the clearance of urea is affected by urine flow.

Recently, radioactively labeled substances, which are easy to measure, have been increasingly used to measure GFR both experimentally and clinically. Some of these substances are Vitamin B_{12} (cyanocobalamine), EDTA, and sodium iothalamate. Like inulin, these substances are excreted exclusively by glomerular filtration.

C. Permselectivity of the Glomerular Capillary Wall

Recent studies of the mechanisms of permeation of large molecules through the glomerular capillary wall have shown that filtration of such molecules depends on three factors: the *size*, the *shape*, and the *net electric charge* of the molecule.

1. Molecular Size

Molecules of the size of inulin or smaller are present in the glomerular filtrate at the same concentration as in plasma water. With increasing molecular size, concentration in the filtrate decreases progressively and becomes very low for serum albumin. Only the smallest plasma proteins filter across the glomerulus.

The permselectivity of the glomerular capillary wall can be studied by comparing clearances of substances of different molecular sizes which filter and are not reabsorbed or secreted by the tubules. Comparison of the U/P ratio of such a substance with the U/P of inulin yields

$$(U/P)_x / (U/P)_{in} \leq 1$$

If the ratio is 1, x filters "freely," like inulin. If the ratio is less than 1, filtration of x is restricted. Molecular radius, above about 25 Å, correlates negatively with $(U/P)_x$, or with $(U/P)_x / (U/P)_{in}$.

2. Molecular Shape

The above considerations are somewhat complicated by the effect of the shape of the molecule on filtration. At equal molecular weight, filtration of globular molecules such as proteins is less than that of random coil molecules such as dextran.

3. Net Electric Charge

Protein filtration is restricted as compared to that of uncharged, inert molecules such as dextrans. This shift can be explained by protein reabsorption, and by the fact that at the pH of body fluids proteins are polyanions. Filtration of negatively charged dextran sulfate is also restricted, as compared to that of neutral dextran, whereas filtration of cationic (positively charged) dextran is favored. Therefore, at constant molecular size, negative charge of the solute restricts and positive charge accelerates its filtration. Glomerular filtration can be phenomenologically treated as if it occurred through pores lined with negative charges. The charge in the pore exerts effects on mobility and local concentration of the filtering molecule. Cations are more concentrated than anions inside the pore. Their mobility decreases because of the electrostatic interaction with the pore wall. However, it has been shown for other systems that the effect on concentration is dominant. Therefore, a charged channel facilitates the flux of counterions and restricts the flux of coions.

D. Structural Basis of Glomerular Filtration

The limiting barrier for permeation across the glomerular capillary has been studied by intravenous administration of electron-dense particles of varying molecular size, shape, and electric charge. By transmission electron microscopy, the site at which they are trapped has been identified. It has been shown that the three barriers of the glomerular capillary wall, i.e., endothelium, basement membrane, and foot processes, contain negatively charged glycoproteins. This fact could explain the selective restriction of permeation of anionic macromolecules, described above.

No specific structure in the glomerular capillary wall appears to act as the sole barrier for filtration of macromolecules. Polyanions such as albumin are restricted by endothelium and internal surface of the basement membrane, whereas polycations are trapped in the external portion of the membrane or the slit diaphragm of the foot processes of the epithelial cell. Neutral macromolecules appear to be restricted essentially by the basement membrane.

V. TUBULAR TRANSPORT

A. Introduction

In this section we will study the essential aspects of reabsorption and secretion by the renal tubule under physiologic conditions. The mechanisms of regulation of these processes and their pathophysiological alterations will be treated in detail elsewhere in this text. We will restrict our description to transport of salt and water and substances which exert effects on them. The physiology of transport of other solutes will be described within the context of the respective pathophysiological alterations.

Our present understanding of transport by the renal tubule has been obtained mainly with three experimental techniques: (1) *micropuncture* of identified segments of renal tubules in anesthetized animals (rat, hamster, dog), to obtain samples of tubular fluid, or to measure electrical parameters (e.g., luminal or cellular electrical potential); (2) *microperfusion* of isolated tubule segments *in vitro*, which allows study of segments not accessible to micropuncture, permits a wider variety of experimental perturbations, and in addition prevents the effect on tubule function of systemic parameters difficult to identify or control; and (3) *transport studies in isolated membrane vesicles*, in which uptake or extrusion of particular substances by specific membranes such as the brush border (luminal membrane) of the proximal tubule, can be measured *in vitro*.

Our present knowledge of the transport functions of the renal tubule permits its division into three major segments: (1) the proximal tubule, (2) the loop of Henle, and (3) the distal nephron. Even though there are subdivisions of these segments, from both a morphological and a physiological viewpoint, it is possible to establish a clear correlation of each of them with a general function.

B. Proximal Tubule

The proximal tubule is a typical leaky epithelium. It transports at a high rate salt, several other solutes, and water. Active Na^+ transport appears to be the essential process, to which transport of Cl^-, several organic solutes, and water are coupled by a variety of mechanisms. Fluid transport is isoosmotic, and solute concentration differences across the wall are small.

The proximal tubule can be divided in three segments on the basis of their intrinsic properties, the different composition of their luminal fluids, or both.

1. Description of Transport Processes

a. Early Proximal Convoluted Tubule

i. Na Reabsorption. Na reabsorption is *active* because it occurs with no transtubular Na concentration difference and against a small transtubular electrical potential (1–5 mV, lumen negative: $V_L = -1$ to -5 mV). Since the cell interior is electrically negative to the lumen, by about 70 mV, and the intracellular Na activity is lower than the luminal activity, Na entry is a downhill process. Studies in a variety of species indicate the existence of several parallel mechanisms of Na transport at this membrane: diffusional entry, carrier-mediated cotransport (with glucose, amino acids, lactate, phosphate, and, at least in amphibian proximal tubule, chloride), and carrier-mediated countertransport (Na^+ uptake coupled to H^+ extrusion). Most of this information comes from studies in brush border vesicles. From these data it is difficult to estimate the quantitative importance of each pathway.

In isolated mammalian tubules it appears that about one third of the Na entry is coupled to glucose and amino acids. Sodium transport from cell to extracellular fluid is an uphill process driven by the sodium–potassium pump.

Intercellular transport of Na is presumed to occur by water flow from lumen to intercellular spaces (because of the osmotic pressure difference generated by salt transport into the intercellular spaces). Since the junctions are highly permeable to NaCl, the salt would be dragged by the water flux (solvent drag). Although reasonable, this mechanism has not been unequivocally demonstrated.

ii. Anion Reabsorption. HCO_3^- is reabsorbed preferentially to Cl^-. HCO_3^- reabsorption is coupled to H^+ secretion into the lumen, which occurs by Na^+-H^+ exchange. As a result of this titration, the bicarbonate concentration in the lumen decreases, whereas the chloride concentration increases, with their sum remaining constant. Cl^- transport from lumen to blood is downhill (both because of its higher concentration in the lumen and the negative transtubular electrical potential difference). However, entry from lumen to cells seems to be coupled to Na (secondary active transport); transport from cells to peritubular space is downhill.

iii. Water Reabsorption. Water reabsorption is coupled to salt transport, probably by the hyperosmotic lateral intercellular space mechanism (see Chapter 1).

iv. Reabsorption of other Substances. Glucose and amino acid reabsorption is uphill, coupled to Na^+ transport and essentially complete in this segment. As described before, glucose and amino acids accumulate in the cell by a Na^+-dependent secondary active transport. Transport from the cell to the extracellular fluid is downhill, and at least in part carrier mediated. Some permeant solutes, such as urea, are partially reabsorbed, by a passive mechanism, because of the increase in their luminal concentration as water is being reabsorbed.

The essential transport properties of the proximal convoluted tubule and the transcellular mechanism of Na transport are summarized in Figure 6.

b. Late Proximal Convoluted Tubule

The luminal fluid of the late proximal convoluted tubule is characterized by a low HCO_3^- and a high Cl^- concentration and by the absence of glucose and aminoacids. The tubule fluid remains isoosmotic to plasma and has the same Na^+ concentration as the filtrate.

The luminal electrical potential (V_L) in this segment is $+1$ to $+3$ mV. This potential is caused by the different anionic composition of tubular and peritubular fluids (lumen: high Cl^-, low HCO_3^-; peritubular fluid: high HCO_3^-, low Cl^-). The tubule is more permeable to Cl^- than to HCO_3^-. Thus, the CL^- concentration gradient across the wall generates a lumen-positive diffusion potential (Figure 7).

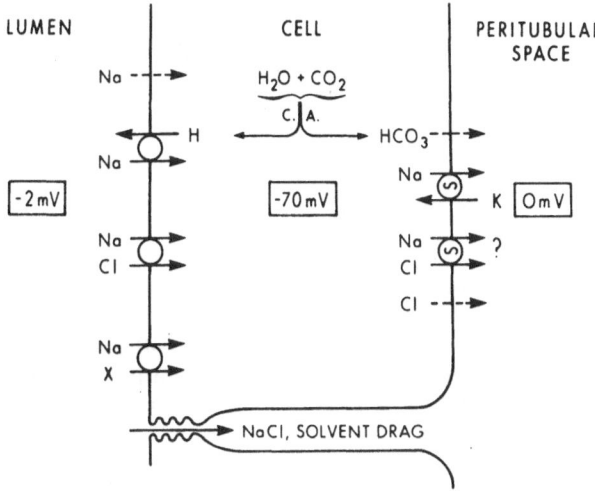

Figure 6. Mechanisms of salt transport by the proximal convoluted tubule. This figure summarizes current hypotheses of transport at the two cell membranes and across the intercellular pathway. Segment arrows indicate simple electrodiffusion across cell membranes; C.A., carbonic anhydrase. Na^+ can enter the cell by simple electrodiffusion (uniport), by exchange with H^+ (antiport), or by cotransport (symport) with Cl or a number of organic or inorganic substrates (X, which can be glucose, amino acids, lactate, or phosphate). Na^+ transport from cell to peritubular fluid occurs by the operation of the Na,K pump and probably also by means of a NaCl neutral pump. Finally, a portion of salt reabsorption can occur bypassing the cells, by solvent drag. Mean values of electrical potentials are also shown. See text.

In experiments *in vitro*, in which luminal and peritubular fluids have identical composition, active Na transport has been shown to occur. A fraction of the Na flux *in situ* is downhill, because of the positive luminal potential, and a third fraction is also passive, by solvent drag, as in the early proximal convoluted segment. The driving forces for Cl^- reabsorption (Cl^- concen-

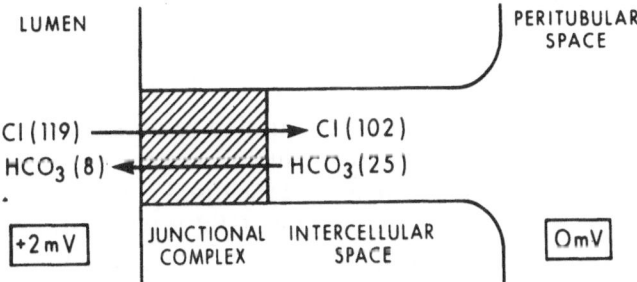

Figure 7. Effect of asymmetric anion concentrations across the late proximal convoluted tubule and pars recta on electrical potential difference. Preferential bicarbonate reabsorption results in low HCO_3^- and high Cl^- concentrations in the lumen, as compared to interstitial fluid (mean values, millimolar, shown in parentheses). Since Cl^- is more permeant than HCO_3, a lumen-positive diffusion potential is generated. This potential can drive part of Na^+ reabsorption. In addition, the permeability difference causes an effective osmotic pressure difference which drives water flow from lumen to peritubular space.

tration difference and solvent drag) can account for passive Cl reabsorption, even though V_L is positive, because of the high Cl permeability and the higher Cl^- concentration in the lumen. The mechanisms of transport at the cell membrane level appear to be similar to those described for the early proximal convoluted tubule.

The late proximal convoluted tubule is the main site of organic acid secretion (PAH, penicillin, uric acid).

c. Proximal Straight Segment (Pars Recta)

The pars recta has intrinsically different transport properties when compared with the convoluted segments. The main ones are that (1) the rates of Na and fluid transport are slower, and (2) the capacities for glucose and amino acid reabsorption are minimal.

As in the late proximal convoluted segment, V_L is positive (by about the same amount), and Na and Cl appear to be transported by the same mechanisms.

In the late proximal convoluted tubule and in the straight segment, the anion concentration gradients can drive water reabsorption in the absence of a total osmotic gradient across the wall, because of the higher HCO_3^- reflection coefficient as compared to Cl^- (see Chapter 1, Section V).

2. Modulation of Reabsorption by the Proximal Tubule

Proximal reabsorption is essentially an obligatory mechanism designed to save most of the filtered fluid and all of a number of essential solutes. Regulation of the final composition of the urine is achieved in the tighter distal and collecting segments of the tubule. Nevertheless, some factors do modulate the transport rate at the proximal tubule and therefore influence the performance of later segments by altering their load.

a. Glomerulo-tubular Balance

Changes in the rate of glomerular filtration result in changes of the rate of proximal tubule fluid reabsorption in the same direction. Hence, the delivery of fluid to the loop of Henle and the distal nephron, and eventually urinary output, vary only moderately when GFR is primarily altered. Glomerulo-tubular balance is a very important adaptive mechanism. If the rate of fluid reabsorption by the tubule did not change with GFR, a 10% increase in GFR (from 120 to 132 ml/min, or equivalently from 180 to 198 liters/day) would cause an increase in urine output of 18 liters/day.

The mechanism of glomerulo-tubular balance, in spite of much research, remains unknown. One possible explanation is a GFR-dependent change in physical factors acting across the tubule wall, as explained below.

b. Transtubular "Physical Factors"

Hydrostatic (P) and colloid-osmotic (π) pressure differences across the tubular wall can influence directly the bulk flow rate from the tubule lumen to the capillary lumen. In addition, changes of P or π in tubule lumen and peritubular capillary can influence indirectly the reabsorption rate by changing the permeability of the intercellular pathway. When π falls or P rises in the peritubular capillaries, the limiting junctions become leakier and backflux (from intercellular spaces to tubular lumen) occurs. The opposite change of π_c and P_c seem to exert opposite effects. The reduced fluid reabsorption observed during ECF expansion could depend in part on this mechanism. Glomerulo-tubular balance has been ascribed to changes of protein concentration (and colloid-osmotic pressure) in the peritubular circulation, directly related to primary GFR changes ($\uparrow$GFR $\rightarrow$ $\uparrow\pi$ efferent arteriole $\rightarrow$ $\uparrow\pi$ peritubular capillaries). A strong argument against this possibility is the demonstration of filtration pressure equilibrium in rats with superficial glomeruli. If this is true in man as well as in rat, π at the efferent arteriole is constant regardless of GFR.

c. Hormones

The possibility of a natriuretic hormone has been suggested from experiments in which expansion of the ECF volume was shown to result in a natriuretic and diuretic response under conditions in which GFR and plasma aldosterone were kept constant. Another condition attributable to a natriuretic hormone is the "escape" (natriuretic response) observed a few days after continuous administration of mineralocorticoids (see Chapter 4). A possible site of action of this hypothetical substance is the proximal tubule. There is no conclusive proof, as yet, of the existence of this hormone.

Parathyroid hormone (PTH) affects mainly Ca and phosphate transport by the tubule. In addition, it reduces proximal Na and fluid reabsorption.

Some authors have claimed that aldosterone increases proximal tubule Na reabsorption, but careful later studies have shown that the elevation of the rate of Na transport was probably caused by a rise of GFR, secondary to the positive Na balance produced by the hormone.

d. Catecholamines

Recent experimental results suggest that catecholamines stimulate fluid reabsorption by the proximal tubule. The physiological significance of these observations has not been established.

C. Loop of Henle

The thin segments of the loop of Henle contribute to the generation of interstitial hyperosmolality in the renal medulla. This hyperosmolality is the driving force for water reabsorption from the collecting ducts, in a regulated mode dependent on the action of antidiuretic hormone (ADH). The gradient for water reabsorption is always present (under physiologic conditions), but water is reabsorbed only if ADH is available to produce an increase of cortical collecting tubule and medullary collecting duct water permeability.

1. Transport Mechanisms at the Thin Segments of the Loop of Henle

There is no clear-cut evidence for active salt transport by the thin segments of the loop. The essential transport properties of the descending and ascending segments are their passive permeabilities to water and solutes. The descending limb has a high water permeability and a low solute permeability, whereas the ascending segment has a low water permeability and a relatively high solute permeability ($P_{NaCl} > P_{urea}$).

In normal mammals the interstitial fluid is hyperosmotic because of high concentration of both urea and NaCl, which ultimately result from NaCl transport by the thick ascending limb of the loop (see below). The composition of the luminal fluid, and the properties of the two segments of the loop, result in quite specific transport processes. At the descending limb, net water flow occurs from lumen to interstitium, with a progressive rise in luminal osmolality toward the papilla (and tip of the loop). At the ascending limb, because the lumen contains mostly NaCl, whereas in the interstitium [urea] > [NaCl], NaCl diffuses outward (J_{NaCl}) and urea inward (J_{urea}). Since NaCl permeability is greater than urea permeability, the net effect is $J_{NaCl} > J_{urea}$, or net addition of solute to the interstitial fluid, in the absence of active transport at this level. The ascending limb fluid becomes diluted, as compared to interstitial fluid at the same level (Figure 8).

2. Transport Mechanisms at the Thick Ascending Segment of the Loop of Henle

The thick ascending segment of the loop is the site of active salt transport responsible for the countercurrent multiplication mechanism in the renal medulla. This segment is essentially impermeable to water and unresponsive to ADH. Therefore, salt transport from lumen to interstitial fluid results in a reduction of the osmolality of the luminal fluid. At the beginning of the distal tubule, the luminal fluid is hypoosmotic as compared to cortical plasma.

When this segment is exposed *in vitro* to the same solution in lumen and bath, it develops a lumen-positive electrical potential difference of about 6 mV. From this observation it has been postulated that Cl^- is the ion actively transported from lumen to ECF, and that Na^+ follows passively, driven by the electrical gradient. Alternatively, Cl entry at the luminal membrane could be coupled to Na entry, and Cl transport from cell to ECF could be a downhill process, whereas Na^+ would be extruded from the cell uphill by the operation of the Na^+ pump. A role of Na^+ in Cl^- transport is strongly

Figure 8. Transport mechanisms in the loop of Henle (thin segments). Luminal fluid entering the loop is isoosmotic to cortical plasma. The descending segment has a high water permeability. Luminal osmolality increases progressively because of a net water flow from lumen to the hypertonic intestitial fluid. At the bend of the loop the fluid in the lumen has the same osmolality that the surrounding interstitial fluid, and is hyperosmotic to cortical plasma. However, the compositions of luminal and interstitial fluid differ: urea predominates in the interstitium because of reabsorption at the collecting ducts. The ascending segment is water impermeable and more permeable

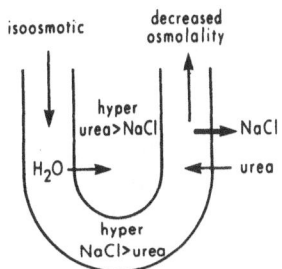

for NaCl than for urea. Therefore, the net NaCl flux from lumen to interstitium is larger than the net urea flux in the opposite direction. The interstitial osmolality is thus increased and the luminal osmolality decreased. See Kokko and Rector (1972).

suggested by the dramatic effect of Na^+ pump inhibitors on Cl^- transport. This matter is unresolved at the present time.

The value of V_L appears to be sufficient to drive downhill reabsorption of K^+ and Ca^{2+} if one considers the permeability of the tubule wall. The pathway for transport of these ions is uncertain.

The rate of salt transport by this segment, as in the proximal tubule, increases when the load rises, providing therefore a compensation for changes in filtration rate or proximal reabsorption.

3. Mechanism of Generation of Renal Medullary Hyperosmolality: Countercurrent Multiplication and Exchange

The hairpin shape of the loop of Henle, in conjunction with the different transport properties of its three segments, permits its operation as a *countercurrent multiplier*. In addition, the medullary blood vessels, or vasa recta, operate as *countercurrent exchangers*.

Countercurrent multiplication results from transport of sodium chloride from lumen to interstitial fluid by the thick and thin ascending segments of the loop. This process establishes a small local osmotic gradient because solute transport is not coupled to water transport. The interstitial fluid osmolality rises, and causes water reabsorption from the thin descending limb, because of the high water permeability of this segment. The local osmotic gradient, or *single effect*, is *multiplied longitudinally* because of the hairpin shape of the loop. This notion can be understood intuitively by considering the operation of the system when transport starts. At time = 0 fluid in both limbs has an osmolality of 300 and the single effect is a difference of osmolality of 20. In the first cycle, fluid enters the loop at 300 mOsm/kg, but leaves at 280 mOsm/kg. The osmolality of interstitial fluid and luminal fluid of the descending segment rises to 320. Therefore, in the next cycle fluid enters the ascending limb at 320 mOsm/kg, and transport rises interstitial osmolality to 340 mOsm/kg. Further operation of the system results in a progressive increase of osmolality of the interstitial fluid and the luminal fluid until a steady state is reached. This equilibrium is characterized by isoosmotic inflow, hypoosmotic outflow, and a progressive rise in osmolality of luminal fluid and interstitium from the cortex to the bend of the loop. It has been shown that the osmolality rises hyperbolically as a function of the distance along the loop, from cortex to medulla. At any level, interstitial fluid and luminal fluid in the descending limb have the same osmolality, but luminal fluid in the ascending limbs has a lower osmolality. The difference is the single effect.

The steady state operation of the countercurrent mechanism requires a precise balance between solute accumulation and solute removal, which is effected by the vasa recta. The rate of removal is small, making the system

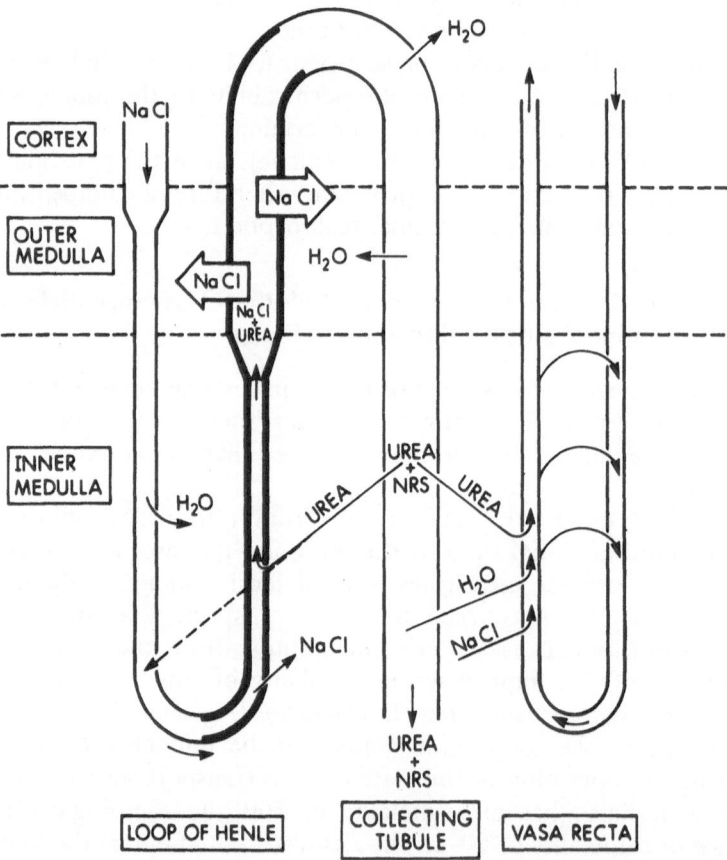

Figure 9. Operation of the countercurrent mechanism. The scheme is based on the model proposed by Kokko and Rector (1972), in which NaCl transport by the thin ascending limb is proposed to be passive. The only active transport mechanism is NaCl reabsorption by the thick ascending segment. Thick wall of ascending segments and distal tubule indicates water imperme-ability. NRS stands for nonreabsorbable solute. See text for details.

highly efficient, because the vasa recta operate as countercurrent exchangers. Since these vessels are highly permeable to NaCl, urea, and water, as blood flows from cortex to medulla its osmolality increases, reaching a maximum at the papilla, and decreases progressively in the ascending limb of the vessel, therefore minimizing solute loss.

In the presence of ADH (antidiuresis), water is reabsorbed in the collecting segments. Since urea permeability is very low in the cortical cellecting tubule, and unchanged by ADH, this results in an increase of luminal urea concentration. In the medullary collecting tubule, ADH increases both water and urea permeability, and therefore both water and urea are reabsorbed. Urea, as stated above, contributes a large fraction of the interstitial osmolality, and enters the tubules, mostly the ascending thin limb of the loop. The end result of this process is trapping of urea in a circuit constituted by ascending limb, distal tubule, cortical collecting tubule, medullary collecting tubule, and medullary interstitium. Cycling of urea contributes to interstitial hyperosmolality and permits net NaCl transport by the thin ascending limb of the loop without the need to postulate active salt transport. In water diuresis (absence of ADH), the lack of urea reabsorption in the medullary collecting tubules causes a decrease of medullary osmolality. This explains, at least in part, the fact that the maximum concentration of the urine in response to exogenous ADH is less in subjects on a high water intake. The operation of the countercurrent mechanism is summarized in Figure 9.

The countercurrent mechanism establishes a hyperosmotic renal medullary interstitium. This compartment is separated from the luminal fluid of the collecting segments by the tubule wall, whose water permeability can be regulated, according to homeostatic needs, by ADH. Under all normal conditions, fluid reaching the distal tubule is hypoosmotic (100–200 mOsm/kg). In the absence of ADH, solute reabsorption continues in distal and collecting segments and the urine becomes more hypoosmotic, to a limit of ~50 mOsm/kg. In the presence of ADH, water is reabsorbed, down the osmotic gradient, in cortical and medullary collecting tubules, and can reach a maximum osmolality equal to that of the papillary interstitium (~1200 mOsm/kg).

Further discussion on the mechanism of water excretion by the kidney is presented in Chapter 6.

D. Distal Nephron (Distal Convoluted Tubule, Cortical Collecting Tubule, and Medullary Collecting Duct)

1. Distal Convoluted Tubule

The distal convoluted tubule is defined here as the segment which extends from the macula densa to the site of transition from homogenous cells to a mixture of dark and light cells (typical of the collecting tubule). This transition occurs before the junction with other "distal" segments.

Within this definition, the distal convoluted tubule is, in some respects at least, functionally similar to the thick ascending segment of the loop of Henle. Some authors have proposed to call these two sections the "diluting segment." As the thick ascending segment of the loop, the distal convoluted tubule is essentially impermeable to water and unresponsive to ADH. NaCl is reabsorbed at a slower rate than in the proximal tubule or in the loop, but against large concentration gradients. The rate of reabsorption, as in the loop of Henle, is directly proportional to the load. Therefore, increases in the rate of fluid delivery by the proximal tubule can be compensated for, at least in part, by these segments.

The electrical potential between the lumen and the peritubular fluid varies along the length of the distal tubule. In the early portion some authors have even found a slightly lumen-positive value. At the end of the segment, V_L is about -45 mV. The cell membrane potential, admittedly difficult to measure because of the small size of the cells, appears to be quite constant (about 70 mV, cell negative) across the basolateral membrane, independently of the distance along the length of the segment.

The magnitude of V_L is clearly related to the concentration of Na in the lumen. High Na concentration results in a greater lumen negativity, presumably by increased Na entry into the cells, and increased pumping at the basolateral membrane. The mechanism of Na^+ entry is not fully understood, since the Na^+ permeability of the membrane appears to be quite low. The possibility of coupled NaCl transport has been proposed. K^+ seems to be more permeant than Na^+ at both the luminal and the peritubular membrane. K^+ secretion by the distal tubule, as discussed in detail in Chapter 7, could then result from uphill uptake at the basolateral membrane (Na pump) and downhill flux from the cell to the lumen, driven by the high K^+ concentration difference, which offsets the opposing effect of the electrical potential (cell negative to the lumen). Two complicating features of this scheme are the experimental demonstrations, under some conditions, of uphill Cl and uphill K reabsorption. As in the case of the thick ascending segment of the loop, uphill Cl transport could be due to either a primary active mechanism (i.e., a Cl^- pump) or a secondary active transport mechanism (coupled to Na^+ transport). Uphill K^+ reabsorption is currently thought to be caused by an inwardly oriented K^+ pump located at the luminal membrane. The net result of K^+ transport at this level can be absorption or secretion, according to homeostatic requirements (see Chapter 7).

Another important transport process at the distal tubule is acidification of the luminal fluid, which has been ascribed to an active H^+ transport mechanism located at the luminal membrane.

The distal tubule, as the collecting segments, is responsive to aldosterone. The net result of the action of this hormone is to increase Na^+ reabsorption and K^+ secretion.

2. Cortical Collecting Tubule

The cortical collecting tubule is defined as the nephron segment which extends from the end of the distal tubule (transition to clear and dark cells) to the cortico-medullary junction.

This segment has a negligible basal water permeability, that increases dramatically by the action of ADH. NaCl is reabsorbed at this level. Therefore, in the absence of ADH the luminal fluid osmolality can drop further. In the presence of ADH, the osmolality equilibrates with that of the cortical interstitial fluid; in other words, the luminal fluid becomes isoosmotic with plasma. ADH increases the osmotic water permeability but not the urea permeability. Therefore, water reabsorption at this level results in an increase of luminal urea concentration.

The luminal electrical potential is on the average about -35 mV, but varies widely according to the status of mineralocorticoid secretion, which in turn is determined by salt intake. Administration of DOCA results in an increase of V_L (lumen more negative) that reaches a maximum in about six days. As in the distal segment, K^+ can be reabsorbed or secreted at this level, and H^+ is secreted.

Na^+ transport is uphill and thought to occur by downhill luminal entry, which can be blocked by the diuretic amiloride, and active transport at the basolateral membrane (Na pump). The mechanism of Cl^- transport, as in the case of the distal segment, is probably active, or secondarily active, at one of the cell membranes. This segment is tighter than the distal tubule.

3. Medullary Collecting Duct

The medullary collecting duct starts at the cortico-medullary junction. It can be divided in an outer and an inner medullary segment. Their limit is the junction between inner and outer medulla. The large papillary ducts (ducts of Bellini) open on the surface of the papilla.

The transport properties of the medullary collecting duct are similar to those of the cortical collecting tubule. In the absence of ADH, the collecting duct has very low water and urea permeability. Since NaCl is reabosrbed at this level, the luminal osmolality can drop further in the absence of the hormone. ADH causes an increase of water permeability and consequently a net water flow from the lumen to the medullary interstitial fluid, which is hyperosmotic. Under the maximum effect of ADH, the luminal fluid equilibrates with the papillary interstitial fluid, and the urine becomes maximally hyperosmotic. The effect of ADH at this segment, in contrast with the one in the cortical collecting tubule, includes an increase in urea permeability. Therefore, in the presence of the hormone the net water flow from lumen to interstitial fluid causes an increase in urea concentration in the lumen and a net urea flux toward the interstitium.

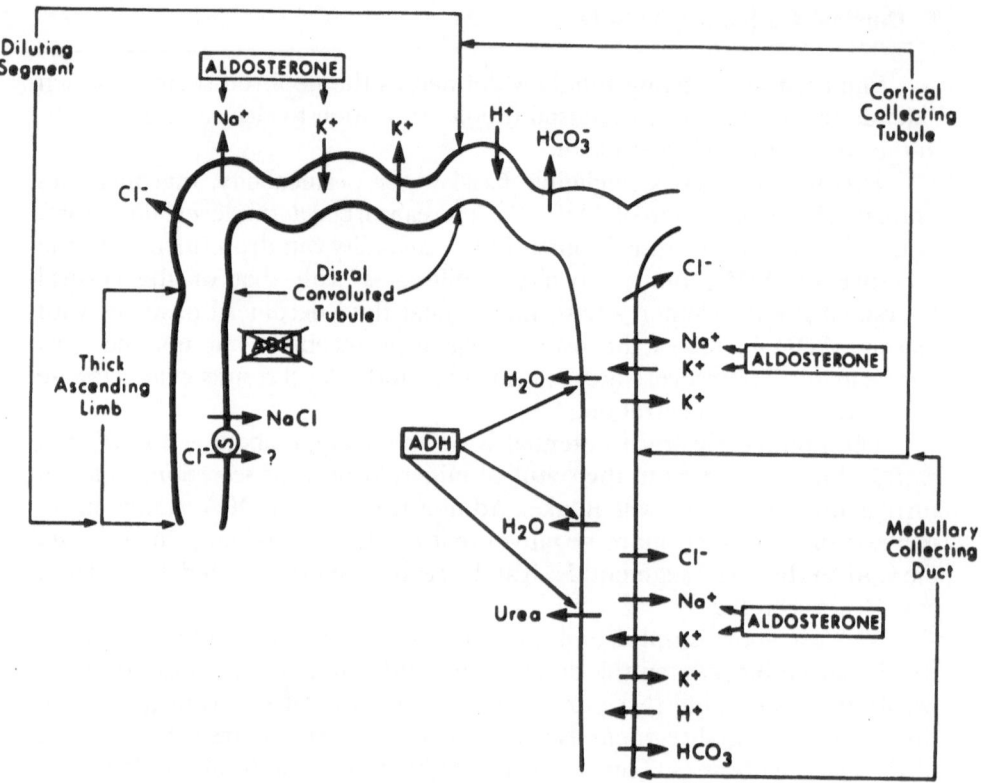

Figure 10. Summary of transport mechanisms in the distal nephron. The "diluting segment" (thick ascending segment of the loop of Henle and distal convoluted tubule) is water impermeable and unresponsive to ADH (thick line). The cortical collecting tubule and medullary collecting tubule are water tight in the absence of ADH, but increase their water permeability in presence of the hormone (thin line). ADH also stimulates reabsorption of urea by the papillary collecting duct. Overall ion transport mechanisms are indicated by arrows. Na^+ reabsorbed (aldosterone stimulates reabsorption); K^+ can be reabsorbed or, usually, secreted (aldosterone stimulates secretion); H^+ is normally secreted against a steep electrochemical gradient. All of these segments are tight epithelia.

The mechanisms of transport of electrolytes and the actions of mineralocorticoids appear to be similar to those described for the cortical collecting tubule.

The transport properties of the distal nephron are summarized in Figure 10.

E. Summary of Renal Tubule Transport Mechanisms

The rate, mechanism of control, and physiological significance of salt and water transport are different in the three essential portions of the renal tubule.

Table I. Summary of Transport Properties of the Renal Tubule

	Solutes reabsorbed	Solutes secreted	Luminal potential (mV)[a]	Permeability		Sodium transport rate (% of filtered)
				Water	Ions	
Proximal tubule						
Convoluted	Na^+, Cl^-, HCO_3^-, K^+, organic solutes, etc.	H^+	-4	High	High	75
Straight	Na^+, Cl^-, HCO_3^-, K^+	H^+, organic acids	-2	High	High	20
Loop of Henle						
Thin descending	—	—	0	High	Low	
Thin ascending	NaCl	—	0	Low	High	
Thick ascending	NaCl, K^+, Ca^{2+}	—	$+6$	Low	High	
Distal nephron						
Distal convoluted tubule	Na^+, Cl^-, HCO_3^-, K^+	H^+, K^+	-45	Low	Low	4
Cortical collecting tubule	Same	Same	-35	Low; ADH: high	Low	
Medullary collecting duct	Same, urea	Same		Low; ADH: high	Low	

[a] Luminal potential measured with the same solution on both sides. *In vivo*, the value in the straight segment is $+2$ mV.

In the *proximal tubule*, typical leaky epithelium, salt and water are transported at high rates, in isotonic proportions. Bulk reabsorption of most of the filtrate (~75%), and virtually complete reabsorption of essential solutes (glucose, amino acids) are the main results of proximal tubular function.

The *loop of Henle and the diluting segment* are a complicated arrangement of three diverse sections with strikingly different properties concerning active transport, water permeability, and solute permeability. Because of these properties, hyperosmolality is built up in the medullary interstitium, and acts as the driving force for final water reabsorption. The loop reabsorbs additional Na and water (~20% of filtrate) and leaves rather small amounts for the last segments of the tubule.

The *distal convoluted tubule and the collecting tubule* are tighter epithelia: water impermeable in the absence of ADH, the collecting tubules increase their osmotic permeability in response to the hormone. It is at these segments that the volume and osmolality of the urine is controlled. Salt transport occurs at slow rates, but against large gradients. The small amount of NaCl delivered to the distal nephron is handled appropriately to the necessities of the body by the regulatory action of aldosterone. K^+ excretion and H^+ excretion are also regulated at these segments.

The main functional characteristics of the different segments of the renal tubule are summarized in Table I.

SUGGESTED READINGS

Aukland, K.: Renal blood flow, in Thurau, K. (ed.): *International Kidney and Urinary Tract Physiology II*. University Park Press, Baltimore, 1976, p. 23.

Beeuwkes III, R., Ichikawa, I., and Brenner, B. M.: The renal circulations, in Brenner, B. M., and Rector, F. C. (eds.): *The Kidney*. W. B. Saunders, Philadelphia, 1981, p. 495.

Boulpaep, E. L.: Electrical phenomena in the nephron. *Kidney Int.* 9:88, 1976.

Boulpaep, E. L.: Electrophysiology of the kidney, in Giebisch, G., Tosteson, D. C., and Ussing, H. H. (eds.): *Membrane Transport in Biology*, Vol. IVA. Springer-Verlag, Berlin, 1979, p. 97.

Brenner, B. M., Boehreer, M. P., Baylis, Ch., and Deen, W. M.: Determinants of glomerular permselectivity: insights derived from observations *in vivo*. *Kidney Int.* 12:229, 1977.

Brenner, B. M., Ichikawa, I., and Deen, W. M.: Glomerular filtration, in Brenner, B. M., and Rector, F. C. (eds.): *The Kidney*. W. B. Saunders, Philadelphia, 1981, p. 289.

Burg, M. B.: Renal handling of sodium, chloride, water, amino acids, and glucose, in Brenner, B. M., and Rector, F. C. (eds.): *The Kidney*. W. B. Saunders, Philadelphia, 1981, p. 328.

Frömter, E.: Solute transport across epithelia: what can we learn from micropuncture studies on kidney tubules? The Feldberg Lecture, 1976. *J. Physiol. (London)* 288:1, 1979.

Hebert, S. H., Schafer, J. A., and Andreoli, T. E.: Principles of membrane transport, in Brenner, B. M., and Rector, F. C. (eds.): *The Kidney*. W. B. Saunders, Philadelphia, 1981, p. 116.

Jamison, R. L.: Urine concentration and dilution. The roles of antidiuretic hormone and urea, in Brenner, B. M., and Rector, F. C. (eds.): *The Kidney*. W. B. Saunders, Philadelphia, 1981, p. 495.

Jamison, R. L., Sonnenberg, H., and Stein, J. H.: Questions and replies: role of the collecting tubule in fluid, sodium and potassium balance. *Am. J. Physiol.* 6:F247, 1979.

Kokko, J. P., and Rector, F. C., Jr.: Countercurrent multiplication system without active transport in inner medulla. *Kidney Int.* 2:214, 1972.

Lameire, N. H., Lifschitz, M. D., and Stein, J. H.: Heterogeneity of nephron function. *Annu. Rev. Physiol.* 39:159, 1977.

Maude, D. L.: Mechanism of tubular transport of salt and water, in Guyton, A. C., and Thurau, K. (eds.): *MTP International Review of Science. Kidney and Urinary Tract Physiology. Physiology Series I*, Vol. 6. Butterworths, University Park Press, Baltimore, 1974, p. 39.

Pitts, R. F.: *Physiology of the Kidney and Body Fluids*, Third edition. Year Book Medical Publishers Inc., Chicago, 1974.

Reineck, H. J., and Stein, J. H.: Regulation of sodium balance, in Maxwell, M. H., and Kleeman, C. R. (eds.): *Clinical Disorders of Fluid and Electrolyte Metabolism.* McGraw-Hill, New York, 1980, p. 89.

Sachs, G.: Ion pumps in the renal tubule. *Am. J. Physiol.* 2:F359, 1977.

Valtin, H.: *Renal Function: Mechanisms Preserving Fluid and Solute Balance in Health.* Little, Brown and Co., Boston, 1973.

Windhager, E. E.: Sodium chloride transport, in Giebisch, G., Tosteson, D. C., and Ussing, H. H. (eds.): *Membrane Transport in Biology*, Vol. IVA. Springer-Verlag, Berlin, 1979, 145.

3

Nonexcretory Functions of the Kidney

SAULO KLAHR

I. INTRODUCTION

The kidney contributes to body homeostasis not only through its excretory functions but also through important metabolic activities of the tubular epithelial cells. The latter are related not only to tubular transport mechanisms (e.g., reabsorption of sodium, chloride, glucose, and amino acids; secretion of hydrogen, potassium, organic acids, and bases) but also to synthesis of hormones, degradation of low-molecular-weight proteins and peptides, and metabolic interconversions aimed at the conservation of energy and the regulation of the composition of body fluids (e.g., maintenance of normal blood concentration of substrates and hydrogen ion activity). This chapter reviews the nonexcretory functions of the kidney, their role in the homeostasis of body fluids, and the changes in these functions brought about by disease.

II. SUBSTRATE UTILIZATION BY THE KIDNEY

A substantial amount of the metabolic work and substrate utilization by the kidney is devoted to functions unrelated to transport, such as gluconeo-

SAULO KLAHR • Department of Medicine, Washington University School of Medicine, St. Louis, Missouri 63110.

genesis, protein synthesis and degradation, excretion of drugs and its metabolites, and maintenance of cell structure.

III. CARBOHYDRATE METABOLISM

A. Glucose: Oxidative and Anaerobic Glycolysis

There is net utilization of glucose by the kidney, and oxidation of this substrate accounts for 13%–25% of renal oxygen consumption. Net glucose utilization occurs despite simultaneous renal glucose production (gluconeo-genesis). Oxidative metabolism and gluconeogenesis occur in the cortex, whereas glycolysis takes place at the papillary tip. The red outer medulla demonstrates both oxidative and anaerobic glycolytic activity. Approximately 60% of the glucose utilized by the kidney *in vivo* is converted to CO_2; most of the remainder is converted to lactate in the medulla. Changes in acid–base balance affect the renal metabolism of glucose.

B. Hexose–Monophosphate Shunt

Glucose oxidation by the hexose–monophosphate shunt pathway (Figure 1) accounts for less than 1% of the energy utilized by the kidney. However, this shunt may be important as a source of NADPH and pentoses required for certain biosynthetic activities (nucleic acids, fatty acids) and in the tubular process of hydrogen secretion. Metabolic acidosis, sodium depletion, and renal growth, following reduction of renal mass, enhance the activity of the hexose–monophosphate shunt in the kidney.

C. Glucose–Xylulose Pathway

This pathway is important in nucleotide and mucopolysaccharide syn-thesis, detoxification of drugs, and biosynthesis of inositol. Inositol synthesis (Figure 1) and conversion to phosphatidyl inositol may influence the prop-erties of tubular cell membranes and its transport characteristics.

D. Renal Gluconeogenesis

Liver and kidney cortex have the capacity for both glucose synthesis from noncarbohydrate precursors (gluconeogenesis) and glucose degradation via the glycolytic pathway (Figure 2). Gluconeogenesis is important when the

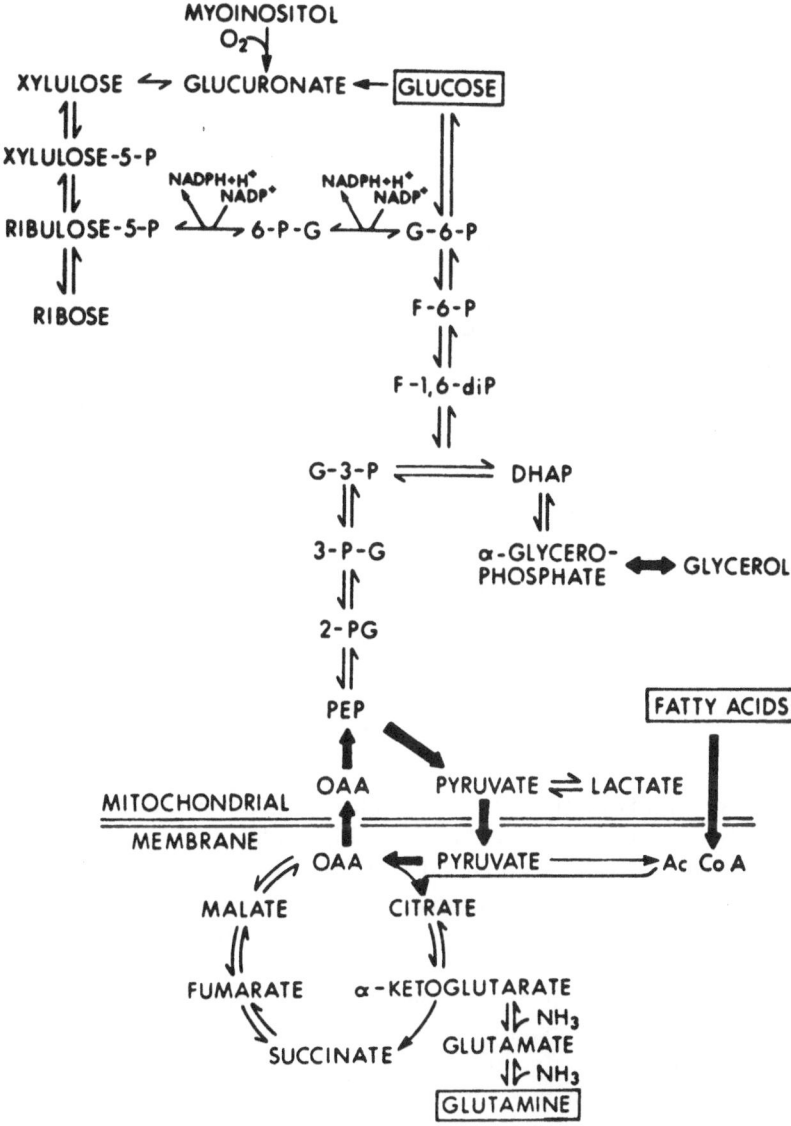

Figure 1. Metabolic pathways for glucose utilization by the kidney. The thick arrows denote rate-limiting steps in the various pathways. Anaerobic glycolysis leads to the production of pyruvate and lactate and takes place in the cytoplasm of tubular cells. Oxidative metabolism of pyruvate and fatty acids (as acetyl CoA) in the tricarboxylic acid cycle (TCA cycle) are intramitochondrial events. Conversion of G-6-P to 6-PG (hexose–monophosphate shunt) and of glucose to glucuronate and xylulose (glucose–xylulose cycle) are the other two important pathways of glucose utilization. Abbreviations: NADP, nicotinamide adenine dinucleotide phosphate; NADPH, reduced form of NADP; G-6-P, glucose-6-phosphate; F-6-P, fructose-6-phosphate; F-1,6-diP, fructose-1,6-diphosphate; G-3-P, glyceraldehyde-3-phosphate; DHAP, dihydroxyacetone phosphate; 3-PG, 3-phosphoglycerate; 2-PG, 2-phosphoglycerate; PEP, phosphoenolpyruvate; OAA, oxaloacetate; NH3, ammonia. (Adapted from Newsholme, E. A., and Gevers, W.: *Vitam. Horm.* 25:1, 1967.)

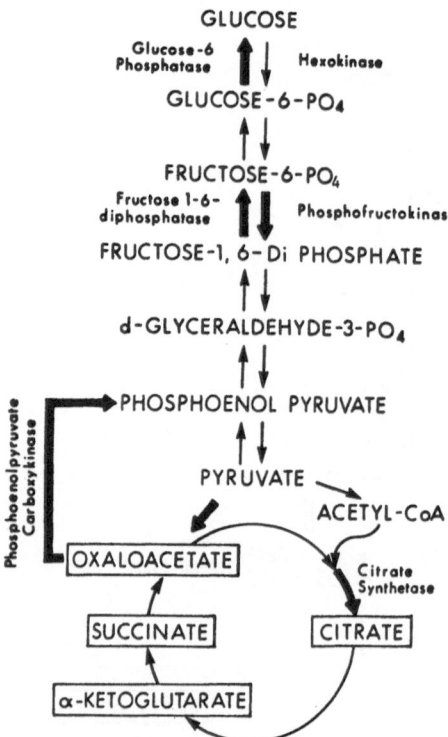

Figure 2. Pathways for renal glycolysis and gluconeogenesis. The thick arrows denote rate-limiting steps. Gluconeogenesis from glutamine proceeds via conversion to α-ketaglutarate (see Figure 1), oxaloacetate, and phosphoenolpyruvate. Phosphoenolpyruvate carboxykinase (PEPCK) is the rate-limiting enzymatic step in this conversion. (Adapted from Goorno, W. E., *et al.: Am. J. Physiol.* 213:969, 1967.)

metabolic demands of the animal for glucose are not met (i.e., starvation, low-carbohydrate diet); under these conditions glucose is required by tissues (central nervous system, red blood cells) which cannot meet their energy requirements from oxidation of fatty acids or ketone bodies. Gluconeogenesis may be important also in removing excessive quantities of certain substances from the blood (i.e., lactic acid after severe exercise). The ability of the kidney to convert certain organic acids (α-ketoglutaric, lactic) to glucose, a neutral substance, is an example of a nonexcretory mechanism in the kidney for pH regulation of body fluids. The major substrates for renal gluconeogenesis are pyruvate, lactate, citrate, α-ketoglutarate, and glutamine. When the rates of gluconeogenesis are increased (fasting, experimental diabetes, administration of glucocorticoids, or intracellular acidosis), there is enhanced activity of the gluconeogenic enzymes of renal cortex, particularly of phosphoenolpyruvate carboxykinase. The activity of this enzyme (which catalyzes the conversion of oxaloacetate to phosphoenolpyruvate) plays a key role in the rate of renal gluconeogenesis *in vivo*. The increased gluconeogenesis observed during fasting or diabetes is due to the development of acidosis since glucose production by the kidney is not increased when the acidosis is prevented by alkali administration. Acidosis increases the rate of renal gluconeogenesis only from those substrates which form oxaloacetate but not from substrates such as glycerol and fructose which enter the gluconeogenic pathway above phosphoenolpyruvate.

E. Control of Renal Gluconeogenesis *in Vivo*

In the intact animal renal gluconeogenesis is influenced not only by the factors discussed above but also by the substrate composition of the blood perfusing the kidney. For example, the increased renal gluconeogenesis during fasting may be due in part to a rise of plasma glycerol. Elevations in plasma lactate (prolonged exercise) may also lead to increased gluconeogenesis. Enhanced conversion of lactate and glycerol to glucose when their plasma concentrations rise is an example of the energy-conserving function of the kidney in which an excess of substrate in arterial plasma is converted to another substrate which may then be utilized or stored in other organs.

F. The Role of the Kidney in the Maintenance of Glucose Homeostasis

The quantitative contribution of renal gluconeogenesis to the maintenance of blood glucose in humans has not been defined. The balance between renal gluconeogenesis and utilization of glucose by the kidney determines whether there is net glucose release or uptake by this organ. During starvation in man the kidney may contribute as much as 50% of the glucose produced daily. Studies in animals suggest that the kidney may play a role in maintaining the basal output of glucose, a process which may not be greatly affected by hormonal changes.

IV. LIPID METABOLISM

The kidney extracts and utilizes fatty acids from plasma. A large fraction of the fatty acids extracted are incorporated into neutral lipids and only a small fraction is oxidized to CO_2. In the intact animal oxidation of palmitate, oleate, and stearate accounts for only 15% of renal oxygen consumption. Free fatty acids inhibit renal glucose oxidation and stimulate gluconeogenesis from lactate or glycerol (Figure 1). The relative contribution of renal fatty acid oxidation to Na transport has not been clearly defined. It appears, however, that the major role of fatty acids in the kidney is the regulation of gluconeogenesis and the maintenance of cell membrane integrity.

The kidney is also involved in the metabolism of mevalonate, a major precursor of cholesterol synthesis. The kidney converts circulating mevalonate to sterols and sterol precursors or oxidizes it to CO_2 (nonsterol or "shunt" pathway). The sterol pathway accounts for 75% and the nonsterol or "shunt" pathway for 25% of the mevalonate metabolized by the kidney. The major end product of mevalonate metabolism in the kidneys is cholesterol. Impaired clearance of blood mevalonate by the kidney could account for the hypercholesterolemia associated with some renal diseases, since such impairment might lead to increased hepatic synthesis and augmented release of cholesterol into the blood.

V. RENAL METABOLISM OF PLASMA PROTEIN AND PEPTIDE HORMONES

The kidney is an important catabolic site for low-molecular-weight plasma proteins (molecular weight below 50,000) but not for proteins with a molecular weight exceeding 68,000 (e.g., albumin, immunoglobulins). Filtration of proteins is apparently necessary for their renal catabolism. For example, a light (L) chain, a component of γ-globulin, is a plasma protein with a molecular weight of 22,000. Its filtration rate is about 8% of the GFR. The amount of L chains filtered is about 5 mg/kg body weight per day. Less than 1% of this amount appears in the urine, indicating a tubular reabsorption of approximately 5 mg/kg per 24 hr, an amount similar to the fractional metabolic rate. These observations suggest that the kidney catabolizes all of the light chains that are filtered and reabsorbed by the renal tubules. Nephrectomy reduces the fractional metabolic rate of L chains by 90%. In certain patients with renal tubular abnormalities, low-molecular-weight proteins may appear in the urine in the absence of albuminuria, owing to their decreased tubular reabsorption. Conversely, in patients with reduced GFR the fractional metabolic rate for light chains is decreased and plasma levels of light chains are elevated. Other low-molecular-weight proteins are handled in a similar manner. Thus, nephrectomy prolongs the half-life or the disappearance from plasma of lysozyme, ribonuclease, β_2-microglobulin, insulin, proinsulin, glucagon, parathyroid hormone, and Bence Jones protein. The kidney is also involved in the catabolism of retinol-binding protein and growth hormone.

A. Renal Handling of Intermediate and High-Molecular-Weight Proteins

The fractional catabolic rate for albumin (molecular weight 68,000), γ-globulins, and larger plasma proteins is relatively low, the kidney accounting for less than 5% of the fractional catabolic rate of these proteins, unless the nephrotic syndrome is present, in which case albumin catabolism can be significantly increased.

B. Products of Renal Protein Catabolism

The plasma proteins reabsorbed and catabolized by the kidney presumably are broken down to amino acids or polypeptides and returned as such into the renal venous blood.

C. Peritubular Uptake of Plasma Proteins

The information summarized above suggests that catabolism of plasma proteins by the kidney is inversely proportional to their molecular weight and proportional to the levels of GFR. Peritubular uptake of albumin and other large proteins presumably does not occur. There is evidence, however, for peritubular uptake of other plasma proteins. Peritubular uptake seems to play a role in the metabolism of hormones with specific receptors in the kidney (parathyroid hormone, glucagon, insulin). Studies of the extraction of β-microglobulin, molecular weight 12,000, also provide evidence for its peritubular uptake.

In summary, low-molecular-weight proteins are filterable, and therefore in the absence of tubular reabsorption will be excreted in the urine. The kidney, by reabsorbing these proteins, prevents their urinary loss, thus conserving the nutritionally important components of these proteins. It has been demonstrated that some of these proteins are catabolized by the kidney, and are not reabsorbed intact across the tubular epithelium. The kidney, therefore, contributes to the regulation of their plasma concentration without loss of the protein components in the urine. Many of these low-molecular-weight proteins and polypeptides are enzymes and hormones and control of their plasma concentration by the kidney underscores the role of renal metabolism in the regulation of body fluid composition.

D. Kidney Metabolism of Peptide Hormones

1. Insulin

The major sites of insulin degradation are the kidney and the liver. Since insulin binds minimally to larger plasma proteins and has a molecular weight of 5800, its glomerular filtration should be similar to that of inulin. In man, less than 1% of the filtered insulin is excreted in the urine. Renal catabolism of insulin involves both filtration and reabsorption and peritubular uptake. The kidney also catabolizes proinsulin and C peptide. The renal extraction of these two peptides and insulin seems to be directly proportional to their arterial concentration. In rats ligation of the renal pedicle results in a 75% rise in plasma insulin levels and a 300% increase in proinsulin and C peptide levels (Figure 3). Therefore, while proinsulin and C peptide are catabolized principally by the kidney, this organ accounts for only 33% of the plasma disappearance rate of insulin while extrarenal sites (mainly liver) account for 67% of its disappearance rate. With decreased renal mass the increased levels of immunoreactive insulin measured in plasma may represent a greater contribution of proinsulin and C peptide than of the active insulin molecule per se. Consequently, a dissociation between insulin levels, as measured by radioimmunoassay and biologically active insulin, may occur in the presence of decreased renal mass. In addition, in diabetics with advancing renal disease decreased degradation of insulin may lower the amount of exogenous insulin required for adequate control of blood glucose. Furthermore, exogenous insulin requirements will increase in diabetic patients with end stage renal disease following renal transplantation.

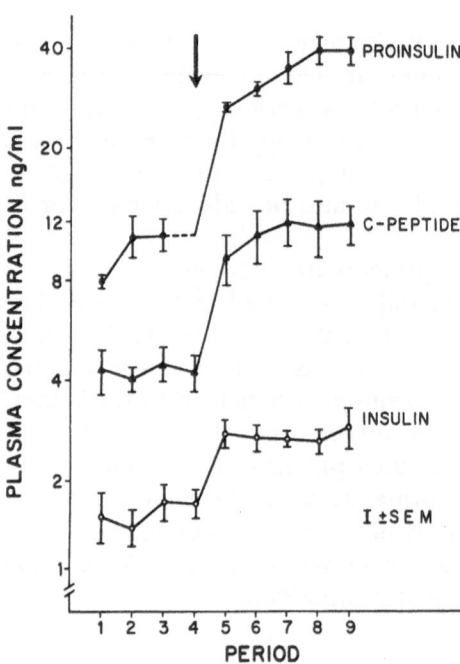

Figure 3. Effect of exclusion of the kidneys from the circulation on the plasma levels of proinsulin, insulin and C-peptide. Periods 1–4 preceded and periods 5–9 followed ligation of both renal pedicles (arrow) in rats infused with equimolar amounts (5 pmol/min) of the three compounds. (Reproduced with permission from Katz, A. I., and Rubenstein, A. H.: *J. Clin. Invest.* 52:1113, 1973.)

2. Glucagon

The kidney is an important site of degradation of this hormone. Elevated plasma levels of glucagon are found in patients with chronic renal failure. This hyperglucagonemia is apparently not due to hyersecretion but to a decreased (approximately 60%) metabolic clearance rate of glucagon in patients with chronic renal failure. The elevation in immunoreactive glucagon observed in chronic renal failure is due, in part, to species of glucagon devoid of biological activity.

3. Parathyroid Hormone

Although parathyroid hormone (PTH) secretion increases in chronic renal disease (due to hypocalcemia), most of the accumulation of immunoreactive PTH in uremia relates to its decreased renal degradation. PTH is catabolized by the kidney by both filtration and peritubular uptake (Figure 4). The peritubular uptake is selective for the biologically active forms of parathyroid hormone and presumably involves specific receptor binding. Filtration rate is responsible for the catabolism of carboxy terminal (biologically inactive) PTH fragments and for a portion of the catabolism of the amino terminal fragments (biologically active) and the intact hormone. A large portion of the elevated immunoreactive PTH in uremia relates to the accumulation of carboxy-terminal fragments which are handled exclusively by filtration. Renal transplantation, in the absence of changes in hormone secretion, will decrease immunoreactive PTh levels to 20% of pretransplantation values within 24 hours when the kidney functions immediately following implant (Figure 5).

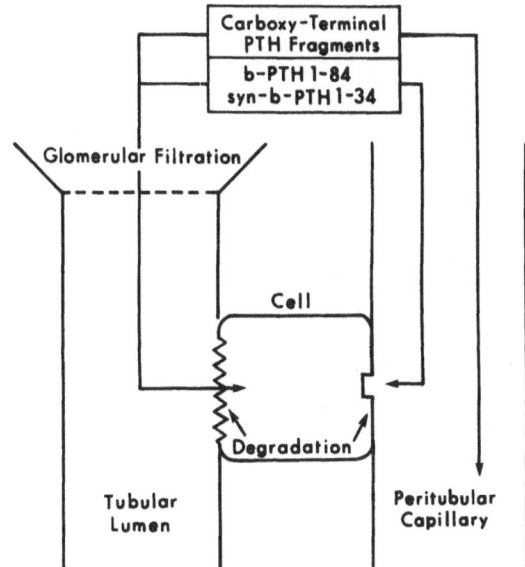

Figure 4. Schematic representation of the renal mechanisms of PTH uptake. Biologically active fragments of PTH (b-PTH 1-84 and syn b-PTH 1-34) are handled by peritubular uptake and by glomerular filtration with subsequent reabsorption and degradation. On the other hand, biologically inactive PTH fragments (carboxy terminal PTH fragments) appear to be dependent exclusively for degradation upon glomerular filtration and reabsorption by renal tubular cells.

Figure 5. Changes in levels of serum iPTH in two different uremic patients in relation to time after a successful renal transplant in one (●——●) or following parathyroidectomy in the other (O---O). The results are expressed as a percent of the preoperative values in the upper panel and in absolute values in the lower panel. (Reproduced with permission from Freitag *et al.*: *N. Engl. J. Med.* 298:29, 1978.)

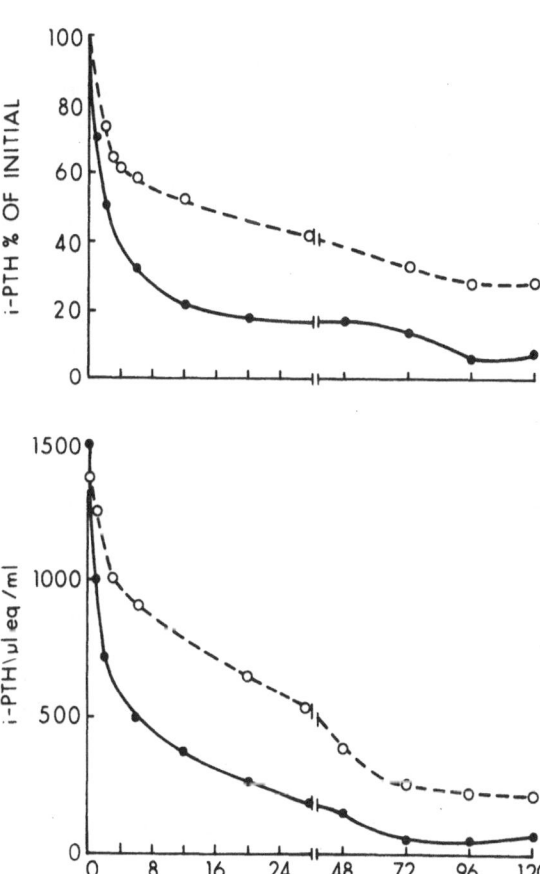

4. Other Peptide Hormones

The heptadecapeptide gastrin is extracted by the isolated perfused dog kidney and the plasma concentration of gastrin in man is increased by nephrectomy. Therefore, the hypergastrinemia present in renal failure is due to reduced degradation of this hormone by the kidney. The kidney is also a site for the degradation of ACTH, growth hormone, angiotensin II, and antidiuretic hormone (vasopressin). As is the case for insulin, vasopressin inactivation by the kidney occurs in direct proportion to its concentration in arterial blood. Although the kidney is a determinant of the half-life of vasopressin, its plasma level is primarily regulated by its secretion.

In summary, the kidney is an important organ in the catabolism of peptide hormones and the increased plasma levels of these hormones seen in chronic renal failure may be due in part to their decreased renal catabolism. Accumulation of these hormones in chronic renal failure may contribute to the pathophysiology of the uremic syndrome.

VI. ROLE OF THE KIDNEY IN THE REGULATION OF VITAMIN D METABOLISM

There are two naturally occurring precursors of vitamin D: ergosterol, which is present in plants, and 7-dehydrocholesterol, which is found in animals including man. After exposure to ultraviolet irradiation, ergosterol is converted into ergocalciferol (calciferol or vitamin D_2) and 7-dehydrocholesterol is converted into cholecalciferol (vitamin D_3).

The main source of vitamin D in man is endogenous vitamin D_3 produced by the ultraviolet irradiation of 7-dehydrocholesterol in the skin. The main source of exogenous vitamin D in the United States is milk. The daily requirement of vitamin D in infants is about 400 units; in older adults the requirement is as low as 70 units per day.

The kidney regulates mineral homeostasis not only by modifying the excretion of phosphate, calcium, and magnesium but also by its role in the metabolism of vitamin D. Vitamin D_3 is metabolized first to 25-hydroxy vitamin D_3 in the liver and subsequently to a number of dihydroxylated derivatives by the kidney (see Figure 6). Of these derivatives, 1,25-dihydroxy D_3 and 24,25-dihydroxy D_3 appear to be the most significant with the former being the calcemic hormone produced in the kidney during hypocalcemia or hypophosphatemia and the latter being elicited under normal mineral conditions. 1,25-dihydroxy D_3 increases intestinal calcium and phosphate transport and bone mineral resorption. The role of 24,25-dihydroxy D_3 is less well defined.

A. The 1,25-Dihydroxy Vitamin D₃

1,25-dihydroxy D_3 is a potent sterol hormone. Its biosynthesis in the kidney and its plasma levels are closely regulated by the mineral needs of the

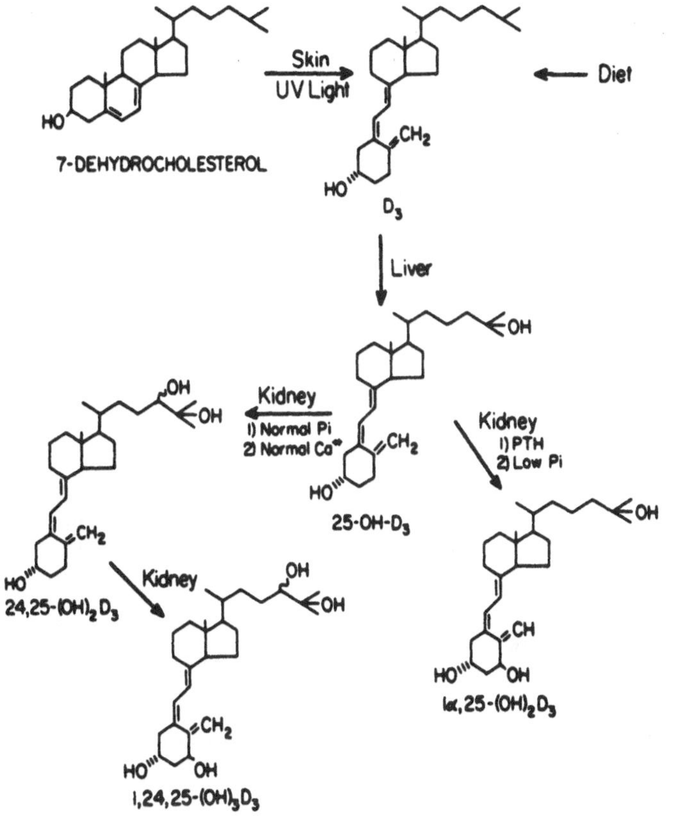

Figure 6. Metabolism of vitamin D_3. Vitamin D_3 formed in the skin by ultraviolet radiation or originating from the diet is metabolized first to 25-hydroxyvitamin D_3 in the liver and subsequently to 1,25-dihydroxy D_3 or 24,25-dihydroxy D_3 in the kidney. Increased levels of parathyroid hormone or decreased levels of phosphorus stimulate the renal production of 1,25-dihydroxy D_3. Conditions of normal mineral balance favor the formation of 24,25-dehydroxy D_3. 1,24,25(OH)$_3$D$_3$ may represent a degradative metabolite.

individual. Thus, low calcium (via PTH), low phosphate, and a number of hormones (estrogens, prolactin, growth hormone) all act *in vivo* to stimulate the production of 1,25-dihydroxy D_3 (Figure 7). Presumably, these latter endocrine factors modulate 1,25-dihydroxy D_3 during physiologic situations of calcium need like growth, pregnancy, and lactation. Conversely, 1,25-hydroxy D_3 biosynthesis is suppressed by hypercalcemia (via calcitonin), by hyperphosphatemia, and by 1,25-dihydroxy D_3 itself. When the production of 1,25-dihydroxy D_3 is suppressed, the renal 24-hydroxylase enzyme is induced and 24,25-dihydroxy D_3 becomes the predominant metabolite of 25-hydroxy D_3. An extrarenal site of production of 1,25-dihydroxyvitamin D_3 has also been suggested. In its target tissues 1,25-dihydroxy D_3 functions in the same way as the classic steroid hormones. It is thought that 1,25-dihydroxy D_3 binds to the genome, influences DNA transcription, and stimulates messenger RNA synthesis. The proteins formed are then functional in mineral translocation. 1,25-dihydroxy D_3 has its major effect in three target organs (see Chapter 9): (1) intestine (increases calcium and phosphate absorption), (2) skeleton (stimulates osteoclastic activity leading to

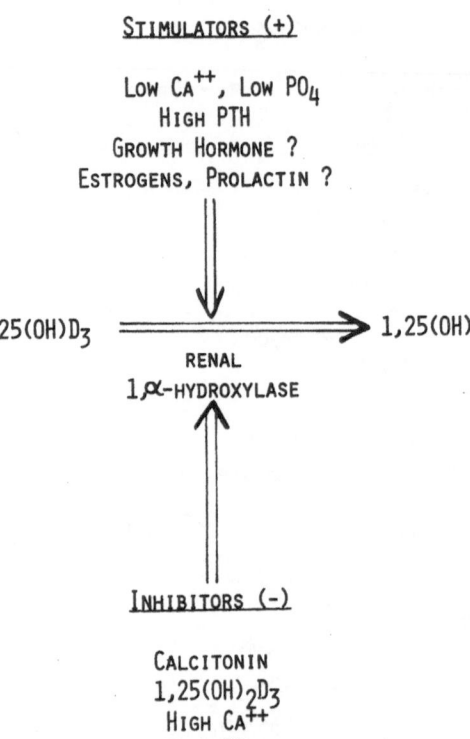

STIMULATORS (+)

Low Ca^{++}, Low PO$_4$
HIGH PTH
GROWTH HORMONE ?
ESTROGENS, PROLACTIN ?

25(OH)D$_3$ ⟶ 1,25(OH)$_2$D$_3$

RENAL
1α-HYDROXYLASE

INHIBITORS (-)

CALCITONIN
1,25(OH)$_2$D$_3$
HIGH Ca^{++}
HIGH PO$_4$

Figure 7. Factors which have been proposed in the control of 1-α-hydroxylase activity in the kidney. This mitochondrial enzyme is responsible for the conversion of 25-hydroxy D$_3$ to 1,25-dihydroxy D$_3$. Substances that accelerate the formation of 1,25(OH)$_2$D$_3$ are shown as stimulators (+) and substances that decrease the renal formation of 1,25(OH)$_2$D$_3$ have been labeled as inhibitors (−).

bone resorption and calcium mobilization), and (3) kidney tubule (stimulates reabsorption of calcium and phosphate).

Based upon the above information several syndromes involving vitamin D antagonism, resistance, or hypersensitivity have been defined. Table I summarizes the diseases currently thought to involve an abnormal level of one or more of the active vitamin D metabolites.

B. The 24-Hydroxylated D Vitamins

In addition to the renal 1-α-hydroxylase, which catalyzes the biosynthesis of the 1,25-dihydroxy D$_3$ hormone from 25-hydroxy D$_3$, there is another enzyme which hydroxylates the 25-hydroxy D$_3$ at carbon-24. Although the 24-hydroxylase is also present in kidney mitochondria, there is evidence for extrarenal production of 24,25-dihydroxy vitamin D$_3$ in rat and man. The exact role of 24-hydroxylation is not completely defined. The fact that 24,25-dihydroxy D$_3$ is less active than 1,25-dihydroxy D$_3$ in stimulating intestinal calcium and phosphate absorption and bone calcium resorption suggests that 24-hydroxylation is part of a breakdown pathway. On the other hand, small doses of 24,25-dihydroxy D$_3$ are very effective in restoring normal calcium metabolism in uremic subjects. Also, this metabolite suppresses PTH secretion

Table I. Plasma Levels of Vitamin D and Its Metabolites in Disorders of Mineral Metabolism[a,b]

Vitamin D	25(OH)D$_3$	1,25(OH)$_2$D$_3$
↑ Hypervitaminosis D	↑ Hypervitaminosis D	↑ Primary hyperparathyroidism
↓ Nutritional osteomalacia	↓ Anticonvulsant therapy	↑ Idiopathic hypercalciuria[c]
↓ Malabsorption	↓ Hepatobiliary disorders	↑ Sarcoid[c]
	↓ Nephrotic syndrome	↓ Chronic renal failure (advanced)
	↓ Nutritional osteomalacia	↓ Hypoparathyroidism
		↓ Pseudohypoparathyroidism
		↓ Vitamin-D-dependent rickets[c]
		↓ Postmenopausal osteoporosis[c]

[a] ↑, increased.
[b] ↓, decreased.
[c] Not all patients exhibit these changes in 1,25(OH)$_2$D$_3$ levels.

and is active in stimulating the synthesis of proteoglycans in chondrocytes. Recent data also indicate that 24,25-dihydroxy D$_3$ is required for normal bone formation in chicks. These activities of 24,25-dihydroxy D$_3$ would suggest that it is the form of vitamin D which promotes bone mineralization.

C. Alterations of Vitamin D Levels in Disease States

The levels of 1,25-dihydroxy D$_3$ have been measured in a number of disorders of mineral metabolism (see Table I). High plasma levels of 1,25-dihydroxy D$_3$ have been reported in patients with primary hyperparathyroidism and some forms of idiopathic hypercalciuria. The levels of this metabolite are markedly reduced in end stage renal failure but are restored to normal after a successful renal transplantation. The lack of 1,25-dihydroxy D$_3$ in patients with renal failure may be one cause of renal osteodystrophy and an excess of the hormone certainly contributes to the hyperabsorption of calcium and resulting nephrolithiasis of primary hyperparathyroidism and some forms of idiopathic hypercalciuria. In vitamin-D-dependent rickets, a disease in which there is an inherited defect in the renal 1-α-hydroxylase enzyme, the plasma levels of 1,25-dihydroxy D$_3$ are markedly decreased. In postmenopausal osteoporosis 1,25-dihydroxy D$_3$ levels are also reduced, perhaps due to estrogen deficiency. Since PTH stimulates the 1-α-hydroxylase and increases the plasma levels of 1,25-dihydroxy D$_3$, it is not suprising that 1,25-dihydroxy D$_3$ is subnormal in hypoparathyroidism and pseudohypoparathyroidism. 1,25-dihydroxy D$_3$ is either suboptimal or "normal" in patients with vitamin D resistant rickets.

The possible alterations of 24,25-dihydroxy D$_3$ in diseases of bone and calcium metabolism are currently controversial. Thus, both normal and undetectable serum levels of 24,25-dihydroxy D$_3$ have been reported in anephric patients. Most workers agree that serum 24,25-dihydroxy D$_3$ is slightly diminished in chronic renal failure patients who retain their diseased kidneys. In primary hyperparathyroidism 24,25-dihydroxy D_3 has been reported to be elevated but the metabolite is apparently unchanged in calcium stone formers without hyperparathyroidism.

VII. ROLE OF THE KIDNEY IN THE REGULATION OF RED BLOOD CELL MASS: ERYTHROPOIETIN

Erythropoietin is a glycoprotein with a molecular weight of approximately 40,000 which is thought to be formed by the kidney. Erythropoietin promotes the differentiation, proliferation, and maturation of red blood cell precursors in the bone marrow. The exact cellular site of synthesis has not been defined (juxtaglomerular cells?). Progress in this area of renal biochemistry has been hampered by the failure to obtain a pure preparation of erythropoietin and the need to rely on bioassays (i.e., ^{59}Fe utilization by polycytemic mice). When renal erythropoietin production is abolished by bilateral nephrectomy, and the patient is kept alive by regular dialysis, profound anemia ensues. Initially, erythropoietin levels are undetectable but small amounts are detected after several months owing to nonrenal production (liver?).

The stimulus to increased erythropoietin production by the kidney appears to be decreased renal oxygen tension or decreased renal perfusion. This may arise from anemia, hypoxia, renal ischemia, or the effect of vasoactive agents such as norepinephrine, angiotensin, or vasopressin. Increased erythropoietin is also seen occasionally in association with renal artery stenosis, renal cysts, renal cell carcinoma, hydronephrosis, and with a transplanted kidney. Erythropoietin production decreases when the kidney is subjected to hyperoxia or an excess red cell volume. Transfusions reduce erythropoietin production. Advancing chronic renal disease leads to a progressive decrease in renal erythropoietin production; this is an important factor in the development of the anemia of uremia. The disease kidney in chronic renal failure may also produce, or fail to excrete, inhibitors or inactivators of erythropoietin; the plasma of azotemic patients decreases the stimulating action of erythropoietin on red cell precursors in the bone marrow.

In summary, the anemia that accompanies chronic renal disease (Chapter 14), although multifactorial in origin, is in part due to decreased erythropoietin production as renal mass decreases. Secondary polycythemia with an increase in red cell mass is frequently associated with conditions in which erythropoietin production is augmented, notably hydronephrosis, renal cysts, and hypernephroma. Patients with polycystic kidney disease may have higher hematocrit values at a given level of renal insufficiency when compared with other patients with chronic progressive renal disease.

VIII. THE HORMONAL ROLE OF THE KIDNEY IN THE REGULATION OF EXTRACELLULAR FLUID VOLUME AND BLOOD PRESSURE

A. The Renin–Angiotensin–Aldosterone System

Renin is a proteolytic enzyme secreted by the granular cells of the juxtaglomerular apparatus. It acts in plasma on a substrate of hepatic origin, angiotensinogen, to form the decapeptide, angiotensin I. In the presence of converting enzyme, two amino acids are split from angiotensin I to form the active octapeptide, angiotensin II. The next split product is a seven-amino-acid peptide, angiotensin III, which also has important physiologic effects. Angiotensin II is a potent hormone, central to the regulation of salt and water balance. It produces vasoconstriction, stimulates aldosterone secretion, antidiuretic hormone secretion, thirst, and the renal reabsorption of sodium. Aldosterone, in turn, increases sodium reabsorption and potassium excretion by the distal nephron. Through the renin–angiotensin–aldosterone system, the kidney plays a role in blood pressure regulation and sodium and potassium homeostasis (see Figure 8). The renin system is but one of several renal systems (prostaglandins, the kallikrein system) that act interdependently in sodium homeostasis and blood pressure regulation (see Chapter 10).

Renin secretion is inhibited by angiotensin II and antidiuretic hormone. These two inhibitory influences constitute a negative feedback system. In addition, renin secretion is controlled by three other important inputs: intravenal baroreceptors, the macula densa, and sympathetic nerves.

1. Intrarenal Baroreceptors

If renal perfusion pressure is lowered, renin secretory rate is increased. This occurs even in a nonfiltering kidney, suggesting that under these conditions the increased release of renin is unrelated to changes in the filtered load of sodium. Cells in the afferent arteriole (presumably juxtaglomerular cells) sense changes in perfusion pressure and regulate the output of renin accordingly.

2. Macula Densa

If sodium delivery to the early distal tubule is changed, independent of perfusion pressure, renin output is altered. Any circumstance leading to increased sodium delivery to the distal tubule (osmotic diuresis, sodium loading, increased GFR) causes an increase of renin secretion. This mechanism serves as a feedback loop to adjust single-nephron GFR. The increase in renin release and the local generation of angiotensin will lead to a decrease in single-nephron GFR. The cells which sense these changes are thought to be macula densa cells of the distal tubule. How these cells signal the juxtaglomerular cells to increase renin output is unknown. Since the ascend-

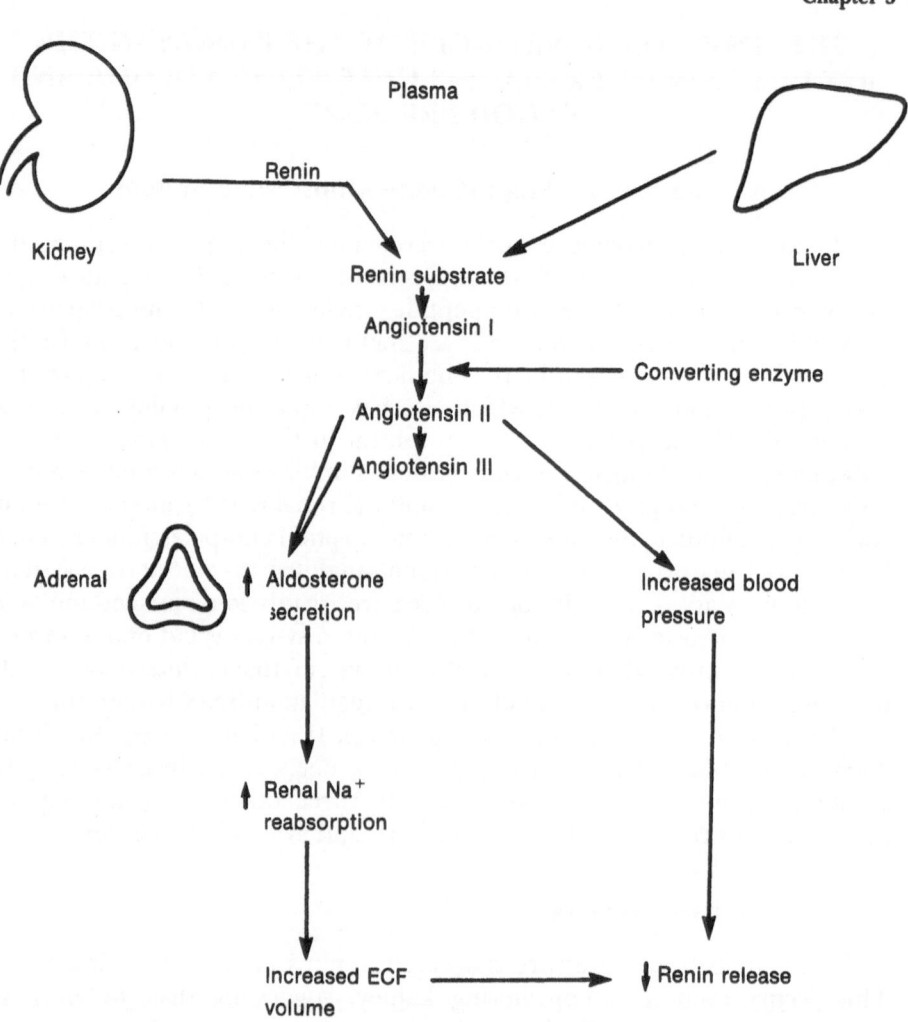

Figure 8. Renin produced in the kidney acts in plasma on a substrate of hepatic origin (renin substrate or angiotensinogen) to form angiotensin I (a decapeptide). Converting enzyme splits two amino acids of angiotensin I to form angiotensin II (an octapeptide). Loss of an additional amino acid from angiotensin II results in the formation of a heptapeptide (angiotensin III). Both angiotensins II and III stimulate the secretion of aldosterone by the zona glomerulosa of the adrenal. Increased aldosterone secretion, through sodium retention and ECF volume expansion and increased blood pressure as a consequence of angiotensin II, inhibit renin release.

ing limb of Henle's loop has an active transport of chloride rather than sodium, it is possible that the macula densa cells respond to changes in chloride delivery rather than to sodium.

3. Sympathetic Nerves

Renin secretion may be increased by stimulation of renal sympathetic nerves. If renal sympathetic nerve activity increases, afferent arteriolar vasoconstriction occurs which indirectly stimulates both the baroreceptors (decreased pressure) and the macula densa (decreased GFR and sodium load). In addition, the sympathetic nerves end at both the juxtaglomerular and macula densa cells. Thus they are capable of stimulating renin release directly.

B. Factors Affecting Renin Release

It is clear, then, that several factors affect renin release: (1) Renal vascular receptors which respond to changes in wall tension may account for the increased renin release that occurs with suprarenal aortic constriction, hemorrhage, and sodium depletion. Since in some of these conditions hypotension is present, the increased renin release may be regarded as a compensatory mechanism to restore blood pressure to normal. (2) Stimulation of renal nerves increases and denervation decreases renin release. This effect is a direct one because it is not inhibited by papavarine that blocks the pressure receptors. The renal nerves are involved in the increased renin release after assuming the upright posture, exercise, and hemorrhage. (3) The status of the extracellular fluid volume is an important regulatory mechanism of renin release. Volume contraction markedly increases, whereas volume expansion inhibits renin release. The effects of changes in ECF volume may be partially mediated by the baroreceptor mechanisms and the renal nerves but there seems to be an effect of the sodium or chloride ions per se at the level of the macula densa. (4) Potassium loading decreases and potassium restriction increases renin release. (5) β-Adrenergic stimulation (norepinephrine or isoproterenol) increase renin release. In certain forms of hypertension, β-adrenergic blockers (propranolol) have been effective in reducing blood pressure in part due to their effects on renin secretion. (6) Angiotensin II can mediate a direct feedback inhibition of renin release. This may explain the rise in renin release observed after blockade of the effects of angiotensin II with competitive inhibitors such as SAR-1-ALA-8 angiotensin II (saralysin). (7) Administration of inhibitors of the converting enzymes result in an increase in renin release.

The angiotensin II produced as a consequence of increased secretion of renin produces peripheral vasoconstriction resulting in increased blood pressure. Renal vasoconstriction with a decrease in both glomerular filtration rate and renal blood flow results. These effects are transient, presumably due to intrarenal release of prostaglandins (PGE_2) that attenuate the vasoconstrictive action of angiotensin II. Angiotensin II is the major physiological regulator of aldosterone secretion and it may have direct effects on sodium reabsorption in the nephron, which may be masked in part by concomitant effects mediated by aldosterone.

Aldosterone, a potent mineralocorticoid, is antinatriuretic and kaliuretic and its secretion from the zona glomerulosa of the adrenal cortex is mediated by the renin–angiotensin system (via angiotensin II or angiotensin III or both), ACTH, and changes in plasma sodium and potassium concentrations. Potassium has an important dual role in the renin–angiotensin–aldosterone system. It stimulates aldosterone secretion and inhibits renin secretion both by direct actions. Aldosterone secretion is also stimulated by ammonium, cessium and rubidium, cyclic AMP, and serotonin.

The renin–angiotensin system seems to play the major role in the control of aldosterone secretion. Increased levels of angiotensin account for hypersecretion of aldosterone after acute hemorrhage, during sodium depletion, experimental malignant hypertension, heart failure, cirrhosis of the liver, the nephrotic syndrome, and in pregnancy. ACTH itself causes only a transient increase in aldosterone secretion but it plays an important permissive effect which is required to demonstrate increases of the hormone produced by other stimuli. Aldosterone acts on the cortical collecting tubule to promote reabsorption of sodium and secretion of potassium. The effect of aldosterone then is to increase potassium excretion and retain sufficient sodium to increase the extracellular fluid volume measurably to induce hypertension, and via these two effects indirectly to inhibit renin release. In some states of secondary hyperaldosteronism these effects are modified so that the aldosterone "escape phenomenon" (restoration of external balance of salt and water after expansion of the ECF space) may not occur and hypertension may not result (as in heart failure and the nephrotic syndrome). When aldosterone levels are high and ECF volume is expanded, there may be an inhibition of renin and angiotensin production and renin and angiotensin levels may be low. In such cases the secretion of aldosterone is usually primary in nature (primary aldosteronism) and not secondary to increased release of renin and formation of angiotensin II.

C. Pathophysiology of the Renin–Angiotensin System

Angiotensinogen (renin substrate) is a glycoprotein produced in the liver. Its plasma concentration is decreased in Addison's disease and severe liver disease and increased after bilateral nephrectomy, in Cushing's syndrome, in pregnancy and after administration of glucocorticoids, ACTH, or estrogens. Glucocorticoids and oral contraceptives can increase renin substrate concentration sufficiently to increase plasma renin activity *in vitro*.

Plasma renin concentration is measured by adding renin substrate in excess to a plasma sample. The mixture is then incubated in the presence of inhibitors of converting enzyme and angiotensinase. The angiotensin I generated is measured by radioimmunoassay. The term *concentration* is used because the addition of substrate in excess renders the kinetics zero order and this makes the angiotensin I liberated solely dependent on the concentration of renin in the plasma sample. The measurement of *plasma renin activity* has a wider clinical applicability. The result of the test depends on both renin concentration and angiotensinogen concentration. The renin substrate reaction is based on first-order kinetics but this is of physiologic

Table II. Levels of Plasma Renin Activity in Different Clinical Entities

I. Decreased Levels	II. Increased Levels
A. Expanded ECF volume	A. Contracted ECF volume
1. Salt loading	1. Salt restriction
2. Primary mineralocorticoid	2. Fluid loss (vomiting, diarrhea, diuretics)
excess	B. Decreased "effective" plasma volume
B. Hyperkalemia	1. Cirrhosis
C. Catecholamine deficiency	2. Nephrotic syndrome
	3. Congestive heart failure
	4. Adrenal insufficiency
	C. Catecholamine excess
	1. Pheochromocytoma
	2. Hyperthyroidism
	D. Hypokalemia
	E. Renal diseases
	1. Renovascular and malignant hypertension
	2. Renin-secreting tumors
	3. Juxtaglomerular hyperplasia (Bartter's syndrome)
	F. Increased renin substrate
	1. Pregnancy
	2. Estrogen therapy ("the pill")
	3. Corticosteroid therapy

importance only when substrate levels are distinctly elevated (administration of estrogen or corticosteroids) or decreased (severe liver disease). Plasma renin activity is affected by many clinical conditions. Table II lists some of them.

D. The Kallikrein–Bradykinin System

The kallikrein system (see Figure 9) has many similarities to the renin system. Kallikrein is a peptidase which acts on a species-specific plasma α-2-globulin substrate (kininogen) to split off a peptide, kinin. The active kinin is rapidly destroyed by plasma and tissue peptidases (kinininases). Kallikreins are widely distributed and are found in plasma, granulocytes, in the salivary, lacrimal and sweat glands, in the gut, and in the kidney. The plasma and glandular enzymes appear to be different.

The term *kinin* refers to three distinct biologically active peptides, methionyl-glycyl-bradykinin (11 amino acids), lysil bradykinin (ten amino acids), and bradykinin (nine amino acids). The kinins are potent vasodilators whose action is not inhibited by adrenergic blocking agents. The action of bradykinin in some tissues may depend on prostaglandin synthesis. Bradykinin may be inactivated in the lung by the converting enzyme which is also responsible for the conversion of angiotensin I to angiotensin II.

The renal kallikrein system may constitute a local hormonal system involved in the regulation of renal blood flow and sodium excretion. Whether

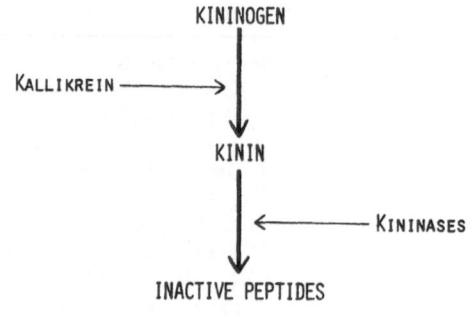

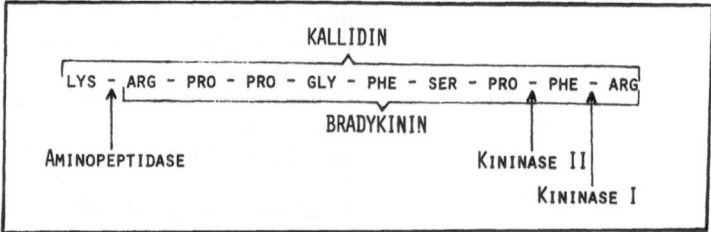

Figure 9. Schematic representation of the kallikrein–kinin system. Kallikrein is a peptidase which acts on a species specific plasma substrate (kininogen) to split off a peptide, kinin. The active kinin is rapidly destroyed by plasma and tissue peptidases (kinininases). The term *kinin* refers to different active peptides such as the decapeptide kallidin or the nonapeptide bradykinin (see insert in lower part of the figure).

renal kallikrein is secreted into the peripheral circulation in sufficient amounts to have physiological effects is unknown. Renal kallikrein is probably produced by the cortex and is excreted in considerable amounts into the urine. It acts on a kinogen substrate to produce the potent vasodilator decapeptide kallidin. Kallidin, when injected into the renal artery, has natriuretic effects. Changes in sodium intake alter the urinary excretion of kallikrein. Reduced sodium intake increases whereas a high sodium intake decreases kallikrein excretion. Mineralocorticoid administration increases kallikrein excretion. Spironolactone (which antagonizes the renal effects of aldosterone; see Chapter 17) decreases the elevated kallikrein excretion when given during low sodium intake (high aldosterone levels). Kallikrein excretion may be related to the levels of circulating mineralocorticoid hormones. Urinary kallikrein excretion may be normal or decreased in patients with essential hypertension. The excretion of subnormal amounts of kallikrein by patients with essential hypertension may represent a defect in the vasodilator system. Such a defect could possibly play a role in the increased renal vascular resistance seen in hypertensive patients. In patients with primary aldosteronism, urinary kallikrein excretion is elevated. Excretion is not affected by sodium intake but is diminished by spironolactone administration. These findings strongly suggest that aldosterone per se influences the urinary excretion of kallikrein. The exact role of the renal kallikrein system requires further study. It is known, however, that renal kallikrein is released by high arterial pressure, vasodilators (bradykinin, acetycholine, prostaglandin E_1, dopamine), low doses of norepinephrine, angiotensin II, mineralocorticoids, and rapid volume expansion.

E. Renal Prostaglandins

Renal prostaglandins are synthesized from free arachidonic acid, which is converted by the cyclooxygenase enzyme to the cyclic endoperoxides, PGG_2, and PGH_2 (Figure 10). The cyclic endoperoxides are then metabolized to a number of prostaglandins which include prostaglandin E_2 (PGE_2), PGF_2, PGD_2, thromboxane A_2, and prostacyclin or PGI_2. Synthesis of prostaglandins occurs in both the cortex (arteries, glomeruli) and medulla (medullary interstitial cells, collecting duct cells). Prostaglandins formed in the cortex are rapidly metabolized.

Renal synthesis of PGE_2 is stimulated by angiotensin II, bradykinin, and vasopressin. Prostaglandin synthesis in the renal papilla can be increased by angiotensin II and hyperosmolar solutions. The enhanced prostaglandin synthesis by the above is due to increased liberation of arachidonic acid from renal lipids by an acyl hydrolase. Prostaglandins are excreted in the urine

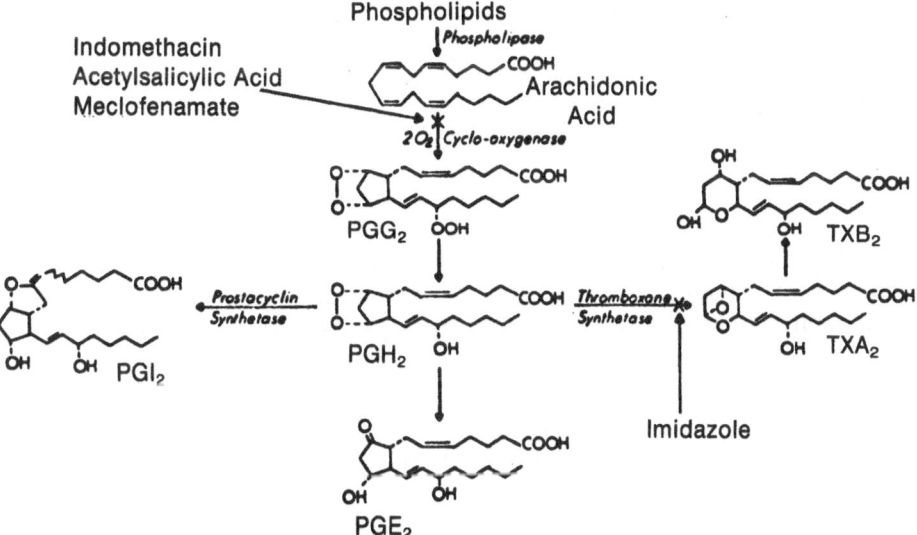

Figure 10. Prostaglandins are synthetized from free arachidonic acid which is liberated from phospholipids by a phospholipase. Arachidonic acid is converted by the enzyme cyclooxygenase to the cyclic endoperoxides (PGG_2 and PGH_2). The cyclic endoperoxides are then metabolized to a number of prostaglandins of the E series (PGE_2), to prostacyclin (PGI_2), or thromboxanes (TXA_2 and TXB_2). The different enzymes responsible for these conversions are shown, as well as those substances capable of inhibiting the activity of such enzymes.

and appear also in the renal venous blood. Clamping of the renal artery, infusion of angiotensin, and stimulation of the renal nerves increase renal venous PGE_2 levels. PGE_2 and $PGF_{2\alpha}$ are present in human urine. The kidney itself is the major source of urinary prostaglandins and evidence has been obtained for PGE_2 secretion into tubular fluid via the organic acid pathway.

The renal vasodilation which may occur in response to decreased renal perfusion appears to be mediated in part by increased synthesis of prostaglandins (PGE_2 is an important vasodilator) since it may be blocked by indomethacin and aspirin, known inhibitors of the cyclooxygenase. When renal blood flow is reduced, as in hemorrhagic shock, the blood flow to juxtamedullary structures is better preserved, a phenomenon which may be dependent on prostaglandin synthesis. Glomerular filtration during diminished perfusion may also be influenced by prostaglandins. In clinical syndromes where renal hemodynamics are disturbed, inhibitors of the cyclooxygenase have profound effects on GFR. For example, individuals on a low salt diet show a significant drop in GFR when given indomethacin. Indomethacin also may reduce GFR in patients with Bartter's syndrome, patients with cirrhosis, and infants with patent ductus arteriosus. These observations suggest a participation of prostaglandins in the maintenance of renal vascular resistance and GFR and suggest that these effects are greatest when renal hemodynamics are perturbed.

1. Prostaglandins and the Renin–Angiotensin System

Renal synthesis of prostaglandins and the renin–angiotensin system are interrelated: (1) Angiotensin II increases renal venous concentrations of PGE_2 and $PGF_{2\alpha}$ and their urinary excretion. The renal vasoconstriction produced by angiotensin II is potentiated by blockers of prostaglandin synthesis. (2) Renal prostaglandins both increase and decrease renal production of renin. Arachidonic acid, PGE_2, endoperoxides, and prostacyclin (PGI_2) stimulate renin release. Indomethacin blocks arachidonic-acid-stimulated renin release, and markedly reduces basal and stimulated renin levels in man and animals. The effects of furosemide on renin production may be due to increased arachidonic acid release and prostaglandin synthesis. $PGF_{2\alpha}$ inhibits renin synthesis and/or release. In conclusion, endoperoxides and PGE_2 stimulate and $PGF_{2\alpha}$ inhibits renin synthesis and/or release. The physiologic meaning of these effects may depend on a sodium-mediated control of conversion of PGE_2 and $PGF_{2\alpha}$.

2. Prostaglandins and the Regulation of Renal Blood Flow

Arachidonic acid and most prostaglandins, when administered intrarenally, increase renal blood flow with greater changes in the inner cortex than in the outer cortex. The contribution of renal prostaglandins to basal renal blood flow may not be as important as it is under conditions of compromised perfusion (hypotension, anesthesia). Inhibition of prostaglandin synthesis with indomethacin does not reduce basal renal blood flow in conscious dogs or in normal human subjects. Autoregulation of renal blood flow and GFR when perfusion pressures are varied between 80 and 150 mm Hg is also not impaired by inhibition of prostaglandin synthesis. In summary, the kidney produces more prostaglandins, especially PGE_2 and PGF_2, in response to ischemia and vasoconstriction. PGE_2 decreases renal vascular resistance (vasdilatory effect). The thromboxanes increase renal vascular resistance (vasoconstrictors). The factors regulating the renal synthesis of thromboxane A_2, a profound vasoconstrictor, and the relative rates of production of vasodilatory prostaglandins (PGE_2 and prostacyclin—PGI_2) vs. vasoconstrictor substances (thromboxanes) are not clearly understood.

3. Blood Pressure Control

Prostaglandins and thromboxanes may influence peripheral vascular resistance and blood pressure by their actions as vasodilators, vasoconstrictors, natriuretic substances, inhibitors of adrenergic neurotransmission, and activators or inhibitors of the renin–angiotensin system. Direct local action of these compounds on vascular smooth muscle and on the renal vascular resistance could significantly alter systemic arterial blood pressure. The potential role of prostaglandin synthesis in the control of blood pressure has been inferred from studies in normotensive and hypertensive animals in which prostaglandin synthesis has been inhibited. Indomethacin administered acutely increases blood pressure. Chronic dosage also increases blood pressure in normal rabbits. Indomethacin augments the hypertension in Goldblatt rats, with a unilaterally constricted kidney (Goldblatt kidney), in rabbits, and in spontaneously hypertensive rats. Chronic use of prostaglandin synthetase inhibitors in man may increase blood pressure slightly and it does enhance the pressor response to angiotensin II. In conclusion, there is evidence that the renal prostaglandins may be involved either primarily or secondarily in many types of hypertension.

4. Prostaglandins and Erythropoiesis

Renal artery constriction and decreased renal blood flow to 30% of normal causes an increase in renal venous erythropoietin and PGE_2 concentrations. These effects are blocked by indomethacin. Infusion of PGE_2 into an isolated hypoxic dog kidney increases erythropoietin production apparently via cyclic AMP. PGE_2 also has a direct stimulatory effect on marrow erythropoiesis and potentiates the action of small amounts of erythropoietin on the incorporation of ^{59}Fe into red cells in marrow culture. It appears, therefore, that prostaglandins influence erythropoietin action on the bone marrow.

5. Effects of Prostaglandins on the Renal Handling of Salt and Water

PGE_2 may influence the renal excretion of sodium and water. Prostaglandins apparently decrease sodium reabsorption and inhibition of their synthesis may result in decreased sodium excretion. Infusion of PGE_2 into the renal artery increases free-water clearance and indomethacin reduces water excretion. Indomethacin reduces free-water clearance in primary nephrogenic diabetes insipidus and in lithium-induced diabetes insipidus, suggesting a prostaglandin effect on water elimination that is independent of antidiuretic hormone. On the other hand, the renal effects of ADH in humans and animals is enhanced by indomethacin. This action has been ascribed to the known antagonism by PGE_2 of the vasopressin-induced increased permeability to water. This effect has been demonstrated in the toad bladder and rabbit collecting duct in association with an inhibition of the increased synthesis of prostaglandins produced by vasopressin.

F. Neutral Lipids

Implantation of renal medullary or renal medullary interstitial cells from cultures will reduce the blood pressure of dogs, rats, and rabbits with diverse types of hypertension. Since indomethacin did not block the vasodepressor effects of this implant, and there was no change in sodium balance, it has been postulated that a nonprostaglandin lipid accounts for the decrement of blood pressure observed in these experiments.

G. Pathophysiology

1. Bartter's Syndrome

This relatively uncommon syndrome is characterized by juxtaglomerular hyperplasia, high plasma renin, hyperaldosteronism, and hypokalemic alkalosis. In spite of very high plasma renin values, the blood pressure is normal. Prostaglandin excretion in the urine, especially PGE_2, has been shown to be very high. Urinary kallikrein excretion has been shown to be extremely high. The primary abnormality in this syndrome is unknown, but a defect of chloride reabsorption in the ascending limb of Henle's loop has been postulated.

Treatment with indomethacin or other prostaglandin synthetase inhibitors has been shown to reduce the renin levels, decrease aldosterone, PGE_2, and kallikrein excretion in the urine and correct the hypokalemic alkalosis. Part of the renin control mechanism involves stimulation by PGE and angiotensin stimulates the kallikrein–kinin system with PGE as an intermediate. Both of these mechanisms would be inhibited by suppression of PGE synthesis by the kidney. The fall in angiotensin would allow the aldosterone levels to decrease to normal and the hypokalemic alkalosis would be corrected.

2. Urinary Tract Obstruction

The effects of ureteral obstruction on renal blood flow have been studied in experimental animals. Following acute obstruction of the ureter to one kidney there is a progressive increase in renal blood flow to that kidney for the first 2–3 hr after obstruction. Thereafter, renal blood flow decreases in such a manner that by 5–6 hr after obstruction the values are comparable to those obtained prior to ligation of the ureter. There is a subsequent and progressive decrease in renal blood flow such that by 24–48 hr after obstruction values approximate 30%–40% of those obtained under control conditions before ligation. Hydronephrotic kidneys perfused *in vitro* have been shown to demonstrate increased production of prostaglandins of the E_2 series. This augmented synthesis of prostaglandins may underlie the increased renal blood flow seen initially after obstruction since administration of indomethacin, an inhibitor of prostaglandin synthesis, will prevent the increase in renal blood flow following ligation. In addition, it has been shown that 18–24 hr after the production of obstruction there is increased synthesis of thromboxane A_2 by the kidney. Thromboxane A_2 is a powerful vasoconstrictor which may be responsible in part for the increased renal vascular resistance and decreased renal blood flow observed at later stages of obstruction.

3. Acute Renal Failure

Increased renal production of thromboxanes has been demonstrated in the glycerol model of acute renal failure (see Chapter 13). This vasoconstrictor may be responsible for the decreased renal plasma flow due presumably to afferent arteriolar vasoconstriction observed in this model.

IX. SUMMARY

The kidney has, in addition to its excretory function, important nonexcretory functions. Progressive renal disease leads to a series of alterations in these nonexcretory functions of the kidney. These alterations, in turn, may contribute to the symptoms and signs of the uremic state.

SUGGESTED READINGS

Brenner, B. M., and Stein, J. H. (eds.): *Hormonal Function and the Kidney.* Contemporary Issues in Nephrology Series, Vol. 4. Churchill Livingstone, New York, 1979.

Carone, F. A., and Peterson, D. R.: Hydrolysis and transport of small peptides by the proximal tubule. *Am. J. Physiol.* 238:F151–F158, 1980.

Carretero, D. A., and Scicli, A. G.: The renal kallikrein–kinin system. *Am. J. Physiol.* 238:F247–F255, 1980.

Dunn, M. J., and Hood, V. L.: Prostaglandins and the kidney. *Am. J. Physiol.* 233:F169, 1977.

Dunn, M. J.: Renal prostaglandins, in Klahr, S., and Massry, S. (eds.): *Contemporary Nephrology*, Vol. 1. Plenum, New York, 1981, pp. 123–164.

Haussler, M. R., and McCain, T. A.: Basic and clinical concepts related to vitamin D metabolism and action. *N. Engl. J. Med.* 297:974, 1041, 1977.

Katz, A. I., and Rubenstein, A. H.: Metabolism of proinsulin, insulin and C-peptide in the rat. *J. Clin. Invest.* 52:1113, 1973.

Levinsky, N. G.: The renal kallikrein–kinin system. *Circulat. Res.* 44:441, 1979.

Martin, K. J., Hruska, K., Freitag, J. J., Klahr, S., Slatopolsky, E.: The peripheral metabolism of parathyroid hormone. *N. Engl. J. Med.* 301:1092, 1979.

Peach, M. J.: Renin–aniotensin system. Biochemistry and mechanisms of action. *Physiol. Rev.* 57:313, 1977.

Rodriguez, H. J., and Klahr, S.: Renal cell metabolism, in Massry, S. G., and Glassock, R. (eds.): *Textbook of Nephrology*. Elsevier-North Holland, New York, in press.

Rubin, A. L., Cheigh, J. S., and Stenzel, K. H.: Symposium on the endocrine functions of the kidney. *Am. J. Med.* 58:1, 1975.

Schoolwerth, A. C.: Renal metabolism, in Klahr, S., and Massry S. (eds.): *Contemporary Nephrology*, Vol. 1. Plenum, New York, 1981, pp. 87–122.

Sherwin, R. S., Bastl, C., Finkelstein, F. O., Fisher, M., Block, H., Hendler, R., and Felig, P.: Influence of uremia and hemodialysis on the turnover and metabolic effects of glucagon. *J. Clin. Invest.* 57:722, 1976.

II

Pathophysiology of Fluid and Electrolyte Disorders

This section comprises six chapters, all of which deal with the pathophysiology of fluid and electrolyte disorders. Alterations in volume regulation and sodium metabolism (dehydration, volume expansion, and edema) are considered in Chapters 4 and 5. The subjects covered in these two chapters represent disturbances of the volume control system. A closely related chapter (Chapter 6) deals with alterations in the control of water balance. The mechanisms of retention or loss of water in excess of solute are considered and the subjects of hyponatremia and hypernatremia are discussed in detail. Chapter 7 describes alterations in the control of potassium balance and the mechanisms leading to the development of hypokalemia and hyperkalemia. Chapter 8 summarizes the alterations of hydrogen ion balance and the mechanisms responsible for the development of metabolic acidosis or alkalosis and respiratory alkalosis or acidosis. Many aspects covered in this chapter interrelate closely with some of the areas covered in Chapter 7. Chapter 9 summarizes the abnormalities of calcium, phosphorus, and magnesium metabolism and deals with the entities of hypocalcemia, hypercalcemia, hyperphosphatemia, hypophosphatemia, hypomagnesemia, and hypermagnesemia. In each one of the chapters an appropriate review of normal control mechanisms is presented.

Pathophysiology of Volume Regulation and Sodium Metabolism

ELSA BELLO-REUSS

I. SODIUM BALANCE AND EXTRACELLULAR FLUID VOLUME

The human body contains approximately 60 mEq of Na per kg. As illustrated in Figure 1, in a 70-kg individual this represents a total body Na content of 4200 mEq. About 40%–45% of total body Na (~1800 mEq) is contained in bone. Of the remaining 2400 mEq, about 2100 mEq are contained in the extracellular fluid (ECF) and only about 300 mEq are contained in the intracellular fluid (ICF) of soft tissues. About 70% of total body Na is exchangeable. The remaining 30% is most likely adsorbed to hydroxyapatite crystals in long bones. Exchangeable Na, therefore, includes all of the Na contained in the ECF and ICF of soft tissues, and a fraction of the Na present in bone. Exchangeable Na is in dynamic equilibrium with ECF Na, and represents a reservoir that can in part compensate for decreases of ECF Na concentration.

The cell membranes, which separate the ECF from the ICF, are highly permeable to water, and effectively exclude sodium (because of the operation of the sodium pump, see Chapter 1). Available evidence indicates that water movement across cell membranes is passive, driven by osmotic pressure

ELSA BELLO-REUSS • Departments of Medicine, and Physiology and Biophysics, Washington University School of Medicine and The Jewish Hospital of St. Louis, St. Louis, Missouri 63110.

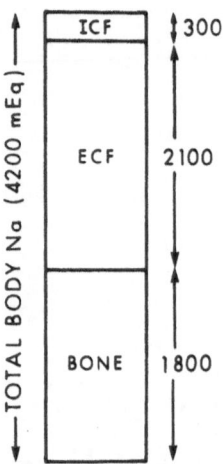

Figure 1. Total body sodium and its distribution.

differences. Normally, the total osmotic pressure of the ECF is equal to that of the ICF, and there is no net water flux across the cell membranes. The total osmolality of a solution is a function of the total concentration of particles in that solution. In the case of the ECF, the sodium salts, essentially NaCl and NaHCO$_3$, represent 90%–95% of the total concentration of particles. Changes in the concentration of Na salts are, thus, the main causes of changes of ECF osmolality. A decrease of NaCl concentration, for instance, causes a fall of ECF osmolality and a net water flux from ECF to ICF. Therefore, the ECF volume falls, even though in the preceding example total body water remained initially unchanged.

In addition to the mechanism outlined above, a primary reduction of ECF NaCl concentration and ECF osmolality results in (1) cessation of the sensation of thirst, and thus in reduced water intake, and (2) inhibition of ADH secretion, and thus in increase of water excretion by the kidney. Both mechanisms tend to decrease ECF volume.

Increases of ECF Na concentration produce the opposite effects: (1) net water flow into the ECF, (2) thirst, and hence increased water intake, and (3) ADH secretion, and thus water retention by the kidneys.

In sum, as illustrated in Figure 2, Na mass in the ECF is the main determinant of ECF volume.

The relationship of extracellular Na mass and ECF volume is not as simple as the diagram shows because more complex feedback mechanisms operate: e.g., ADH secretion is not only affected by osmolality but also by ECF volume changes (see Chapter 6).

Serum concentration does not provide unequivocal information on total Na mass, or the status of Na balance. Water balance deviations can cause changes in ECF Na concentration independently of the sodium content of the ECF. An increase of volume (expansion) of the ECF can be accompanied by either a reduction, an increase, or no change in Na concentration.

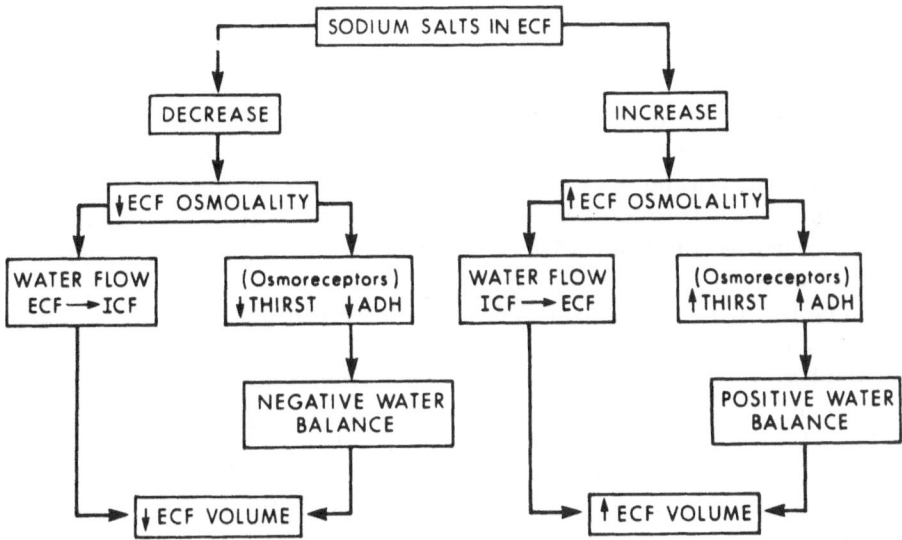

Figure 2. Mechanisms of the relationships between sodium content and extracellular fluid (ECF) volume. The amount of sodium salts in the ECF compartment is the main determinant of the volume of the ECF.

Conversely, a decrease in the extracellular space volume (contraction) can occur also with normal, increased, or decreased ECF Na concentration.

Although interrelated in a complicated fashion, the mechanisms of regulation of ECF osmolality and volume can be separated for didactic reasons. The negative feedback control mechanisms that regulate osmolality, i.e., thirst and ADH secretion, are designed to maintain water balance. Their

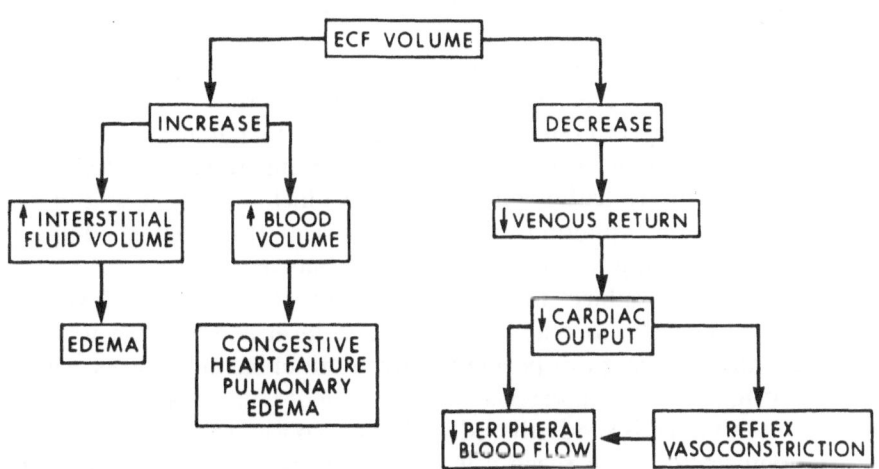

Figure 3. Pathophysiologic effects of changes in ECF volume. Increase of extracellular fluid (ECF) volume causes edema and/or congestive heart failure. Decrease of ECF volume causes reduction of peripheral blood flow.

simplest mode of operation is in response to initial alterations of total body water, and their end point is to restore body water to normal levels. The regulation of extracellular fluid volume is primarily associated with Na balance. Primary changes in ECF volume activate feedback mechanisms which tend to keep the total mass of Na salts in the ECF constant, by either reducing or increasing the rate of urinary Na excretion. The mass of Na salts determines, in turn, the volume of the ECF because of its effects on water exchange between ICF and ECF and because of the effects of ECF osmolality on Na balance (see Figure 2).

The maintenance of a normal ECF volume is essential for the function of the circulatory system. Large increases of ECF volume cause fluid accumulation in the interstitial space, i.e., edema, and/or an increase in plasma and blood volume that can precipitate or accentuate congestive heart failure. Large decreases of ECF volume result in a reduction of venous return and cardiac output, reflex vasoconstriction in many vascular beds, and eventual insufficiency of peripheral blood flow. These pathophysiological alterations are summarized in Figure 3.

II. RENAL REGULATION OF SODIUM BALANCE

A. General Considerations

Normally, the kidney regulates sodium balance in a very efficient way. Teleologically, this makes unnecessary a control mechanism of Na intake analogous to thirst. For cultural reasons, salt intake is very high in humans as compared to any other species. Essentially all of the daily intake of Na is excreted in the urine; under normal conditions, extrarenal Na excretion is very small (Chapter 1).

The average intake of sodium in the Western World is about 170 mmoles per day, of which about 165 mmoles are excreted in the urine and approximately 5 mmoles appear in the feces. Sources other than ingestion, important in therapeutic situations, include intravenous administration, peritoneal and extracorporeal dialysis. Pathological losses of Na include increases of urinary and fecal excretion, vomiting, skin losses (sweat, transudates), drainage, fistulae, and fluid sequestration in normal or abnormal cavities.

When a normal subject increases the intake of salt, sodium excretion increases progressively, to reach a steady state level equal to the intake in about three days. During this period positive sodium balance occurs, with an accompanying retention of water and a consequent gain in body weight.

When salt intake is suddenly reduced, the opposite effects are observed: Na excretion decreases to reach a level equal to the intake in about three days; the brief period of negative Na balance results in a reduction of total body water and therefore in body weight. In normal people, these deviations from normal Na and water balance in response to changes of the diet are rather small. The new balance can be maintained indefinitely, either with a high or a low salt intake.

The regulation of Na balance, and therefore ECF volume, depends on changes in the rate of Na excretion by the kidneys. In man there is no salt appetite, which seems to be well developed in some herbivorous animals. There are reports, however, of preference for high-salt-content foods in patients with adrenal insufficiency, and of the development of "salt thirst" after intracranial infusions of angiotensin II. In essence, however, changes of Na balance are compensated for only by changes, in the appropriate direction, of the rate of Na excretion in the urine.

Sodium filters freely in the glomerulus and is partially reabsorbed by all segments of the renal tubule (proximal, loop of Henle, distal, and collecting). There is no evidence for tubular secretion under normal conditions. Uremic plasma, however, induces Na and fluid secretion by the straight portion of the proximal tubule. In the normal kidney, therefore, the amount of Na excreted per unit time equals the amount filtered minus the amount reabsorbed in that time:

$$E(Na) = F(Na) - R(NA)$$

The amount filtered is the product of the volume of filtrate per unit time (i.e., the glomerular filtration rate, GFR) and the Na concentration in the filtrate (approximately equal to the plasma concentration, P_{Na}):

$$E(Na) = GFR \cdot P_{Na} - R(Na)$$

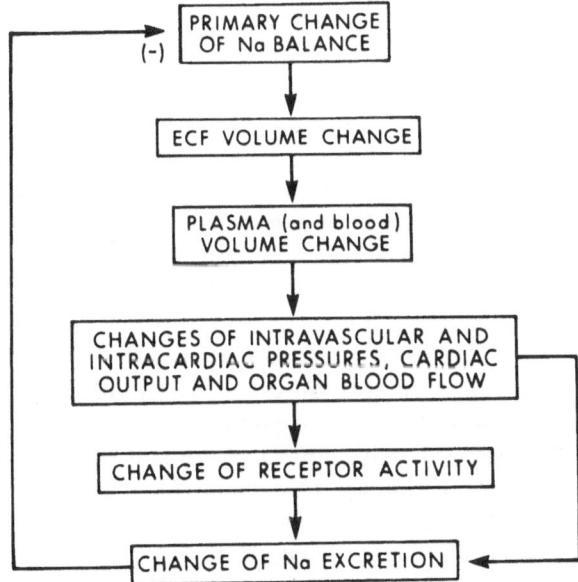

Figure 4. Negative feedback mechanisms in the control of sodium balance.

In theory, E(Na) could change by alterations in any of the three variables on the right-hand side of the equation. However, P_{Na} varies little, even during large alterations of Na balance, because of concomitant water imbalances or compensatory water fluxes from or toward the ICF. Therefore, the important control variables are the rate of glomerular filtration and the rate of tubular sodium reabsorption.

Several mechanisms control GFR and the rate of sodium reabsorption in ways appropriate for the maintenance of the total Na mass in the ECF (and the body). Changes in Na mass are not sensed as such, but as secondary changes of ECF volume. Total ECF volume changes are not sensed directly either, but through their effects on circulatory dynamics. The alterations of flow and/or pressure in the cardiovascular system are finally sensed by specific receptors, as illustrated in Figure 4.

The receptors involved in the mechanisms of regulation of Na balance seem to be primarily baroreceptors located in the high-pressure side (arterial system) of the circulation. They include aortic and carotid stretch receptors and the juxtaglomerular apparatus. Low-pressure baroreceptors (e.g., atrial baroreceptors) appear to be related more to the control of ECF osmolality (see Chapter 3).

B. Control of Glomerular Filtration Rate

The amount of sodium filtered each day in the glomeruli is enormous when compared to the amount excreted in the urine. Very small changes in the rate of glomerular filtration would result in large changes in Na excretion if the rate of Na reabsorption did not change. For instance, a 1% increment in GFR (from the normal value of 125 ml/min, or 180 liters/day) would result in an increase of the filtered load of Na of about 240 mEq/day. If Na reabsorption remained the same, Na excretion would more than double, even though the GFR change would probably be unmeasurable by clearance techniques. Conversely, a 1% reduction of GFR would result—if Na reabsorption did not change—in total Na reabsorption, and therefore the excretion of Na in the urine would fall to zero. These changes do not take place because Na reabsorption is a function of the load, i.e., the rate of Na reabsorption changes in the same direction as GFR. This phenomenon, discussed in Chapter 2, is commonly referred to as *glomerulo-tubular balance*. Its precise mechanism has not been determined. However, it is known to occur essentially in all segments of the renal tubule, but mostly in the proximal segments and in the loop of Henle.

The main physiological mechanism of control of GFR is sympathetic. The renal vasculature is highly responsive to renal nerve activity and circulating catecholamines. In the case of a negative Na balance, these mechanism operate as illustrated in Figure 5.

Catecholamines increase the resistance of both afferent and efferent glomerular arterioles. This results in a large reduction in renal blood flow

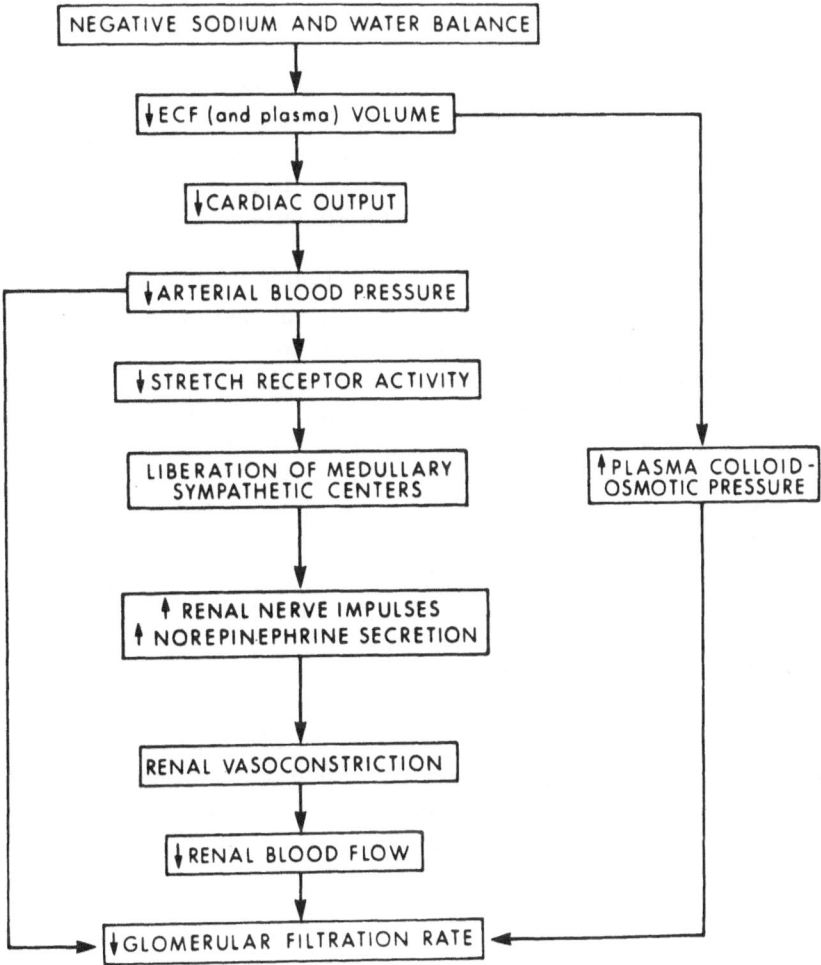

Figure 5. Mechanisms underlying the decrease of glomerular filtration rate in response to a primary negative balance of salt and water.

and a small increase in glomerular capillary pressure, indicating that the primary action of catecholamines is efferent vasoconstriction. Contraction of the afferent arteriole, seen only if aortic blood pressure rises, is probably a secondary myogenic response. The decrease of GFR produced by catecholamines is secondary to the reduction of renal blood flow, which is offset in part by the elevation of glomerular capillary pressure.

In case of a primary positive Na balance with ECF volume expansion, cardiac output, renal perfusion pressure, and renal blood flow tend to increase, and GFR rises. The role of the sympathetic system in this mechanism appears to be minimal or nonexistent. The renal nerves do not exert a tonic effect on renal hemodynamics under basal conditions, i.e., they are inactive when arterial pressure is normal. Therefore, increases in pressure do not result in effects on the renal circulation or GFR mediated by the sympathetic system. The effects are directly related to the changes of renal hemodynamics, particularly the high renal blood flow.

Hemodynamic and sympathetic effects on renal blood flow and glomerular filtration rate are "buffered" by the mechanisms of autoregulation of RBF and GFR. Because of these adaptive responses of the glomerular vasculature, the changes of GFR are smaller than if the renal circulatory system were entirely passive. Changes in sympathetic tone reset autoregulation at a new level.

As illustrated also in Figure 5, changes of plasma colloid-osmotic pressure can play a role in the control of GFR. If salt and water are lost (e.g., gastrointestinal losses) the plasma colloid-osmotic pressure rises and thus GFR decreases, a homeostatically adequate response. However, if protein is also lost (for instance in burns or hemorrhage) and drop in systemic capillary pressure causes bulk flow from interstitial fluid to plasma and hemodilution results. Therefore, the colloid-osmotic pressure falls, tending to increase GFR, a homeostatically inadequate response. Since the fall of arterial pressure and the sympathetic reflex are dominant in this situation, GFR falls, regardless of the decrease of colloid-osmotic pressure.

Changes in glomerular filtration rate have effects on the rate of Na excretion, but these effects are less important than primary alterations of tubular Na reabsorption. Two lines of evidence support this view, which is especially valid for ECF volume expansion. First, sizable increases of GFR not accompanied by ECF volume expansion do not result in large natriuresis. Second, the natriuretic response to ECF volume expansion occurs even if GFR is experimentally maintained constant, or even decreased.

C. Control of Tubular Sodium Reabsorption

As stated above, tubular reabsorption is more important than GFR as a control mechanism of Na excretion. Several agents are known to influence Na reabsorption. The best known is the adrenocortical hormone *aldosterone*, which exerts effects on Na reabsorption by the distal and collecting segments of the nephron. Recent experimental observations have shown that extracellular volume expansion can be accompanied by natriuresis (increased urinary Na excretion) under conditions in which both GFR and aldosterone activity are kept constant. It is likely that this effect is caused by a rather heterogeneous group of mechanisms, some hypothetical, whose precise roles have not been entirely clarified.

1. Aldosterone

Aldosterone, the hormone produced by the *zona glomerulosa* of the adrenal cortex, exerts a potent sodium-retaining effect on the cortical collecting tubule and perhaps other segments of the distal nephron. Secretion of aldosterone is mainly controlled by sodium balance and ECF volume.

Acute decreases of ECF volume, reductions in venous return, and low-salt diet stimulate aldosterone secretion. Increases of ECF volume or venous return, and high-salt diet, inhibit the secretion of the hormone.

a. Mechanisms of Secretion

The level of secretion of aldosterone is determined by at least four inputs:

i. Angiotensin II. This octapeptide is produced in plasma by a series of reactions normally rate-limited by the plasma renin concentration. Renin acts on its substrate, angiotensinogen, to produce the decapeptide angiotensin I. The converting enzyme catalyzes the production of the octapeptide angiotensin II, which has vasoconstrictor effects on arterioles and is the trophic hormone of the zona glomerulosa. Aldosterone secretion is stimulated by an increase of the renin secretion by the juxtaglomerular apparatus in response to a decrease in renal perfusion pressure (baroreceptor) and probably in the amount of salt that reaches the macula densa (chemoreceptor). A detailed description of the renin–angiotensin–aldosterone system can be found in Chapter 3. See also Chapter 2, for a discussion of the separate mechanisms of systemic renin secretion and hypothetical local renin secretion as a mechanism of autoregulation of renal blood flow.

ii. Plasma Sodium Concentration. Aldosterone secretion increases in response to a decrease in plasma sodium concentration. This stimulus appears to be less important than angiotensin.

iii. Plasma Potassium Concentration. Increases in plasma potassium concentration cause increases in the secretion of aldosterone by a local action in the zona glomerulosa. Conversely, hypokalemia (low plasma potassium concentration) results in a decrease of aldosterone secretion. These effects of potassium are opposed, in the intact animal, by actions on the rate of renin secretion: high K^+ decreases renin secretion, whereas low K^+ has a stimulating effect. In terms of secretion of aldosterone, the direct adrenal effect of K^+ dominates.

iv. Secretion of ACTH. ACTH has a permissive effect on the secretion of aldosterone. This action is quantitatively less important than those of angiotensin, plasma sodium, and plasma potassium concentration.

b. Site and Mechanism of Action

Aldosterone binds to the cells of the distal and collecting segments of the renal tubule and produces an increase of Na reabsorption, mediated by synthesis of RNA and one or more specific proteins. It is not entirely clear if the final effect is (1) direct stimulation of the active sodium transport mechanism, (2) increase of Na permeability at the luminal cell membrane, which would make more Na available to the pump, or (3) stimulation of metabolism, which would increase the availability of energy for the transport mechanism. Recent evidence suggests that the effect on luminal membrane

Na permeability is dominant. The increase in Na reabsorption is accompanied by an increase of K secretion into the tubular lumen, and therefore by an increase in urinary K excretion. The Na/K concentration ratio in the urine is an excellent index of aldosterone activity. Similar effects are exerted by aldosterone at the level of the colon, salivary glands, and sweat glands. These are unimportant as a mechanism of regulation of Na balance, although useful for diagnostic purposes.

In the distal tubule, only a small fraction of the filtered sodium load remains in the luminal fluid, since most is reabsorbed by both proximal tubule and loop of Henle. Although the fraction of the filtered Na load under aldosterone control is only about 2%, this mechanism is highly efficient in the control of Na excretion. Under conditions of maximum secretion of aldosterone, Na excretion is virtually zero, while in the absence of the hormone it is about 2% of the filtered load: if GFR and plasma Na concentration are normal, Na excretion can in principle be as high as 500 mEq/day, or near 30 g of NaCl. This is, of course, well beyond any reasonable intake. Therefore, the efficiency of the aldosterone control mechanism of Na excretion is, in theory, very high.

Even though the renin–angiotensin–aldosterone system plays an important role in the maintenance of Na balance and ECF volume, its function cannot be considered separate from other regulatory mechanisms. This is illustrated by the two following observations. In the total absence of aldosterone, as seen in patients in which the adrenal cortex is destroyed, a moderate increase of dietary salt content suffices to compensate for the modest urinary losses characteristic of the syndrome. This indicates that the natriuresis expected from the total absence of aldosterone is compensated in chronic situations, at least in part, by other mechanisms. A second illustration of the interplay between the mechanisms of regulation of Na balance is the *escape* from the action of aldosterone. Animals receiving continually exogenous mineralocorticoids and patients afflicted by excessive aldosterone secretion (hyperaldosteronism) retain salt and water for a few days and then undergo, spontaneously, natriuresis and diuresis, in such a way that a new steady state is reached, i.e., a null balance is achieved at a higher ECF volume. It is believed that the escape phenomenon is triggered, after fluid retention and ECF volume expansion, by factors other than GFR or aldosterone itself.

2. Other Mechanisms of Regulation of Na Reabsorption

As explained above, expansion of the ECF volume can result in natriuretic and diuretic responses even if GFR (first factor) and aldosterone (second factor) are controlled. The precise mechanism of this effect is unknown. Several possible factors have been invoked. These are usually referred to as the *third factor* in the control of sodium excretion. Some reasonable possibilities, based on experimental studies, are (1) a natriuretic hormone, (2) a change in driving forces and/or permeability of the proximal tubule produced by alterations of hydrostatic or colloid-osmotic pressures in the lumen and/or the capillaries, (3) redistribution of renal blood flow, (4) a direct effect of catecholamines on salt and fluid reabsorption, and (5) effects of prostaglandins and kinins on renal hemodynamics and probably tubular transport. It is possible that the third factor is the result of more than one of these mechanisms, and presumably others, as yet unidentified.

a. Natriuretic Hormone

The existence of such a hormone has been postulated on the following bases: (1) the demonstration, in cross circulation experiments, of natriuresis in the recipient animal when the donor is volume expanded, and (2) the isolation from nervous tissue, plasma, or urine of factors that exhibit physiological effects consistent with the possibility of an inhibitory action on renal tubular sodium reabsorption. Although research in this field has been very active in recent years, no unequivocal demonstration of a natriuretic hormone has been provided.

b. Physical Factors across the Tubular Wall

Fluid transport from the interstitial peritubular spaces into the capillary lumen is governed by Starling forces, i.e., hydrostatic and oncotic pressure differences, acting across the capillary wall. In addition, this flow depends on the rate of peritubular capillary blood flow and the permeability of the tubular wall. All of these parameters can influence the rate of fluid reabsorption.

Increases in peritubular plasma oncotic pressure result in an increased reabsorption. It has been shown that during volume expansion, in which proximal reabsorption is decreased, efferent arteriolar protein concentration and colloid-osmotic pressure are also decreased. Proximal reabsorption is corrected by perfusion of the capillaries with a solution of normal oncotic pressure. The opposite mechanism would operate in the case of increased peritubular capillary oncotic pressure.

The influence of physical factors on fluid reabsorption by the proximal tubule appears to be important and well documented. However, it has also been shown that the inhibition of reabsorption in the proximal tubule can be "compensated" for by more distal segments as occurs after systemic infusions of hyperoncotic albumin solutions, which are followed by much smaller natriuresis than saline infusions despite comparable effects on proximal fluid reabsorption. It is clear now that other mechanisms, acting in the distal nephron, must be fundamental in determining the natriuresis of volume expansion.

c. Intrarenal Blood Flow Redistribution

The mammalian kidney has two nephron populations: superficial ("cortical") and deep ("juxtamedullary"). It seems certain that the latter have a higher Na reabsorptive capacity. Increased renal nerve activity, for instance during Na depletion, has been claimed to reduce mainly outer cortical blood flow. In relative terms, then, blood flow, and glomerular filtration, would increase in the deep cortex, as compared to superficial blood flow and filtration. Sodium excretion would then decrease because of the intrinsically higher rate of reabsorption by the tubules of the deep nephrons. The opposite mechanism would operate in case of positive Na balance. The overall experimental evidence in favor of this hypothesis is not conclusive.

d. Catecholamines

There is anatomical evidence that the renal tubules are innervated by adrenergic fibers. Acute renal denervation produces natriuresis and diuresis, and renal nerve stimulation increases sodium and water reabsorption. These effects take place in the proximal tubule, under experimental conditions in which RBF and GFR do not change. Additional effects on more distal segments have not been established. Consistent with these results, norepinephrine and isoproterenol stimulate fluid transport by the isolated proximal convoluted tubule, an effect that is inhibited by propranolol. The experimental data on the effects of chronic renal denervation are controversial. The physiological significance of this effect of the sympathetic system on salt and water reabsorption is uncertain at the present time.

e. Prostaglandins and the Kallikrein–Bradykinin System

As explained in detail in Chapter 3, renal prostaglandins and kinins are vasodilators and increase sodium excretion. It seems clear that they play a role in the control of renal vascular resistance. Direct effects on tubular transport have also been proposed. Prostaglandins exert an effect on water excretion by antagonizing the effect of ADH. The importance of these substances in the regulation of Na excretion has not yet been established.

III. SODIUM DEPLETION AND ECF VOLUME CONTRACTION

Because of the high efficiency of the mechanisms for renal sodium conservation, it is very difficult to produce sodium deficiency by the mere restriction of sodium intake in normal people.

In healthy volunteers, chronic experiments of sodium deprivation combined with increased losses by sweating in a hot box result in a simultaneous decrease in total body sodium and water content during the first three days. At this time, ECF volume is reduced, whereas ECF osmolality remains normal. Later on, the weight stabilizes while both total body sodium content and plasma sodium concentration continue to decrease with the expected fall of ECF osmolality. In this phase, control of ECF volume acquires priority over control of ECF osmolality. The mechanisms involved in this response are not completely understood. It has been shown that the presence of ADH is not a requisite for the retention of water.

A. Mechanisms of Production of Negative Sodium Balance

A significant negative sodium balance always results from a continued period in which the sodium losses are greater than the total gains. As explained above, if renal function is normal a reduction of sodium intake will not result, by itself, in sizable negative sodium balance. This condition requires an increase of sodium losses.

It is convenient to classify abnormal sodium losses as *extrarenal* or *renal*.

1. Extrarenal Causes of Sodium Depletion

The most frequent conditions in which sodium depletion occurs due to excessive extrarenal losses are listed in Table I. The two most important groups are gastrointestinal and cutaneous losses.

The composition of fluids lost from the gastrointestinal tract varies according to the segment from which the fluid is lost. Most gastrointestinal secretions are approximately isotonic to plasma. Therefore, usually no change in ECF osmolality occurs, unless fluid replacement is incorrect. For instance, if the isotonic salt solution lost by vomiting and diarrhea is replaced with isotonic glucose, hypotonicity will result.

The composition and volume of the fluid secreted by the main segments of the digestive system are summarized in Table II. It should be noted that potassium concentration is higher at all levels of the gastrointestinal tract than in plasma. Thus, excessive GI losses tend to cause potassium depletion (see Chapter 7). Gastric fluid has normally a high hydrogen ion concentration. Therefore, its loss by vomiting or suction or its sequestration is equivalent to a loss of fixed acid and causes metabolic alkalosis. Intestinal secretion, pancreatic secretion, and bile have in general a higher bicarbonate concentration than plasma. If the predominant fluid losses occur at this level, the net loss of bicarbonate, equivalent to gain of fixed acid, results in metabolic acidosis.

The rates of secretion shown in Table II are those observed in normal humans. Under pathological conditions they can increase severalfold. A typical example is the stimulation of fluid secretion by the jejunum and ileum in cholera. Cholera toxin binds to intestinal epithelial cells and stimulates adenylate cyclase. The resulting increase of intracellular cyclic AMP is responsible for the stimulation of secretion, primarily due to Cl and HCO_3 transport from ECF to lumen. Enterotoxins of a number of bacteria (for instance *E. coli*) also stimulate intestinal secretion.

In summary, excessive losses of gastrointestinal fluids are equivalent to

Table I. Extrarenal Causes of Sodium
Depletion

I. Gastrointestinal sodium losses
    A. External
        1. Vomiting
        2. Diarrhea
        3. Suction
        4. Fistula
    B. Sequestration
        1. Small bowel obstruction
        2. Pancreatitis
        3. Peritonitis
II. Skin sodium losses
    A. Normal skin barrier
        1. Heat exposure
        2. Cystic fibrosis
    B. Altered skin barrier
        1. Burns
        2. Inflammation
III. Miscellaneous sodium losses
    A. External
        1. Severe hemorrhage
        2. Paracentesis
    B. Sequestration
        1. Extensive limb trauma
        2. Peripheral vaso/venodilatation

an isoosmotic reduction of ECF volume. K depletion is an accompanying feature. According to the segments involved, metabolic alkalosis or acidosis ensue.

The most frequent causes of cutaneous sodium losses are sweating and burns (see Table I). Both differ pathophysiologically from the negative balance of isotonic salt solution generated by excessive gastrointestinal losses. Sweat is hypotonic: the water losses are proportionally greater than the sodium losses, and the end result is ECF hyperosmolality, with consequent

Table II. Volume and Electrolyte Concentrations[a] of Gastrointestinal Fluids

	Mean volume (ml/day)	Na^+	K^+	Cl^-	HCO_3^-	H^+
Saliva	1300	56	16	16	53	
Gastric secretion	1200	47	13	100	—	33
Bile	700	183	8	100	29	
Pancreatic secretion	800	153	7	80	73	
Jejunal secretion	2500	144	7	120	29	
Ileal secretion	1500	127	6	70	71	
Stools	50	196	9	103	—	

[a] Concentrations in mEq/liter. H^+ concentration in all fluids but gastric secretion is negligible as compared to other electrolytes.

reductions of both ECF and ICF volumes. Burns and other extensive lessions of the skin are accompanied by an increase in capillary permeability, which causes a loss of plasma proteins in addition to salt and water. This, because of the decrease in plasma colloid-osmotic pressure, results in a contraction of the intravascular compartment which is disproportionately large for the magnitude of the negative sodium balance.

2. Renal Causes of Sodium Depletion

As shown in Table III, excessive sodium losses in the urine can occur because of abnormal influences on otherwise normal kidneys or because of renal disease.

a. Renal Sodium Losses in the Absence of Renal Disease

A normal kidney can excrete more sodium than appropriate for homeostasis because of a defect in the normal mechanisms of regulation of sodium reabsorption or because of inhibition of Na transport by the renal tubule. The latter condition can occur by direct pharmacological effects (diuretic drugs) or by a large increase of the filtered solute load (osmotic diuresis).

i. Hypoaldosteronism. Hypoaldosteronism, e.g., as a component of Addison's disease, results in moderate but persistent salt losses in the urine because of the lack of stimulation of Na reabsorption by the distal nephron. The most likely explanations for the common observation that the increase of urinary Na excretion is rather modest are the fall in GFR that follows the initial negative balance of salt and water, and the compensatory effect of other factors involved in the control of sodium balance (see above). Usually,

Table III. Renal Causes of Sodium Depletion

I. Normal kidney
    A. Osmotic diuresis/nonreabsorbable anion diuresis
        1. Endogenous (urea, glucose)
        2. Exogenous (mannitol, dextran, urea, glycerol,
            radiocontrast material)
    B. Diuretic administration
    C. Mineralocorticoid deficiency
        1. Steroidogenesis deficiency
        2. Renin secretion deficiency
II. Abnormal kidney
    A. Chronic renal failure
    B. Nonoliguric acute renal failure; recovery from oliguric acute
        renal failure
    C. Salt wasting nephropathy
        1. Relief of obstructive uropathy
        2. Nephrocalcinosis/interstitial nephritis
        3. Medullary cystic disease
        4. Bartter's syndrome

a moderate increase in dietary NaCl intake suffices to maintain these patients in balance. However, extrarenal pathologic losses can result in large depletion of the ECF volume because of the lack of appropriate renal compensation.

ii. Diuretic Drugs. Drugs which act on the renal tubule and decrease Na reabsorption can produce negative Na balance if salt intake is less than total excretion. This is the basis for the therapeutic use of diuretics, for instance in hypertensive and edematous patients. However, abuse of diuretic drugs can result in complications derived from an excessive reduction of ECF volume. Patients under prolonged diuretic therapy can experience severe ECF volume depletion if another mechanism of salt loss develops (vomiting or diarrhea). The normal renal response to the renin–angiotensin–aldosterone mechanism will be absent or reduced because of the action of the drug.

iii. Osmotic Diuresis. This is a condition that can arise with a normal or an abnormal kidney when the amount of solute presented to the lumen of the proximal tubule per unit time or the nature of the solute limits the capacity of this segment to reabsorb salt and water. Osmotic diuresis can then result from (1) excessive filtered load of solute(s) normally reabsorbable, e.g., glucose, or (2) presence in the lumen of nonreabsorbable solute, e.g., mannitol.

Normally, the composition of the luminal fluid at the end of the proximal tubule is quite similar to the one of the filtrate, indicating that water and most solutes are reabsorbed at similar rates. If an effectively nonreabsorbable solute is present in the lumen at a significant concentration water reabsorption is reduced, even if the capacity for salt transport is not primarily altered. This process may be understood by considering that as salt is reabsorbed water follows passively, and the concentration of the nonreabsorbable solute in the lumen rises. This increase in concentration has two effects: (1) it limits the rate of water reabsorption, and (2) it causes a decrease in salt concentration in the lumen, therefore generating a gradient that limits salt transport. The underlying explanation of these effects is the high water permeability of the proximal tubule epithelium, which makes the luminal fluid always isoosmotic with respect to the peritubular fluid. Osmotic diuresis results in an increased delivery of fluid to the loop of Henle. In many cases, the total amount of salt entering the loop per unit time is also increased, in spite of the lower luminal concentration because of the high flow rate. The increase in volume of the urine and the inappropriately high rate of sodium excretion characteristic of osmotic diuresis are due to the excessive load offered to the loop of Henle and the distal nephron. These segments of the nephron have a relatively low transport capacity, and cannot handle excessive loads even if they are subject to hormonal influences which promote sodium retention (aldosterone) and water retention (antidiuretic hormone).

Osmotic diuresis can be *endogenous* or *exogenous*. Endogenous osmotic diuresis results from increases in the filtered load of solute normally present in plasma, such as glucose, bicarbonate, and urea. These solutes are normally transported by the proximal tubule: glucose and bicarbonate by uphill mechanisms and urea by passive transport (see Chapter 2). When the load is greater than the maximal transport rate, large amounts of the solute remain in the lumen and trigger the sequence of events described above. The most typical example is decompensated diabetes mellitus, in which hyperglycemia results in an increased filtered load of glucose which exceeds the tubular transport maximum (T_m) for this solute.

The expression *anion diuresis* is sometimes used to describe a situation similar to osmotic diuresis that takes place when the effectively nonreabsorbable solute is an anion, such as ketoacid anions, in diabetic acidosis or fasting, or bicarbonate, administered or ingested in amounts larger than the tubular maximum reabsorptive capacity. In both cases, the large filtered load results in "incomplete reabsorption." Renal tubular acidosis with normal or low filtered load of bicarbonate is another example of "incomplete reabsorption." The high luminal concentration of the anion limits the rate of sodium reabsorption, mostly because of a negative luminal electrical potential (see Chapter 2) with the end result of reduced salt and therefore water reabsorption.

b. Renal Sodium Losses in Renal Disease

Renal losses of sodium can take place in a variety of renal diseases, as shown in Table III. All of these will be discussed in detail elsewhere in this text. The common characteristic of these conditions is that the renal tubular epithelium is unable to reabsorb sodium with the normal efficiency, even when subject to maximal hormonal stimulation. This can be due to intrinsic defects of the transport mechanisms, for instance because of lesion of the cells during nonoliguric acute renal failure or during the diuretic (postoliguric) phase of acute renal failure. In chronic renal failure it has been postulated that the surviving nephrons retain their transport properties, but are subject to an increased filtered load, i.e., glomerular filtration per nephron is increased. The large load results in osmotic diuresis, as described above. In addition, there is some experimental evidence which suggests that in chronic renal failure there is an increase in plasma concentration of natriuretic substances (third factor). It should be stressed that even when glomerular filtration rate is severely reduced in chronic renal failure the rate of Na excretion can stay relatively high and, most important, will not change significantly by the influence of the normal control mechanisms. In other words, Na excretion remains fixed, and therefore increases of extrarenal losses can result in severe negative Na balance.

B. Pathophysiological Consequences of Negative Sodium Balance (Sodium Depletion)

1. General Considerations

Once a sizable sodium depletion has resulted from any of the mechanisms discussed above, the effects on organ function will depend mostly on the reduction of the ECF volume. Frequently, however, ECF volume contraction will by accompanied by (1) disproportionate changes of water balance as compared to salt balance, and therefore osmolality changes, (2) changes in K balance that can result in hyperkalemia or, more frequently, hypokalemia, and (3) acid—base alterations. The nature and magnitude of these effects depend on the composition of the fluid losses and the amount and composition of the intake and therapeutically administered fluids. Our discussion will refer to the simplest condition: isotonic ECF volume contraction. We will not discuss alterations in K or acid—base balance. These subjects, and osmolality changes, are treated in detail in Chapters 7 and 8 of this book.

If losses of salt and water are not adequately compensated by intake or administration, the extracellular fluid volume is reduced. In the absence of concomitant changes of ECF osmolality, no net flux of water takes place across the cell membrane and therefore the ICF volume remains unchanged. Because of the fluid exchange mechanisms at the capillary walls, contraction of the ECF will ultimately result in a reduction of both plasma volume and interstitial fluid volume. The magnitude of the reduction of each compartment depends on their initial volumes and on whether plasma proteins are lost or sequestered. In the case of a primary loss of sodium chloride and water from plasma, the fall in blood volume causes a decrease in mean capillary filtration pressure. Since plasma proteins are concentrated by the loss of salt and water, the plasma colloid-osmotic pressure rises. Both events (the fall in hydrostatic pressure and the increase in colloid-osmotic pressure) displace the equilibrium at the capillary endothelium, resulting in net bulk flow of interstitial fluid toward the intravascular compartment. A new steady state condition is achieved in which both extracellular fluid subcompartments are contracted. When the fluid losses include significant amounts of plasma proteins (for instance, burns) the increase in plasma colloid-osmotic pressure will not occur and the fall in plasma volume will be larger than if only salt and water are lost.

The central issue in ECF volume contraction is the reduction in plasma volume. The decrease in mean filling pressure of the heart causes a drop of cardiac output. This, in turn, results in a reduction in the supply of oxygen and nutrients to peripheral tissues and in reflex vasoconstriction of some vascular beds, among them the kidney.

2. Compensatory Mechanisms

ECF volume depletion, because of the hemodynamic effects mentioned above, turns on compensatory mechanisms which (1) tend to restore ECF volume by reducing urinary losses of salt and water, and (2) tend to maintain arterial blood pressure and therefore to preserve blood flow to vital organs. We will discuss these two mechanism separately.

a. Mechanisms of Restoration of ECF Volume

As shown in Figure 6, the drop of Na excretion observed during negative Na balance in subjects with normal kidneys and an intact renin—angiotensin—aldosterone system is a consequence of the reduction of GFR,

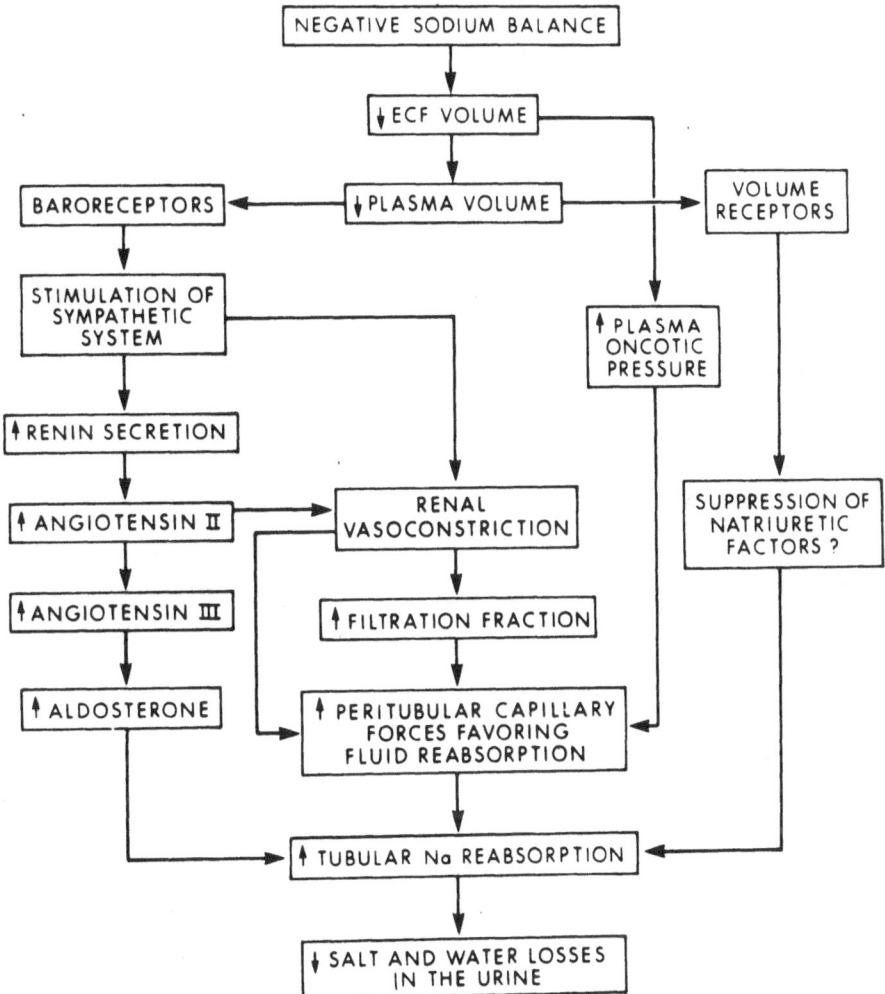

Figure 6. Mechanisms responsible for increased Na reabsorption by the renal tubule in response to negative sodium balance. These mechanisms and the accompanying stimulation of thirst and ADH secretion tend to restore the ECF volume.

secretion of aldosterone, and possibly changes in other factors which control Na reabsorption.

In addition, large reductions of plasma volume result, by themselves, in thirst and secretion of ADH. Angiotensin II (which is elevated because of the reduction in plasma volume) also stimulates thirst and ADH secretion. The net result, if the kidney is normal, is a reduction in urine volume and an increase in urine osmolality.

b. Mechanisms of Preservation of Arterial Blood Pressure

When plasma volume is not corrected by the mechanism described above, cardiac output falls, the level of stimulation of the baroreceptors decreases, sympathetic medullary centers are released, and sympathetic tone

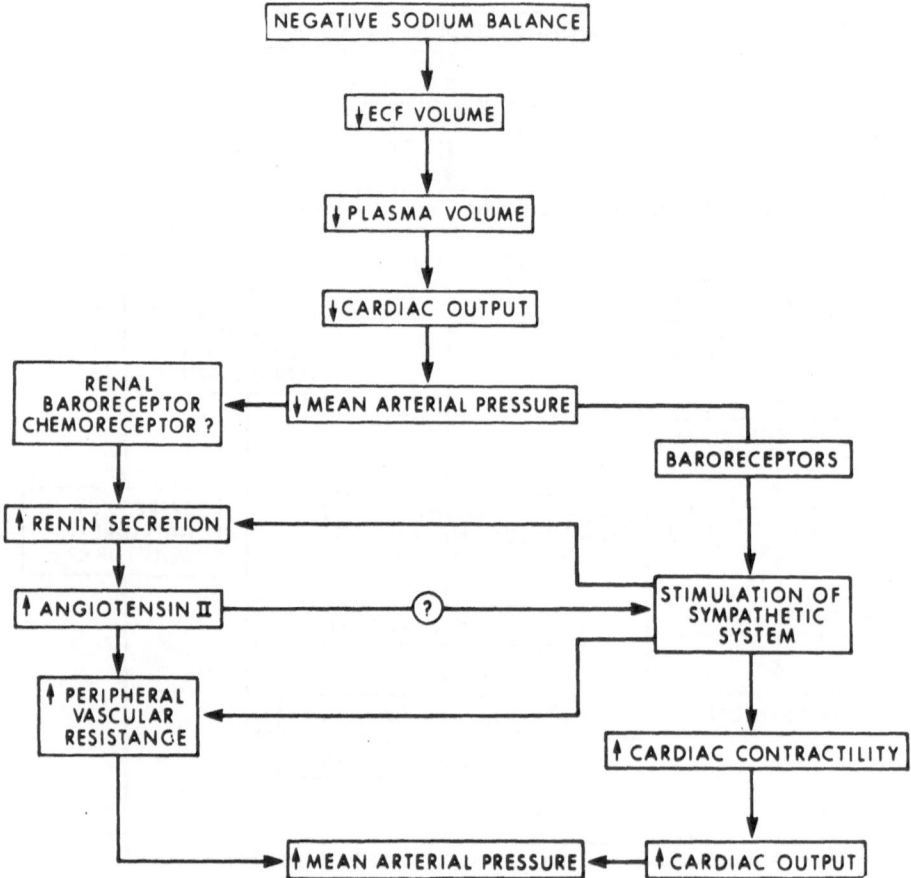

Figure 7. Mechanisms responsible for the preservation of arterial blood pressure in negative sodium balance.

increases. This mechanism result in tachycardia, increased cardiac contractility, and vasoconstriction of small arteries innervated by the sympathetic system. Thus, blood flow to a number of organs (kidney, skin, gastrointestinal tract) is decreased, as a trade-off to maintain perfusion of the myocardium and the central nervous system. Another mechanism of vasoconstriction in sodium depletion states is the increase in the production of angiotensin II, in response to the decrease in arterial blood pressure and to the stimulation of renin production caused by the elevated sympathetic tone (see Figure 7). It has been postulated that angiotensin II also activates the sympathetic nervous system. Furthermore, the peptide potentiates the vasoconstrictor effect of norepinephrine.

3. Mechanisms of the Clinical Manifestations of ECF Volume Depletion

In previously healthy adults, signs and symptoms of chronic sodium depletion appear when the Na deficit amounts to 200–400 mEq. Of course,

Table IV. Most Common Symptoms
and Signs of ECF Volume Depletion

1. Thirst, weakness, cold
2. Dryness of mucous membranes
3. Decreased skin turgor
4. Decreased sweating
5. Sunken eyes and cheeks
6. Orthostatic decrease in blood pressure
7. Tachycardia
8. Hypothermia
9. Decreased venous pressure
10. Circulatory insufficiency

the previous state of health of the patient and the rapidity of the alteration can change this threshold. The most frequent symptoms and physical signs of this disorder are listed in Table IV. Since rarely isotonic ECF volume contraction occurs in the absence of associated disorders in potassium and hydrogen ion balance, it is difficult to ascribe all of these manifestations to the alteration of sodium balance per se.

The most important physical signs of Na depletion are the circulatory ones. In general, the demonstration of orthostatic hypotension and/or orthostatic tachycardia are early signs of this disorder. Severe volume depletion is accompanied by peripheral vasoconstriction. In extreme cases, circulatory insufficiency ensues. Among other effects, this pathophysiologic condition can produce acute renal failure, with or without tubular necrosis.

With the exception of the measurement of exchangeable sodium or of ECF volume, there are no pathognomonic laboratory signs of sodium depletion. Since plasma Na concentration depends not only on the amount of Na in the ECF, but also on the volume of water, it can remain within the normal range, increase, or decrease, according to the relative magnitudes of Na and water negative balance. Severe depletion is usually accompanied by hyponatremia and a reduction of plasma osmolality. The changes in potassium and bicarbonate concentrations and pH in plasma are variable, depending on the cause of depletion. The reduction in plasma volume results in hemoconcentration: the hematocrit rises and, if protein losses are relatively small or nonexistent, plasma protein concentration rises as well.

The urinary laboratory signs of Na depletion provide useful means to distinguish between normal (adequate) renal homeostatic response and an etiologic role of the kidneys in the pathogenesis of the disorder. When the source of depletion is extrarenal, the compensatory mechanisms illustrated in Figure 6 are evidenced by decreased urinary volume, decrease of urinary sodium concentration, increase of urinary potassium concentration, and high U/P values for creatinine and urea. Of these indices, which reflect the hormonal responses to the reduction of ECF volume, the most useful one is the reduction of sodium concentration in the urine. It is commonly accepted that if the renal response to sodium depletion of extrarenal origin is normal, urinary sodium is less than 10 mEq/liter, whereas sodium depletion of renal origin is characteristically associated with higher urinary Na concentrations (20 mEq/liter or more). Accordingly, the fraction of the filtered load of sodium excreted, $(U/P)_{Na}/(U/P)_{cr}$, is less than 1% in the absence of renal disease and higher in renal failure. For calculations of the magnitude of the sodium deficit in pathophysiologic conditions, see Chapter 6.

IV. POSITIVE Na BALANCE AND ECF VOLUME EXPANSION

In normal people, an increase in the amount of salt in the diet results in an increase of the urinary excretion of sodium in such a way that sodium balance is restored in less than five days. When Na excretion is impaired, by renal disease or persistent stimulation of Na reabsorption, the increased sodium load causes positive sodium balance, water retention, and expansion of the ECF.

ECF volume expansion can cause an increase in plasma volume and/or an increase in interstitial volume. The final distribution of the fluid retained depends on the forces which govern exchange across the capillary wall.

A. Mechanisms of Production of Positive Sodium Balance

As shown in Table V, positive sodium balance can occur because of structural renal disease, most frequently characterized by low GFR, or because of a primary extrarenal disorder which results in renal sodium retention inappropriate for the homeostatic requirements. Significant, persistent positive sodium balance is always accompanied by renal sodium and water retention.

In the acute nephritic syndrome, in acute renal failure (particularly the oliguric phase), and in terminal chronic renal failure the positive sodium balance is clearly related to the decrease in glomerular filtration rate.

Table V. Causes of Positive Sodium Balance

I. Proportionally distributed in intravascular and interstitial compartments
  A. Acute nephritic syndrome
  B. Oliguric phase of acute renal failure
  C. Iatrogenic overload (i.e., in obstructive uropathy, tubular necrosis)
II. Predominantly in interstitial compartment
  A. Chronic heart failure
  B. Nephrotic syndrome
  C. Hepatic cirrhosis
  D. Protein deficiency states
  E. Lymphatic obstructions
  F. Hormonal edema (estrogen, aldosterone)
  G. Idiopatic edema

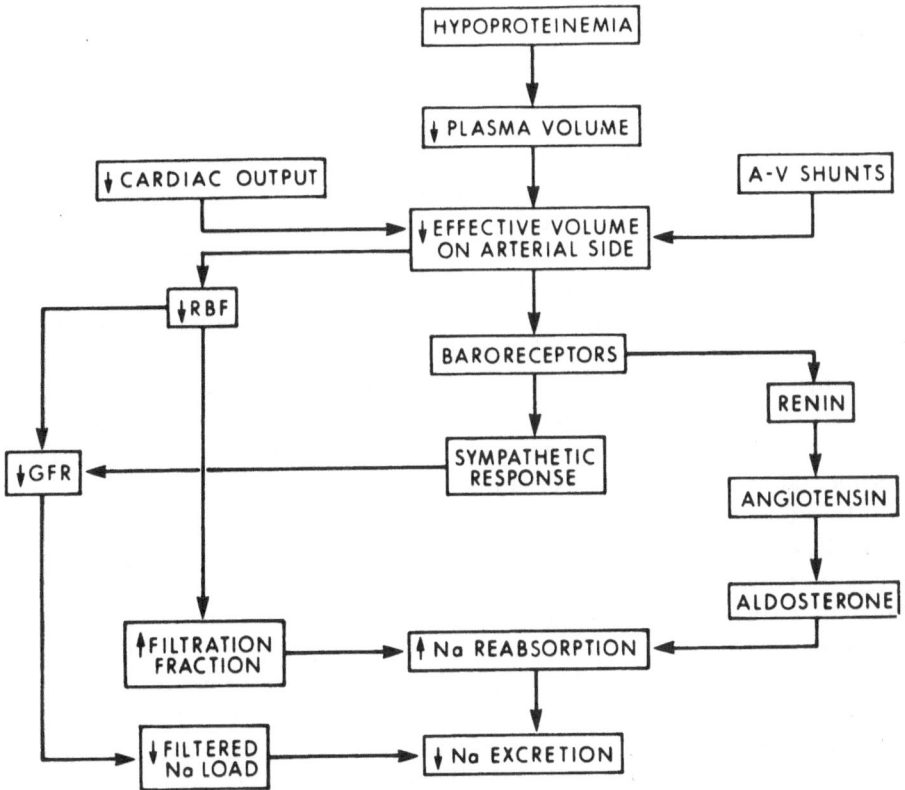

Figure 8. Mechanisms of production of positive sodium balance in generalized edema syndromes (see text). The decrease in the filtered load of sodium and the increase in sodium reabsorption ultimately depend on a reduction in effective blood volume on the arterial side of the systemic circulation.

The extrarenal causes of ECF volume expansion usually result in generalized edema, i.e., accumulation of fluid in the interstitial compartment, and sometimes also in serosal cavities. The pathophysiology of edema in these conditions is described in Chapter 5. Here, we will restrict the discussion to the mechanisms of retention of salt and water by the kidney.

Edema of congestive heart failure, hepatic cirrhosis, and hypoproteinemia have as a central common feature a reduction of the effective blood volume on the arterial side of the systemic circulation. This is due to the fall of cardiac output in heart failure, reduction of plasma volume in hypoproteinemic conditions such as malnutrition and the nephrotic syndrome, and to the development of hepatic and systemic arteriovenous shunts in cirrhosis. In some of these conditions, notably in cirrhosis, total blood volume is in fact increased. Nevertheless, the abnormal distribution of blood in the systemic circulation has pathophysiologic consequences similar to those which obtain in hypovolemia.

As illustrated in Figure 8, the hemodynamic alterations described above result in both decreased filtered load of sodium, because RBF and GFR decrease, and increased sodium reabsorption. In congestive heart failure there is evidence that the rate of sodium reabsorption is increased in all segments of the nephron: proximal tubule, loop of Henle and distal nephron. It is thought that the effects on the proximal tubule and the loop are mediated by factors other than GFR and aldosterone. Physical factors operating at both segments might explain the increased reabsorption, since the filtration fraction is increased and therefore the peritubular plasma oncotic pressure is elevated. Increased Na reabsorption by the distal nephron may be due to augmented aldosterone secretion.

Other mechanisms which could control sodium reabsorption, such as a natriuretic hormone, prostaglandins, and kinins, may play a role in sodium-retaining conditions, but this has not been conclusively proven. Redistribution of renal blood flow to deep nephrons was also thought to occur in congestive heart failure and other sodium-retaining conditions. However, recent experimental observations do not support this hypothesis.

In some of the syndromes of generalized edema, mechanisms other than those described above can contribute to the renal retention of sodium. Among these, we should mention the decrease of hepatic clearances of hormones such as aldosterone and renin, which occurs in cirrhosis and in congestive heart failure, and the effect of increased systemic venous pressure on sodium reabsorption. The latter effect has been attributed to activation of low-pressure baroreceptors which would stimulate aldosterone secretion.

Na retention is accompanied by water retention. This is mainly due to an increase in the secretion of ADH. There is evidence in favor of a role for low-pressure baroreceptors (located in atria and large veins) and high-pressure baroreceptors (carotid artery) in ADH secretion. These control mechanisms are stimulated by hypovolemia or diminished effective arterial volume in the conditions listed in Table V. In addition, ADH secretion is stimulated by angiotensin II, and the plasma concentration of this peptide is usually increased in generalized edema. Thirst is also stimulated by the mechanisms just described. A tendency to increase water intake accompanies, then, the renal retention, resulting in positive water balance. Finally, the reduction of GFR and the increase in filtration fraction result in a large fractional reabsorption of water in the proximal tubule and hence in a diminished delivery to the distal segments of the nephron. The mechanisms of positive water balance in generalized edema are summarized in Figure 9.

B. Pathophysiological Consequences of Positive Sodium Balance

The effects of ECF volume expansion depend on whether the mechanisms of fluid exchange across the capillary wall are altered. Positive balance of salt and water tend to increase both plasma volume and interstitial fluid volume. If the initial condition of the patient includes normal plasma and interstitial volumes, and preserved permeability and driving forces across the capillary endothelium, ECF volume expansion will expand plasma and

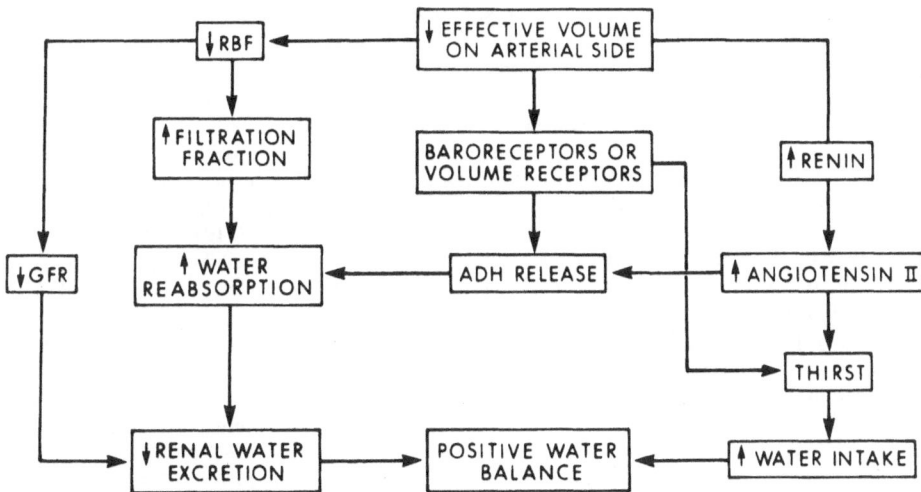

Figure 9. Mechanisms of production of positive water balance in generalized edema syndromes.

interstitial compartments in proportion to their initial volumes: roughly, 1 : 4. In this case, illustrated by acute nephritic syndrome and oliguric phase of acute or chronic renal failure, the main pathophysiologic effect is hypervolemia, which can cause congestive heart failure. When the driving forces across the capillary wall favor filtration, because of increased capillary hydrostatic pressure [generalized (congestive heart failure) or localized (hepatic cirrhosis with portal hypertension)], or decreased plasma colloidosmotic pressure (malnutrition, nephrotic syndrome), the end result of salt and water retention is a dominant expansion of the interstitial compartment (see Chapter 5). In fact, the mechanisms of positive balance of salt and water tend to correct the deficit in blood volume on the arterial side, but such correction is not achieved because of the altered tissue–capillary fluid exchange mechanisms.

SUGGESTED READINGS

Anderson, R. J., and Linas, S. L.: Sodium depletion states, in Brenner, B. M., and Stein, J. H. (eds.): *Sodium and Water Homeostasis, Contemporary Issues in Nephrology*, Vol. 1. Churchill Livingstone, New York, 1978, p. 154.

Berl, T., and Schrier, R. W.: Water metabolism and the hypo-osmolar syndromes, in Brenner, B. M., and Stein, J. H. (eds.): *Sodium and Water Homeostasis. Contemporary Issues in Nephrology*, Vol. 1. Churchill Livingstone, New York, 1978, p. 1.

Blair-West, J. R.: Renin angiotensin system and Na metabolism, in Thurau, K. (ed.): *International Review of Physiology*, Vol. 11. *Kidney and Urinary Tract Physiology II*. University Park Press, Baltimore, 1976, p. 95.

Davis, J. O., and Freeman, R. H.: Mechanisms regulating renin release. *Physiol. Rev.* 56:1, 1976.

De Wardener, H. E.: The control of sodium excretion. *Am. J. Physiol.* 4:F163, 1978.

Humes, H. D., Gottlieb, M. N., and Brenner, B. M.: The kidney in congestive heart failure, in

Brenner, B. M., and Stein, J. H. (eds.): *Sodium and Water Homeostasis. Contemporary Issues in Nephrology*, Vol. 1. Churchill Livingstone, New York, 1978, p. 51.

Kaloyanides, G. J.: Pathogenesis and treatment of edema with special reference to the use of diuretics, in Maxwell, M. H., and Kleeman, C. R. (eds.): *Clinical Disorders of Fluid and Electrolyte Metabolism.* McGraw-Hill, New York, 1980, p. 647.

Kopple, J. D., and Blumenkrantz, M. J.: Total parenteral nutrition and parenteral fluid therapy. Section II. Parenteral fluid therapy, in Maxwell, M. H., and Kleeman, C. R. (eds.): *Clinical Disorders of Fluid and Electrolyte Metabolism.* McGraw-Hill, New York, 1980, p. 459.

Oberg, B.: Overall cardiovascular regulation. *Annu. Rev. Physiol.* 38:537, 1976.

Phillips, S. F.: Water and electrolytes in gastrointestinal disease, in Maxwell, M. H., and Kleeman, C. R. (eds.): *Clinical Disorders of Fluid and Electrolyte Metabolism.* McGraw-Hill, New York, 1980, p. 1267.

Reineck, H. J., and Stein, J. H.: Regulation of sodium balance, in Maxwell, M. H., and Kleeman, C. R. (eds.): *Clinical Disorders of Fluid and Electrolyte Metabolism.* McGraw-Hill, New York, 1980, p. 89.

Seely, J. F., and Levy, M.: Control of extracellular fluid volume, in Brenner, B. M., and Rector, F. C. (eds.): *The Kidney.* W. B. Saunders Company, Philadelphia, 1981, p. 371.

Valtin, H.: *Renal Dysfunction: Mechanisms Involved in Fluid and Solute Imbalance.* Little, Brown and Company, Boston, 1979.

5

Edema and Edema-Forming States

ALAN M. ROBSON

I. INTRODUCTION

Edema occurs when the volume of fluid in the tissue space is increased from normal. It may be the consequence of numerous diseases which can affect the kidneys, the cardiovascular system, the liver, or the endocrine system, or it may result from the administration of certain drugs or a variety of other disorders (Table I). Edema may be localized to a very circumscribed area of the body, to one limb or to one region of the body such as the lungs. More often, it is generalized. Even generalized edema may not be detected by the patient or the physician if it is modest in amount. However, when interstitial fluid volume is increased by approximately 15%, or 2 liters in a 70-kg man, the edema becomes clinically apparent. Because, as is discussed below, intracapillary hydrostatic pressure and tissue pressure are two of the important factors which regulate interstitial fluid volume, generalized edema usually presents in areas where venous pressure is the highest or tissue pressure is the lowest. Thus, it may be seen first in the ankles if the patient has been upright for any length of time, over the sacrum if the patient has been supine or around the eyes or in the scrotum or labia where skin is lax. Alternately, generalized edema may present as pulmonary edema because of

ALAN M. ROBSON • Department of Pediatrics, Washington University School of Medicine, St. Louis, Missouri 63110.

Table I. Some Diseases Associated with the Formation of Generalized Edema

I. Diseases of the kidney
  A. Those producing nephrotic syndrome (see Chapter 11)
  B. Acute and chronic glomerulonephritides
  C. Acute and chronic renal failure
II. Diseases of the cardiovascular system
  A. Low output failure: myocardial infarction, congenital heart disease, pulmonary disorders causing congestive heart failure
  B. High output failure: anemias, thyrotoxicosis, beri-beri
  C. Venous diseases: obstruction of either the superior or inferior vena cava
III. Diseases of the liver
  A. Cirrhosis, obstruction of hepatic vein
IV. Diseases of endocrine system
  A. Hypothyroidism, mineralocorticoid excess, diabetes mellitus, inappropriate ADH syndrome
V. Drug administration
  A. Estrogens and oral contraceptives
  B. Diazoxide, minoxidil
  C. Rapid intravenous administration of saline and comparable solutions
VI. Other causes
  A. Pregnancy: toxemia
  B. Idiopathic cyclical edema of women
  C. Chronic malnutrition
  D. Edema of the neonate

the marked symptoms which result from fluid retention in the lungs. If generalized edema is massive in amount, it is referred to as anasarca.

Although numerous diseases can result in edema, they do so through a limited number of mechanisms. The same basic mechanism may result in either localized or generalized edema depending on the site and nature of the primary disease. Thus, edema will be analyzed according to the pathophysiologic mechanism responsible rather than by individual disease states causing the problem. This approach results in a better understanding of the cause for expansion of tissue fluid, and, when taken in conjunction with the disease state responsible, provides a rational approach to determine optimum management.

II. NORMAL PHYSIOLOGY

A. Regulation of Body Fluid Spaces

Prior to discussing the pathophysiologic mechanisms responsible for edema, the factors which maintain interstitial fluid volume relatively constant in amount in health will be reviewed.

After the first year of life, water represents between 55% and 60% of body weight. Approximately two thirds of this fluid (40% body weight) is intracellular and one third (20% body weight) extracellular. The distribution of water between the intracellular and extracellular fluid spaces is determined by osmotic forces operating across cell membranes which are freely permeable to water. In health, intracellular osmolar content and, therefore, intracellular fluid (ICF) volume are maintained relatively constant primarily by the active transport of potassium into, and sodium out of, cells. As a consequence, intracellular sodium concentrations are maintained at low levels and intracellular potassium concentrations at high levels. Indeed, potassium, with an average intracellular concentration of around 150 mEq/liter, is responsible alone for approximately 45% of intracellular osmolality.

If the osmolalities in the ICF and extracellular fluid (ECF) differ, there is net movement of water down its concentration gradient so that the ratio of fluid in the ICF to that in the ECF is altered. Thus hypernatremia, which causes a relative increase in ECF osmolality, results in the net movement of water into the ECF space and decreases ICF volume. Conversely, hyponatremia causes a net movement of water into cells and an increased ICF volume. If a change in the ECF osmolality is accompanied by a comparable change in ICF osmolality, there is no osmotic gradient across the cell walls and there will be no net fluid shift. This occurs when blood urea nitrogen levels are elevated. Although the urea increases ECF osmolality, urea enters the cells freely so that ICF osmolality increases in proportion to that in the ECF. There is no net movement of water across the cell walls.

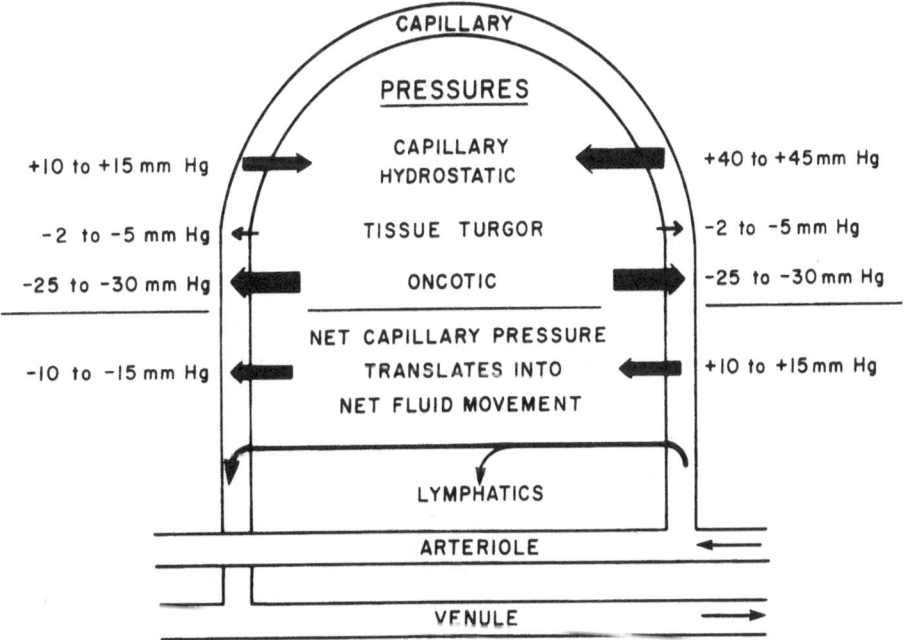

Figure 1. A schematic representation of Starling's forces, which regulate, at the capillary level, the distribution of extracellular fluid between the interstitial and vascular spaces. The size and direction of the arrows indicates the relative magnitude and direction of each of the forces.

Although discussed so far as a fluid space, ECF does not represent a homogeneous entity. It is composed of three major components. The largest is interstitial fluid, which comprises approximately 15% of body weight; intravascular water amounts to approximately 5% of body weight and transcellular water represents an even smaller volume of fluid. There is a constant flux of water between the interstitial and intravascular spaces, with the volume of fluid in the intravascular space being maintained by a balance between hydrostatic and osmotic forces operating at the level of the peripheral capillaries (Figure 1). Although total osmotic pressure regulates fluid shifts between the ECF and ICF spaces, it does not affect the distribution of ECF between its intravascular and interstitial components. This is because the crystalloid solutes, which are responsible for most of the total osmotic pressure of about 5100 mm Hg, are able to penetrate the capillary wall

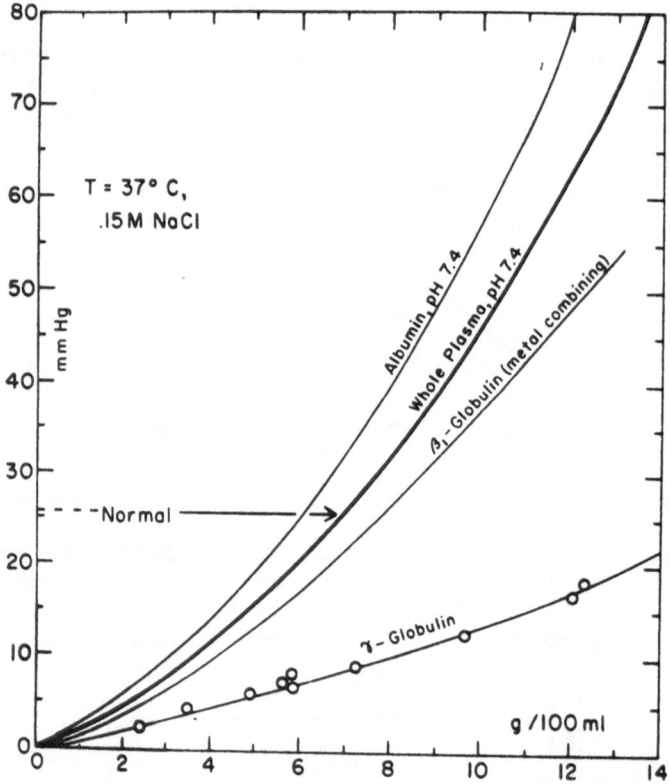

Figure 2. The effect of varying the concentration of either selected plasma proteins or whole plasma (horizontal axis) on oncotic pressure (vertical axis). Because molecules of albumin are smaller than those of globulins, any given amount of albumin contains more molecules and exerts a greater oncotic pressure than does an equal weight of globulin. (Reprinted with permission from Landis, E. M., and Pappenheimer, J. R.: Exchange of substances through the capillary walls, in Hamilton, W. F., and Dow, P. (eds.), *Handbook of Physiology*, Section 2, Circulation, Vol. II, Chap. 29, American Physiological Society, Washington, D.C., 1963, pp. 961–1034.)

completely. Having similar concentrations on the two sides of the capillary walls, they exert no net osmotic force across these membranes and, therefore, cannot modify net movement of fluid between the intravascular and interstitial fluid spaces.

In contrast to the crystalloid solutes, the plasma proteins and other colloidal solutes are confined almost completely to the capillary lumen in health. The osmotic pressure exerted by these solutes, colloid osmotic pressure or oncotic pressure, amounts to only 25–30 mm Hg or less than 1% of total osmotic pressure. However, being virtually limited to the vascular space, oncotic pressure exerts a net force across the capillary wall and is a major factor in maintaining vascular fluid volume. Because of its relative abundance and small molecular size, albumin is the protein primarily responsible for oncotic pressure (Figure 2).

Not only oncotic pressure but hydrostatic forces regulate the distribution of fluid across the capillary wall too (Figure 1). Blood enters the arteriolar end of the capillary under a mean hydrostatic pressure of 40–45 mm Hg. The equivalent pressure in the interstitial space is less than 5 mm Hg so that there is a net hydrostatic pressure of approximately 40 mm Hg driving fluid out of the capillaries into the interstitial space. This net hydrostatic pressure opposes oncotic pressure and, being the larger force, results in movement of plasma ultrafiltrate from the arteriolar end of the capillary into the interstitial space. Intracapillary hydrostatic pressure is dissipated along the length of the capillary. In addition, the loss of ultrafiltrate at the arteriolar end of the capillary results in a minor degree of hemoconcentration with a small increase in both plasma protein and oncotic pressure. By the distal or venous end of the capillary, oncotic pressure exceeds hydrostatic pressure. Thus, there is an effective net force for the return of ultrafiltrate into the capillary. The amount of fluid leaving the arteriolar end of capillaries is slightly in excess of that returning at the venous end. This excess fluid, along with any colloid that penetrates the capillary walls, is removed from the interstitial space through the lymphatic vessels and is returned to the vascular space as lymph.

This analysis of interstitial volume regulation may be too simplistic and may place too much emphasis on Starling forces, which were first described a century ago. Thus, not all patients with analbuminemia, a congenital defect caused by a major decrease in the rate of albumin synthesis, are edematous even though they have virtually no serum albumin. Presumably there are several additional regulatory mechanisms. One, which has been suggested by careful anatomic studies, is the presence of anastomoses between arterioles and venules supplying capillary beds. Dilation or contraction of such anastomotic channels would modify blood flow through the capillaries and could play an important role in regulating fluid movement into tissue spaces.

B. Characteristics of Peripheral Capillaries

From the preceding discussion, it is obvious that the normal distribution of ECF between its intravascular and interstitial fluid components depends on the maintenance of oncotic pressure across the capillary walls. This requires that the walls of these vessels prevent significant loss of colloid into the interstitial space. The peripheral capillaries function as though they contain pores smaller than those in the glomerular capillaries. The functional size of these pores, 65 Å in diameter, prevents significant movement of protein and explains why normal interstitial fluid is virtually protein free.

In contrast to the glomerular capillaries which function as though pores constitute 5% of surface area, the density of pores in peripheral capillaries is much lower, representing only 0.1% of capillary surface. Because of this and of the lower hydrostatic pressure in the peripheral capillaries, the rate of fluid movement across the peripheral capillaries is much lower than that in the glomeruli. Indeed, it has been calculated that fluid movement across all the capillaries contained in 100 g of tissue in the human forearm amounts only to about 0.003 ml/min or 4.0 ml/day. This rate of movement of plasma ultrafiltrate is inadequate to meet the nutritional needs of the tissue. Such observations indicate that, in addition to bulk movement of fluid through pores, there must be a significant diffusion across peripheral capillary walls.

C. Interstitial Fluid Sodium

Body sodium amounts to approximately 58 mEq/kg body weight, of which 70% is in the exchangeable sodium pool. Although sodium is the major ECF cation and is the principal osmotic solute responsible for the maintenance of ECF volume, less than 50% of total body sodium is present in this space. Most of the remainder is in bone where it is either nonexchangeable or only slowly exchangeable. The factors which regulate total body sodium content and distribution of sodium between the various components of body fluid are incompletely understood and are discussed in Section I, Chapter 1, and Section II, Chapter 4. Sodium in the ECF can diffuse freely across the peripheral capillaries so that its concentration in the interstitial and vascular fluid spaces are similar. The slightly lower values in the interstitial space are due to the restriction of proteins to the vascular space and the resulting Gibbs–Donnan effect. Regulation of ECF sodium concentration is primarily through the osmoregulatory mechanisms involving secretion of antidiuretic hormone. Thus, the amount of sodium present in the interstitial space is the product of the ECF sodium concentration and the volume of interstitial fluid.

III. EDEMA FORMATION

A. General Considerations

Reviewing the regulation of interstitial fluid volume (Figure 1), it is apparent that edema might result from several basic abnormalities. These are (1) a decrease in capillary oncotic pressure, (2) an increased capillary permability to protein, permitting leak of colloid into interstitial fluid and reducing the effective oncotic pressure in the capillary, (3) an increase in capillary mean hydrostatic pressure, and (4) obstruction of lymph flow preventing removal of fluid and colloid filtered but not reabsorbed at the capillary level. That most of these mechanisms can result in either generalized or localized edema is depicted in Table II, where diseases causing edema are classified according to the major factor contributing to the edema formation.

Most systemic disorders result in generalized edema. Total body contents of both sodium and water are increased. When first seen by their physician, the majority of patients with generalized edema are in positive sodium and water balance. In some, however, a new steady state has been established by the time the patient seeks medical advice so that the excretion of sodium and water matches the intakes. Typically, the retention of sodium and water are in proportion to one another so that plasma, and therefore interstitial fluid sodium concentration, remains within the normal range. Less frequently, sodium and water retention are not proportional so that hypo- or hyperna-tremia can result. Even edematous patients with hyponatremia, however, have an increase in total body sodium content. Some patients with edema secondary to nephrotic syndrome may have pseudohyponatremia if their lipid levels are markedly elevated. Sodium concentrations measured in the plasma or serum of such patients appear low, but concentrations in plasma water are normal. Treating pseudohyponatremia with the measures usually used to correct true hyponatremia, fails to return the serum sodium concentration to normal.

Table II. Some Causes of Edema Classified According to Pathophysiologic Mechanisms

I. Decreased plasma oncotic pressure
    1. Generalized: nephrotic syndrome, cirrhosis, malnutrition
II. Increased vascular permeability to colloids
    1. Generalized: angioneurotic edema, anorexia (especially newborns)
    2. Localized: burns, local release of enzymes from damaged tissue, histamine (wheals), inhalation of toxins (pulmonary edema)
III. Increased hydrostatic pressure
    A. Increased transmission of arteriolar pressure
        1. Generalized: diazoxide, minoxidil
        2. Localized: exercise
    B. Increased venous pressure
        1. Generalized: congestive heart failure
        2. Localized: venous thromboses
IV. Obstruction of lymph flow
    1. Localized: tissue irradiation, surgery, filariasis, metastases
V. Other causes
    A. Inappropriate renal retention of sodium and water
        1. Generalized: acute glomerulonephritis, estrogen administration, primary aldosteronism, cyclic idiopathic edema
    B. Myxedema
        1. Generalized: hypothyroidism

Localized edema may be so limited in extent that total body sodium and water are not significantly increased in amounts nor is serum sodium concentration affected.

B. Causes of Edema

1. Decreased Plasma Oncotic Pressure

Hypoalbuminemia reduces plasma oncotic pressure and, if severe, will result in generalized edema formation as long as the patient has a continuing sufficient intake of sodium and water to permit significant positive balance. In general, clinical edema does not appear until the plasma albumin concentration falls to 2 g/dl or less. However, there are many exceptions to this general rule. Some patients become edematous with plasma albumin concentrations above 2 g/dl, and others remain edema free despite very low albumin concentrations.

Because of the mathematical relationship between plasma albumin concentration and oncotic pressure (Figure 2), a decrease in plasma albumin concentration results in an even greater decrease in plasma oncotic pressure. The large size of globulin molecules results in their oncotic effect being much less for any given plasma concentration so that hyperglobulinemia cannot compensate for the decreased albumin concentration. Thus, hypoalbuminemia results in a decrease in oncotic pressure irrespective of changes in plasma globulin concentrations.

The decrease in plasma oncotic pressure increases the net driving force for fluid movement out of the arteriolar end of capillaries (Figure 3). More importantly, it decreases the force available for reabsorption of fluid at the venous end of the capillary. In consequence, fluid accumulates in the interstitial space and results in small amounts of edema as well as in some decrease in blood volume. This mechanism alone, i.e., redistribution of extracellular fluid with net movement of fluid from the vascular to the interstitial space, cannot account for the amount of edema present in most edematous patients. For example, a normal 70-kg man has a plasma water volume of approximately 3.5 liters (5% of body weight) and an interstitial fluid volume of 10.5 liters (15% of body weight). Edema would not become apparent in such a person until interstitial fluid space had been expanded by at least 2 liters. To accumulate this volume of edema by transfer of fluid from the vascular to the interstitial compartments would require blood volume to be reduced by more than 50%—a situation that may not be compatible with life. It obviously is a physiologic impossibility for the 5 or more liters of edema characteristically seen in many edematous patients to accumulate by this mechanism alone. Indeed, measurements of blood volume in patients with either mild, moderate, or severe amounts of edema have failed to show consistent or marked decreases.

Equally important in the formation of edema are the physiologic changes precipitated by the initial reduction in plasma volume. These changes result

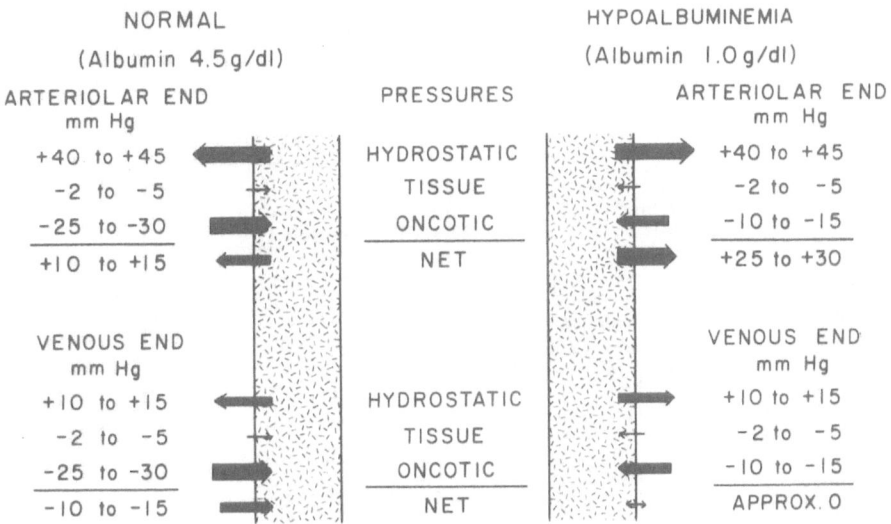

Figure 3. A schematic representation of the effects of hypoalbuminemia on the forces regulating fluid movements at the level of the capillary.

in sodium and water retention by the kidneys (Figure 4), and are designed to return blood volume to normal. The major mechanisms which have been proposed include a reduction in glomerular filtration rate and an increased secretion of both antidiuretic hormone and renin, the latter stimulating increased secretion of aldosterone. Although plasma renin and aldosterone levels frequently are elevated in patients with this form of edema, aldosterone secretion is not always increased. As a result of such observations, it has been postulated that the increased renin secretion is needed in many edematous patients to maintain arterial blood pressure, but that the secondary increase in aldosterone which occurs is not the primary cause of the sodium retention. Recent tantalizing observations have suggested a decreased secretion of the proposed natriuretic hormone may contribute to the sodium retention and edema formation too. This thesis has not been proven, however. Other as yet ill-defined changes almost certainly contribute to the retention of sodium and water and to the formation of edema.

Depending on circumstances and the underlying disease state, some of the retained sodium and water may remain in the vascular space. Thus, plasma volume may or may not be returned to normal when anasarca and new equilibrium conditions have been established. However, because of the low plasma oncotic pressure, much of the retained sodium and water does not remain in the vascular space. It enters the interstitial space and results in increasing amounts of edema.

A decrease in plasma oncotic pressure is thought to be a major factor responsible for edema formation in nephrotic syndrome, in certain diseases of the liver, and possibly in malnutrition. The pathophysiology of the nephrotic syndrome is discussed in Section IV, Chapter 11, and will not be

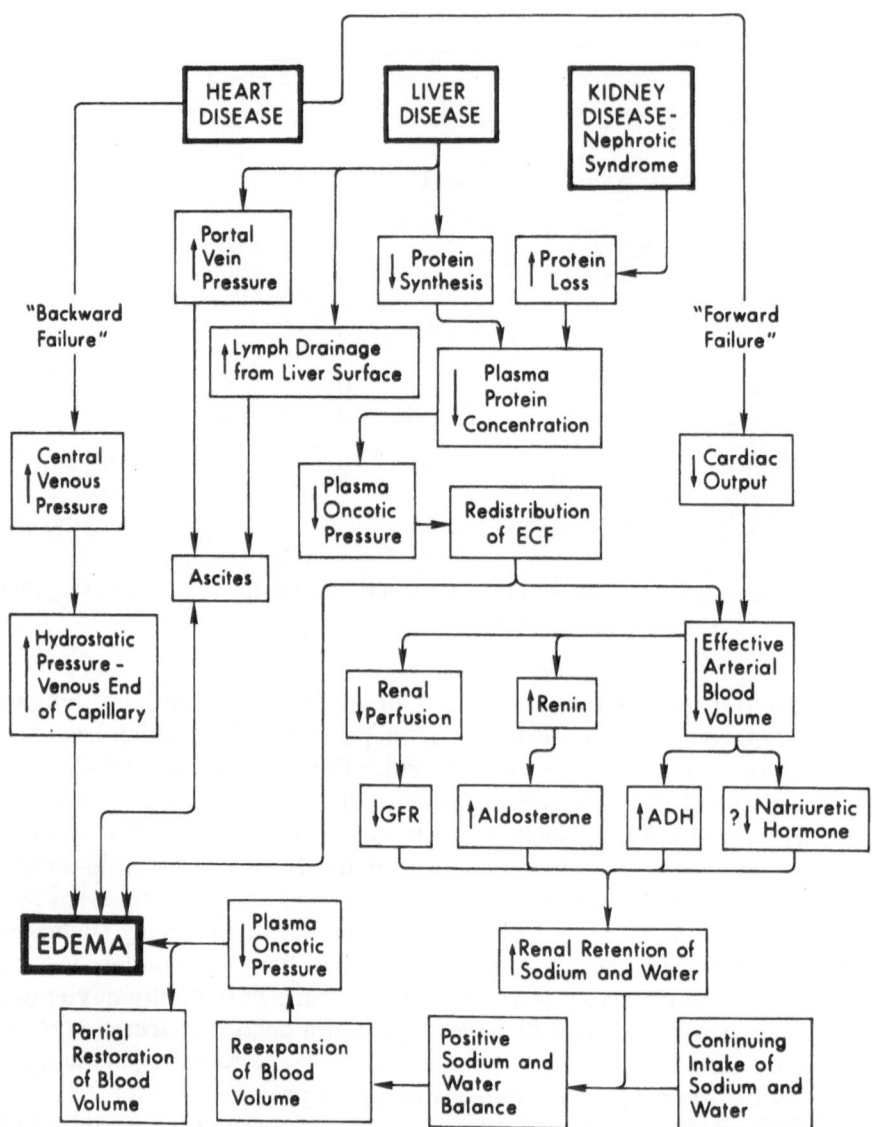

Figure 4. The interaction of factors responsible for the genesis of edema seen in certain diseases of the heart, liver, and kidneys.

reiterated here. In patients with edema secondary to cirrhosis of the liver, total plasma volume may be increased rather than decreased. Much of this extra blood volume is present in the splanchnic bed because hepatic scarring impedes return of blood from this segment of the circulation to the right side of the heart. As a consequence, there is decreased cardiac output with reduced renal perfusion. This, along with the effects of hypoalbuminemia which results from liver damage, stimulates aldosterone production and renal tubular retention of sodium. At the same time, the elevated portal pressure increases fluid transudation from the splanchnic capillaries contributing, along with excess lymph drainage from the liver, to the accumulation of edema fluid and ascites in the abdomen.

The hypoproteinemia seen in severe protein-calorie malnutrition almost certainly contributes to the formation of edema in these patients. The degree of edema, however, does not always correlate with the level of decrease in albumin concentration. Furthermore, an improved dietary intake by malnourished subjects may be followed by loss of edema before serum protein concentrations have increased. It has been shown that as the serum protein concentration falls in malnutrition, there is a fall in colloid in the interstitial fluid, too. The resulting decrease in interstitial fluid colloid osmotic pressure appears to compensate, at least in part, for the decreased plasma oncotic pressure. In many malnourished patients, the hypoproteinemia is potentiated by vitamin deficiency which may cause beri-beri, and by multiple deficiencies which cause anemia. Both result in high output congestive heart failure. Indeed, these and other mechanisms concerned with retention of sodium and water may play an important role in precipitating the appearance of edema in severe malnutrition.

2. Increased Vascular Permeability

An increase in capillary permeability with extravasation of protein into the interstitial space will reduce net oncotic pressure and decrease the ability of the capillaries to retain fluid. This may be a generalized phenomenon secondary to circulating capillary toxins, but more often is a localized one. Thus, local edema may result from physical damage to capillaries secondary to heat (burns) or to exposure to ultraviolet light (sunburn). In the lungs it may result from inhalation of toxins such as the oxides of nitrogen, oxygen in high concentrations, smoke, and corrosive chemicals such as phosgene, from ingestion of the herbicide paraquat, from aspiration of gastric juice or certain hydrocarbons, from prolonged exposure to high altitudes, from infections, or from many other causes. An even more localized form of edema is seen with wheal formation.

The mechanisms responsible for edema due to increased vascular permeability are being unraveled slowly. Histamine, 5-hydroxytryptamine, and bradykinin all increase vascular permeability. Histamine probably exerts its action through the H_1 receptors, which have been found to play a part in the early transient phase of increased vascular permeability after injury. In contrast, H_2 receptors do not appear to be involved in altering vascular permeability. Prostaglandin E_1 increases vascular permeability directly. Prostaglandin I_2 (PGI_2) has no direct effect on vascular permeability, but potentiates the action of both histamine and bradykinin. The effect of locally infused histamine to increase vascular protein efflux is antagonized by catecholamines, probably due to both α- and β-adrenoreceptor-mediated actions.

It has been proposed from these observations that there are direct mediators of increased vascular permeability such as histamine and bradykinin. Substances such as PGI_2, which have no direct action but which potentiate the direct mediators of vascular permeability, are thought to act as vasodilators, increasing blood flow and increasing plasma exudation from the altered capillary walls. According to this view, catecholamines oppose the action of histamine by decreasing blood flow. Similarly, the nonsteroidal antiflammatory compounds suppress inflammatory swelling and edema formation by inhibition of vasodilatation.

A variety of mechanisms are responsible for localized increases in vascular permeability and edema. Histamine release may be the prime mediator of the edema in a wheal. In other situations, alternate factors are operative. For example, in burns, anoxia and release of proteolytic enzymes from damaged tissue increases capillary permeability to protein and cause transudation of fluid with local edema formation. In addition, the increased adherence of white blood cells to blood vessels in burned tissue has been shown to reduce markedly the effective diameter of these vessels. This may increase postcapillary resistance and hydrostatic pressure in the capillaries, causing or aggravating edema in the burn.

Hereditary angioneurotic edema is a fascinating syndrome associated with intermittent attacks of localized edema caused by increased vascular permeability. First described by Quincke, this syndrome is now recognized not to be as rare as was thought at one time, and may have an incidence as high as $1:150,000$. Episodes of edema occur with greatest frequency in childhood and disappear by age 60 years. Typically, they are initiated by physical and emotional stress and may occur in several locations in the body. In the skin they present as circumscribed, noninflammatory subepithelial swellings. In the gastrointestinal tract they may cause colic or even obstruction. In the airway they have resulted in death from suffocation.

Although usually familial, the pattern of inheritance of the syndrome remains to be delineated completely. The pathology of the lesion shows increased vascular permeability in the absence of inflammatory changes. The site of the abnormality is the postcapillary venules where the endothelial cells are contracted with leaks present between these cells. Similar changes have been observed following the experimental administration of histamine, serotonin, and bradykinin. However, the elevated levels of bradykinin and histamine reported in patients with hereditary angioedema are thought to be secondary rather than primary events.

The importance of this syndrome in defining mechanisms responsible for edema is that it has been linked to a deficiency of C1 esterase inhibitor. This protein regulates the action of both the activated first component of complement and kallikrein. In consequence, plasma levels of both the C2 and C4 components of complement are decreased, especially during episodes of the syndrome. Even more exciting is the observation that the plasma of patients with hereditary angioedema contains a polypeptide kinin, distinct from bradykinin, which has permeability-enhancing activity. This could activate contractile proteins within the endothelial cells and cause the observed contraction of these cells.

3. Increased Capillary Hydrostatic Pressure

Increasing hydrostatic pressure inside the capillaries will increase net filtration of fluid out of the arteriolar end of the capillary and decrease return at the venous end. If the resulting accumulation of fluid in the interstitial space is sufficiently great, edema will develop.

This form of edema can result from one of two basic mechanisms. In the first, dilatation of the arterioles and precapillary sphincters results in increased transmission of arterial blood pressure to the capillaries. This is the mechanism for the troublesome and undesirable edema which sometimes occurs when certain vasodilator drugs, such as diazoxide and minoxidil, are used to treat hypertension for protracted periods of time. Arteriolar vasodilation is responsible also for the edema observed in exercise, in exposure to a high environmental temperature, and it contributes to the edema at the site of localized inflammation.

The second basic mechanism causing this form of edema is increased resistance in venous outflow tracts. This results in increased venous pressure. A generalized increase in venous pressure most often is secondary to a decreased cardiac output and heart failure secondary to various heart diseases. If the left ventricle fails, for example from an arrythmia, a myocardial infarct, hypertension, or valvular heart disease, pressure in the pulmonary veins increases so that pulmonary edema is the initial manifestation. Persistence of the heart failure will result in generalized edema when the elevated venous pressure results in an increased central venous pressure and is transmitted to the systemic venous circulation and capillaries. This is only one of the mechanisms responsible for the edema observed in congestive heart failure. It is sometimes referred to as the "backward" component of such failure. Equally important is the "forward" component in which a decreased cardiac output and decreased renal perfusion result in renal retention of sodium and water by mechanisms discussed already.

Localized increases in venous resistance such as that which occurs with venous thrombosis will result in more circumscribed areas of edema, the site of the edema depending on the site of venous occlusion. For example, deep vein thrombosis occurring in one leg produces edema in that limb alone; if the thrombosis extends to the inferior vena cava, then both lower limbs will become edematous.

4. Obstruction of Lymph Flow

Disruption of the lymphatics may result in edema when the normal drainage through these lymph vessels is obstructed. The excess fluid and any colloid that leaks out of the capillaries is not returned to the vascular system and accumulates in the interstitial space. This usually results in localized edema. It may occur after tissue irradiation, following surgery, with filariasis where the adult worms inhabit and occlude the lymph vessels, or with metastases from malignant tumors.

5. Decreased Tissue Pressure

It is theoretically possible that decreased tissue pressure could predispose to edema formation. Since tissue pressure is low compared to intracapillary pressure, it is unlikely that an abnormality in tissue pressure is the primary cause of edema in any patient. However, low tissue resistance in the periorbital regions, in the scrotum, or in the labia is presumed to be the explanation for why these sites often are the first at which edema appears. In addition, reduced tissue resistance may account for the observation that once edema has caused extensive tissue stretching at any site, this location is more susceptible to develop edema subsequently.

6. Other Causes

The role of plasma volume in the genesis of some forms of edema remains controversial. It is uncertain whether the volume of fluid in the vascular space varies in health, paralleling changes in dietary intakes of sodium and water. If this occurs, serious physiologic consequences might be prevented by compensating mechanisms. For example, an increase in vascular volume could be compensated for by a decrease in peripheral venous tone, which would cause blood to pool in the peripheral venous system. This would maintain central venous volume and central venous pressure at normal levels. Alternately, there could be shifts of blood to localized segments of the circulation with pooling in areas such as the spleen or the splanchnic bed.

A second alternative is that vascular capacity normally is limited and that blood volume must be maintained within rather narrow limits. According to this theory, maintenance of a relatively constant blood volume would be accomplished by shifts of fluid between the intravascular and interstitial compartments of ECF. This would allow compensation for altered dietary intakes of sodium and water and prevent major changes in blood volume. For example, if blood volume was to be expanded acutely, a net shift of fluid from the intravascular to interstitial fluid compartment would minimize the change in blood vlomue at the expense of an expanded interstitial fluid volume and edema.

Such a physiologic mechanism could explain the edema seen in several clinical situations, the pathophysiology of which has not been fully understood previously. Each is known to be characterized by inappropriate sodium and water retention by the kidney. For example, patients with acute glomerulo-nephritis have proteinuria and hypoproteinemia. However, the urinary loss of protein is relatively modest in amount and the hypoproteinemia charac-teristically is moderate in degree. Rather than being the primary cause of the edema, the hypoproteinemia is thought to be secondary to fluid retention and volume expansion. In the acute phase of glomerulonephritis, the urinary excretion of sodium and water is reduced, probably due to an acute reduction in GFR and the patient is in positive sodium and water balance. Prevention of excessive blood volume expansion by storage of much of this retained sodium and water in the interstitial space would account for the edema observed in this disease.

A similar sequence of events, i.e., inappropriate sodium and water retention with storage of retained sodium and water in the interstitial fluid space, may be responsible for the edema seen in patients with primary aldosteronism, escape mechanisms preventing it from becoming too severe. It may also explain the edema which occurs with estrogen administration as well as that observed in the syndrome of idiopathic edema.

Idiopathic edema is unlikely to be an entity but rather results from a variety of disorders. For example, some patients labeled as having idiopathic edema have been found subsequently to be hypothyroid. In others, excessive amounts of sodium and water are retained after the patient has discontinued medication with diuretics or laxatives. It is proposed that this form of idiopathic edema is due to a rebound phenomenon, that plasma renin levels are elevated during the period of therapy and remain inappropriately elevated for a protracted period of time after the drugs have been discontinued, causing sodium and water retention. The classical syndrome of idiopathic edema, however, is typically observed in women who develop recurrent episodes of edema of unknown etiology. The edema shows a diurnal variation with excessive retention of sodium and water occurring when the patients assume an upright position. This appears to be an important contributing etiologic factor in the majority of patients. Although a variety of abnormalities, including inappropriate sodium retention by the kidneys and abnormal regulation of arginine vasopressin, has been described in such patients, none has been proven to be the primary cause.

Certain endocrine abnormalities are associated with edema, too. The pathophysiologic mechanisms are not fully understood in all of them. A unique type of edema, myxedema, occurs in patients with hypothyroidism. It is characterized by binding of salt and water in large amounts to anionic mucopolysaccharides in the subcutaneous tissues. Edema occurs also in some hyperthyroid patients. It is not related to myxedema, but usually is the consequence of high output heart failure. Transient edema may also develop in diabetic patients shortly after starting treatment with insulin. This complication has been described in some series in up to 3.5% of diabetic patients. The cause is not known.

IV. TREATMENT OF EDEMA

A. General Approach

The treatment of edema has been revolutionized by the development of modern diuretic drugs. Indeed, the use of these drugs has markedly improved the well being of most edematous patients. It must be remembered,

Table III. Basic Approach to Treatment of Edema

   I. Treatment of disease causing the edema
  II. Increased excretion of sodium and water
      A. Diuretics
      B. Other measures
         1. Bed rest, local pressure, ultrafiltration
         2. Special measures in specific disease states
 III. Decreased sodium and water intake
      A. Dietary restrictions
      B. Restrictions of parenteral fluid administration

---

however, that use of these drugs should constitute only part of a three-pronged approach to the mangement of edema (Table III). Before starting diuretics, one must attempt to determine the cause of the edema and treat the primary disease. With most cases of localized edema and in many patients with mild degrees of generalized edema, this may be all that is necessary. This aspect of management is beyond the scope of the present chapter and will not be discussed in detail.

In patients with more severe generalized edema or in those in whom localized edema is associated with marked swelling of tissues, additional measures are required. These are designed to increase the urinary losses of both salt and water by the use of diuretics alone or in conjunction with other methods, and to decrease the amount of salt and water available for absorption from the gastrointestinal tract by appropriate dietary restrictions. Both of these approaches to treatment will be presented in detail.

B. Increasing Urinary Salt and Water Losses

1. Diuretics

Since modern diuretics are such potent drugs, it is tempting to rely solely on their use for control of edema. There are many reasons for not taking this approach, however. One is that the use of these drugs alone may not result in satisfactory resolution of the edema. The reductions in plasma volume which occur after a diuretic-induced diuresis, produce secondary physiologic changes. These include a further decrease in renal perfusion with further reduction in glomerular filtration rate, even greater stimulation of both ADH and renin release with increased production of angiotensin and aldosterone, and an increase in plasma protein concentration with an accompanying relative increase in peritubular oncotic pressure. All of these changes contribute to even more avid retention of sodium and water by the kidney. Under these circumstances, any diuretic-induced increases in renal losses of sodium and water will not result in negative balances for the patient unless dietary and other restrictions of sodium and water intake are imposed simultaneously.

Another reason for not relying solely on diuretic therapy when treating edema is that edema represents expansion of the interstitial fluid space; diuretics, however, do not decrease the size of this space initially. Rather, they result in losses of salt and water from the vascular space. Unless there is subsequent movement of fluid and solute from the interstitial into the vascular space, the patient may develop symptoms of hypovolemia, even in the presence of anasarca. This can occur in the nephrotic syndrome if massive amounts of edema fluid are removed too quickly. Plasma volume becomes markedly contracted during the period of negative fluid balance. Since hypoproteinemia limits the return of edema fluid into the vascular space, hypotension and shock can develop. Similarly, if too brisk a diuresis is established in patients with cirrhosis and ascites, vascular collapse may occur even though marked ascites remains.

Yet another problem with the use of diuretics alone to control edema is illustrated by the management of congestive heart failure. These drugs are very beneficial in the treatment of heart failure. For example, reduction in the amount of edema improves tissue perfusion, as well as the patient's morale. Too great a reduction in the vascular volume, however, may reduce significantly the venous filling pressure. This will cause further decreases in the efficiency of the failing heart and further reduce the decreased cardiac output. Therefore, when treating patients with heart failure, it is necessary to attempt to increase cardiac output too, using appropriate measures such as the administration of digoxin.

Finally, it must be remembered that almost any diuretic has unwanted side effects. Limiting the number of drugs taken by a patient reduces the number of potential complications that may develop.

Despite these limitations, modern diuretics are powerful and extremely useful drugs. Since different groups of diuretics act at different segments of the nephron (Table IV), optimal use of these drugs requires an understanding of renal physiology and of the sites in the nephron at which each works. Such knowledge permits selection of the appropriate diuretic(s) to be used alone or in combination. The present chapter discusses the principles of use

Table IV. Sites of Diuretic Action in the Nephron

Site in nephron	Diuretics acting at site
Proximal tubule	Major action: acetazolamide, mannitol
	Minor action: furosemide, ethacrynic acid, mercurials, thiazides
Thick ascending loop of Henle	Major action: furosemide, ethacrynic acid, mercurials
	Minor action: mannitol decreases sodium and water absorption in Henle's loop
Cortical diluting segment/early distal nephron	Thiazides, chlorthalidone, metolazone
Distal nephron	Spironolactone, triamterene

of diuretics. A more detailed analysis of drug action is presented in Section VII, Chapter 17. The recommended doses of drugs given here are meant as guidelines only. Responses of patients to diuretics varies so that an individual regimen must be developed for each patient. In general, patients with congestive heart failure have a greater response to the use of these drugs than do patients with nephrotic syndrome, renal failure, or cirrhosis.

a. Sulfonamide Diuretics

These are the most numerous of the popular diuretics. They consist of two groups, the thiazides such as hydrochlorothiazide, and the nonthiazides such as chlorthalidone and metolazone. Most of the sulfonamide diuretics are capable of inhibiting carbonic anhydrase and do have an effect on the proximal tubule. Their major action, however, is on the early portion of the distal nephron referred to as the cortical diluting segment. They inhibit the active transport of sodium, and accompanying transport of chloride at this site (Figure 5). The specific mechanism responsible for their action remains unknown. Inhibition of Na–K ATPase and inhibition of glycolysis, an energy supply for transport, have been suggested.

The dose of a typical thiazide, hydrochlorothiazide, that is usually recommended to initiate a diuresis in an adult patient is 50 to 200 mg/day (2–3 mg/kg body weight in children). Occasionally higher doses are required. They are given by mouth, either in a single dose or in two divided doses. Typically, a lower dose can be utilized for maintenance therapy once a diuresis has been established. The drug is a modestly potent diuretic and may induce a maximal natriuresis equal to about 10% of the filtered load of sodium. The onset of diuresis occurs about two hours after administration and can last for 12 hr or more.

Thiazides are well tolerated by patients with the incidence of adverse side effects or hypersensitivity reactions being low. Troublesome nocturia can be limited by giving no dose later than early afternoon. Prolonged use of the drug may result in hypokalemia, in metabolic alkalosis, or in hyponatremia. Hypokalemia typically is mild but can be symptomatic and, in patients with liver disease, can precipitate hepatic coma. Hyponatremia occurs less frequently with thiazides than with the use of loop diuretics. In addition to these side effects, thiazide administration causes a reduction in glomerular filtration rate and can result in hyperglycemia and in hyperuricemia. Indeed, frank attacks of gout can be precipitated. Although thiazides are used to treat hypertension, hypotension is not a complication when the drugs are given to normotensive subjects not receiving other hypotensive drugs.

Structurally somewhat different, the nonthiazide sulfonamide diuretics, chlorthalidone and metolazone, have similar potencies, actions, and side effects to those described for the thiazides. Chlorthalidone has a more prolonged action of up to 48 hr and metolazone, when given in the upper

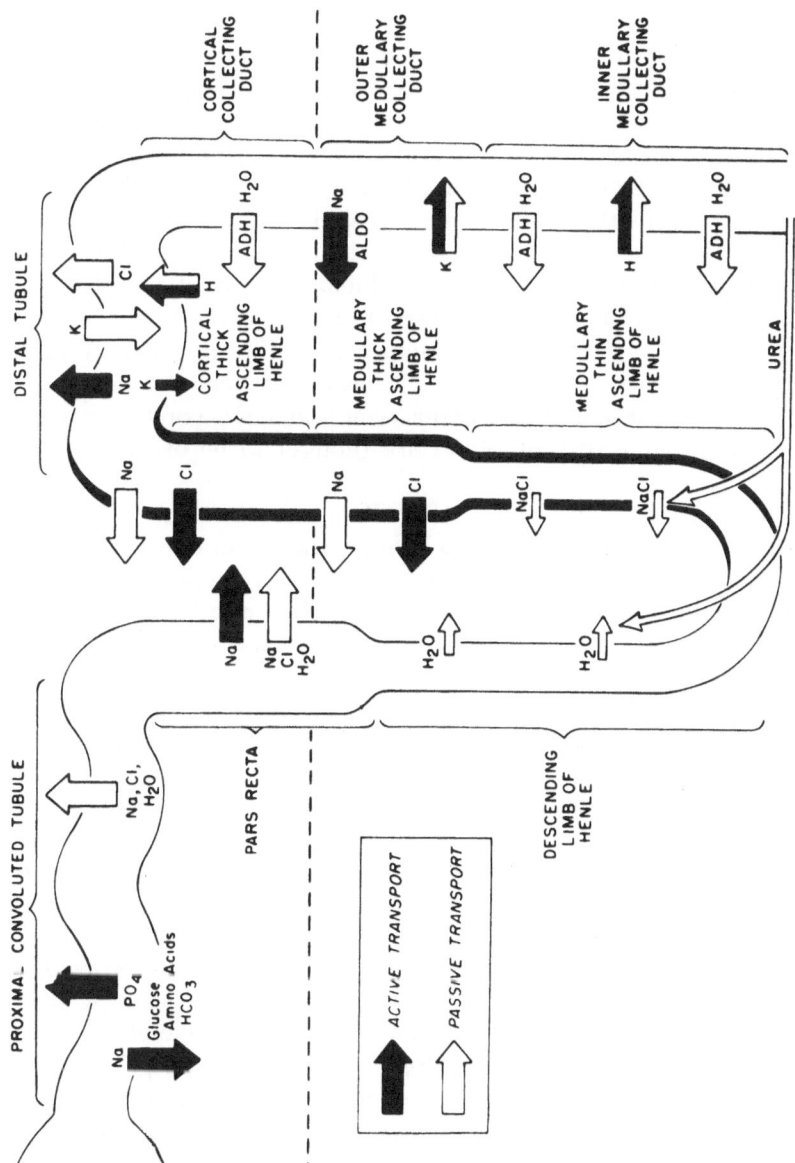

Figure 5. A schematic representation of the major transport processes in the nephron that may be affected by diuretics. (Reprinted with permission from Jacobsen, H.R., and Kokko, J.P.: Diuretics: sites and mechanisms of action. *Annu. Rev. Pharm. Toxicol.* 16:201–214, 1976.)

range of recommended dosage, may result in a diuresis and saliuresis for up to 24 hr.

b. Loop Diuretics

These drugs include furosemide, ethacrynic acid, and two newer agents, bumetanide and triflocin. They are the most potent diuretics available for clinical use and may increase urinary sodium excretion to as high as 20%–30% of the filtered load of sodium.

The major action of these drugs is thought to be inhibition of active chloride transport in the thick ascending limb of the loop of Henle. Sodium transport and that of other cations is decreased secondarily. It has been proposed that these drugs may act by inhibition of Na–K ATPase, by inhibition or displacement of cAMP or by inhibition of glycolysis. The exact mode of action at a cellular level, however, is still being elucidated. In addition to their action in the loop of Henle, these diuretics exert some of their natriuretic activity by alteration of intrarenal hemodynamics, and furosemide, bumetanide, and possibly ethacrynic acid may act on the proximal tubule too. These latter sites of action are thought to be of little clinical significance.

The loop diuretics exert their effects from the luminal side of the membrane. They are largely bound to serum proteins so that little can be filtered. Thus, most of the drug reaches its site of action by being transported in the tubular fluid following active secretion by the organic acid transport pathway in the proximal tubule. This physiology explains why the drugs are so potent but have few systemic side effects, and why, as discussed below, the effect of the loop diuretics is influenced by other organic acids.

Furosemide may be administered by the oral or intravenous route. The usual initiating oral dose is 80 mg (2 mg/kg body weight in children) and can be repeated after 6–8 hr. A diuretic effect typically occurs within one hour and lasts for 6–8 hr. Higher doses can be given to patients who have an unsatisfactory initial response. With careful titration, doses of 500 mg or more per day have been utilized without any major problems having been encountered. When given intravenously, a diuresis often begins within 5 min, reaches a peak after 30 min, and lasts for 2 hr. The usual intravenous dose is 0.5–1 mg/kg body weight given over 1–2 min. It can be repeated 2 hr later in higher dosage if necessary. The drug is well tolerated by this route. Indeed, very large intravenous doses of up to 0.5–1.0 g have been used in some patients in an attempt to abort the development of acute renal failure without untoward side effects being reported.

Chronic use of furosemide may induce the same changes in serum electrolytes that were described with chronic thiazide administration, namely, hypochloremic alkalosis, hypokalemia, and hyponatremia. Hyperglycemia and hyperuricemia occur, too. Probably reflecting relative diuretic potency, the electrolyte changes tend to occur more frequently and to be more severe with furosemide than with thiazides. If the serum potassium falls below 3 mEq/liter, dietary supplementation with an oral potassium preparation is required. When such supplemental therapy is given, serum potassium levels should be monitored regularly, especially in patients in whom renal function is impaired. Hyponatremia is very common and has several causes. The major reason relates to the loop diuretic's effect of impairing the ability of the kidney to generate and excrete solute-free water. If excess amounts of water are ingested, the patient is unable to excrete a sufficiently dilute urine and hyponatremia results. Also contributing to the hyponatremia is the contraction in vascular volume which often occurs with use of loop diuretics. This stimulates ADH release and further impairs the ability of the kidney to excrete free water. In addition to its natriuretic action, the drug increases urinary excretion of calcium, an important point to be remembered if treating a patient with a past history of nephrolithiasis. Prolonged use of furosemide in high dosage may result in deafness. Unlike thiazides, the use of furosemide does not cause an acute decrease in GFR.

The variability of response to furosemide that is observed in individual patients can be explained by the physiology of the renal handling of the drug. In patients with elevated plasma levels of other organic acids, e.g., patients with renal failure, these acids compete with the loop diuretics for the proximal tubular transport sites. Thus, even though plasma levels of furosemide are adequate, the amount reaching the site of action is reduced, as is the diuretic response. Much higher plasma levels and, therefore, larger doses, are required to ensure adequate amounts being transported to the tubular fluid in the loop of Henle. Conversely, and also because of competition for the organic acid transport sites, the administration of furosemide decreases salicylate excretion and increases the potential for salicylate toxicity. Other drugs such as indomethacin may reduce the diuretic response to furosemide, too. This has been attributed to inhibition of prostaglandin synthesis by indomethacin, although the exact interaction between prostaglandins and furosemide is not yet known.

The use, as well as most of the side effects, of ethacrynic acid and other loop diuretics is similar to that described for furosemide. Individual patients may tolerate one of these agents better than the others, providing an advantage in having more than one potent diuretic in this group.

c. Potassium-Sparing Diuretics

The two major drugs in this group are spironolactone and triamterene. Although structurally dissimilar and having different modes of action, these two drugs act at a similar site in the nephron, the distal tubule, and result in similar changes in urinary electrolyte excretion. Both are relatively weak diuretics, increasing sodium excretion to between 2% and 3% of the filtered sodium load. In contrast to the sulfonamide and loop diuretics, they decrease rather than increase urinary excretion of both potassium and hydrogen ions.

Spironolactone has been shown to be a specific inhibitor of aldosterone. It is effective only when aldosterone is present and inhibits competitively at the initial step in aldosterone binding to the cell. Since aldosterone has been shown to exert its effect in the cortical collecting duct, spironolactone is assumed to work at this site, too. The usual dose in adults is 100–200 mg/day (3 mg/kg body weight per day in children) given in divided doses. The drug may take 3–5 days to exert its effects, since it takes this long to block aldosterone binding sites. Side effects are few. Hyperkalemia may occur if the patient has a high potassium intake or has impaired renal function. Troublesome gynecomastia may occur and may persist after the drug is stopped.

Triamterene acts at a similar segment of the nephron and has the same effects on urinary electrolyte excretion as does spironolactone. It is not, however, a competitive inhibitor of aldosterone. Rather, it appears to inhibit exchange of sodium for potassium in the cortical collecting duct.

d. Other Diuretics

Acetazolamide is a potent inhibitor of carbonic anhydrase and will reduce bicarbonate reabsorption in the proximal tubule. Reabsorption of salt and water are decreased secondarily. Carbonic anhydrase inhibitors affect hydrogen ion secretion in the distal nephron, too, but they do not have a direct diuretic effect at this site. Although the proximal tubule is the site in the nephron where most of the filtered sodium and water are reabsorbed, acetazolamide is not a potent diuretic. Much of the increased salt and water that it causes to be delivered out of the proximal tubule is reabsorbed by more distal segments of the nephron. Furthermore, carbonic anhydrase inhibitors induce bicarbonaturia and a systemic acidosis. As the plasma bicarbonate concentration falls, the drug becomes progressively less effective because the filtered load of bicarbonate falls in parallel to the decrease in plasma bicarbonate.

Osmotic diuretics such as mannitol have several mechanisms of action. Through their osmotic effect, they decrease by 5% and 10%, respectively, the fractional reabsorption of sodium and water in the proximal tubule. They also inhibit water absorption in the loop of Henle. This action accounts for most of their diuretic effect. In addition, they increase renal plasma flow and glomerular hydrostatic pressure secondary to vasodilatation of the afferent arterioles. However, as with other drugs which act primarily in the proximal segment of the nephron, compensating changes in function of the distal nephron limit the clinical effectiveness of mannitol as a diuretic.

Organomercurials were the first potent diuretic drugs available to clinicians. One, mercaptomerin sodium, is still available. The drug must be administered parenterally. Early studies, which used high concentrations of these drugs, suggested that their site of action was the proximal tubule. Subsequent observations with more appropriate doses have shown that the major site of action is in the thick ascending limb of the loop of Henle. The mechanism of action at the cellular level has not been defined. The advent of the powerful loop diuretics, which can be taken orally, has limited the use of organomercurials to patients who, for some reason, are unable to tolerate the loop or sulfonamide diuretics. The efficacy of the organomercurials, when taken for a prolonged time, can be potentiated by the simultaneous administration of an acidifying agent such as ammonium chloride.

e. Choice of Diuretics

For reasons already enumerated, diuretics which act primarily on the proximal tubule have limited clinical usefulness. It is preferable to begin therapy with either one of the sulfonamide or loop diuretics. A sulfonamide is chosen if a milder diuresis is required, one of the thiazides usually being the preferred drug. For a more potent diuresis, a loop diuretic, usually furosemide, is administered. This drug has the added advantage in patients with renal failure of not decreasing GFR—sometimes a problem with the thiazides.

Since loop diuretics bind strongly to plasma proteins, their effectiveness is related in part to the peak plasma concentration of free drug. Thus, it is better to give only one of the loop diuretics in large dose than to give two drugs in smaller dosages. Any dose given once a day is likely to be more effective than half the dose given twice a day. As discussed already, other organic acids may decrease the effectiveness of a loop diuretic by competing for the transport sites in the proximal tubule. If a loop diuretic is not effective, the patient's entire therapy should be reviewed to determine whether other organic acids, such as penicillins or salicylates, are being given.

If high doses of a single drug do not induce a diuresis, a second drug can be prescribed. Sulfonamides and loop diuretics can have additive effects. It is more usual, however, to add one of the potassium-sparing drugs to the patient's drug regimen. These act on a more distal segment of the nephron and usually potentiate, significantly, the diuretic effect of a loop diuretic. Spironolactone is the favored drug, especially if the patient has a reason for secondary hyperaldosteronism. Beneficial effects are not always seen immediately since this drug takes three or more days to block the aldosterone receptors.

This combination of drugs, given in adequate dosages, is usually effective. If it is not, one can consider adding acetazolamide, which has a primary site of action in the proximal tubule. However, before adding a third drug one should reexamine whether the primary disease process could be treated more effectively, whether adjuncts to diuretic therapy (see next section) are indicated and whether dietary and other intakes of both sodium and water are being controlled appropriately.

2. Adjuncts to Diuretic Drugs

Most patients labeled as being "resistant to diuretics" either have not been given adequate doses of drugs or an appropriate combination of drugs has not been utilized. Alternately, the drug's effectiveness has been limited by competition from organic acids or the drug may have been poorly absorbed because of edema in the intestinal mucosa or at its site of injection. After these possibilities have been excluded, a small number of edematous patients are found to be truly resistant to diuretics and respond poorly to even the most aggressive and appropriate diuretic therapy. Such patients can be helped by a variety of maneuvers.

Institution of strict bed rest often will improve the response to diuretics. It is presumed that this works by improving renal perfusion. Wrapping the legs or other edematous areas with elastic bandages or surgical elastic stockings can reduce the edema markedly. This is an old therapeutic approach which has been recently rediscovered. It has been shown that this maneuver will induce a diuresis and natriuresis, correct the hemodynamic abnormalities due to diuretic induced plasma volume contraction, and elevate endogenous creatinine clearance. Ultrafiltration dialysis can be very beneficial in some patients who have massive amounts of edema, those who have accumulated edema rapidly, those who are resistant to diuretics, or those in whom rapid removal of edema is vital, for example, to prepare them for urgent cardiac surgery. It should be stressed, however, that few patients require this therapeutic approach.

Fortunately, with the advent of potent diuretics, mechanical removal of edema fluid by means such as aspiration of pleural fluid or ascites is rarely needed. Insertion of tubes into subcutaneous tissue planes to drain edema from the patient is an obsolete practice.

C. Restriction of Sodium and Water Intakes

Dietary restriction of sodium and water intake represents an important component of any comprehensive plan to control edema. Such restrictions alone rarely will result in loss of edema. The reasons for this are readily apparent when sodium balance is analyzed in the typical edema-forming patient. The average American diet contains about 160 mEq of sodium a day. Typically, edema-forming patients have extremely low urinary sodium concentrations of 10 mEq/liter or less. In consequence, the urinary sodium losses in these patients amount to 5 mEq or less per day. Extrarenal sodium losses, i.e., those in the sweat and stools, average around 10 mEq/day so that total losses of sodium in the edema-forming patient amount to only 15 mEq/day. Therefore, on a regular diet, the edema-forming patient will be in positive sodium balance of about 145 mEq/day. This will result in retention of about 1 liter of edema fluid per day. To ensure a negative sodium balance, dietary sodium intake would have to be limited to under 15 mEq/day. However, the most sodium-restricted diets that are practical contain approximately 0.5 g (22 mEq) sodium. Thus, even these severely restricted diets, sometimes referred to as 1-g salt diets, contain an amount of sodium equal to the patient's losses. Their use will prevent edema from becoming more marked, but will not cause any lessening of the amount of edema. Even if the edema-forming patient had a sodium-free intake, the maximum negative sodium balance would amount to only 15 mEq/day and it would take 10 days to lose 1 liter of edema.

Contrary to what has just been stated, an occasional edematous patient will show a reduction in the amount of edema when treated only with a salt-restricted diet and no diuretics. This usually is due to an improvement in the disease process that caused the edema in the first place. Typically in such patients, the urinary excretion of sodium increases and a significant negative sodium balance results. Examples include patients with glomerulonephritis in whom there is a spontaneous and marked acute increase in glomerular filtration rate, or those with congestive heart failure in whom cardiac function and cardiac output are increased by digoxin. Loss of edema in such patients may be gradual at best. Since 1 liter of edema fluid contains about 135 to 145 mEq of sodium, it takes 3 days of negative sodium balance of approximately 50 mEq/day before the amount of edema is reduced by 1 liter.

Diets with a severely restricted sodium content, even those designed by a dietician, are not well tolerated by most patients. Only a very few patients, e.g., those with severe left ventricular heart failure, warrant the use of such diets for a protracted period of time. Even in this instance, one would attempt to use the diet only during the acute phase of the illness. It is preferable to manage most of the remaining edematous patients with less severe restriction of sodium intake, using diuretics or other measures to increase sodium loss in the urine. This approach is better accepted by the patient and can be followed at home as well as in the hospital. The usual intake of sodium permitted is around 50–60 mEq/day—equivalent to between 3 and 4 g of salt. This is sometimes referred to as a "no-added-salt" diet. The patient should not cook with salt, should not add table salt to the food, and must avoid salty foods. Foods with a high sodium content include cheeses, cured meats such as ham and frankfurters, soups, sardines, soy sauce, tomato ketchup, and many preprepared foods. Those preparing food should be reminded that baking soda contains sodium too. Many detailed, low-sodium diets are readily available, usually in pamphlet form. It is preferable, however, for a dietician to develop each diet on an individual basis according to the patient's likes and dislikes and to be available to answer the myriad of questions which usually arise once the patient returns home. This results in better compliance.

In most instances, salt substitutes are permitted in the diet. Indeed, they often can be encouraged as a convenient and palatable method to increase potassium intake, replacing diuretic-induced urinary losses. The exception is the patient with renal failure. Use of salt substitutes in these patients, if not monitored by blood chemistries, may result in hyperkalemia and severe metabolic acidosis, the latter from metabolism of the ammonium chloride contained in several salt substitutes.

Most patients in whom dietary intake of sodium is controlled regulate their own intake of water appropriately. There are exceptions, however.

Such patients probably develop a marked thirst secondary to plasma volume contraction. Unless water intake is restricted in these patients, they develop dilutional hyponatremia which can be severe. To avoid such problems, it usually is advisable to recommend some restriction of fluid intake. As with sodium, patients require some intake of fluid. This is necessary if they are to eat solid foods with needed calories and ingest medications. We usually allow approximately 300–350 ml/day per m^2 body surface area, which amounts to 500–600 ml/day for the average adult. This amount of fluid is somewhat less than insensible fluid loss. However, after making allowances for the amount of water ingested in "solid" foods and for the water generated from the metabolism of carbohydrates, this amount of fluid will efffectively replace the amount lost as normal insensible losses, i.e., as sweat and through the lungs. Such a regimen will result in negative fluid balance in an amount approximately equal to the volume of urine passed during the day. If the patient has a high urine output, a more generous intake of water can be permitted. However, if the fluid intake equals the sum of urine output and insensible fluid loss, the patient will lose neither weight nor edema.

Regulating dietary intake alone can be futile if the patient is receiving intravenous fluids—even if it is "just as a vehicle for administration of medications." Saline given intravenously at a rate of only 10 ml/hr amounts to an intake equivalent to a quarter of a liter of edema in a 24-hr period. If the patient requires restriction of sodium and water intake, every aspect of intake must be controlled.

D. Special Therapeutic Approaches to Specific Disease States

Certain forms of edema may be particularly difficult to treat. Ascites secondary to cirrhosis often is resistant to diuretic therapy, especially if it is present in the absence of peripheral edema. Vigorous efforts to remove the ascitic fluid with diuretics may result in hypovolemia and even in acute ischemic renal failure. The usual approaches of bed rest, dietary sodium restriction, and cautious use of diuretics may be supplemented in patients with gross ascites by reinfusion of ascitic fluid concentrated by ultrafiltration. This procedure is well tolerated by most patients. Another approach is to use the LeVeen peritoneal-jugular shunt detailed in the references cited.

Nephrotic edema may also prove refractory. Infusions of salt-poor albumin given in conjunction with diuretics may trigger a diuresis in patients with severe hypoproteinemia, even though the increase in plasma albumin concentration is small and transient. This is discussed in more detail in Section 4, Chapter 11. Once the diuresis is initiated, the dose of diuretics needed to maintain the diuresis usually can be reduced substantially.

Patients with advanced renal failure may appear to be "diuretic resistant," but often will respond to these drugs providing adequate doses are used. Indeed, large doses of furosemide have resulted in the excretion of up to 87% of the filtered load of sodium in patients with advanced renal insufficiency.

The treatment of edema in patients with congestive heart failure can be facilitated by taking appropriate steps to increase cardiac output. In those patients resistant to more conventional approaches, the use of aminophylline in continuous infusion along with small doses of furosemide may induce a good diuretic response, as may the infusion of furosemide in doses of 4–6 mg/hr. This has resulted in satisfactory diuresis at blood concentrations below those at which extrarenal toxic effects have been reported. There is increasing evidence that pharmacologic interruption of the renin–angiotensin–aldosterone system with the oral inhibitor of angiotensin converting enzyme inhibitor, Captopril, is very beneficial in patients with severe congestive heart failure. Increased cardiac output, a diuresis with weight loss, improvement in orthopnea and exertional dyspnea and reduction in or loss of edema, correction of hyponatremia, and decreased azotemia have all been described in patients following use of this drug. Demeclocycline, which inhibits anti-diuretic hormone, has also been shown to be of some value in the therapy of resistant edema in advanced heart failure, too.

Effective treatment for patients with idiopathic edema can prove to be remarkably difficult. Some may be helped by spironolactone. An inhibitor of angiotensin converting enzyme (Captopril) has been used in others, based on the thesis that alterations in the renin–angiotensin–aldosterone system are responsible for the salt and water retention in some women with idiopathic edema. Preliminary observations have been encouraging. The confusion surrounding the management of the syndrome of idiopathic edema is apparent in that both metoclopramide, a dopaminergic inhibitor, and brom-ocriptine, a central dopamine agonist, have been reported to benefit some patients with this syndrome. Based on the observation that metoclopramide increased urinary sodium excretion in some patients with idiopathic edema, it was proposed that dopaminergic control of renin and aldosterone was altered in the syndrome. Whether metoclopramide corrected this defect or had a direct effect on the kidney could not be determined. Bromocriptine may also result in increased renal excretion of sodium and water in idiopathic edema. This could be due to its action in depressing prolactin release from the pituitary, or from a direct action on renal vasculature as a dopaminergic agonist. Unfortunately it has many side effects which limit its usefulness.

Of the several drugs which have been shown to benefit patients with angioneurotic edema, use of the synthetic anabolic androgen Danazol is most consistently beneficial. Its use will increase the serum C1 inhibitor level three- to fivefold. More recently, successful treatment of acute episodes of angioedema has been reported with replacement therapy using a partly purified preparation of the C1 inhibitor.

In summary, most edema can be treated effectively using the basic approach outlined. Only an occasional patient requires the special therapeutic maneuvers referred to in this section. If edema proves to be resistant to diuretics and to the additional modes of treatment, it suggests that the underlying disease is terminal.

SUGGESTED READINGS

Reviews

Kaloyanides, G. J.: Pathogenesis and treatment of edema with special reference to the use of diuretics, in Maxwell, M. H., and Kleeman, C. R. (eds.): *Clinical Disorders of Fluid and Electrolyte Metabolism*, Third edition. McGraw-Hill, New York, 1979, pp. 647–701.

Levy, M., and Seely, J. F.: Pathophysiology of edema formation, in Brenner, B. M., and Rector, F. C., Jr. (eds.): *The Kidney*, Second edition. W. B. Saunders, Philadelphia, 1981, pp. 723–776.

Pitts, R. F.: Volume and composition of body fluids, in, *Physiology of the Kidney and Body Fluids*, Third edition. Year Book Medical Publishers, Chicago, 1974, pp. 11–35.

Seely, J. F., and Levy, M.: Control of extracellular fluid volume, in Brenner, B. M., and Rector, F. C., Jr. (eds.): *The Kidney*, Second edition. W. B. Saunders, Philadelphia, 1981, pp. 371–407.

Pathophysiology of Edema

Bernard, D. B., and Alexander, E. A.: Edema formation in the nephrotic syndrome: pathophysiologic mechanisms. *Cardiovasc. Med.* 4:605–625, 1979.

Chonko, A. M., Bay, W. H., Stein, J. H., and Ferris, T. F.: The role of renin and aldosterone in the salt retention of edema. *Am. J. Med.* 63:881–889, 1977.

Dorhout Mees, E. J., Roos, J. C., Boer, P., Yoe, O.H., and Simatupang, T. A.: Observations on edema formation in the nephrotic syndrome in adults with minimal lesions. *Am. J. Med.* 67:378–384, 1979.

Eriksson, E., and Robson, M. C.: New pathophysiologic mechanism explaining the generalized edema after a major burn. *Surg. Forum* 28:540–543, 1977.

Fiorotto, M., and Coward, W. A.: Pathogenesis of oedema in protein-energy malnutrition: the significance of plasma colloid osmotic pressure. *Br. J. Nutr.* 42:21–31, 1979.

Golden, M. H. N., Golden, B. E., and Jackson, A. A.: Albumin and nutritional oedema. *Lancet* 1:114–116, 1980.

Klahr, S., and Alleyne, G. A. O.: Effects of chronic protein-calorie malnutrition on the kidney. *Kidney Int.* 3:129–141, 1973.

Kruck, F., and Kramer, H. J.: Third factor and edema formation. *Contrib. Nephrol.* 13:12–20, 1978.

Little, R. A., Savic, J., and Stoner, H. B.: H_2 receptors and traumatic edema. *J. Pathol.* 125:201–204, 1978.

MacGregor, G. A., Markandu, N. D., Roulston, J. E., Jones, J. C., and DeWardener, H. E.: Is "idiopathic" oedema idiopathic? *Lancet* 1:397–400, 1979.

Marciniak, D. L., Dobbins, D. E., Maciejko, J. J., Scott, J. B., Haddy, F. J., and Grega, G. J.: Antagonism of histamine edema formation by catecholamines. *Am. J. Physiol.* 234:H180–H185, 1978.

Solomon, L. M., Juhlin, L., and Kirschenbaum, S.: Prostaglandin on cutaneous vasculature. *J. Invest. Dermatol.* 51:280–285, 1978.

Thibonnier, M., Marchetti, J., Corvol, P., Menard, J., and Milliez, P.: Abnormal regulation of antidiuretic hormone in idiopathic edema. *Am. J. Med.* 67:67–73, 1979.

Ullrich, I., and Lizarralde, G.: Amenorrhea and edema. *Am. J. Med.* 64:1080–1083, 1978.

Williams, T. J.: Oedema and vasodilation in inflammation: the relevance of prostaglandins. *Postgrad. Med. J.* 53:660–662, 1977.

Special Forms of Edema

Bleach, N. R., Dunn, P. J., Khalafalla, M. E., and McConkey, B.: Insulin oedema. *Br. Med. J.* 2:177–178, 1979.

Donaldson, V. H.: Hereditary angioneurotic edema. *Disease a Month* 26, No. 2, 1–37, 1979.

Editorial: Exercise oedema. *Lancet* 1:961–962, 1979.

Sitprija, V.: Heat oedema: a clinical study. *Postgrad. Med. J.* 55:728–729, 1979.

Streeten, D. H. P.: Idiopathic edema: pathogenesis, clinical features and treatment. *Metabolism* 27:353–383, 1978.

Treatment—Diuretics

Dirks, J. H.: Mechanisms of action and clinical uses of diuretics. *Hosp. Pract.* 14, No. 9, 99–110, 1979.

Eknoyan, G.: Understanding diuretic therapy. *Drug. Ther.* 11:47–58, 1981.

Treatment—Other Methods

Allison, M. E. M., and Kennedy, A. C.: Diuretics in chronic renal disease: a study of high dosage frusemide. *Clin. Sci.* 41:171–187, 1971.

Asaba, H., Bergestrom, J., Furst, P., Shaldon, S., and Wiklund, S.: Treatment of diuretic-resistant fluid retention with ultrafiltration. *Acta Med. Scand.* 204:145–149, 1978.

Bank, N.: External compression for treatment of resistant edema. *N. Engl. J. Med.* 302:969, 1980.

Davison, A. M., Lambie, A. T., Verth, A. H., and Cash, J. D.: Salt poor human albumin in management of nephrotic syndrome. *Br. Med. J.* 1:481–484, 1974.

Dent, R. G., and Edwards, O. M.: Bromocriptine in idiopathic edema. *Clin. Endocrinol.* 11:75–80, 1979.

Gadek, J. E., Hosea, S. W., Gelfand, J. A., Santaella, M., Wickerhauser, M., Triantaphyllopoulos, D. C., and Frank, M. H.: Replacement therapy in hereditary angioedema. Successful treatment of acute episodes of angioedema with partly purified C1 inhibitor. *N. Engl. J. Med.* 302:542–546, 1980.

Hollenberg, N. K., and Williams, G. H.: The renin–angiotensin system in congestive heart failure (use of Captopril). *J. Cardiovasc. Med.* 6:359–369, 1981.

Lawson, D. H., Gray, J. M. B., Henry, D. A., and Tilstone, W. J.: Continuous infusion of furosemide in refractory oedema. *Br. Med. J.* 2:476, 1978.

Mimran, A., and Targhetta, R.: Captopril treatment of idiopathic edema. *N. Engl. J. Med.* 301:1289–1990, 1979.

Moult, P. J. A., Parbhoo, S. P., and Sherlock, S.: Clinical experience with the Rhone-Poulenc ascites reinfusion apparatus. *Postgrad. Med. J.* 51:574–576, 1975.

Norbiato, G., Bevilacqua, M., Raggi, U., Micossi, P., Nitti, F., Lanfredini, M., and Barbieri, S.: Effect of metoclopramide, a dopaminergic inhibitor, on renin and aldosterone in idiopathic edema: possible therapeutic approach with levodopa and carbidopa. *J. Clin. Endocrinol. Metab.* 48:37–46, 1979.

Snell, J. A., Schweigger, M., and Quinlan-Watson, S.: Elastic stockings in the control of hand edema. *Med. J. Aust.* 1:461, 1979.

Wapnick, S., Grosberg, S., Kinney, M., and LeVeen, H. H.: LeVeen continuous peritoneal-jugular shunt. Improvement of renal function in ascitic patients. *J. Am. Med. Assoc.* 237:131–133, 1977.

6

The Pathophysiologic Bases for Alterations in Water Balance

JOHN BUERKERT

I. PHYSIOLOGIC CONSIDERATIONS

In man and other terrestrial animals, a highly developed physiologic system maintains the tonicity of body fluids within a relatively narrow range (± 2 mOsm/kg H_2O in man). The efficiency of this system is reflected in the relative constancy of the concentration of sodium in plasma (normal values are between 136 and 145 mEq/liter in man). Thus, under most circumstances alterations in plasma sodium concentration reflect changes in the tonicity of total body water (TBW). Figure 1 depicts the relationship between total body water and sodium under normal (A) and pathologic conditions. A fall in plasma sodium concentrations below the normal range, that is, *hyponatremia*, is either a consequence of a relative or an absolute excess in TBW. A relative excess in total body water in relation to sodium may be seen under conditions of dehydration where there is a deficit of both sodium and water (B). Hyponatremia may also be a consequence of an absolute excess of water and a sodium deficit as when vasopressin release is inappropriate (C). Finally, it may be seen in edema-forming states where both sodium and water are in excess (D). Similarly, an increase in the concentration of sodium in plasma,

JOHN BUERKERT • Department of Medicine, Washington University School of Medicine and The Jewish Hospital of St. Louis, St. Louis, Missouri 63110.

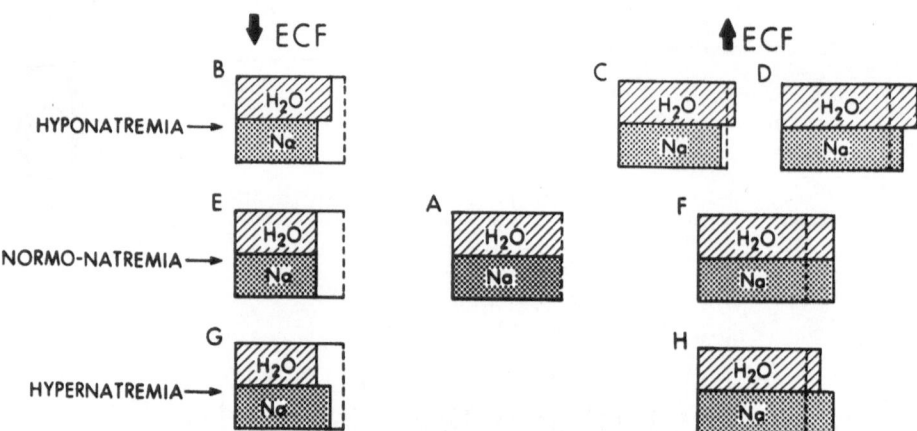

Figure 1. How alterations in serum sodium concentration may occur independently of ECF volume. Part A illustrates the relationship between ECF water and sodium under normal conditions. To the left, alterations are shown in the relationship between water and sodium when ECF volume is reduced (B, E, and G). To the right, these relationships are shown when ECF volume is increased (C, D, F, H).

hypernatremia, may be seen in conditions in which TBW is either decreased (G) or increased (H).

The major sites for the control of fluid tonicity lie in the hypothalamus. There are two target organs: (1) the cerebrum, which by control of thirst or drinking, regulates water intake, and (2) the kidney, which by a humoral mechanism (the secretion of vasopressin), and perhaps through nervous stimulation, controls the excretion of water and sodium. It is postulated that within the hypothalamus two kinds of receptors, thirst and osmoreceptors, are present. Both seem to respond to similar stimuli although there are some differences. Verney noted more than 30 years ago that drinking was stimulated in dogs when hypertonic solutions of either NaCl or sucrose, which are confined to the extracellular space, were infused into the carotid arteries (that is, these substances were dipsogenic). This response was associated with a marked decline in urine output (these solutions were antidiuretic). When substances not confined to the extracellular space (urea or glucose) were infused, neither response was elicited. These studies suggested that an alteration in cellular hydration was the initial step in eliciting the dipsogenic and antidiuretic response. Other investigators have shown that the site of the effect of hypertonic NaCl or sucrose is in the third ventricle. Thus when hypertonic solutions were instilled into this ventricle a dipsogenic and antidiuretic response was elicited, an effect which could not be produced when certain areas within the third ventricle were ablated.

A. Mechanisms Involved in the Control of Thirst

The process of drinking can be either primary or secondary. *Secondary* drinking is also termed *anticipatory*. Man drinks water as he takes in food and therefore is usually in a state of water excess, that is, he drinks water in *anticipation* of his needs. Under normal conditions, the total solute excretion is the sum of urea, which is a consequence of protein breakdown, and electrolytes excreted in the urine (approximately 700 mOsm/24 hr). If the maximal urine osmolality is 1000 mOsm/kg, the total urine volume required per 24 hr to excrete this osmolar load is 700 ml. This amount of urine is frequently referred to as *obligatory* urine volume. It is apparent from these measurements that this component of total urine volume will depend on protein intake and the catabolic state of the individual. From Table I, it can be seen that man usually exceeds the obligatory urine volume by an additional liter of so-called *facultative* urine. Thus, under normal circumstances water intake exceeds demands and the stimulus for thirst is suppressed. The stimuli for thirst are only evoked when free water intake falls below the sum of insensible water losses (i.e., through respiration, sweating, and stool) and the amount necessary to excrete the solute load.

In *primary* or need-induced drinking, there appear to be two main regulatory signals. One emanates from the cellular compartment and the other from the extracellular compartment. By far, the most important of these is the former (i.e., changes in cellular hydration). Stimuli for thirst are evoked under conditions of cellular dehydration and may be a consequence of (1) water deprivation, (2) hypertonic states resulting from either the endogenous production of excess solute (e.g., hypercalcemia) or the administration of hypertonic solutions, and (3) depletion of the intracellular cation, potassium. While the studies of Verney indicate that a change in osmolality within the intravascular space is a stimulus for thirst, the mechanism by which this occurs is not clear. Two theories have been put forth: (1) A portion of the third ventricle lies in direct contact with the intravascular space and is sensitive to changes in osmolality, or (2) receptors for thirst are controlled not by changes in plasma osmolality, but by changes in the sodium concentration of the cerebral spinal fluid, which in turn reflect changes in intravascular osmolality.

Table I. A Balance for Water in Normal Man[a,b]

	Water intake (g)			Water output (g)	
	Obligatory	Facultative		Obligatory	Facultative
Drink	650	1000	Urine	700	1000
Preformed	750		Skin	500	
Oxidative	350		Lungs	400	
			Feces	150	
Subtotals	1750	1000		1750	1000
Total	2750			2750	

[a] From A. V. Wolf: *Thirst*. Charles C. Thomas, Springfield, Illinois, 1958. Reprinted with permission.
[b] A rounded off, 24-hr water balance statement for normal man at 15°C and 40% relative humidity, based upon a particular 3000-calorie diet and energy expenditure. The diet contained 98.8 g of protein, 163.3 g of fat, and 294.3 g of carbohydrate, yielding 377.6 g of oxidative and 755.6 g of preformed water in "solid" food (1910.8 g of preformed water if fluid foods such as orange juice, milk, etc., have been considered). The pulmonary water loss is based upon the assumptions that oxygen extraction in the lungs is 6%, and that expired air is saturated at 35°C.

The second regulatory signal comes from a decrease in the volume of the extracellular fluid compartment and is a consequence of two mechanisms. The first is from distension of receptors located in the left atrium and pulmonary veins and from the arterial baroreceptors. This signal is the most difficult to evaluate and is probably seen only under conditions of profound volume loss (approximately 30%). It is difficult to differentiate this effect from humorally mediated stimuli for thirst. The second mechanism by which volume changes in the extracellular compartment stimulate thirst involves the production of angiotensin II. As shown in Figure 2, angiotensin II stimulates thirst when placed in the third ventricle. The site of this action is located in the anterior wall of the third ventricle near the subfornical area and the organum vasculosum of the lamina terminalis. In this region there appears to be a system which is capable of producing angiotensin II by the same sequence of chemical events which occur in plasma. Thus when, renin, or renin substrate are introduced into the third ventricle, thirst will be stimulated as a consequence of the local production of angiotensin II. The subfornical area and the organum vasculosum are highly vascular organs. It is postulated that the dipsogenic action of angiotensin II is mediated by an effect on the

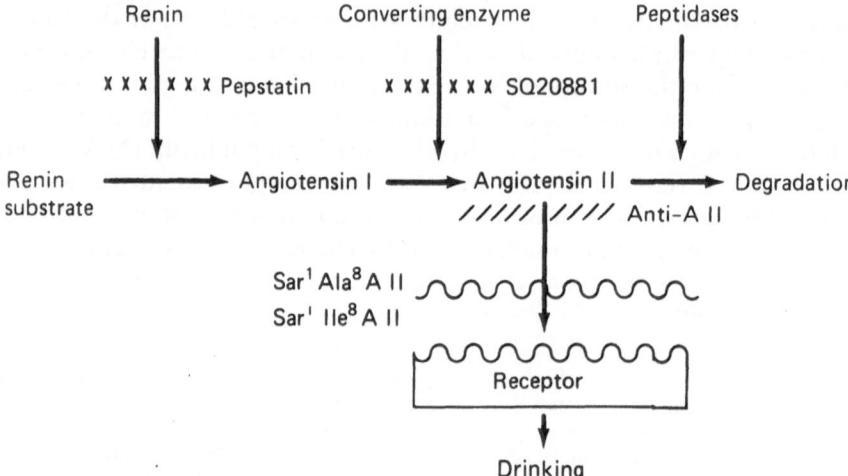

Figure 2. Evidence supporting the hypothesis that stimulation of thirst can be evoked by activation of the renin–angiotensin system. If renin substrate is placed in the third ventricle, angiotensin II is produced and thirst is stimulated. The following experimental maneuvers suggest that angiotensin II directly stimulates thirst centers and that the mechanism by which angiotensin II is produced is similar to that found in plasma. When pepstatin, an inhibitor of the renin–angiotensinogen reaction is placed in the third ventricle, substrate-induced drinking is abolished. If angiotensin I is then added, angiotensin II is produced and drinking is stimulated. If angiotensin I or its precursor renin–substrate are added in the presence of the converting enzyme inhibitor SQ 20881, angiotensin II is not produced and drinking is not stimulated. Finally, if the competitive antagonist of angiotensin II, saralasin acetate, is placed in the third ventricle, the stimulus for drinking is blocked. Similarly, if antisera to angiotensin II are added, angiotensin-II-induced drinking is attenuated. (Reprinted with permission from Fitzsimons, J. T.: The renin–angiotensin system and drinking behavior. *Progr. Brain Res.* 42:215–233, 1975.)

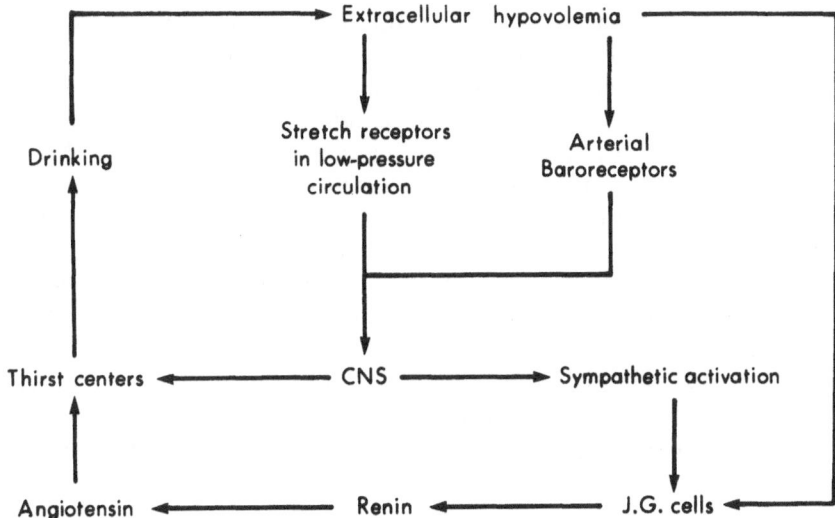

Figure 3. Mechanisms by which thirst is stimulated when ECF volume is reduced. Note that these centers may be stimulated directly through receptors in the venous or arterial system and through stimulation of juxtaglomerular (JG) cells, which ultimately leads to the production of angiotensin II. (Reprinted with permission from Martini, L., and Motta, M. (eds.): *The Hypothalamus.* Academic Press, New York, 1970, pp. 195–212.)

blood vessels in these structures. In fact, vasoplegic substances (papaverine, $NaNO_2$, sodium nitroprusside, and prostaglandin E_2) block the dipsogenic action of angiotensin II. Other agents in pharmacologic doses can also stimulate thirst. Most interesting of these is isoproterenol, which is both dipsogenic and antidiuretic. This β-adrenergic agent is thought to work secondarily through the stimulation of the renin–angiotensin system. The relationship between the humoral and nervous stimulation of thirst is graphically depicted in Figure 3. Again, the relative importance of these two systems in the overall maintenance of volume is not well delineated. Studies to date have only elicited such changes when circulating concentrations of angiotensin II and its precursors are in the pharmocologic range or under circumstances when volume is drastically reduced. Further, it appears that the stimuli for thirst may arise not only from centers in the third ventricle but also from an area near the septum polonium and in the fourth ventricle.

B. Mechanisms Which Control Antidiuretic Hormone Release

The anatomical site of those receptors which give rise to the secretion of the antidiuretic hormone (ADH), arginine vasopressin, are more clearly delineated than those for thirst. They are located in the hypothalamus near the optic chiasm and extend into the anterior infundibular wall of the third ventricle. Cells in this zone can stimulate the paraventricular and supraoptic nuclei to synthesize and transport ADH to the neurohypophysis from where the hormone is released. As with thirst, the major stimulus for the secretion of vasopressin is an increase in the plasma osmolality (see Figure 4). These receptors are exquisitely sensitive to changes in osmolality and serve to maintain the tonicity of plasma within a standard deviation of ±2.0 mOsm/kg (a change of less than 1%). While changes in osmolality are the most sensitive, and therefore the primary regulator of vasopressin synthesis and secretion, alterations in ECF volume can both modulate and override the tonicity control system. However, stimulation of vasopressin secretion seldom occurs unless volume loss is greater than 10%. The relationship between changes in osmolality, ECF volume, and vasopressin levels is shown in Figure 5.

Baroreceptor stimulation is thought to be the mechanism by which changes in volume can evoke an increase in ADH secretion. This effect is potentiated and may be partially a consequence of elevated levels of circu-

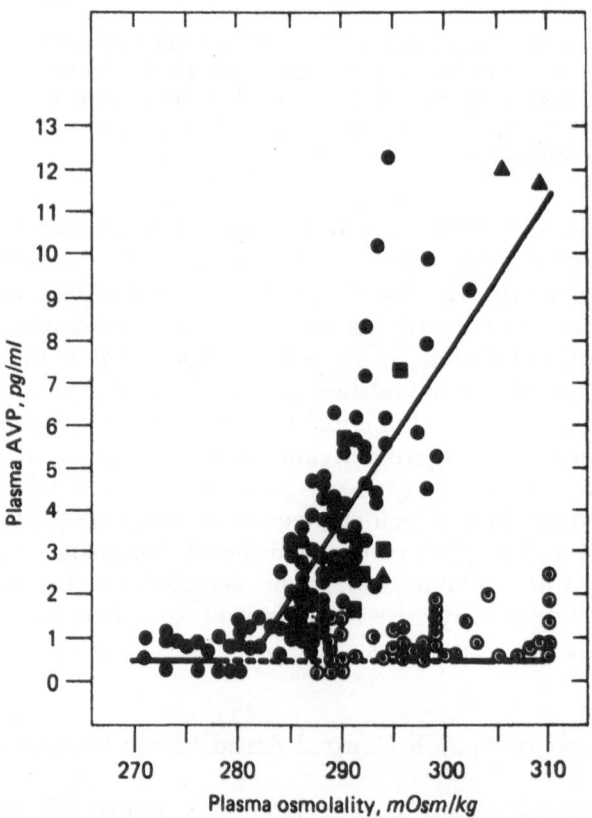

Figure 4. Relationships between plasma osmolality and the concentration of vasopressin in the plasma of healthy adults (●), patients with primary polydipsia (■), and patients with vasopressin-resistant (▲) and vasopressin-deficient (○) diabetes insipidus. (Reprinted with permission from Robertson, G. L., Mahr, E. A., Athar, S., and Sinha, T.: Development and clinical application of a new method for the radioimmunoassay of arginine vasopressin in human plasma. *J. Clin. Invest.* 52:2340–2352, 1973.)

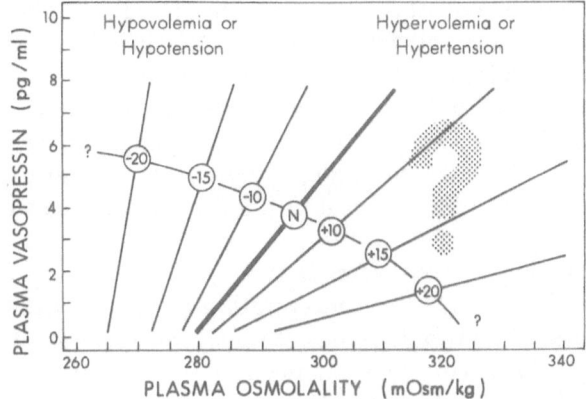

Figure 5. Relationship between effective intravascular volume, plasma osmolality, and vasopressin levels in the blood. The numbers inside the circles indicate the magnitude of the hemodynamic change required to cause a shift in the corresponding regression line. (Reprinted with permission from Robertson, G. L., Shelton, R. L., and Athar, S.: The osmoregulation of vasopressin. *Kidney Int.* 10:25–37, 1976.)

lating catecholamines which act directly on these receptors. Angiotensin II, prostaglandins, and nicotine also exert their effects on ADH release through their action on arterial baroreceptors.

C. Renal Regulation of Water Excretion

The GFR of normal man is approximately 120 ml/min, thus roughly 170 liters of water are filtered in a 24-hr period. Of this amount, less than 2 liters of urine or approximately 1% of the amount filtered is excreted. Except for setting an upper limit for the amount of water that can be excreted per unit time, GFR is not involved in the regulation of water excretion. This upper limit assumes importance only when GFR is profoundly reduced as in acute renal failure or end stage chronic renal disease. In the normal setting, the tubule is the major site for the renal regulation of water excretion.

The tubular reabsorption of water is due to the passive diffusion of water down its concentration gradient into a region of higher osmolality. In the proximal tubule, this gradient is established in the basolateral and intercellular spaces and is a consequence of the active transport of sodium out of the tubular lumen and ultimately into these spaces. Water flows rapidly through this highly permeable segment of the renal tubule and as a consequence fluid osmolality is not different from plasma. Hence, reabsorption of water in the proximal tubule is said to be *isoosmotic*. Water reabsorption in this segment is frequently termed *obligatory* since in the presence of high water permeability, water *must* follow sodium out of the tubular lumen. About 60% of the filtered water is reabsorbed by the end of the proximal tubule. The control of water reabsorption in this segment is intimately related to those factors which control the reabsorption of sodium. These factors are discussed elsewhere and will be mentioned only briefly in this section in reference to abnormalities in plasma sodium concentration.

By the end of the proximal tubule the relationship between water and sodium reabsorption is lost. In the remaining nephron segments water reabsorption is, to a large extent, independent of the reabsorption of solute. It is therefore referred to as the reabsorption of solute free water, or more simply *free water*.

The reabsorption of free water is largely dependent on the interrelationship of four factors: (1) the concentration of solute in the interstitium through which the renal tubule passes, (2) the concentration of solute in the tubular fluid, (3) the permeability of the renal tubule to water and solute, and (4) the circulating levels of ADH.

It is well known that the concentration of solute or the osmolality of renal tissue increases progressively from the corticomedullary junction to the tip of the renal papilla. In the cortex, the interstitial osmolality is equal to that of plasma. Near the tip of the papilla tissue osmolality may be four times greater than that of plasma. This progressive rise is the result of the deposition of solute, chiefly NaCl and urea, in the renal interstitium and is a consequence of *countercurrent multiplication*.

Countercurrent multiplication is graphically depicted in Figure 6. From this illustration it is apparent that three factors are essential for the mechanism to function. First, there must be flow through two channels in opposing directions (countercurrent flow). Second, there has to be a force (frequently referred to as the "single effect") that will result in the net movement of solute out of the tubular lumen of the limb leaving this environment. Finally,

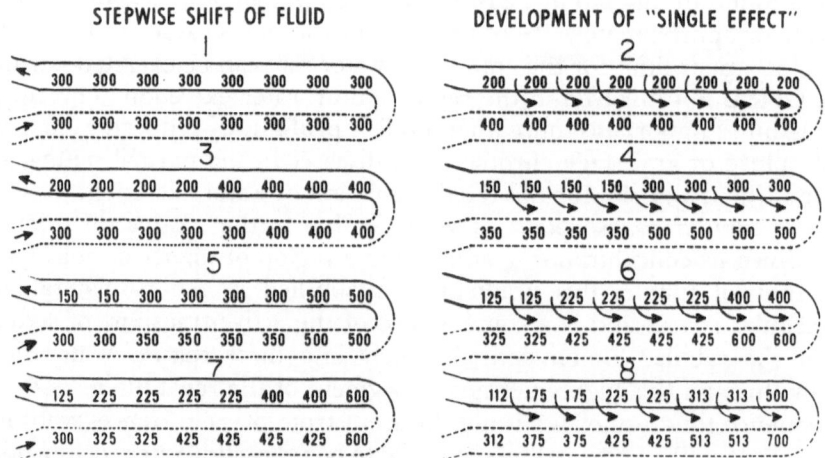

Figure 6. The principle of countercurrent multiplication of concentration, based on the assumption that, at any level along the loop of Henle, a gradient of 200 mOsm/liter can be established between ascending and descending limbs by active transport of ions. (Reprinted with permission from Pitts, R. F.: *Physiology of the Kidney and Body Fluids,* Third edition. Yearbook Medical Publishers, Chicago, 1974.)

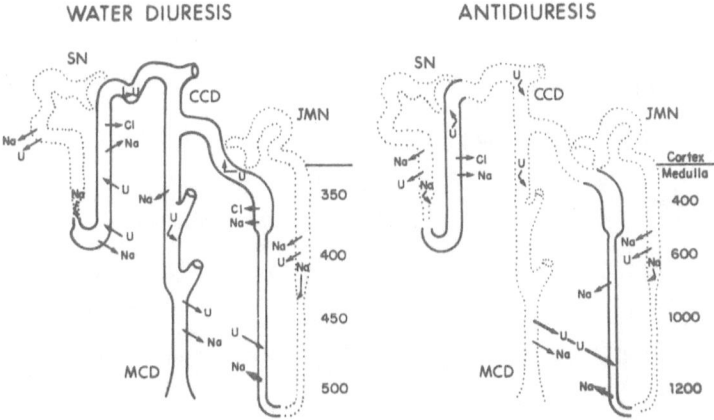

Figure 7. The movement of sodium (Na) and urea (U) out of the highly water permeable (······) proximal tubule of both superficial nephrons (SN) and juxtamedullary nephrons (JMN), with no movement of Na out of the equally water-permeable thin descending limb of the loop of Henle. At the bend of the loop of Henle, the characteristics of the epithelium change. The thick and thin acending limbs are impermeable to water (——) but highly permeable to sodium. Sodium moves out of this segment into the interstitium, and to a lesser extent, urea moves into the tubular fluid and hypertonic medullary interstitium. The outward movement of sodium is potentiated by active chloride transport in the thick ascending limb of the loop of Henle. In the absence of ADH the distal tubule, the cortical collecting duct (CCD), and the medullary collecting duct (MCD) are only slightly permeable to water, and the free water formed is excreted in the urine (water diuresis). In the presence of ADH (antidiuresis), part of the distal tubule and the cortical collecting duct are rendered highly permeable to water. Permeability of these segments to urea is not significantly altered, but the medullary collecting duct is rendered highly permeable to both water and urea.

this limb must be relatively *impermeable* to water while the limb by which fluid enters this area must be *freely permeable* to water. The net effect is the establishment of a progressive increase in interstitial osmolality and the production of an effluent that is hypotonic with respect to fluid entering.

In man, nephrons whose glomeruli are located at the corticomedullary junction, called juxtamedullary nephrons, are responsible for countercurrent multiplication. These nephrons are morphologically distinct from those whose glomeruli lie just below the cortical surface, called superficial or cortical nephrons. One important difference is that juxtamedullary nephrons possess long thin loops of Henle which extend deep into the inner zone of the medulla. Superficial nephrons have only short thin descending limbs which extend into the outer medullary areas. The thin descending and ascending limbs of juxtamedullary nephrons lie in close proximity to each other as they enter and leave the medulla; hence flow through them is countercurrent. Further, the limbs of the loop of Henle are functionally distinct (see Figure 7). The descending limb is highly permeable to water. It is probably only slightly permeable to urea and highly *impermeable* to sodium. On the other hand, the thin ascending limb is highly *permeable* to sodium, moderately permeable to urea, but not at all permeable to water. The

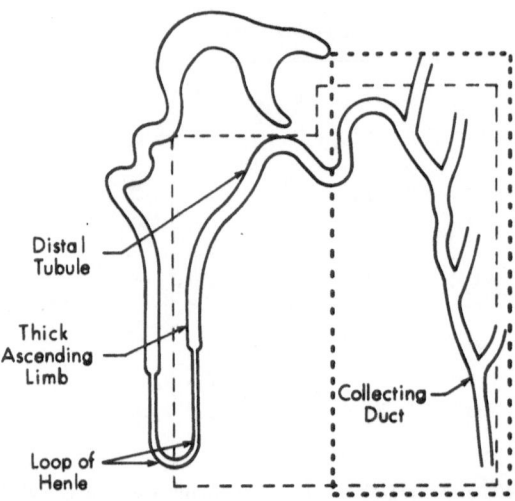

Distal
Tubule

Thick
Ascending
Limb

Collecting
Duct

Loop of
Henle

Figure 8. The nephron and part of the collecting duct system. Those portions that contribute to the production of free water (diluting segment) are circumscribed by the thin broken line (– – –) and that part responsible for the reabsorption of free water (concentrating segment) is outlined by the thicker line (---). Note that the collecting duct and distal tubule are involved in both processes.

osmolality of fluid in the ascending limb gradually decreases, becoming hypotonic with respect to the interstitium and the descending limb. Hence, solute is being extracted from the ascending limb in excess of water. The mechanism responsible for the decline is osmolality, that is, the single effect, is not clear. It is thought by some that the decline in osmolality is due to the active reabsorption of sodium or chloride along the water-impermeable thin ascending limb. Others have suggested that the dilution of fluid in the ascending limb is a result of differences in permeability of this segment to sodium and urea. They have proposed that the sodium concentration of fluid entering the ascending limb is greater than that of the papillary interstitium. Hence, sodium will diffuse passively out of this segment. On the other hand, the concentration of urea in the tubular fluid is lower than that of the papillary interstitium. Thus, there is a tendency for urea to move into the tubular lumen, but at a rate slower than the efflux of sodium, since this segment is considerably less permeable to urea than to sodium. The net effect would be an increase in the solute content of the medulla and the production of tubular fluid that is hypotonic with respect to the surrounding interstitium.

The process of tubular fluid dilution continues in the thick ascending limb of both superficial and juxtamedullary nephrons. As in the thin ascending limb this segment is permeable to sodium chloride but not to water. In addition, the thick ascending limb actively reabsorbs sodium and chloride, thus enhancing the rate of tubular fluid dilution. The production of hypotonic tubular fluid is frequently referred to as the formation of solute free water (or simply free-water formation). It occurs wherever solute reabsorption exceeds that of water. In the absence of antidiuretic hormone, free-water formation continues along the distal tubule and throughout the length of the collecting duct. These sites of free-water formation are collectively referred to as the *diluting segment* (see Figure 8). The amount of free water excreted per minute is called free-water clearance and may be calculated by the following formula:

$$C_{H_2O} = V - C_{osm}$$

where V is urine flow per unit time and C_{osm} is the osmolar clearance (U_{osm} V/P_{osm}) and is equal to the fraction of the urine produced, which is required to excrete the solute cleared from the plasma in an isotonic state. Therefore, when free water is excreted, the osmolality, or solute concentration of the urine, will be below that of the plasma. In man, maximum free-water clearance approaches 18 ml/min or 25 liters/day. This is roughly 15% of the filtered water. Thus the ability to excrete free water far exceeds the normal intake. Further, patients with impaired renal function are not likely to have difficulty with excretion of excess free water until their GFR falls below 10 ml/min. At this level of GFR, one could maximally excrete 2 liters of free water. This amount is still in excess of the normal physiologic intake of water.

The capacity to reabsorb the free water that is formed is largely dependent on the circulating levels of arginine vasopressin. In the presence of ADH, the distal tubule and collecting ducts are rendered highly permeable to water, which will then diffuse out of the tubular lumen (Figure 8). As a result, the tubular fluid becomes isoosmotic with respect to the surrounding interstitium. Thus by the end of the distal tubule fluid osmolality is the same as that of plasma. The change in the osmolality of tubular fluid from approximately 60 to 280 mOsm/kg indicates that nearly 80% of the free water formed was reabsorbed. The remaining free water will be extracted as fluid passes through the medulla where the osmolality of the interstitium progressively rises. From these considerations, it is readily apparent that the bulk of free water is reabsorbed in the distal tubule and cortical collecting ducts and is therefore not dependent on the production of a hypertonic renal medulla. The efficiency with which the remaining 20% of the free water is extracted from the lumen depends on the degree to which solute is concentrated in the medullary interstitium. Besides the presence of the normally functioning juxtamedullary nephrons, three other factors are involved in the generation of high solute concentration in the renal medulla.

One is the manner in which urea is handled by the distal tubule and collecting duct system. Unlike water, the urea permeability of the distal tubule and cortical collecting duct is increased only slightly by ADH; hence the concentration of urea in these segments rises as water is extracted in the antidiuretic state. On the other hand ADH renders the medullary collecting duct highly permeable to urea. Thus the high concentrations of urea generated in the cortical segments during antidiuresis result in the deposition of urea in the medullary interstitium and a total increase in the osmolality of the medulla.

The second factor is medullary blood flow. The blood supply to the medulla is through the long loops of the vasa recta. These vessels not only supply nutrients to the medullary structures but also carry off water that has

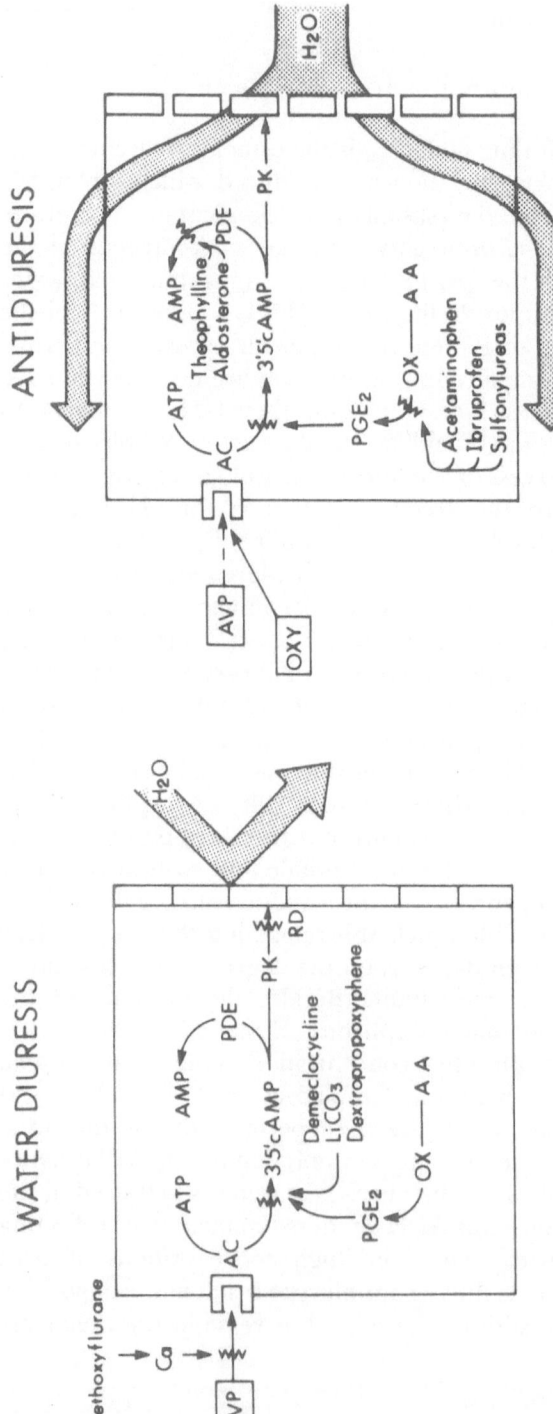

Figure 9. The mechanism by which arginine vasopressin (AVP) evokes an increase in water permeability in a collecting duct cell. AVP combines with a receptor site located on the peritubular side of the collecting duct cell and activates adenylate cyclase (AC), which results in the formation of $3'5'$-cAMP from adenosine triphosphate (ATP). This reaction is modulated by prostaglandins of the E_2 series (PGE_2). Ultimately, protein kinase (PK) is activated and evokes an alteration in the luminal cell wall, which increases its permeability to water. The response of the collecting duct cell to AVP can be blocked (left) at the receptor site, perhaps by calcium (Ca) or methoxyflurane. Demeclocycline, lithium carbonate ($LiCO_3$), and dextropropoxyphene block the formation of $3'5'$-cAMP by AC. Renal disease (RD) may affect the cell wall response to PK. However, it may also alter the intracellular biochemical reactions previously described. An inappropriate increase in water reabsorption may occur by a number of mechanisms (right). Analogs like oxytoxin (OXY) may activate AC activity. Inhibitors of prostaglandin synthesis antagonize the regulatory or modulating effect of PGE_2 on AC activity. Thus, acetaminophen inhibits cyclo-oxygenase activity (OX) and therefore blocks the conversion of arachidonic acid (AA) to PGE_2. Those substances that block the breakdown of cAMP to AMP by phosphodiesterase (PDE) may also enhance water reabsorption.

been reabsorbed. The configuration of the vasa recta is such that they tend to preserve the osmolality generated by the loops of Henle and they are frequently referred to as *countercurrent exchangers*. An increase in medullary blood flow would result in an increased rate of removal of NaCl and urea from the medulla and ultimately dissipate the osmotic gradient established by countercurrent multiplication.

A final important factor relates to alterations in the sensitivity of the collecting duct to ADH. Arginine vasopressin is a low-molecular-weight polypeptide which increases the permeability of collecting duct cells to water by initiating a series of intracellular biochemical reactions through the activation of the enzyme adenylate cyclase. The function of adenylate cyclase is to transform ATP into $3'5'$-cyclic AMP, which induces an increase in water permeability through the activation of a protein kinase. Protein kinase is thought to act through phosphorylation of the luminal membrane. This alteration in biochemical structure is thought to induce a change in water permeability (see Figure 9). Clearly any factor which affects this series of biochemical events may effect a change in the response of the collecting duct cell to ADH. This may occur as a consequence of a disease state which specifically affects collecting duct cell structure or as a consequence of a number of pharmacologic and humoral agents which may either enhance or block the action of ADH. Some of these agents are listed in Tables V and VII and will be discussed subsequently.

Those structures involved in the extraction of free water from the tubular lumen are collectively referred to as the *concentrating segment* (Figure 8). The capacity of this segment to reabsorb free water in the antidiuretic state ($T^c_{H_2O}$) can be quantitated with the formula for C_{H_2O} but the result will be a negative number:

$$T^c_{H_2O} = V - C_{osm}$$

II. PATHYOPHYSIOLOGIC CONSIDERATIONS

A. Hyponatremia

1. Symptoms of Hyponatremia

Although hyponatremia is usually defined as a serum sodium concentration below 135 mEq/liter, patients seldom become symptomatic until the concentration falls below 130 mEq/liter. The development of symptoms depends not only on the degree, but also on the rapidity of onset of the hyponatremic state. When the serum sodium concentration falls below 120 mEq/liter in less than a 12-hr period, symptoms may progress from anorexia, confusion, headaches, and muscle cramps to convulsions, coma, and death. These symptoms are related to the development of cerebral edema, and are the consequence of the relatively normal osmolality of CNS tissues and the hyposmolality of plasma. Thus a gradient is established for the movement of water into the cells.

In patients who develop hyponatremia gradually the symptoms may be subtle or absent. Usually, however, patients complain of lethargy, loss of appetite, periods of confusion, headaches, and muscle cramps. When hyponatremia is profound (below 120 mEq/liter) a variety of neurologic symptoms may be seen, most common of which are dementia, acute psychosis, hemiparesis, convulsions, and coma. In chronic hyponatremic states, symptoms do not correlate well with the serum sodium concentration. The neurologic symptoms seen during chronic hyponatremia may be a consequence of a decrease in intracellular sodium and an impairment in the sodium-dependent metabolic activities of these cells. Experimentally it has been shown that in this setting tissue and serum osmolality are the same.

2. Disorders of Tonicity Associated with Hyponatremia

a. Hyponatremia Not Accompanied by a Reduction in Osmolality

Under normal circumstances, serum sodium concentrations range from 136 to 145 mEq/liter. This sodium is distributed only in the aqueous phase of serum. Thus an increase in the nonaqueous, that is, the lipid portion, of serum will artifactually reduce the measured concentration of sodium. This is frequently referred to as *factitious hyponatremia*. An estimate of serum water can be obtained from the following formula:

$$W_s = 99.1 - 1.03\text{Ls} - 0.73\text{Ps}$$

where W_s is the milliliters of water in 100 ml of serum, 99.1 the volume of serum minus crystalline (nonlipid and nonprotein) solids, Ls the total lipid concentration, and Ps the total protein concentration (g/100 ml) serum. On the average, serum water is 94% of the total volume. Thus, the concentration of sodium in serum water is about 154 mEq/liter. When sodium concentrations are found to be low, the total osmolality of the serum should be measured. Measurement of osmolality is made by determining the depression of the freezing point. This parameter is not as influenced by the presence of displacing substances and therefore reflects the concentration of solute in serum water. The osmolality may be calculated from the following formula:

$$\text{Total osmolality} = 2(\text{Na} + \text{K}) + \frac{\text{glucose}}{18} + \frac{\text{blood urea nitrogen}}{2.8}$$

The difference between this calculated value and the measured value should be less than 10 mOsm/kg H_2O. This difference is frequently termed the *osmolar gap*. A gap greater than 10 should make one suspect a high lipid or protein concentration in the serum or the presence of unmeasured solute.

The most common cause of factitious hyponatremia is hyperlipidemia, which may develop during diabetic ketoacidosis and acute pancreatitis. In Figure 10, the clinical course of a patient with diabetic ketoacidosis and hyponatremia is shown. Laboratory data obtained in this patient on admission included a serum sodium concentration of 89 mEq/liter. The osmolality of the plasma was 340 mOsm/kg H_2O. Plasma glucose was 600 mg/100 ml. The calculated osmolality and osmolar gap were 219 and 121 mOsm/kg, respectively. Subsequently it was noted that the plasma was turbid. Plasma triglyceride levels were then measured and found to be 1600 mg/100 ml (normal 60–160). In these studies, serum water was measured and found to be 71% of the serum (normal = 94%). When the serum sodium concentration was divided by this value, the actual concentration of sodium in serum was 125 mEq/liter. Thus, although the patient was hyponatremic, the fall in serum sodium concentration was not as severe as suggested by the initial measurements. Factitious hyponatremia may also be seen when plasma protein concentrations rise above 10 g/100 ml. This is most commonly seen in multiple myeloma and less frequently seen in *Sjögren's syndrome* and in *macroglobulinemia*.

Hyponatremia may not be accompanied by a reduction in osmolality when nonsodium solute accumulates in the extracellular fluid. This is frequently seen in patients with hyperglycemia due to insulin deficiency. In this setting, glucose remains in the extracellular space and will draw water out of the intracellular space until both compartments have the same osmolar concentration. The osmolar gap is *normal*. In such patients, fluid replacement is dependent to some extent on calculated estimates of the sodium concentration in plasma after correction of the hyperglycemia. The fraction of total

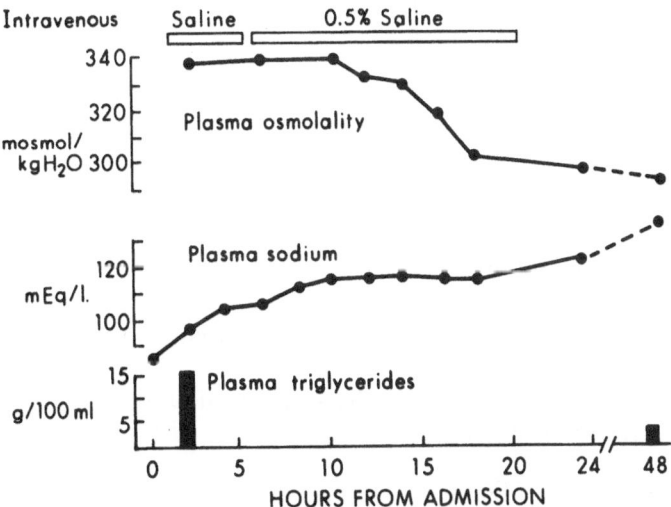

Figure 10. Changes in plasma osmolality, measured plasma sodium, and triglycerides in a patient with diabetic ketoacidosis and hypertriglyceridemia. (Reprinted with permission from Bell, J. A., Hilton, P. J., and Walker, G.: Severe hyponatraemia in hyperlipaemic diabetic ketosis. *Br. Med. J.* 4:709–710, 1972.)

plasma osmolality contributed by plasma glucose (P_G) can be estimated by dividing the plasma glucose concentration in the blood (usually expressed in mg/dl) by its molecular weight ($P_G \times 10/180$) and is approximately 5.5 mOsm/kg H_2O for every 100 mg/dl of glucose. If it is assumed that for every increase of 5.5 mOsm contributed by glucose, the osmolality generated by sodium and chloride will fall proportionately and therefore the sodium concentration will decline by 2.8 mEq, an overestimate of sodium needs will be made. This estimate fails to take into acount fluid shifts which occur between the intra- and extracellular space as the plasma concentration of glucose falls. For example, assume that 1000 mOsm of glucose are added to the total body water of a 70-kg man, who has a plasma glucose of 100 mg/dl, osmolality of 285 mOsm/kg, and Na of 140 mEq/liter. Since total body water is approximately 60% of body weight or 42 liters, the added glucose will increase the osmolal content of the TBW from 11,970 (285×42) to 12,970 mOsm and plasma osmolality will increase to 309 mOsm/kg (12,970/42). However in the absence of insulin almost all of the glucose will stay in the ECF compartment and this change in osmolality will cause a shift of fluid out of the intracellular space. If 66% or 28 liters of the TBW were present in the intracellular space before glucose was given, the volume shift can be calculated as follows:

$$285 \times 28 = 7980 = \text{osmolal content of ICF before glucose is added}$$
$$7980/309 = 25.8 \text{ volume of ICF after the fluid shift}$$
$$28 - 25.8 = 2.2\text{-liter shift}$$

Therefore the ECF volume increased from 14 to 16.2 liters. The final concentration of glucose in the ECF will be equal to

$$[1000 + (5.5 \times 14)]/16.2 = 66.5 \text{ mOsm/kg } H_2O$$

or

$$[66.5 \times 180]/10 = 1197 \text{ mg/100 ml}$$

the concentration of sodium will be

$$[140 \times 14]/16.2 = 121 \text{ mEq/liter}$$

The relationship between the fall in Na concentration (ΔP_{Na}) and the rise in glucose concentration (ΔP_G) is

$$\frac{\Delta P_{Na}}{\Delta P_G} = \frac{140 - 121 \text{ mEq/liter}}{1197 \text{ mg/100 ml}} = \frac{19 \text{ mEq/liter}}{1197 \text{ mg/dl}} \times 100 = \frac{-1.6 \text{ mEq/liter}}{100 \text{ mg/dl}}$$

This estimate may be in error to the extent that the space that glucose enters in insulin deficiency is greater than the ECF. Recent studies indicate that a better estimate is that the sodium concentration will drop 1.33 mEq/liter for each increase in glucose of 100 mg/dl. Thus, sodium replacement based on the figure of 2.8 mEq/liter would result in a twofold overestimate of sodium needs and in the development of hypernatremia.

Other solutes may also depress sodium concentrations while total osmolality remains normal or high. These substances are unmeasured and will therefore result in an *increase* in the osmolar gap. These are listed in Table II. Of these, the infusion of hypertonic mannitol is the most important clinically. This can occur in patients with congestive heart failure who are given mannitol as a diuretic and in patients with oliguric renal failure who are given hypertonic mannitol as a therapeutic trial. The effects of mannitol will be similar to those of glucose in terms of its effect on decreasing the sodium concentration in the ECF.

b. Hyponatremia and Decreased ECF Volume

Volume depletion is an uncommon cause of hyponatremia. When it occurs, it is a consequence of significant loss of sodium either through the gastrointestinal tract (diarrhea, biliary drainage, or vomiting), excessive sweating, or inappropriate loss of sodium in the urine (see Table II). These patients have a deficit of both sodium and free water and, in all instances, volume replacement has been attempted with an excess of free water. In each of these cases, the major stimulus in the development of hyponatremia is a decrease in effective arterial volume which stimulates the release of antidiuretic hormone through increased sympathetic discharge of the baroreceptors. Of secondary importance is the production of angiotensin II, which may stimulate the thirst centers. Thus, in addition to the usual symptoms of hyponatremia these patients may also complain of thirst. In these patients, the physical findings of dehydration (i.e., poor skin turgor, sunken eyes, and weight loss) are present. In every case, the patient is hypotensive and tachycardic on standing and will complain of symptoms related to these hemodynamic events. Blood studies are characterized by a greater rise in BUN than in creatinine (i.e., prerenal azotemia). When sodium and water losses are nonrenal, urine output is sharply reduced and there is evidence of avid water and Na reabsorption. Urine sodium concentration is low (less than 10 mEq/liter) and fractional excretion of water (FE_{H_2O}) and fractional excretion of sodium (FE_{Na}) are less than 1%. An important subset of these patients are those who have "salt-losing nephropathy." These patients have renal insufficiency which is usually a consequence of an interstitial disease (most commonly they have obstructive nephropathy). In such individuals, the ability to conserve sodium is impaired. Thus, when extrarenal sodium losses are in excess of sodium intake (illness, strenuous exercise, or after surgery) and the individual is allowed to drink freely, dehydration with hyponatremia may develop. Patients with Addison's disease do not efficiently conserve sodium owing to low aldosterone levels and may develop hyponatremic dehydration under the conditions just described.

Table II. Classification of the Causes of Hyponatremia

I. Hyponatremia not accompanied by a reduction in plasma osmolality
  A. Reduction in aqueous phase of plasma
    1. Hyperlipidemia
      a. Acute pancreatitis
      b. Diabetic ketoacidosis
    2. Hyperproteinemia
      a. Multiple myeloma
      b. Sjögren's syndrome
      c. Macroglobulinemia
  B. Increase in extracellular nonsodium solute
    1. Hyperglycemia
    2. Mannitol therapy
    3. Sodium diatrizoate
    4. Sorbitol (peritoneal dialysis)
    5. Ethanol
    6. Isoniazid
II. Hyponatremia accompanied by a reduction in plasma osmolality
  A. Hyponatremia and decreased ECF volume
    1. Gastrointestinal losses
      a. Vomiting
      b. Biliary drainage
      c. Diarrhea
    2. Excessive sweat loss with only free-water replacement
    3. Renal loss
      a. Diuretic therapy
      b. Intrinsic renal disease (salt-losing nephropathy)
        i. Pyelonephritis
        ii. Obstructive uropathy
        iii. Sickle-cell-induced interstitial nephropathy
      c. Addison's disease
  B. Hyponatremia and normal ECF volume
    1. Resetting of the osmostat
    2. Inadequate sodium replacement
      a. Addison's disease
      b. Chronic renal disease
      c. Diuretic therapy
        i. Chronic hypokalemia
      d. Beer drinkers' potomania
  C. Hyponatremia and increased ECF volume
    1. Absolute sodium deficiency and absolute water excess
      a. Inappropriate ADH secretion
      b. Drug therapy
      c. Increased intake of free water
        1. Iatrogenic
        2. Polydipsia
          (a) Psychogenic
          (b) Drug-induced
      d. Myxedema
    2. Absolute excess of sodium and water (edema-forming states)
      a. Congestive heart failure
      b. Advanced liver disease
      c. Nephrotic syndrome

c. Hyponatremia and Normal ECF Volume

Hyponatremia and euvolemia may arise in four settings: (1) when a sodium deficit occurs in a subject who has a fixed intake of sodium and in whom the renal capacity to conserve sodium is impaired, (2) in patients who are potassium depleted, (3) in chronic disease states where it is postulated that the "osmostat" is reset at a lower level, and (4) when free-water intake exceeds the intake of solute required to excrete it. In each setting there is a deficit of total body sodium but total body water and extracellular fluid volume are nearly normal. Therefore the clinical signs, which include blood pressure measurements, heart rate, and skin turgor, will be within the normal range.

In the first instance patients have sustained a significant salt loss and although allowed unlimited free water, sodium intake is restricted. In these patients renal conservation of sodium is impaired either because of an intrinsic renal lesion (obstructive nephropathy, pyelonephritis, or other chronic interstitial nephritis), diuretic therapy, or mineralocorticoid deficiency. In such individuals sodium intake equals urinary losses and is not sufficient to replace preexisting sodium deficits. In these subjects effective intravascular volume is maintained by two mechanism: (1) increased free-water intake (thirst) partially a consequence of increased circulating levels of angiotensin II, and (2) increased reabsorption of free water due to increased secretion of ADH, a consequence of an increase in sympathetic stimulation. Since these patients are in balance they will respond normally to an increase or decrease in free-water intake. That is, when given a water load urine osmolality will fall appropriately to a value below 100 mOsm/kg H_2O and the serum sodium concentration will remain unchanged. When water is withheld urine osmolality will rise. But renal sodium conservation is impaired and thus urinary sodium concentration will be high and FE_{Na} may exceed 1% of the filtered load. Correction of hyponatremia can be achieved by replacing the Na deficit of such individuals. This can be calculated from the following formula:

$$[\text{Volume of ECF} \times \text{actual } P_{Na}]$$
$$- [\text{Volume of ECF} \times \text{desired } P_{Na}] = \text{Na deficit}$$

Here P_{Na} is the plasma sodium concentration. An illustrative example is that of a 70-kg man with chronic renal disease who comes to the clinic for routine follow-up care and is found to have a serum Na of 121 mEq/liter. He states he has just recovered from the "flu." During that interval he vomited frequently and had a poor appetite. He subsequently resumed his normal diet which allows water *ad lib* but which restricts protein intake and limits sodium intake to 4 g of NaCl (68 mEq) per day. His physical exam was unremarkable, supine and upright blood pressures were not different. A 24-hr urine collection contained 67 mEq of Na. Thus sodium intake was equal to output. This indicates that this patient's obligatory sodium loss or *lower threshold* for sodium conservation is 67 mEq/24 hr. In order to correct his hyponatremic state, sodium intake must exceed this lower threshold. As a first step in calculating this patient's sodium needs, one must determine the volume of the extracellular space:

$$ECF = TBW \times 0.33$$
$$= (0.6 \times 70 \text{ kg}) \times 0.33$$
$$= 13.9 \text{ liters}$$

The sodium deficit is equal to the difference in the sodium contained in the ECF and the desired value (138 mEq/liter):

$$(13.9 \times 121) - (13.9 \times 138) = 1682 - 1918 = -236.3 \text{ mEq}$$

Since 1 g of NaCl has 17 mEq of Na, the amount needed to correct this patient's hyponatremia is

$$[236.3]/17 = 13.9 \text{ g NaCl}$$

Thus if the patient were told to double his salt intake, in 4 days he would have received 16 g of additional sodium chloride and his serum sodium would have returned to normal.

Hyponatremia and euvolemia seen in patients with potassium deficiency is usually the result of taking diuretics on a long-term basis. These patients are always *hypokalemic*. They have both a sodium and potassium deficit. Simply increasing sodium intake is not corrective. Potassium supplements must be given concomitantly. The reasons for the development of hyponatremia in this setting and its resistance to simple sodium replacement are not clear. Two mechanisms may be involved: (1) Intracellular potassium depletion leads to a fall in cellular osmolality. In order to maintain cell volume, extracellular osmolality and the serum sodium concentration are reduced appropriately through increased levels of circulating ADH. (2) Hypokalemia renders the collecting tubules more sensitive to circulating levels of ADH.

The third cause of hyponatremia and euvolemia is only seen in patients with chronic diseases, like tuberculosis, malignancy, and chronic alcoholism. In this group hyponatremia is thought to be a consequence of "resetting of the osmostat." Studies performed in such a patient are presented in Figure 11. The response to water loading and deprivation were appropriate. But serum osmolality and sodium concentration remained low and unchanged. When the patient was infused with saline, a natriuresis ensued. Again serum sodium and osmolality did not change. Circulating levels of ADH were appropriately depressed during the water load and rose when hypertonic saline was infused. In such patients, the mechanism by which hyponatremia

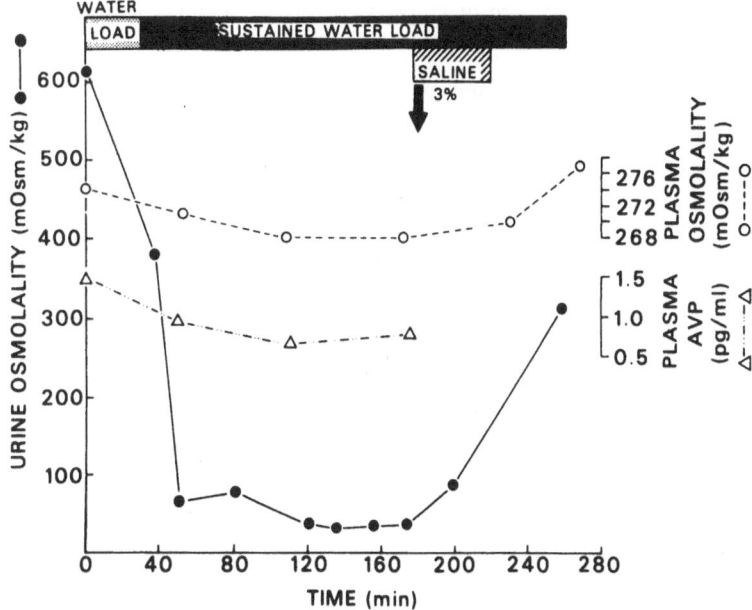

Figure 11. Response of a patient with a "reset osmostat" to a water load. Note that plasma osmolality remains unchanged. There is a prompt decline in plasma arginine vasopressin after an acute water load. Levels remained suppressed during the period of sustained water diuresis. (Reprinted with permission from DeFronzo, R. A., Goldberg, M., and Agus, Z. S.: Normal diluting capacity in hyponatremic patients. *Ann. Intern. Med.* 84:538–542, 1976.)

has developed and is sustained is not clear. One theory is that the cellular content of "osmoregulators" has been altered. A reduction in the cellular protein content and in phosphate esters and in their anionic intermediates would give rise to a reduction in potassium content and in the osmolality of the cell. If it is assumed that cell volume and therefore intracellular osmolality is the primary determinant for the osmolality of body fluids, and if the protein content and therefore osmolality of the cell falls, prevention of cellular distortion must occur through a "resetting of the osmostat."

Finally hyponatremia and euvolemia may occur when solute intake is extremely low and drinking is excessive. One example is *beer potomania*, which commonly occurs in individuals who are eating little and ingesting excessive quantities of beer (usually greater than 5 liters/day). Since beer has no protein and contains only 1–2 mEq of Na/liter, solute loss may exceed intake in these patients. Table III presents the information mathematically. In the illustrative case, it is assumed that the minimal urine osmolality that man can achieve is 60 mOsm/kg. In a 70-kg man the usual solute excretion is approximately 700 mOsm/24 hr; thus urine output and therefore intake may approach 12 liters/day with no real alterations in serum sodium concentration. On the other hand a beer drinker of the same size ingests less than 12 mEq of sodium per day, and the urea excreted results from only endogenous protein breakdown, roughly 0.25 g/kg protein. In this individual daily solute excretion is 304

Table III. Mechanism of Hypoosmolality in Beer Potomania[a]

I. Normal 70-kg subject
  A. Ingests normal diet containing 1 g protein/kg per day and average intake of ions and acid
  B. Urine solutes:
1. Sodium	50 mEq/day	
2. Potassium	70 mEq/day	
3. Ammonium	30 mEq/day	
4. Anions	150 mEq/day	
5. Urea	400 mEq/day	
Total	700 mOsm/day	
  C. If subject ingests and excretes 12 liters of water, urine will be 700 mOsm/12 liters of 60 mOsm/kg.
II. 70-kg Beer potomaniac
  A. Subject ingests only 6 liters of beer/day; assume catabolism of 0.25 g body protein/kg per day
  B. Urine solutes:
1. Sodium	12 mEq/day	
2. Potassium	60 mEq/day	
3. Ammonium	30 mEq/day	
4. Anions	102 mEq/day	
5. Urea	100 mOsm/day	
Total	304 mOsm/day	
  C. If 6 liters of 60 mOsm/kg are excreted, subject will excrete 56 mOsm more solute than were ingested or formed from metabolism.

[a] Modified with permission from *Lancet* 2:245–246, 1975.

mOsm. However, 360 mOsm are required to excrete 6 liters of urine at the lowest osmolality. Thus the patient loses 56 mOsm of solute a day. In this setting profound and symptomatic hyponatremia may develop.

d. Hyponatremia and Increased ECF Volume

This category of diseases falls into two groups: (1) those who have an increased volume but no detectable edema and (2) those who have clear manifestations of increased volume, that is, they have edema. The multiple causes of the syndrome of inappropriate secretion of ADH (SIADH) and conditions characterized by increased intake of free water are examples of the former and congestive heart failure, advanced liver disease, and the nephrotic syndrome are examples of the latter.

i. Hyponatremia and Overhydration, but No Edema. In these pathophysiologic states hyponatremia develops as a consequence of either a decrease in the excretion or an increase in the intake of free water.

The syndrome of inappropriate secretion of ADH is the best example of overhydration due to a decrease in free-water excretion. In this syndrome the secretion and production of ADH occurs independent of the usual osmotic and nonosmotic stimuli. There is maximal free-water reabsorption and serum sodium and osmolality fall below the normal range, while urine osmolality is inappropriately high. Total body water and effective intravascular volume are increased. For example, if an individual who weighs 70 kg and who has SIADH ingests 2 liters of water in excess of insensible losses, TBW will initially increase from 42 to 44 liters. Since 33% of the TBW is ECF, the volume of this compartment would increase from 13.9 to 14.5 liters. If the initial sodium concentration was 138 mEq/liter the decline in sodium concentration could be calculated as follows:

$$138 \times 13.9/14.5 = 1918/14.5 = 132 \text{ mEq/liter}$$

Since effective intravascular volume is expanded, mechanisms involved in the control of volume come into play. Secretion of aldosterone is inhibited and those factors which govern the isoosmotic reabsorption of sodium in the proximal tubule are suppressed. As a consequence a natriuresis would occur and urine output would increase to 2 liters. The urine osmolality would be equal to sum of the plasma osmolality (262 mOsm/kg) and 400 mOsm of solute produced from protein breakdown and distributed in the 2 liters of urine or 462 mOsm/kg. TBW is thus maintained slightly expanded and prevented from further expansion by incurring a sodium deficit. Thus, patients who are hyponatremic because of SIADH have a total body deficit of sodium. Since patients with this syndrome are maximally expanded, serum concentrations of K, HCO_3, uric acid, and urea will fall below the normal range. Such patients may be polyuric and in all cases urinary sodium concentrations are high. Because of the natriuretic state, urine osmolality will be only slightly greater than that of plasma. Under conditions where water or fluid intake is increased significantly, urine flow through the distal segment may be so great that urine osmolality will fall slightly below that of plasma. Thus, patients with SIADH may actually excrete a dilute urine, although in all cases it will not be maximally dilute (50–60 mOsm/kg H_2O). Clearly, the more free water the patient ingests, the more profoundly hyponatremic he will become. Conversely, free-water restriction will correct the hyponatremic state as free water is eliminated through insensible losses. The syndrome can be aggravated by the ingestion or intravenous administration of NaCl. In this setting the TBW of the patient is expanded even more, sodium delivery out of the proximal tubule and to the diluting segment of the nephron is increased. Thus, more free water is made and therefore reabsorbed (see Figure 8).

The causes of SIADH are listed in Table IV. They are divided into two categories: those due to the ectopic production by tumors of peptide substances with antidiuretic activity and those which are the result of an increase in the endogeneous production of ADH. By far the most common causes of this syndrome are associated with diseases of the respiratory system. Carcinoma of the lung, especially of the small or "oat" cell variety, is a frequent cause of SIADH. Of equal incidence is the development of SIADH in the presence of respiratory infections, respiratory distress syndromes, or during positive pressure respiration. It is interesting to note that SIADH

Table IV. Classification of the Causes for the Inappropriate
Secretion of Antidiuretic Hormone

I. Tumors which may produce ADH
  A. Lung
    1. Oat-cell carcinoma
    2. Large-cell carcinoma
  B. Adenocarcinoma of the pancreas
  C. Adenocarcinoma of the duodenum
  D. Adenocarcinoma of the thymus
  E. Myeloid leukemia
  F. Hodgkin disease?
  G. Carcinoma of the ureter?
II. Inappropriate increases in the endogenous production of ADH
  A. Respiratory system
    1. Infection
      a. Pneumonia
      b. Abscess with cavitation
      c. Tuberculosis
      d. Fungus (aspergillosis)
    2. Respiratory distress syndrome in the infant
    3. Cystic fibrosis
    4. Positive pressure respiration
  B. Central nervous system
    1. Infection
      a. Menningitis
        (1). Viral
        (2). Bacterial
        (3). Tuberculosis
      b. Encephalitis
      c. Guillian–Barré syndrome
    2. Tumor
      a. Pituitary adenoma
      b. Glioblastoma
      c. Metastatic invasion of the hypothalamus
    3. Degenerative disease
      a. Cerebral atrophy
      b. Cerebellar atrophy
      c. Pontine myelinolysis
    4. Trauma
      a. Subdural hematoma
      b. Subarachnoid hemorrhage
      c. Cerebral thrombosis
      d. Occlusion of a ventriculo-venous shunt
  C. Metabolic
    1. Acute intermittant porphyria
  D. Idiopathic

---

may occur in association with tuberculosis even when the lesion is not
pulmonic. Almost any disease known to affect the central nervous system has
been associated with SIADH.

Hyponatremia and overhydration may also be a consequence of drugs
which impair free water excretion (see Table V). This can occur by three
mechanisms. (1) Some drugs produce an inappropriate release of ADH:

carbamazepine, clofibrate, nicotine, and narcotics like morphine are the classic examples. (2) Other drugs may enhance the activity of ADH by increasing the rate adenylate cyclase activation (see Figure 9). Although the sulfonylureas may evoke an increase in ADH release, their major effect seems to be through this latter mechanism. They are thought to block the antagonistic effect of prostaglandins. Acetaminophen, aspirin, and indomethacin also enhance adenylate cyclase activation most likely by inhibiting the synthesis of prostaglandin E_2. (3) Finally, drugs which are analogs of ADH may produce hyponatremia. Oxytocin when given in large amounts during the induction of labor may produce profound and symptomatic hyponatremia if water intake has not been carefully controlled.

One characteristic of patients presenting in *myxedema* coma is a profound hyponatremia. Early studies suggested that this was a consequence of either a "resetting of the osmostat" or the syndrome of inappropriate ADH secretion. However, recently it has been demonstrated that thyroid deficiency has profound effects on renal function. In almost all cases of myxedema, GFR is reduced. Thyroid hormone appears to nonspecifically promote sodium transport in all segments of the nephron. Urine osmolality falls appropriately when myxedematous patients are given a water load and is not different from values measured after the patient has become euthyroid or in control subjects. However, the absolute amount of free water excreted is

Table V. Drugs Which Impair Free-Water
Excretion

I. Drugs which increase ADH release
  A. Tricyclics
    1. Carbamazepine (Tegretol)
    2. Amitriptyline (Elavil)
    3. Thiothixene (Navane)
    4. Fluphenazine (Prolixin)
  B. Vincristine
  C. Sulfonylureas
    1. Chlorpropamide
    2. Tolbutamide
  D. Morphine
  E. Barbiturates
  F. Nicotine
  G. Cyclophosphamide
  H. Clofibrate (Atromid S)
II. Analogs of ADH
  A. Oxytocin
III. Drugs which enhance the action of ADH
  A. Sulfonylureas
    1. Chlorpropramide
    2. Tolbutamide
  B. Acetaminophen
  C. Acetylsalicyclic acid
  D. Indomethacin (Indocin)
  E. Ibuprofen (Motrin)

sharply reduced. In hypothyroidism there is an increase in the absolute and fractional delivery of water and sodium out of the proximal tubule. Since delivery to the diluting segment is increased and since free-water excretion is diminished, it is implied that thyroid hormone is necessary to maximize free water formation in the ascending limb of the loop of Henle. Thus in hypothyroidism, hyponatremia is a consequence of an intrinsic defect in ascending limb function resulting in impaired free-water formation.

Increased water intake may occur through other routes. Injudicious intravenous administration of fluids is a common mechanism by which patients can become hyponatremic. This is most likely to occur in the postoperative patient who may have inappropriately elevated levels of ADH due to increased sympathetic discharge and catecholamine release. Excessive use of large tap water enemas also may produce hyponatremia. This is particularly true in children who because of chronic constipation or disease (ulcerative colitis) may have a dilated colon. Overhydration and hyponatremia may occur also in the patient who has undergone a transurethral prostatectomy, and whose bladder is irrigated with hypotonic solutions to maintain patency of the urethra.

ii. Hyponatremia and Edema. Hyponatremia in edematous patients results from a variety of physiologic events designed to correct a decrease in *effective* arterial volume. It is important to emphasize that while effective arterial volume is decreased, all such patients are in both total body water and sodium excess. A decrease in effective arterial volume of 10% or greater evokes both neural and humoral mechanisms. There is augmented sympathetic discharge from arterial baroreceptors which increase not only arterial tone and cardiac output, but stimulate the release of ADH. The humoral limb of this response is an increase in the production of angiotensin II which acts directly to increase arteriolar tone and indirectly by increasing baroreceptor discharge, stimulating the release of aldosterone and the drive to drink (see Figure 3). Thus an essential part of maintaining effective arterial volume is the conservation of water and sodium. In such patients urine volume will be reduced and urinary sodium concentration will be low (less than 10 mEq/liter). Fractional excretion of both water and sodium will be less than 1%. Since thirst is increased and the stimulus for the secretion of ADH is nonosmotically mediated such patients may become hyponatremic.

When cardiac output is severely reduced, the tendency for the development of hyponatremia may be aggravated by intrarenal mechanisms which impair free-water formation. Renal blood flow falls markedly and is associated with a disproportionate increase in resistance at the efferent end of the glomerulus. The net effect is a greater fall in renal blood flow than in GFR and a subsequent increase in filtration fraction. This change in filtration fraction favors an increase in the reabsorption of sodium and water along the proximal tubule (see Chapter 4). Thus, sodium delivery to the diluting segment is reduced owing to both a decrease in the filtered load of sodium (decrease in GFR) and an increase in the reabsorption of sodium in the proximal tubule. The capacity to generate free water will therefore be diminished because of reduced sodium delivery to the diluting segment.

In patients who have congestive heart failure or cirrhosis and edema, the development of hyponatremia is primarily the result of increased free-water reabsorption. It is likely that impaired free-water formation may play a role only when cardiac output is severely compromised and GFR is drastically reduced. Studies in dogs with right heart failure have shown that hyponatremia is corrected and free-water clearance returns to normal after hypophysectomy or when the carotid sinus has been denervated. The role of ADH in the hyponatremia of end stage liver disease (Laennec's cirrhosis) is unclear. There is no evidence that liver disease alters the metabolism of ADH. In most studies, there is no correlation between these measured levels of ADH and whether or not the patients are hyponatremic. Further, when ADH secretion is tested with water loading or deprivation there is an appropriate response. On the other hand, there is considerable evidence to suggest that the capacity to elaborate free water is impaired for the reasons described above. In such patients, there is usually some evidence of progressive decrease in GFR and avid sodium reabsorption. Further when intravascular volume is restored as occurs during whole body water immersion, free-water clearance improves.

3. Therapeutic Approach to Hyponatremia

The therapeutic approach to the treatment of hyponatremia will be dependent on three factors: (1) the presence of hyperglycemia or of an osmolar gap, (2) the symptomatology exhibited by the patient, and (3) the volume status of the individual. A schema for the approach to hyponatremia is presented in Figure 12. The initial step, is to determine whether or not there is an osmolar gap and if measured or unmeasured solute could be depressing the sodium concentration in the blood. Failure to take into account such a possibility may lead to inappropriate sodium replacement and ultimately to the development of hypernatremia. For example, hyperlipidemia should always be considered in hyponatremic patients being treated for diabetic ketoacidosis. In these patients, the true plasma sodium concentration estimated by using the factor mentioned previously in the text (a 1.3-mEq fall in plasma sodium is to be expected for every increase of 100 mg/dl of glucose). If after this correction hyponatremia is still found to be present, then the approach will be dependent upon the volume status and symptomatology of the patient.

Before any therapy is instituted in the treatment of *true* hyponatremia, the volume status of the individual must be assessed. Patients who have evidence of a total body water deficit (i.e., weight loss, postural hypotension, tachycardia, and poor skin turgor) will always be treated by extracellular fluid volume expansion. That is, such patients should be given *only* normal saline or its equivalent until evidence of volume depletion is gone. Once this

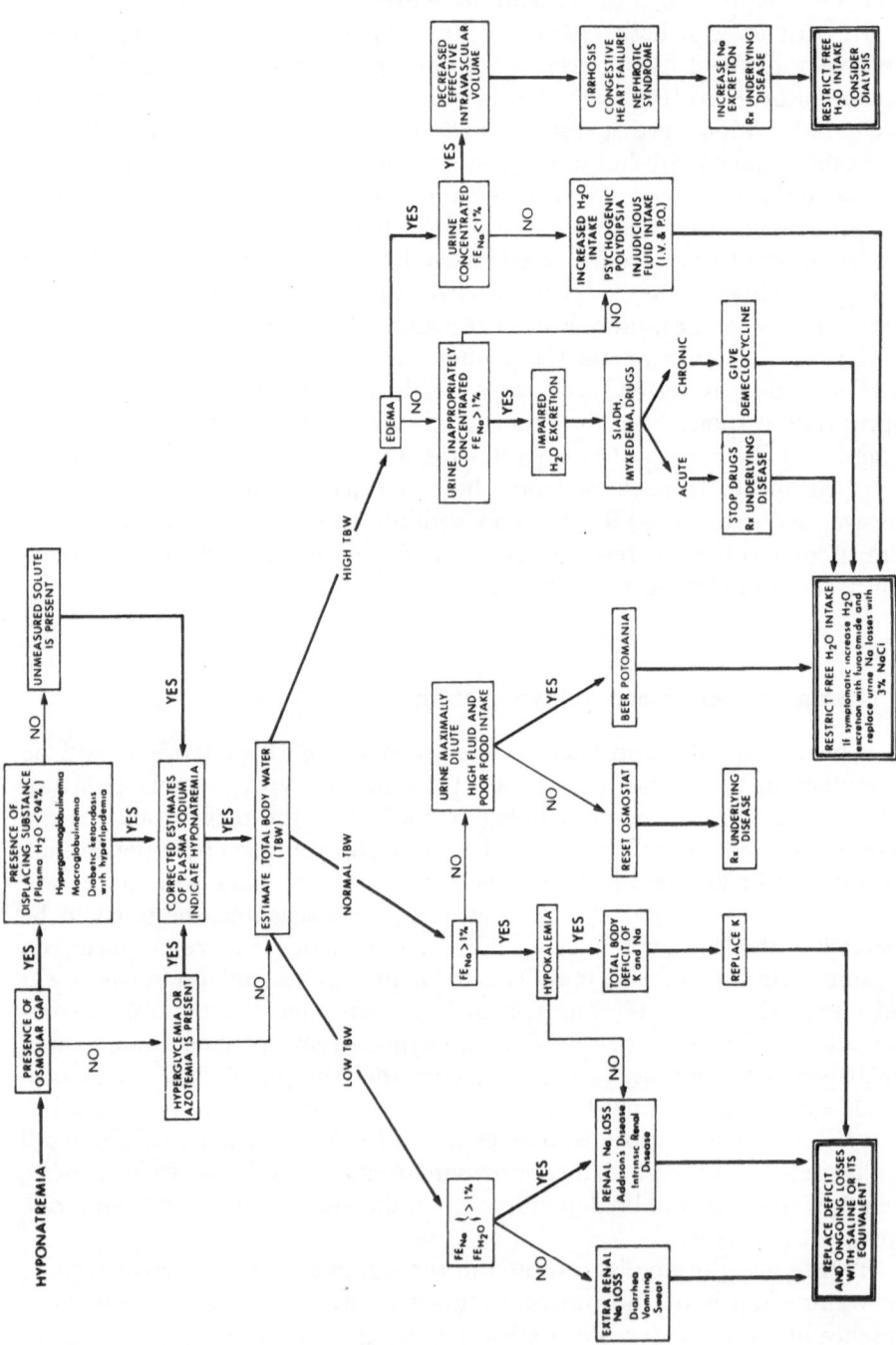

Figure 12. Schema for the diagnostic and therapeutic approach to hyponatremia.

has been done, the patient must be reevaluated and further therapy will be dependent upon the patients natremic state. Equally important in the care of such patients is to determine the route of water and sodium loss. Before volume replacement is attempted, urine samples should be obtained and the fractional excretion of water and sodium should be determined. Patients who have excessive losses of sodium and water from extrarenal sites should exhibit maximal renal conservation of sodium and water (fractional excretion of sodium and water should be less than 1%). In such patients, both historical and clinical evidence of extrarenal loss is usually readily apparent (i.e., diarrhea, nausea, vomiting, high fevers, and excessive sweating). In patients whose sodium and water losses are greater than 1%, intrinsic renal disease should be suspected. In such patients, serum creatinine and blood urea nitrogen will be equally elevated. In those patients where there is little or no evidence of intrinsic renal disease but sodium excretion is high, the diagnosis of Addison's disease or diuretic therapy should be considered. *In all patients fluid replacement has to include not only the patient's deficit at the time of the initial evaluation, but also the ongoing sodium and water losses.*

In patients who are found to be euvolemic and hyponatremic, it is imperative to determine the etiology of the hyponatremic state. Patients on fixed sodium intakes who have an impaired capacity to conserve sodium because of renal disease may only require additional sodium supplements, while those who have hyponatremia due to excessive diuretic therapy may require potassium in addition to sodium replacement. On the other hand, an individual who gives a history of excessive intake of fluid while eating little may require both water restriction and sodium supplementation. In most cases, these patients are only mildly symptomatic and free-water restriction with sodium supplementation given orally will be satisfactory. Occasionally, such patients may be profoundly symptomatic and a more agressive approach may be indicated.

When total body water is increased, as a consequence of either a massive intake of free water or impaired free-water excretion, the patient will appear to be euvolemic. However, blood chemistries indicate clear evidence of dilution. Blood urea nitrogen and serum creatinine concentrations are low or within the normal range. In the syndrome of inappropriate secretion of ADH, the urine osmolality is inappropriately concentrated and sodium excretion is inappropriately high ($FE_{Na} > 1\%$). When hyponatremia is due to an inappropriately high intake of free water the physical findings are similar to those found in patients with SIADH, with the important exceptions that the urine osmolality is always maximally dilute and fractional excretion and absolute sodium excretion are appropriate for the patient's dietary salt intake. In addition, such patients may demonstrate bizzare behavior which will be associated with profound and compulsive polydipsia.

In forms of hyponatremia in which the major problem is excess water, treatment is directed toward increasing the excretion of free water and reducing intake to minimal levels. The approach will depend on the degree of hyponatremia and whether or not the patient is symptomatic. Hyponatremia which is asymptomatic or produces only mild symptoms (i.e., lethargy and dulled sensorium) may be corrected by restricting water to 500 ml/day and allowing the excess water to be eliminated through insensible losses. In patients with SIADH produced by an acute and reversible disease, resolution of hyponatremia may occur when the underlying problem is resolved. At this point, ADH levels will fall rapidly and the urinary excretion of free water will rise abruptly. In patients with symptoms or in whom serum sodium concentrations are below 120 mEq/liter rapid correction is essential. In such patients, the infusion of hypertonic saline (3%) will temporarily correct the abnormality and thus may be life saving. It is imperative that the sodium deficit be calculated such that the amount of sodium given as hypertonic sodium be sufficient *only* to reverse the symptoms. That is, if an individual has a plasma sodium of 110 mEq/liter then hypertonic saline should be given in an amount which is calculated to return the patient's sodium concentration to the 125- to 130-mEq/liter range. The remainder of the sodium deficit can be given either as normal saline or by mouth. A major problem with such patients is that they may be volume expanded and the risk of precipitating acute left heart failure is great in those with borderline myocardial function. To avoid this risk it is useful to increase free-water excretion by giving furosamide and to replace urinary losses of sodium with 3% NaCl. To this replacement solution, potassium chloride must also be added. Using this technique, cation losses but not water losses are replaced and hyponatremia can be corrected within 6–8 hr. Once the hyponatremic state has been corrected, water restriction should be instituted to maintain a normal serum sodium concentration. In those patients who have hyponatremia due to SIADH on a chronic basis (i.e., idiopathic or in association with a malignant disease), free-water excretion may be increased by giving a druglike demeclocycline which blocks the renal effects of ADH (see Table VII and Figure 8).

When hyponatremia is found in association with edema, total body water and sodium are in excess. Therefore, giving sodium in any form is seldom indicated. Rather, increasing water and sodium excretion are the mainstay of treatment, as is restriction of free-water intake. In such patients there is usually a decrease in effective intravascular volume and therapy usually includes an attempt to reverse this. Thus, water and sodium excretion will increase when digitalis and vasodilators are given to patients with congestive heart failure or when albumin is administered intravenously to patients with nephrotic syndrome. Occasionally the hyponatremia is profound and mobilization of excess water is not possible by these conservative measures. In such patients peritoneal or hemodialysis should be considered. Correction of hyponatremia in patients with severe liver disease is the most difficult entity to treat. Free-water restriction, the cautious use of diuretics, and the infusion of albumin are the mainstay of therapy. Peritoneal dialysis in such patients has produced disastrous results.

B. Hypernatremia

1. Symptoms of Hypernatremia

Hypernatremia is said to exist when the serum sodium concentration is greater than 150 mEq/liter. The signs and symptoms of hypernatremia depend somewhat upon degree and the rapidity with which the hypernatremic state develops. The predominant abnormalities are neurologic. When hypernatremia develops rapidly, the initial symptoms include lethargy, irritability, progressive muscle rigidity, tremor, hyperreflexia, ataxia, and convulsions. Ultimately a marked depression in sensorium develops, which may be followed by frank coma. In chronic hypernatremia, symptoms are less marked. Early findings may only be a dulled sensorium and in children increased irritability. Muscle tone is usually normal although some patients may present with hyperreflexia, myoclonus, and seizures. Other neurologic abnormalities described include psychosis, choreoathetoid movements, and hemiparesis. Cerebrospinal fluid is often bloody or xanthochromic and protein content is usually elevated. Electroencephalograms of hypernatremic patients may show generalized slow wave activity and sometimes characteristic epileptic patterns may be observed. Unlike hyponatremia, hypernatremia may be associated with severe brain damage. It is a common disease in children and when it occurs is associated with a substantial mortality and morbidity. Permanent sequelae include profound mental retardation and localizing neurologic defects (hemiplegia and paraplegia).

Several mechanisms are involved in the pathogenesis of symptoms seen in the hypernatremic state. When hypernatremia develops acutely, the abrupt elevation of plasma osmolality creates an osmotic gradient between the ECF and ICF of the brain and leads to a rapid movement of water out of the central nervous system. The loss of tissue water results in a rapid shrinkage of the CNS tissues, causing hemorrhage as bridging vessels between the dura mater and the surface of the brain are torn. The movement of fluid out of the intracellular space into vessels can cause rapid venous dilatation and result in further hemorrhage. And, when hypernatremia is associated with dehydration cerebral venous thrombosis may occur. Finally, it is thought that a high intracellular concentration of sodium impairs the metabolic activity of the cell. In chronic hypernatremia, intracellular concentrations of known solutes, although elevated, are not high enough to account for the measured osmolality. These "idiogenic osmols" are thought to be metabolized from intracellular protein and are designed to maintain lower concentrations of intracellular sodium and potassium while preventing cellular dehydration.

Hypernatremia may be associated with other abnormalities including hyperkalemia, hypocalcemia, elevated plasma glucose levels and a mild metabolic acidosis. In chronic hypernatremia muscular weakness leading to paralysis may occur. This may be due to mobilization of potassium ions from the intracellular to the extracellular space. Indeed when hypernatremia is

Table VI. Classification of Causes for Hypernatremia

I. Hypernatremia due to water loss
  A. Inadequate free-water intake
    1. Impaired conscious state
      a. Postsurgical patients
      b. Comatose patients
    2. Altered thirst mechanism (adipsia)
      a. Hypothalamic lesion
        i. Granuloma
        ii. Tumors
          (a) Germinoma
          (b) Meningioma
          (c) Metastatic Carcinoma
          (d) Pinealoma
          (e) Craniopharyngioma
        iii. Central nervous systen injury
          (a) Postirradiation
          (b) Prolonged hypernatremia?
          (c) Convulsions
        iv. Idiopathic
  B. Increased free-water loss
    1. Insensible losses
      a. Integumental
        i. Increased sweating
          (a) Elevated ambient temperature
          (b) Exercise
          (c) Fever
        ii. Burns
        iii. Generalized dermatologic eruptions
      b. Respiratory
    2. Gastrointestinal losses
      a. Vomiting
      b. Gastrointestinal drainage
      c. Diarrhea
        i. Secretory
          (a) *C. welchii*
          (b) *E. coli*
          (c) *V. cholerae*
        ii. Osmolar
          (a) Improper treatment of infantile diarrhea
            (i) Boiled milk
            (ii) High-glucose solutions
            (iii) Electrolyte solutions
          (b) Tube feedings
          (c) Lactulose therapy in hepatic encephalopathy
      d. Hypertonic enema
        i. Hypertonic phosphate (Fleet or Tudvad)
        ii. Hypertonic sodium bicarbonate (Mayo)
      e. Peritoneal dialysis
    3. Renal losses
      a. Increased excretion, obligate water loss
      b. Increased excretion of free water
        i. Vasopressin deficiency (vasopressin-deficient diabetes insipidus)
        ii. Renal defect (vasopressin-resistant diabetes insipidus)

(Continued)

Table VI. (*Continued*)

II. Hypernatremia due to excess sodium
    A. Reset osmostat
    B. Endocrine
        1. Cushing disease
        2. Primary aldosteronism
    C. Increased Na intake
        1. Increased oral intake
            a. Hypertonic emetics
            b. Improper formula preparation: accidental substitution of NaCl for glucose
            c. Ingestion of salt tablets
            d. Drinking of sea water
        2. Increased parental intake
            a. Administration of $NaHCO_3$

---

severe, rhabdomyolysis may occur and result in acute renal failure. Vascular insufficiency and gangrene may also occur in this setting although profound dehydration may be the major inciting mechanism.

2. Disorders of Tonicity Associated with Hypernatremia

a. Hypernatremia Due to a Water Deficit

i. Inadequate Free-Water Intake. Under normal circumstances obligatory fluid losses, that is, evaporative water losses through the lung and skin plus the amount necessary to excrete the renal solute load in maximally concentrated urine, is approximately 1000 ml/day or 10% of the ECF volume. On the other hand, sodium losses during deprivation are much smaller. As discussed before, the losses of sodium in stool and sweat are usually less than 4 and 10 mEq/day, respectively, while those in urine may be reduced to less than 5 mEq/day when volume is being conserved. Thus, per day, sodium losses from the extracellular pool can be reduced to less than 1%, a tenth of obligate water losses. Therefore when intake is poor and losses of both sodium and water occur, hypernatremia will result. This is likely to develop in individuals who become confined to bed and who are unable to feed themselves and, in hospitalized patients whose intake is inappropriately restricted.

Rarely, hypernatremia may develop because of a failure to stimulate thirst (adipsia) (see Table VI). This may occur in patients with psychiatric disturbances like schizophrenia in whom a high threshold to the normal stimuli for thirst may be present. However, adipsia is usually the result of destruction of thirst centers located in the hypothalamus. In many of these cases, the development of adipsia is preceeded by a period of polyuria and polydipsia. This is due to the initial destruction of the supraoptic nuclei which produce ADH. Then, after an indeterminate period of time, adipsia develops and can result in profound hypernatremia and volume depletion.

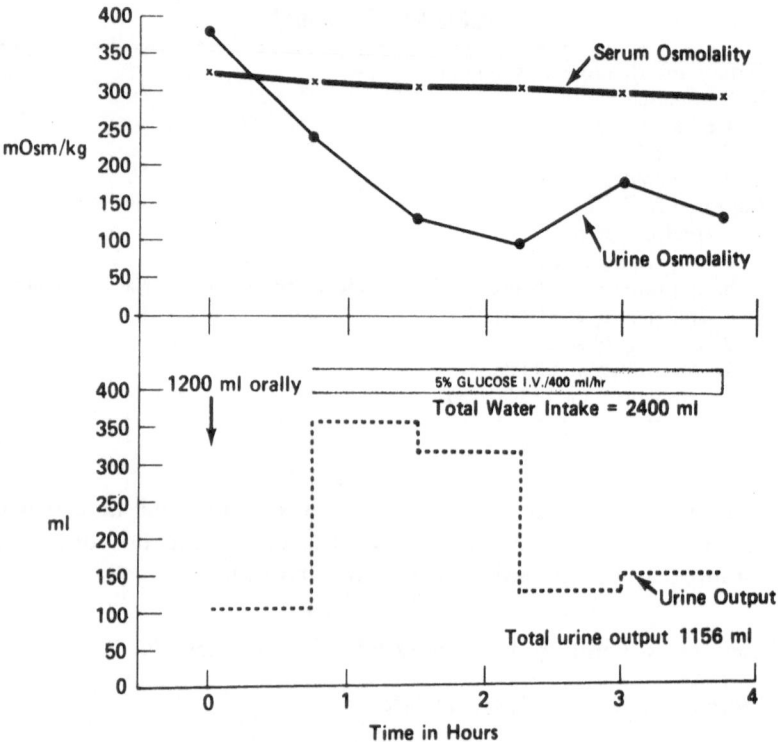

Figure 13. Response of the patient with "essential hypernatremia" to a water load. Note that prior to the initiation of the water load, the patient's serum osmolality is approximately 325 mOsm. When given 1200 ml of water orally followed by an intravenous infusion of 5% glucose and water at 400 ml/hr, the patient's urine output appropriately rises and is associated with a concomitant decline in urine osmolality. Despite this appropriate response to water load, serum osmolality remains virtually unchanged and the hypernatremia persists. (Reprinted with permission from Gossain, V. V., Kinzel, T., Strand, C. V., and Rovner, D. R.: Essential hypernatremia. *Am. J. Med. Sci.* 275:353–358, 1978.)

The development of adipsia in this setting is most likely the consequence of further infiltration and destruction of the hypothalamus. In some instances, hypernatremia per se may cause irreversible damage to the centers for regulation of thirst. This is most likely to occur in patients with preexisting diabetes inspidus who are prone to develop hypernatremia when intake is poor. In many patients with adipsia other evidence of hypothalamic dysfunction is present (i.e., obesity and gonadal dysfunction).

In some patients, it has been proposed that the osmoreceptor has been reset. These patients are said to have *essential hypernatremia*. Their hypernatremic state persists in spite of fluid challenges and remains unchanged during fluid deprivation. Figure 13 presents such a case. These patients have many of the abnormalities seen in cases with pure adipsia. They differ from them in that the stimulus for thirst occurs, but at a level of osmolality higher than normal. If the etiology is unknown, then forced intake of greater amounts of free water is essential. However, if an underlying lesion is found and removed, correction of the hypernatremic state will result.

ii. Increased Insensible Loss of Free Water. When insensible water losses are increased due to fever, or high ambient temperatures, hypernatremia may develop. This is especially true in patients who cannot respond appropriately to the stimuli for thirst because water is restricted or because of an impairment in their conscious state.

Insensible losses may also be increased when the integumental barrier is disrupted, as has been described in infants with disseminated seborrheic dermatitis. Similarly, insensible losses may be profound in patients who have suffered second and third degree burns over large portions of their body. In both of these settings increased insensible water loss may be increased by the use of creams and ointments which are hyperosmotic and will therefore extract water from the exposed dermis.

iii. Renal Losses of Free Water. Hypernatremia may be a consequence of loss of water by the kidney. In these patients urine output is inappropriately increased, that is, they are polyuric. Polyuria is always a reflection of a decrease in renal tubular reabsorption of water and may or may not be appropriate to the individual's water intake. Renal water loss may be *primary* and result from a decrease in the reabsorption of free water per se or it may be *secondary* and be due to an increase in obligate water loss. In Table VII is a partial list of conditions which can result in hypernatremia because of impaired water reabsorption by the kidney.

Hypernatremia due to renal obligate water loss (secondary polyuria). An important cause of secondary polyruia is the glomerular filtration of high concentrations of low-molecular-weight substances that are poorly reabsorbed by the renal tubule. One example is the osmotic diuretic *mannitol*. Mannitol is freely filtered at the glomerulus and poorly reabsorbed by the renal tubule. Because of its small molecular size (mol. wt. 180), it can exert a significant intraluminal osmotic force when present in high concentrations and reduce the isoosmotic movement of water out of the proximal tubule and loop of Henle. Thus, as sodium and water are reabsorbed along the proximal tubule the concentration of mannitol will rise, further increasing the osmotic force it exerts and decreasing the movement of water out of this segments. At first, sodium reabsorption will continue, and there will be a progressive decline in the concentration of sodium in the tubular fluid. When the concentration of sodium falls below 100 mEq/liter, the backflux of sodium into the tubular lumen will equal its active reabsorption and the net movement of sodium out of the proximal tubule will cease. Hence, the presence of a nonreabsorbable solute such as mannitol not only impairs water reabsorption out of the proximal tubule but also reduces the amount of sodium reabsorbed in this segment. This is graphically illustrated in Figure 14. This effect may suppress proximal tubule reabsorption of filtered sodium and water by as much as 10% and 20%, respectively. The movement of water out of the descending

Table VII. Classification of Causes of Hypernatremia Due to Renal Water Loss

I. Increased excretion of solute and obligate water loss (secondary polyuria)
   A. Increased solute load
      1. Osmotic diuretics
         a. Mannitol
         b. Angiographic dyes
      2. Glycosuria–diabetes mellitus
      3. Urea
         a. Recovery phase of acute oliguric renal failure
         b. High protein intake
            i. Tube feedings
            ii. Infant formula preparation
         c. Postobstructive diuresis
      4. Cholestyramine
   B. Impaired renal tubular reabsorption of NaCl
      1. Nonoliguric renal failure
      2. Diuretic therapy
      3. Interstitial disease, e.g., pyelonephritis
II. Impaired reabsorption of free water (primary polyuria)
   A. Vasopressin deficiency (vasopressin-deficient diabetes insipidus)
      1. Idiopathic
      2. Posthypophysectomy
         a. Surgical
         b. Traumatic
      3. Tumor
         a. Metastatic
         b. Primary
      4. Miscellaneous
         a. Granuloma
         b. Histiocytosis
         c. Vascular
         d. Infection
   B. Renal defect (vasopressin-resistant diabetes insipidus)
      1. Congenital
      2. Acquired
         a. Renal tubular damage
            i. Chronic interstitial–infiltrative disease
               (a) Amyloid
               (b) Multiple myloma
               (c) Pyelonephritis
               (d) Sjögren's syndrome
            ii. Distal tubular and/or collecting duct defects
               (a) Sickle cell trait/disease
               (b) Nephrocalcinosis
               (c) Chronic obstructive uropathy
               (d) Hypokalemic nephropathy
               (e) Medullary cystic diseases
               (f) Polycystic diseases
         b. Hormone interference at receptor site
            i. Drugs
               (a) Demeclocycline
               (b) Lithium carbonate
               (c) Methoxyflurane
               (d) Dextropropoxyphene
            ii. Hypercalciuria

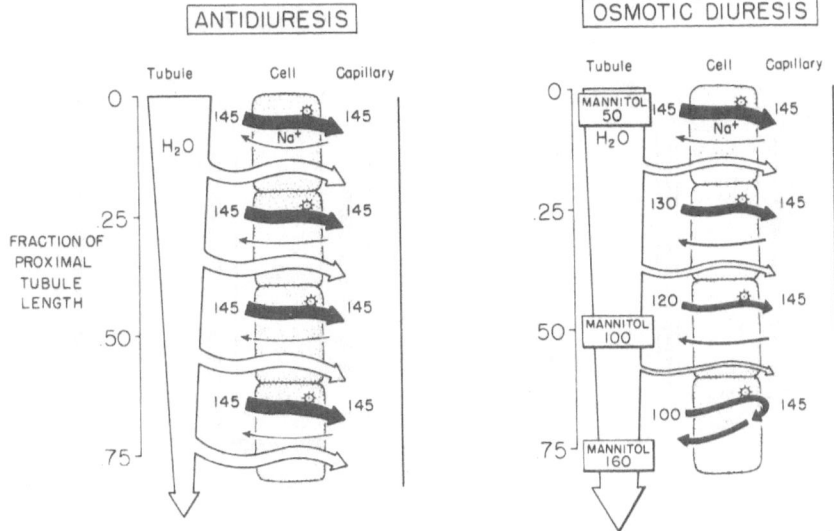

Figure 14. Schematic representation of sodium and water reabsorption in the proximal tubule during antidiuresis and osmotic diuresis. During antidiuresis, the concentration of sodium in the tubular fluid does not change; during osmotic diuresis, the presence of mannitol in the filtrate (50 mM) reduces water reabsorption, and thus as sodium reabsorption proceeds, tubular fluid sodium concentration falls progressively. (Reprinted with permission from Gennari, F. J., and Kassirer, J. P.: Osmotic diuresis. *N. Engl. J. Med.* 291:714–720, 1974.)

limb of the loop of Henle is also impaired during an osmotic diuresis. This is due to a decrease in the osmolality of the medullary interstitium. The decline in medullary osmolality is the result of a number of factors. One factor is that the concentration of sodium in luminal fluid may be reduced by as much as 50%. Thus, the concentration gradient favoring the movement of sodium out of the ascending segment of the loop is significantly decreased, and the mechanism of countercurrent multiplication will be impaired to the extent that this driving force is reduced. Second, medullary blood flow is increased and therefore solute is removed at a greater rate from the medulla. The increase in blood flow is probably the result of a direct effect of mannitol on the blood vessels. A final reason for a decrease in papillary osmolality is a redistribution of SNGFR. During a mannitol diuresis, SNGFR of surface nephrons tends to rise while that of deep nephrons may fall by as much as 50%. Thus, countercurrent multiplication will be diminished due to an absolute reduction in the delivery and therefore the deposition of NaCl and urea in the medullary interstitium. Although the active reabsorption of sodium and chloride out of the thick ascending limb may be impaired during a mannitol diuresis, it has been shown that the concentration of sodium in luminal fluid will fall below 100 mEq/liter in this segment and free water will be formed. However, the reabsorption of this water in the distal and cortical collecting tubule is impaired by the presence of the osmotically active mannitol. That is, the water obligated by the presence of mannitol is not recaptured in these segments. The consequence of these alterations in the

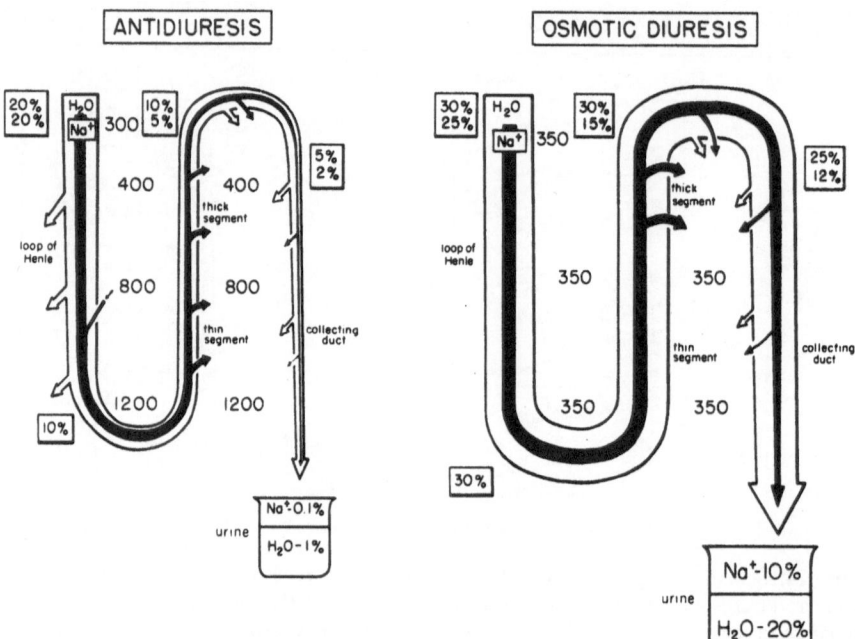

Figure 15. A simplified model of sodium and water reabsorption along the loop of Henle, distal tubule, and collecting duct during antidiuresis and osmotic diuresis. Note that while sodium and water excretion are strikingly increased, water loss is significantly greater than that of sodium, thus making the development of hypernatremia likely.

renal tubular handling of sodium during the infusion of mannitol is that losses of water exceed those of sodium and the individual may become hypernatremic (see Figure 15).

While the infusion of mannitol is the best example of an osmotic diuresis, it is not a frequent cause of secondary polyuria. Probably the most common cause is the development of glycosuria in patients with poorly controlled diabetes mellitus. In this setting, the amount of glucose filtered through the glomerulus per unit time (i.e., the filtered load of glucose) exceeds the reabsorptive capacity of the renal tubule. As in the case of mannitol, the unreabsorbed glucose impedes the isoosmotic movement of water out of the proximal tubule and results in a significant reduction in the reabsorption of sodium and water along the renal tubule.

Angiographic dyes may produce similar results. These dyes are of small molecular size and are not reabsorbed by the renal tubule. Thus hypernatremic dehydration can occur in patients given large intravenous doses of radiographic contrast material during diagnostic procedures. However this is not likely to occur unless the studies are performed in patients who have a restricted sodium and water intake.

Urea is another small molecule that is not well reabosrbed in the proximal tubule. Therefore, high concentrations of urea in blood give rise to an increase of obligate water excretion and hypernatremia may develop. The following example illustrates how hypernatremia can result from a urea-induced diuresis. A 70-year-old man receiving a high-protein tube feeding develops a serum sodium concentration of 154 mEq/liter. The urinary volume is 1500 ml/24 hr and has an osmolality of 520 mOsm/kg H_2O. The tube feeding is given in 1500 ml of water and contains 80 g protein, 50 g glucose, 100 mEq NaCl, and 50 mEq KCl. The metabolism of the protein in the feeding generates 480 mOsm of urea. The sodium plus potassium and accompanying anions add another 300 mOsm of solute. Thus the osmolar load from such an intake is 780 mOsm/24 hr. If the maximal urine osmolality that this patient can achieve in this setting, approximates 500 mOsm/kg H_2O, the minimum volume of urine needed to excrete the solute load is 1500 ml/day. Because of an additional 700 ml of insensible water loss, 2300 ml of water are needed for fluid replacement. On the regimen described, the patient incurred a water deficit of 800 ml/day and became hypernatremic. In infants this is a common mechanism by which hypernatremia develops. It usually occurs as a consequence of an inappropriate intake of high-solute-containing formula preparations. This was particularly true in the early sixties and was an important cause of "crib deaths." The propensity to develop hypernatremia in these patients is worsened during illnesses which result in diarrhea. Another example is patients in the recovery phase of acute oliguric renal failure. This is especially true in those who have been treated conservatively (i.e., without dialysis) and who will therefore have abnormally high circulating levels of urea. Such patients may move rapidly from the oliguric to the polyuric phase and go into a state of negative water balance.

From the above discussion it is apparent that the diagnosis of secondary polyuria can be established rather easily. First, renal water excretion will be inappropriately high in both absolute (>2 liters) and fractional terms (>1%). Second, the concentration of sodium will be in the range of 50–70 mEq/liter, and the fraction of the filtered load of sodium excreted will be greater than 1% and may exceed 10%.

Hypernatremia due to loss of free water by the kidney (primary polyuria). As stated previously, hypernatremia may occur when free water reabsorption is impaired. Since under normal circumstances free-water formation is equal to 15% of GFR or 18–20 ml/min, volume depletion and hypernatremia can develop rapidly when intake is inadequate and water reabsorption is impaired. By definition, the urine is hypotonic when hypernatremia is due to primary polyuria. However, the level of hypotonicity will depend largely on the degree of impairment in the concentrating segment. In contrast to secondary polyuria, sodium excretion will be in the normal range, that is, less than 1% of the amount filtered. Table VII lists the conditions that produce decreased free-water reabsorption or primary polyuria. These conditions can be divided into two groups: (1) those patients in whom free-water loss is due to low or absent circulating levels of ADH (*vasopressin-deficient diabetes insipidus*) and (2) those cases where the loss is due to a defect in the response of the concentrating segment to ADH (*vasopressin-resistant* or *nephrogenic diabetes insipidus*).

Vasopressin-deficient diabetes insipidus is due to inappropriately low or absent levels of circulating ADH. Probably the most frequent cause of a vasopressin deficiency is hypophysectomy either as a consequence of treating diabetic retinopathy or due to traumatic injury in an auto accident. Craniopharyngioma is the tumor most frequently associated with diabetes insipidus with considerably fewer cases being the result of gliomas and vascular tumors. Metastatic tumor is rarely a cause. Pituitary tumors do not cause diabetes insipidus unless they extend beyond the sella turcica and either invade the hypothalamus or destroy the supraoptic nuclei by pressure. In less than 10% of patients, the cause is an infiltrative lesion like histiocytosis, sarcoid, or tuberculosis. Approximately 30% of the patients with vasopressin-deficient diabetes insipidus will have no known etiology. The bulk of these patients are young females who give a history of an abrupt onset of polyuria that may exceed 10 liters per day. Less than 3% of these patients have a familial incidence. And when they do, they will differ from the majority in that the onset of polyuria develops during infancy or early childhood. Aside from the annoyance of the polyuric state, a profound increase in thirst and a particular craving for cold water, such patients will be relatively healthy. In these patients hypernatremia develops only when insensible water loss is increased and/or intake is poor (i.e., gastrointestinal illness and postoperative states). Patients with long-standing polyuria may develop marked bladder and ureteral dilatation that occasionally leads to impaired renal function.

The causes of nephrogenic diabetes insipidus (NDI) are divided into a small group of patients who have an inherited defect in the response of the collecting duct to ADH and a much larger group whose resistance to ADH is a consequence of a wide variety of acquired factors. Congenital NDI is a rare hereditary disease which appears to be sex linked and of dominant inheritance. In its complete form, it is seen only in the male offspring, but may be variably present in female carriers. If the child is to develop normally the diagnosis must be made shortly after birth. Failure to make an early diagnosis is likely to result in multiple episodes of hypernatremia during acute and febrile illnesses. Such episodes are thought to be the reason for the high incidence of mental retardation in children with this disease. In congenital NDI, the defect in collecting duct function appears to be the result of failure to generate cyclic AMP in response to circulating ADH (see Figure 9).

As stated previously, there are great number of causes for acquired NDI. Those renal diseases (medullary cystic disease, chronic obstructive nephropathy, nephrocalcinosis, and polycystic kidney disease) which preferentially affect the distal tubule and the collecting duct segments of the nephron are frequently associated with some degree of unresponsiveness to vasopressin. And, in a broader sense, relative impairment in concentrating ability is likely to be seen in chronic renal disease that preferentially affects tubular and medullary structures. Thus, chronic interstitial and infiltrative diseases like amyloid are likely to be associated with some degree of polyuria. The urinary concentrating defect seen in patients with sickle cell trait or disease is thought to be due to impaired medullary collecting duct function. The relative hypoxia of the medulla is postulated to cause sickling of erythrocytes and increased vascular resistance to blood flow. Medullary blood flow is therefore reduced and oxygen content falls further. Eventually sludging of erythrocytes occurs and gives rise to tissue anoxia and ultimate destruction of medullary structures. Such changes are said to be the pathogenesis of papillary necrosis in these patients and obviously will have a profound effect in maximal urine osmolality achieved by such individuals. In addition, prolonged and profound hypokalemia impairs the renal response to ADH. This state is not immediately improved by potassium repletion, but improvement seems more related to the resolution of the histological lesions found in the distal tubules.

In recent years, a number of pharmacologic agents have been shown to block the response of the collecting duct to arginine vasopressin (see Table VII and Figure 9). This effect is usually reversible shortly after the offending agent is discontinued. It has been shown in animal studies that in the presence of lithium carbonate or demeclocycline, cyclic AMP production by the collecting duct is reduced when ADH is given. It is not known how propoxyphene interferes with the response of the collecting duct to ADH.

A marked increase in the urinary excretion of calcium may impair water reabsorption by the concentrating segment. Acutely, it is thought that hypercalciuria blocks cyclic AMP production in response to circulating ADH and alters the polar structure of water. This effect is rapidly reversible. On the other hand, chronic hypercalciuria may cause irreversible damage to the distal tubule and the collecting duct and lead to the development of nephrocalcinosis. This change results in a permanent concentrating defect. It has been postulated that the reversible NDI seen after the administration of the anesthestic methoxyflurane is a consequence of the hypercalciuria produced by this agent.

iv. Gastrointestinal Losses. The sodium concentration in gastrointestinal fluid is always lower than that of plasma. Thus, when losses occur through this route, water is lost in excess of sodium and hypernatremia may develop. When vomiting is copious, as in pyloric obstruction, hypernatremia develops not only as a consequence of loss of gastric secretions which are low in sodium (10–89 mEq/liter) but because free water intake is impaired. In this setting, hydrogen ion loss is excessive and hypernatremia may be complicated by the development of a metabolic alkalosis (see Chapter 8). On the other hand, duodenal drainage, while still relatively low in sodium content when compared to that of plasma (110–120 mEq/liter), contains higher concentrations of bicarbonate. Thus, duodenal drainage in the absence of replacement will result in a volume deficit characterized by hypernatremia and a normal anion gap metabolic acidosis.

Diarrhea may result in a disproportionately greater loss of water than sodium. The magnitude of the free-water loss will depend on the severity and mechanism by which diarrhea develops. When it is a consequence of osmotic factors, water loss is more likely to be greater than that of sodium. Under normal circumstances, sodium and water absorption begins in the jejunum. Here, absorption is isosmotic due to the high water permeability of the mucosa. In both ileum and colon, sodium absorption continues but in excess of water. And, under normal circumstances, the concentration of sodium in stool water may approach 1 mEq/liter. When poorly absorbed but osmotically active solute is ingested, movement of water out of the lumen of the jejunum is impeded and, as in the proximal tubule, sodium transport is diminished when the concentration of sodium in the lumen falls below the maximal chemical gradient. Thus, delivery of water and sodium to the ileum and colon is increased and while sodium continues to be absorbed, the volume delivered exceeds these segments' absorptive capabilities and diarrhea develops. The net effect is a greater loss of water than sodium. In adults, osmotically induced diarrhea may occur as a consequence of tube feedings with a high solute content. Lactulose, when utilized to treat hepatic encephalopathy, may produce diarrhea and hypernatremia by the same mechanism.

When diarrhea is secretory in origin, the volume deficit may be striking although sodium and water loss are more likely to be proportional. In this case, an enterotoxin produced by a bacterial agent stimulates the small bowel to secrete anions, chiefly bicarbonate. The high content of these anions in luminal fluid creates an electrical gradient for the movement of cations out of the intravascular space and an osmotic gradient for water extraction. As with osmotically induced diarrhea, the effectiveness of electrolyte absorption by the colon will be dependent on the rate of delivery. In childhood, diarrhea is an important cause of hypernatremia. In most instances, the primary mechanism is secretory in nature; however, fluid losses may be compounded when therapy is inappropriate. Large quantities of boiled milk (a home remedy for infantile diarrhea) result in an increased content of osmotically active solute in the stool. When these patients are given solutions containing high concentrations of electrolytes or glucose, losses of free water in the stool may be increased by a similar mechanism.

Despite the fact that the colon is able to maintain high osmotic gradients, hypernatremia has developed in patients given hypertonic enemas. Hypertonic sodium-containing enemas (Fleets and Tudvad) have a sodium concentrations in excess of 2000 mEq/liter and will result in the net movement of water out the intravascular space and into the lumen. This is the basis for their action. However, profound hypernatremia may develop in the patient who has a dilated or chronically diseased colon (e.g., toxic megacolon). Similarly, gastrographin is an osmotically active solute and has occasionally been associated with hypernatremia when used in the radiologic evaluation of the large bowel.

Finally, hypernatremia may develop in patients undergoing peritoneal dialysis. This can occur as a consequence of the relatively higher osmolality of the dialysis fluid when compared to plasma. It is likely to occur when solutions containing greater than 4% glucose are used.

b. Hypernatremia Due to Excess Sodium Intake

When sodium intake is increased in an individual who is in sodium balance, it follows that those mechanisms which maintain ECF volume within a narrow range will come into play and the sodium ingested will be excreted in the urine. Thus, obligate water loss will increase. If water intake is not increased in proportion to sodium intake, hypernatremia will develop. This is most commonly seen in the pediatric age group and occurs when infant formula has been mistakenly prepared with NaCl instead of sugar and when hypertonic solutions are given as emetics. In adults, it is most frequently associated with the ingestion of NaCl tablets by individuals with increased insensible water loss due to sweating but in whom free water intake is not increased appropriately. Similarly, the ingestion of sea water increases obligate water losses. The sodium concentration in sea water is 450–500 mEq/liter and total osmolality may exceed 1200 mOsm/kg. Thus the ingestion of 100 ml of sea water would require the obligate excretion of *greater* than 100 ml of urine.

Similarly, hypertonic saline given parentally results in the extraction of water from the intracellular compartment, an osmotic diuresis results, and hypernatremic dehydration develops. This rare cause of hypernatremia is most commonly associated with the administration of excessive quantities of $NaHCO_3$ in the treatment of cardiac arrest and the acute respiratory distress syndrome. Although, the intra-amniotic instillation of excessive quantities of hypertonic saline (20%) for the mid-trimester termination of pregnancy may become a more common cause of hypernatremia.

Finally, mild elevations in sodium concentrations may occur in Cushings disease and primary aldosteronism. In these patients, the small change in sodium concentration may be due to the more avid distal tubular reabsorption of sodium and to a slight increase in the osmotic threshold. This later effect is a consequence of a more rapid metabolism of cAMP produced by ADH in collecting duct cells (see Figure 9).

3. Therapeutic Approach to Hypernatremia

The three important determinants in the therapeutic approach to hypernatremia are (1) the symptoms exhibited by the patient, (2) the volume status of the individual, and (3) if a water deficit exists whether it is associated with a reduction in total body sodium (see Figure 16). An equally important consideration in the treatment of this electrolyte abnormality is the rate at which the water deficit should be replaced. Although controversial, it is felt that rapid hydration can result in cerebral edema. It is thought that during this process, the dilution of plasma occurs at a rate faster than that of the ICF of cerebral tissue. Thus an osmotic gradient is established which favors the movement of water into the cells of the central nervous system, and as a consequence, coma, convulsions, and permanent neurological damage can result. It has been reported by some, although not substantiated by others,

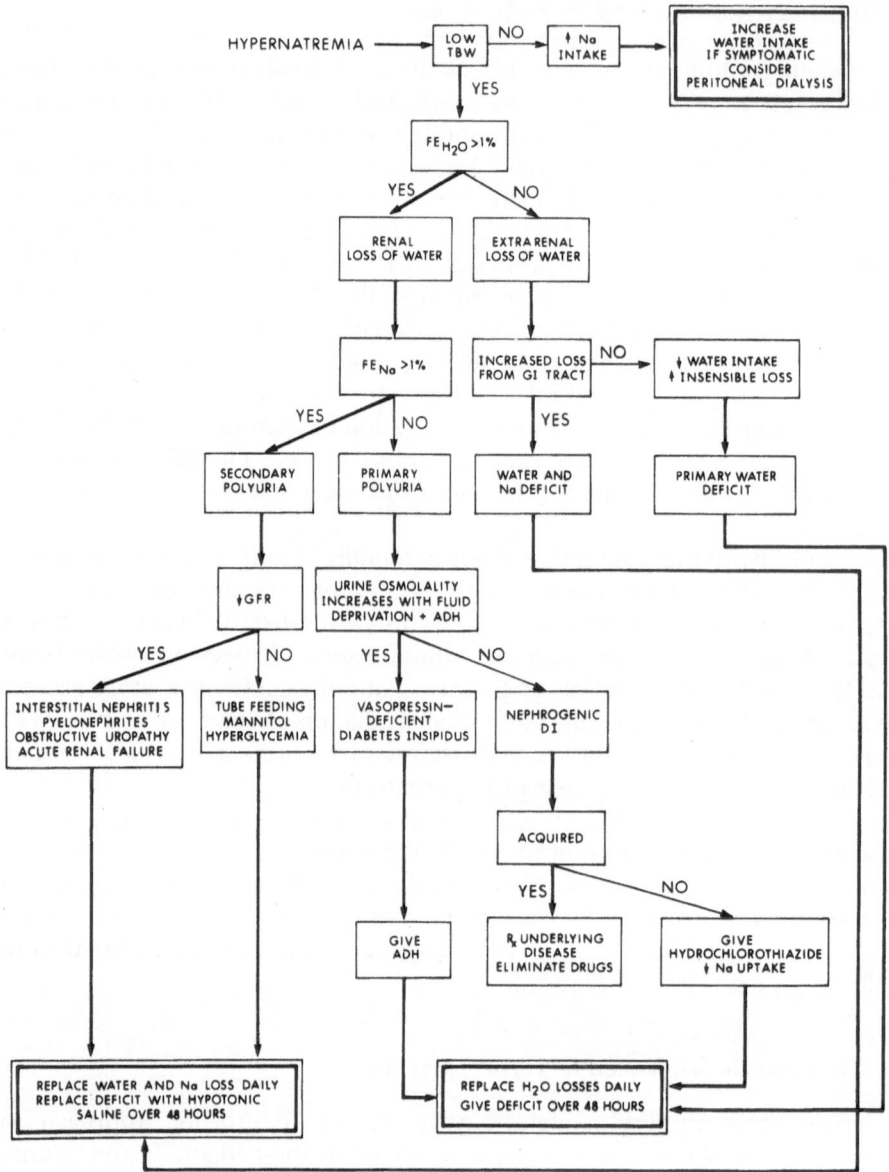

Figure 16. Schema for the diagnostic and therapeutic approach to hypernatremia.

that 40% of hypernatremic children develop neurologic symptoms following rapid replacement of a water deficit (less than 48 hr). Although there are no studies which demonstrate that immediate correction of the hypernatremic state in the adult produces cerebral edema, slow replacement of water losses (over 48 hr) is recommended in both age groups.

In patients who are hypernatremic, because insensible water loss has not been replaced adequately, urine output is sharply diminished and sodium conservation is maximal. The urine sodium concentration is usually less than 10 mEq/liter and the osmolality is substantially greater than that of plasma. These individuals have sustained, primarily, a water loss and more than likely the sodium deficit will be less than 25 mEq/day. In such patients, the difference between the true and present weight can be used as a first approximation of the patient's water deficit. When the initial weight is unknown, the water required to correct the hypernatremic state can be estimated from the following calculation:

$$\text{Water deficit} = \left[\frac{P_{Na} \text{ actual}}{P_{Na} \text{ desired}} \right] \times \text{TBW} - \text{TBW}$$

Where TBW equals 60% of the present weight (kg). For example: a 70-year-old woman found unconscious in her apartment is brought to the emergency room where she is found to have postural hypotension, a temperature of 40°C, and acute pyelonephritis. On admission, her weight was 60 kg. Pertinent laboratory studies included a serum sodium of 165 mEq/liter. In this patient, water loss is the primary deficit and is due to increased insensible losses from fever. Her total water deficit can be estimated as follows:

$$\text{Water deficit} = \frac{165}{140} \times (0.6 \times 60 \text{ kg}) - 0.6 \times 60 \text{ kg}$$
$$= 1.18 \times 36 - 36$$
$$= 42.5 - 36$$
$$= 6.5 \text{ liters}$$

In adipsic patients, regimental water intake is essential and the cautious use of vasopressin analogs may be necessary.

In patients who are hypernatremic because of renal loss of free water, urine osmolality is low and volume will be inappropriately high. If water loss is profound, the patient may be oliguric and urine osmolality will approach that of plasma. In this setting, GFR is markedly reduced and therefore less free water is made. Since tubular flow is reduced, luminal fluid is more likely to come into equilibrium with the surrounding interstitium and more free water is reabsorbed. In these patients, the first clue to the source of water loss may be discovered when rehydration is attempted and there is an inappropriate rise in urine output and decline in urine osmolality.

The therapeutic approach to these patients is threefold: (1) replace the water deficit, (2) keep up with losses, and (3) reduce the renal excretion of free water. To this latter end, it is important to differentiate vasopressin-deficient from vasopressin-resistant diabetes insipidus. The best and most accepted approach to this problem is a fluid deprivation test followed by the administration of vasopressin. The first part of the test is designed to dehydrate the patient and maximally stimulate the endogenous production of ADH. At the onset of the test, urine and plasma osmolality are measured. Then urine osmolality should be determined hourly until the change is less than 50 mOsm/hr. This usually requires 12–16 hr of water deprivation. It is essential to monitor patients carefully during this interval; such patients may become profoundly dehydrated. Hence, this portion of the test should be discontinued when the patient has lost 5% of body weight. Once urine osmolality is stabilized or weight loss is significant, 5 units of aqueous vasopressin should be administered subcutaneously. Plasma and urine are collected for the measurement of osmolality 60 minutes later. When this test is administered to normal subjects, maximal urine osmolality is achieved in 16–18 hr and ranges between 850 and 1,440 mOsm/kg. Plasma osmolality may increase slightly. After the administration of ADH, urine osmolality will either fall slightly or not change. The reason for this is that maximal stimulation of endogenous ADH release (16 hr of fluid deprivation) brings the final urine into equilibrium with the papillary interstitium and thus additional amounts of vasopressin have no effect. Thus, the magnitude of the change in osmolality after ADH administration is usually less than 5%. In patients with vasopressin-deficient diabetes insipidus, urine osmolality will seldom rise above plasma osmolality after fluid deprivation. In most instances, maximal urine osmolality will be less than 200 mOsm/kg. On the other hand, there will be a striking rise in plasma osmolality, frequently above 300 mOsm/kg, and the patient will become hypernatremic. After vasopressin administration, the urine osmolality will rise significantly. However, the osmolality of urine will not be as great as in normal subjects. Most importantly, the increase in urine osmoality, after ADH in vasopressin-deficient diabetes insipidus, is likely to be greater than 180% baseline values. In patients with a partial defect in ADH release, dehydration will produce an increase in urine osmolality, perhaps to 400 mOsm/kg. However, in these patients urine osmolality will increase further after ADH is given, although the magnitude of the increase is considerably less than in those patients with complete absence of ADH (approximately 25%). As is predicted, patients with *vasopressin-resistant* diabetes insipidus continue to produce hypotonic urine after prolonged water deprivation and following the administration of vasopressin.

Other tests have been used to differentiate between these causes of primary polyuria; however, a number of factors might alter the patient's response and frequently make these tests difficult to interpret. One such tests is the use of nicotine to stimulate the release of endogenous vasopressin. This test is frequently associated with profound nausea and vomiting, which may in turn adversely affect renal blood flow and therefore GFR. Infusions of hypertonic saline will increase ADH production but pose a danger to patients with a borderline compensated cardiovascular status. Further, in well-hydrated patients, urine flow may actually increase. Therefore in these patients $T^c_{H_2O}$ must also be measured. Probably the most helpful new diagnostic tool is the measurement, by radioimmunoassay, of plasma arginine vasopressin. Such measurements will obviously be important in differentiating individuals with partial defects in ADH increase and release from those with mild degrees of NDI (see Figure 4). As is depicted in Table VIII, with the use of these studies and other measurements previously mentioned, renal

Table VIII. Systematic Approach to the Differential Diagnosis of Hypernatremia
Due to Renal Water Loss

Polyuric state	PAV^a	$U/P_{osm}^{\ b}$	$FE_{Na}^{\ c}$	P_{osm} after H_2O deprivation^d	
				Before ADH	After ADH
Secondary polyuria (obligate water loss)	↑	> or = 1	10%–15%		
Primary polyuria (free-water loss)			>1.0%		
ADH-deficient	↓	<1		NC	↑
ADH-resistant	↑	<1		NC	NC

^{a} PAV, plasma arginine vasopressin. ^{c} FE_{Na}, fraction of filtered sodium excreted.
^{b} U/P_{osm}, ratio of urine to plasma osmolality. ^{d} P_{osm}, plasma osmolality; NC, no change.

loss of water may be approached systematically and the site of impaired water reabsorption can be ascertained. In some instances, it will be necessary to do additional studies to determine which of the specific causes listed in Table VII is the reason for the resulting polyuria.

While the reason for the development of hypernatremia in this group of patients is readily apparent, management may be complicated in patients who have been subjected to surgical or traumatic hypophysectomy; urine output may exhibit a triphasic pattern that is characterized by an initial marked increase in urine output and thus a propensity toward the development of hypernatremia. This may then be followed, in hours to days, by a period when urine output returns to normal and urine osmolality markedly increases. This interphase is transient, lasting several days, and is proabably due to release of ADH from degenerating nerve fibers located in the hypothalamic stalk. Hence, the level of ADH in plasma during the interphase period is *not* under physiologic control. Careful management is essential in this period since patients are prone to progress from a hypernatremic state to acute water intoxication if fluid intake is not reduced appropriately. Ultimately, the circulating vasopressin is catabolized and these patients enter the third phase characterized by a marked increase in renal free-water loss.

Clearly, if a diagnosis of vasopressin-deficient diabetes insipidus is made, equally important to the replacement of ongoing water losses is the administration of vasopressin or one of its analogs to decrease free-water excretion. These agents may be given either by injections or insufflation. On the other hand, if a diagnosis of vasopressin-resistant diabetes insipidus is made, the mainstay of therapy is directed toward decreasing the formation of free water. This is usually done by administering hydrochlorothiazide and limiting the salt intake of the patient. This should result in decreased intravascular volume and decrease delivery of sodium to the ascending limb and thereby decrease free water formation.

In those patients in whom the water deficit is accompanied by a deficit of sodium, it is important to determine the site of loss. That is, patients who have a renal loss of sodium will have an inappropriately high rate of urine flow associated with a high fractional excretion of sodium. Those with extrarenal losses (i.e., diarrhea and vomiting) will be conserving sodium and water maximally. That is, the fraction of the filtered load of water and sodium appearing in the urine will be less than 1%. In these patients, frequently a first step in the correction of the hypernatremic state is to restore intravascular volume with a solution of hypotonic saline. In acidotic patients part of the sodium deficit should be given as $NaHCO_3$. Once blood pressure and the manifestations of cardiovascular depletion have been corrected, the water deficit can be reestimated and the remaining fluid and sodium deficit replaced over a 48-hr period.

In all patients who have primarily a water deficit, it is important to remember that to correct the hypernatremic state water replacement must include not only the deficit but the amount of the ongoing water loss. Thus if the patient receiving the tube feeding (see page 187) weighs 68 kg, the water deficit would be

$$\text{Water deficit} = \left[\frac{154}{140} (0.6 \times 68) \right] - 0.6 \times 68$$

$$= [1.10 \times 40.8] - 40.8$$

$$= 44.9 - 40.8$$

$$= 4.1 \text{ liters}$$

However, in order to correct the water deficit over 48 hr the patient would require

$$\underset{\text{(Water replacement)}}{2.05 \text{ liters}} + \underset{\text{(Obligate water)}}{2.3 \text{ liters}} = 4.35 \text{ liters of water per day for 2 days}$$

In the rare cases where hypernatremia is a consequence of excess sodium intake and there is no evidence of volume depletion, access to a sufficient amount of free water to allow for the excretion of the excess sodium may be sufficient. However, if hypernatremia is severe and the patient is symptomatic, dialysis, usually peritoneal, is the only effective mode of therapy. In this instance, the dialysate used must have an osmolality greater than that of the patient's plasma. The usual dialysis fluid has an osmolality of 360 mOsm/kg. In patients that are profoundly hypernatremic, plasma osmolality may be greater than this; thus if the usual dialysate is introduced into the peritoneum, fluid may actually leave this space and enter the intravascular space resulting in hypervolemia and cardiac decompensation. Thus, prior to the institution of peritoneal dialysis, it is essential to insure that the osmolality of the dialysate exceeds that of plasma. This can be accomplished by increasing the glucose concentration in the solution. In this setting, the sodium will move down its concentration gradient into the peritoneum and excess sodium can be removed in a relatively efficient fashion.

SUGGESTED READINGS

Physiologic Considerations

Anderson, B.: Regulation of water intake. *Physiol. Rev.* 58:582, 1978.

Fitzsimons, J. T.: Thirst. *Physiol. Rev.* 52:468, 1972.

Jamison, R.: Urinary concentration and dilution, in Brenner, B. M., and Rector, F. C., Jr. (eds.): *The Kidney*, Second edition. W. B. Saunders, Philadelphia, 1981, pp. 495–551.

Schrier, R. W., and Berl, T.: Nonosmolar factors affecting renal water excretion. *N. Engl. J. Med.* 292:81, 1975.

Wolf, A. V.: *Thirst: Physiology of the Urge to Drink and Problems of Water Lack.* C. C. Thomas, Springfield, Illinois, 1958.

Pathophysiologic Considerations

General

Arieff, A. I., and Guisado, R.: Effects on the central nervous system of hypernatremic and hyponatremic states. *Kidney Int.* 10:104, 1976.

Arieff, A. I., Llach, F., and Massry, S. G.: Neurological manifestations and morbidity of hyponatremia: correlation with brain water and electrolytes. *Medicine* 55:121, 1976.

Bay, W. H., and Ferris, T. F.: Hypernatremia and hyponatremia: disorders of tonicity. *Geriatrics* 31:53, 1976.

Berl, T., Anderson, R., McDonald, K., and Schrier, R.: Clinical disorders of water metabolism. *Kidney Int.* 10:117, 1976.

Hays, R., and Levine, S.: Pathophysiology of water metabolism, in Brenner, B. M., and Rector, F. C., Jr. (eds.): *The Kidney*, Second edition. W. B. Saunders, Philadelphia, 1981, pp. 777–841.

Hyponatremia

Anderson, R. J., Cadnapaphornchai, P., Harbottle, J. A., McDonald, K. M., and Schrier, R. W.: Mechanism of effect of thoracic inferior vena cava constriction on renal water excretion. *J. Clin. Invest.* 54:1473, 1974.

Barlow, E. D., and DeWardener, H. E.: Compulsive water drinking. *Q. J. Med.* 28:235, 1959.

Bartter, F. C.: The syndrome of inappropriate secretion of antidiuretic hormone (SIADH), in Dowling, H. F. (ed.): *Disease-a-Month.* Year Book Medical Publishers, Chicago, 1973.

Cannon, P. J.: The kidney in heart failure. *N. Engl. J. Med.* 296:26, 1977.

Cooke, C. R., Turin, M. D., and Walker, W. G.: The syndrome of inappropriate antidiuretic hormone secretion (SIADH): pathophysiologic mechanisms in solute and volume regulation. *Medicine* 58:240, 1979.

DeFronzo, R. A., Goldberg, M., and Agus, Z. S.: Normal diluting capacity in hyponatremic patients. *Ann. Intern. Med.* 84:538, 1976.

Discala, V. A., and Kinney, M. J.: Effects of myxedema on the renal diluting and concentrating mechanism. *Am. J. Med.* 50:325, 1971.

Fichman, M. P., Vorherr, H., Kleeman, C. R., and Telfer, N.: Diuretic-induced hyponatremia. *Ann. Intern. Med.* 75:853, 1971.

Flear, C. T. G., and Singh, C. M.: Hyponatremia and sick cells. *Br. J. Anaesth.* 45:976, 1973.

Forrest, J. N., Jr., Cox, M., Hong, C., Morrison, G., Bia, M., and Singer, I.: Superiority of demeclocycline over lithium in the treatment of chronic syndrome of inappropriate secretion of antidiuretic hormone. *N. Engl. J. Med.* 298:173, 1978.

Hantman, D., Rossier, B., Zohlman, R., and Schrier, R.: Rapid correction of hyponatremia in the syndrome of inappropriate secretion of antidiuretic hormone. *Ann. Intern. Med.* 78:870, 1973.

Macaron, C., and Famuyiwa, O.: Hyponatremia of hypothyroidism. *Arch. Intern. Med.* 138:820, 1978.

Michael, U. F., Kelley, J., Alpert, H., and Vaamonde, C. A.: Role of distal delivery of filtrate in impaired renal dilution of the hypothyroid rat. *Am. J. Physiol.* 230:699, 1976.

Moses, A. M., and Miller, M.: Drug-induced dilutional hyponatremia. *N. Engl. J. Med.* 23:1234, 1974.

Thomas, T. H., Morgan, D. B., and Swaminathan, R.: Severe hyponatraemia. *Lancet*, Saturday, March 25, 1978, pp. 621.

Hypernatremia

Banister, A., Matin-Siddiqi, S. A., and Hatcher, G. W.: Treatment of hypernatraemic dehydration in infancy. *Arch. Dis. Child.* 50:179, 1975.

Bode, H. H., and Crawford, J. D.: Nephrogenic diabetes insipidus in North America—the Hopewell hypothesis. *N. Engl. J. Med.* 280:750, 1969.

Coggins, C. H., and Leaf, A.: Diabetes insipidus. *Am. J. Med.* 42:807, 1967.

Conley, S. B., Brocklebank, J. T., Taylor, I. T., and Robson, A. M.: Recurrent hypernatremia: A proposed mechanism in a patient with absence of thirst and abnormal excretion of water. *J. Pediatr.* 89;898, 1976.

Epstein, M.: Deranged sodium homeostasis in cirrhosis. *Gastroenterology* 76:622, 1979.

Gennari, F. J., and Kassirer, J. P.: Osmotic diuresis. *N. Engl. J. Med.* 291:714, 1974.

Hogan, G. R.: Hypernatremia—Problems in management. *Pediatr. Clin. N. Am.* 23:569, 1976.

Ross, E. J., and Christie, S. B. M.: Hypernatremia. *Medicine* 48:441, 1969.

Pathophysiology of Potassium Metabolism

HECTOR J. RODRIGUEZ and SAULO KLAHR

I. INTRODUCTION

The daily intake of potassium in an average American diet is about 100 mEq. Virtually all of the potassium ingested is absorbed by the gut (less than 10 mEq are excreted in stools) and maintenance of external balance requires the daily renal excretion of an amount of potassium identical to that absorbed from the gut. Potassium is the major cation of the intracellular fluid space. The body distribution of potassium is depicted in Figure 1. Total body content of potassium is approximately 3700 mEq, of which only 50–70 mEq are distributed in the extracellular fluid (ECF), the remainder being confined to the intracellular fluid space (ICF). The bulk of the ICF potassium is contained in muscle cells ($\simeq$2800 mEq) and comparably smaller quantities are distributed in skin ($\simeq$500 mEq), liver cells ($\simeq$100 mEq), and red blood cells ($\simeq$250 mEq).

The predominant intracellular localization of potassium is reflected in the fact that the concentration of this ion in the ICF (about 150 mEq/liter) is substantially greater than the concentration in the ECF (about 5 mEq/liter).

HECTOR J. RODRIGUEZ • Department of Medicine, Washington University School of Medicine, St. Louis, Missouri 63110. *Present address:* 9400 Brighton Way, Beverly Hills, California 90210.   SAULO KLAHR • Department of Medicine, Washington University School of Medicine, St. Louis, Missouri 63110.

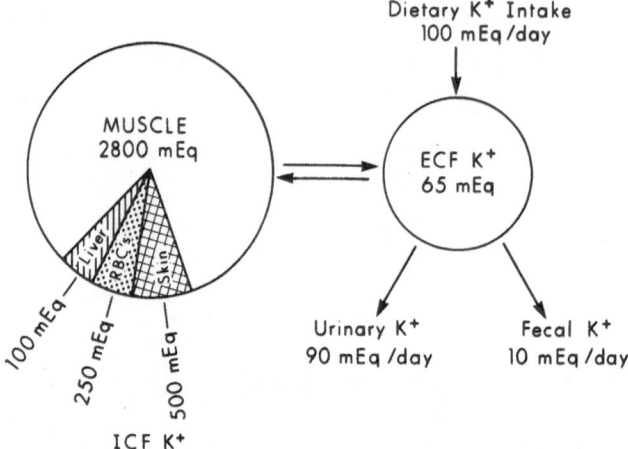

Figure 1. Dietary intake, excretion, and distribution of potassium.

This is in contrast to sodium, whose concentration is higher in the ECF (Table I). The cell membranes, which separate the ECF from the ICF, allow the diffusion of potassium and, to a lesser extent sodium, down their chemical concentrations differences. Thus, the maintenance of these asymmetric ionic concentrations requires the "pumping" of potassium in and sodium out of the cell. It is believed that an enzyme acts as a sodium–potassium pump, and that this enzyme is the membrane-bound Na–K ATPase. This enzyme catalyzes the hydrolyzis of ATP and the free energy of this reaction is utilized to extrude sodium from the cell and to accumulate potassium inside the cell, thus resulting in asymmetric ionic concentrations. Plasma membranes in general possess a high permeability for potassium and a low permeability for

Table I. Normal Ionic Concentrations in Extracellular Fluid (Plasma, Interstitial Fluid) and Intracellular Fluid

	Extracellular fluid (mEq/liter)		Intracellular fluid[a] (mEq/liter)
	Plasma	Interstitial fluid	
Cations			
Na^+	152	143	13
K^+	5	4	157
Ca^{2+}	5	5	—
Mg^{2+}	3	3	28
Anions			
Cl^-	113	117	—
HCO_3^-	27	27	10
PO_4^{2-}	2	2	113
Anionic Proteins	16	2	74
Organic Acids	6	6	—

[a] The values for intracellular electrolytes are the approximate concentrations taken from data available for muscle cells.

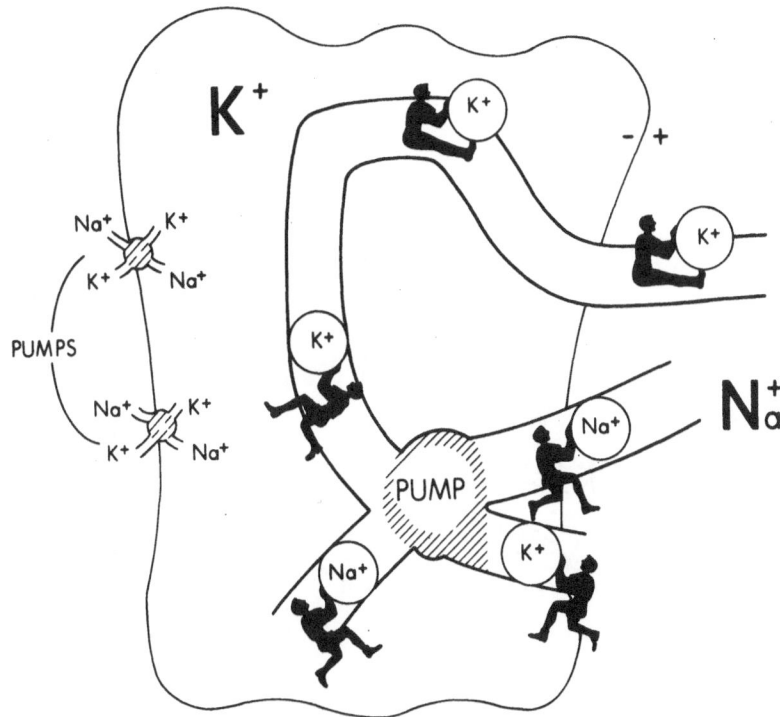

Figure 2. Schematic representation of the Na–K pump (or its enzymatic equivalent, the Na–K ATPase). The diagram depicts a nonepithelial cell (e.g., muscle, erythrocyte) in which Na–K pumps are evenly distributed around the plasma membrane. The pumps accomplish the "uphill" extrusion of Na and influx of K resulting in asymmetric ionic concentrations (high K inside the cell, high Na outside the cell). K diffuses out of the cell readily because of a favorable concentration difference and a high membrane permeability, giving rise to an electrical potential (inside negative) across the plasma membrane. (Na diffusion inward is limited because of low membrane permeability.) In renal tubular cells and other epithelial tissues, the Na–K pump is confined to the antiluminal (peritubular) side of the plasma membrane.

sodium. Because of this property, as potassium accumulates inside the cell and a concentration difference develops, diffusion of this ion out of the cell (outflux) gives rise to an electrical potential (cell interior negative) across the cell membrane (Figure 2). Sodium diffusion into the cell (influx) would tend to make the cell interior positive, and thus it would oppose the potassium-diffusion potential. But owing to the low permeability of the cell membrane to sodium, the magnitude of sodium influx is greatly exceeded by the potassium outflux. Hence for practical purposes it is agreed that the potassium outflux is the major source of the cell membrane electrical potential (Figure 2). Changes in the ECF potassium concentration will be reflected in alterations of the transmembrane concentration difference, which in turn will affect potassium outflux. This will result in changes in the magnitude of the resting membrane potential and will impair the activity of cells whose function is critically dependent on changes in the magnitude of the membrane potential (e.g., nerves, skeletal muscle, cardiac muscle).

The resting membrane potential is about −90 mV (with cell interior

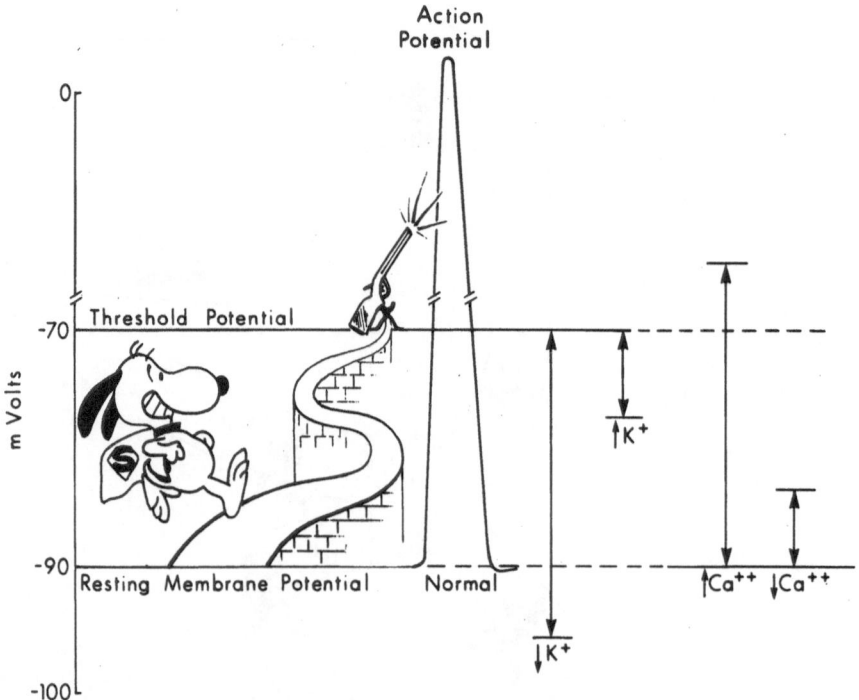

Figure 3. Schematic representation of the effects of K^+ and Ca^{2+} on excitability of muscles and nerves. Impinging stimuli (S) lower (depolarize) the resting membrane potential until a critical value (threshold potential) is reached, at which point an action potential is "fired" and excitation occurs. K^+ affects the resting membrane potential whereas Ca^{2+} has a major influence on the threshold potential. The effects of K^+ and Ca^{2+} on excitability can be explained by changes in the difference between resting membrane potential and threshold potentials. Hyperkalemia decreases (makes less negative) the resting membrane potential and thus decreases the difference between resting and threshold potentials. This increases cell excitability. Hypokalemia has opposite effects. Hypercalcemia decreases the threshold potential and thus increases the difference between resting and threshold potentials. This in turn decreases cell excitability. Hypocalcemia has opposite effects. Notice that the increased excitability from hyperkalemia can be reversed by increasing the serum calcium (hypercalcemia). $\downarrow K^+$, Hypokalemia; $\uparrow K^+$, hyperkalemia. $\downarrow Ca^{2+}$, Hypocalcemia; $\uparrow Ca^{2+}$, hypercalcemia.

electrically negative to the ECF). The effect of physiological stimuli on nerve and muscle cells is to decrease the resting membrane potential (depolarize the cell membrane). This effect is mediated by release of acetylcholine at synaptic junctions and muscle end plates. When the resting membrane potential has reached a critical value (threshold potential) there is an increase in sodium permeability and therefore a large change in the electrical conductance of the cell membrane with the production of an action potential and subsequent excitation of the cell. Hence, how easily nerves and muscles can be excited depends to a large extent on the difference between the resting membrane potential and the threshold potential (Figure 3). In general, a decrease in the steady state concentrations of potassium in the ECF (hypokalemia) results in an increase in the transmembrane concentration difference for potassium. Hence, potassium outflux is enhanced, the cell interior becomes more negative and hyperpolarization (increase of the resting membrane potential) occurs. This, in turn, increases the difference between resting and threshold potentials and decreases excitability of the cell. By contrast, an increase in the ECF potassium concentration (hyperkalemia) depolarizes (decreases) the resting membrane potential and increases cell excitability (Figure 3). The clinical consequences of states of potassium deficiency and potassium excess are essentially determined by the effect of this ion on transmembrane electrical potential. Changes in the ECF concentration of ionized calcium also influence cellular excitability by modifying the levels of the threshold potential (Figure 3).

In clinical practice, it is difficult to ascertain potassium balance. This difficulty stems from two facts: (1) Only the ECF (serum or plasma) concentration of this ion is measured. Since potassium is distributed predominantly in the ICF (cf. Table I), a serum or plasma (ECF) measurement does not reflect ICF potassium or total body stores. (2) Changes in acid–base status (ECF pH) have profound effects on the distribution of potassium across cell membranes without necessarily changing the total body stores of this cation (Figure 4). Furthermore, although increases in total body potassium correlate well with serum potassium concentrations (hyperkalemia), there is a poor correlation between serum potassium concentrations and total body potassium in states associated with potassium depletion (Figure 4).

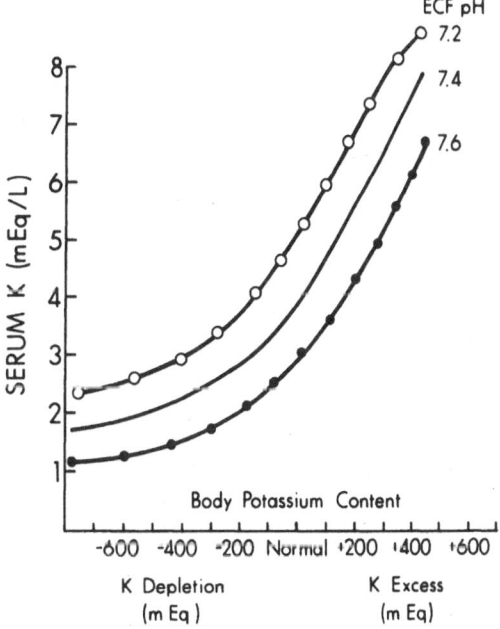

Figure 4. Schematic representation of the changes of serum K as a function of total body K content at different values of ECF pH. Acidosis (pH 7.2) is accompanied by an increase and alkalosis (pH 7.6) by a decrease in serum K. Notice that pH-dependent K shifts occur in the presence of increased or decreased body stores. Also, serum K is a poor index of states associated with depletion of body potassium. (Reprinted with permission from Rosenfeld, M. G. (ed.): *Manual of Medical Therapeutics, Washington University*, Twentieth edition. Little, Brown and Co., Boston, 1971, p. 45.)

II. REGULATION OF ECF POTASSIUM CONCENTRATION

The concentration of potassium in the ECF is basically determined by two factors: (1) the pH of the ECF and (2) renal tubular function.

A. ECF pH

Changes in the hydrogen ion activity (and therefore pH) of the ECF are accompanied by large shifts of potassium between ECF and ICF: a decrease in ECF pH (acidosis) results in shifting of potassium out of cells (as protons move inside cells) and raises the ECF potassium concentration. This shifting may be viewed as a buffering mechanism that enables the cells to accumulate protons during acidosis and thus to prevent large changes in the ECF pH. Likewise, an increase in ECF pH (alkalosis) produces shifting of potassium from the ECF into cells and lowers the ECF potassium concentration. It has been estimated that a pH change of 0.1 unit is attended by a change in the ECF potassium concentration of approximately 0.6 mEq/liter. These shifts occur in states associated with either total body potassium excess or depletion (Figure 4). Thus, *acidosis* is normally accompanied by *hyperkalemia* and *alkalosis* is normally associated with *hypokalemia*.

B. Renal Tubular Function

The kidney excretes approximately 90 mEq of potassium per day. Under normal conditions, essentially all of the potassium filtered is reabsorbed by the proximal tubule. Proximal reabsorption of potassium although "uphill" (see Appendix, Chapter 1) is related to sodium reabsorption. However, there seems to be a fraction of proximal potassium reabsorption that becomes apparent when proximal sodium transport is blocked by acetazolamide and may represent an active potassium transport system.

Distal nephron segments can both reabsorb and secrete potassium.* The balance between distal reabsorption and secretion determines the net urinary excretion of this cation. These two processes are best understood in terms of chemical concentration differences and electrical potential differences across the distal tubular epithelium (see Figure 5). Distal potassium reabsorption

---

* Recently, it has been recognized that rather large amounts of potassium may be secreted within the lumens of the pars recta and/or the thin descending limb of Henle's loop in juxtamedullary nephrons. This secretory process can be affected by maneuvers that modify distal potassium transport (e.g., furosemide, amiloride, changes in dietary potassium content), which suggests that a fraction of potassium reabsorbed in distal nephron segments (distal and collecting tubules) may reenter the pars recta and/or thin descending limb. It is unclear whether this "recycling phenomenon" also occurs in cortical nephrons, and its relative contribution to overall potassium balance has not been defined.

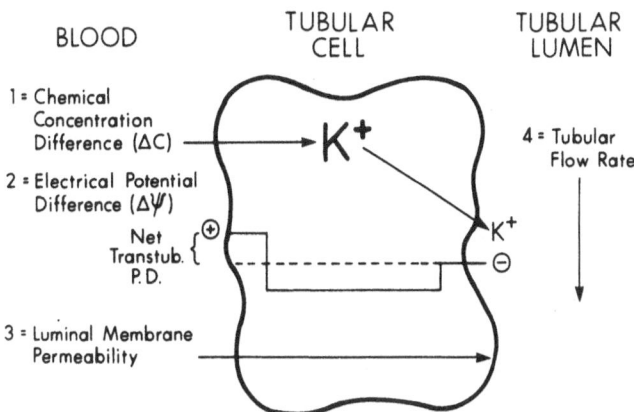

Figure 5. Factors modulating secretion of K by the distal nephron. The net transtubular potential difference (P.D.) is the algebraic sum of P.D. steps at the liminal and peritubular plasma membranes. Notice that the cell is electrically negative to luminal and peritubular fluids, but the step at the peritubular membrane is larger than at the luminal membrane and the net transtubular P.D. is as depicted: lumen negative to the peritubular side. The P.D. of the peritubular membrane is a function of the Na–K pump.

across the tubular luminal membrane is favored by an electrical potential difference (cell interior negative with respect to lumen) (cf. Figure 5). Despite this fact, luminal reabsorption has been considered to represent "uphill" transport because of an unfavorable chemical concentration difference due to the high intracellular concentration of this ion. However, it should be pointed out that the magnitude of this concentration difference cannot be ascertained because the intracellular activity of potassium has not been determined. Thus, if the thermodynamic activity of potassium inside the tubular cells is lower than the chemical concentration, the concentration difference may be offset by the electrical potential difference and reabsorption of potassium may in effect be a passive phenomenon.

Distal tubular secretion of potassium is a multifactorial event. Four major factors are known to modulate distal tubular secretion of potassium (see Figure 5 and Table II). These are (1) the presence of a concentration difference across the luminal membrane (ΔC), (2) the presence of an electrical potential difference across the distal tubular epithelium ($\Delta\psi$), (3) the permeability properties of the tubular luminal membrane, and (4) the tubular flow rate.

From these considerations, it becomes apparent that the contribution of glomerular filtration rate to the renal excretion of potassium is negligible. The proximal tubule does not contribute to the urinary excretion of this cation. The amount of potassium that appears in the urine is essentially a function of the transport activity of distal nephron segments.

Most of the conditions that modify renal potassium excretion can be readily understood by considering the factors presented in Figure 5 and Table II.

Table II. Factors Regulating Renal Tubular Secretion of
Potassium

I. Chemical concentration difference (ΔC)
    A. ECF pH (acidosis–alkalosis)
    B. Glucocorticoid hormones?
    C. Aldosterone
II. Electrical potential difference ($\Delta\psi$)
    A. Distal Na^+ delivery
        1. ECF volume
        2. Diuretics
        3. Aldosterone
        4. Bartter's syndrome
    B. Poorly reabsorbed anions (HCO_3^-; SO_4^{2-}; carbenicillin)
        1. Proximal RTA
        2. Metabolic alkalosis
        3. Carbenicillin therapy
    C. Primary stimulation of distal Na^+ reabsorption: Aldosterone
III. Tubular luminal membrane permeability
    A. Aldosterone
    B. Distal RTA?
IV. Tubular flow rate
    A. ECF volume
    B. Diuretics

---

1. Luminal Membrane Concentration Difference (ΔC)

Under normal conditions there is a chemical concentration difference across the luminal membrane of the tubular epithelium that favors diffusion of potassium from the cells into the lumen. This stems from the fact that the concentration of potassium in tubular epithelial cells is higher than in the tubular fluid. Changes in the intracellular potassium concentration may change the magnitude of this concentration difference and modify the rate of tubular secretion. During alkalosis, potassium shifts into the tubular cells. This increases the intracellular concentration of potassium and increases the concentration difference across the luminal membrane. Hence, tubular secretion of potassium is enhanced, leading to increased urinary excretion of potassium (kaliuresis). Acidosis has opposite effects. The kaliuretic effect of glucocorticoid hormones may be in part mediated by stimulation of the sodium–potassium pump at the peritubular membrane (the luminal membrane lacks sodium–potassium pump) with an increase in the intratubular potassium concentration. Mineralocorticoid hormones (aldosterone) may have a similar effect.

2. Electrical Potential Difference ($\Delta\psi$)

There is now convincing evidence that the distal nephron segments engaged in potassium secretion possess large electrical potential differences across the tubular wall. It is also agreed that the major factor responsible for the maintenance of these potential differences is the active reabsorption of sodium from the tubular lumen. The cell interior appears to be negative with respect to the luminal fluid, whereas the peritubular fluid (blood) is positive with respect to the cell interior. The net transtubular potential difference is the algebraic sum of the steps at the luminal and peritubular membranes and is as depicted in Figure 5: tubular lumen negative with respect to peritubular fluid (blood). The peritubular membrane potential step is essentially determined by the activity of the Na–K pump.

Under normal conditions, the electrical potential difference across the tubular luminal membrane does not favor potassium secretion into the lumen and most of the potassium secreted is driven by the concentration difference. However, if the luminal fluid becomes more negative (e.g., presence of unreabsorbed anions: HCO_3^-, SO_4^{2-}) the tubular luminal membrane electrical potential difference will change in the direction of favoring potassium secretion and enhanced kaliuresis may occur. During contraction of the ECF volume (dehydration) there is an increase in the proximal reabsorption of sodium with a corresponding decrease in the amount of sodium delivered to distal nephron segments. This may decrease the magnitude of the transtubular electrical potential differences and thus decrease the urinary excretion of potassium. By contrast, the kaliuresis associated with volume expansion and diuretic therapy may in part be explained by increases in the delivery of sodium to distal nephron segments. Increased distal delivery also occurs in states associated with excess of mineralocorticoid hormones (aldosterone) owing to increased sodium reabsorption and ECF expansion. In some patients with Bartter's syndrome there appears to be a defect in proximal sodium reabsorption which would lead to increased sodium delivery and kaliuresis. The presence in the tubular lumen of certain anions (e.g., bicarbonate, sulfate) that are poorly reabsorbed by the tubular epithelium increases the electrical gradient (by increasing luminal negativity) and enhances tubular secretion of potassium. This mechanism appears to account for the kaliuresis that accompanies proximal renal tubular acidosis and some cases of metabolic alkalosis, conditions in which the tubular fluid of distal nephron segments contains large concentrations of bicarbonate. Likewise, during therapy with large doses of the antibiotic carbenicillin, high concentrations of the slowly metabolized anion of the drug may be present in the distal tubular lumen leading to kaliuresis. Mineralocorticoid hormones (aldosterone) stimulate sodium reabsorption by the cortical collecting tubule, which results in an increase in the magnitude of the transtubular electrical potential differences and kaliuresis.

3. Tubular Luminal Membrane Permeability

In addition to the chemical concentration differences and electrical potential differences that normally drive potassium secretion by distal tubular segments, the permeability of the luminal membrane to potassium has profound effects on the urinary excretion of this cation. Several lines of experimental evidence indicate that the kaliuretic effect of mineralocorticoid hormones (aldosterone) is largely mediated by a marked increase in the permeability of the luminal membrane to potassium. Likewise, it is possible that changes in membrane permeability explain, in part, the kaliuresis associated with distal renal tubular acidosis.

4. Tubular Flow Rate

Since the chemical concentration difference across the luminal membrane is an important driving force for potassium secretion, changes in tubular flow rate may alter potassium secretion by modifying this concentration difference. An increase in tubular flow rate (e.g., diuretics, volume expansion) enhances the urinary excretion of potassium by lowering intratubular concentrations of the cation, thus maintaining a favorable concentration difference for secretion of potassium from cells into tubular lumen.

5. Other Factors Influencing ECF Potassium Concentration

In addition to the mechanisms described above, the ECF potassium concentration appears to be influenced by humoral and nonhumoral stimuli that act by promoting shifts of potassium between ICF and ECF and/or modifying the tubular handling of this cation. Among these, the most important one is the concentration of insulin. An increase in the concentration of insulin promotes a shift of potassium from the ECF into cells and thus lowers the ECF potassium concentration (Figure 6). This effect of insulin appears to be mediated by stimulation of potassium uptake by muscle cells, via activation of the sodium–potassium pump, and it occurs despite the fact that insulin appears to stimulate potassium reabsorption by the kidney. Likewise, there is some evidence that catecholamines may be important in potassium homeostasis by promoting movement of potassium into the cells. Finally, the kidney is capable of adapting to large increases in the dietary intake of potassium or to decreases in renal mass by increasing the urinary excretion of this cation; the mechanisms responsible for these adaptive responses involve an increase in the activity of Na–KATPase in the kidney. This increased activity is apparently due to a greater density (number) of Na–KATPase in tubular cells, without major changes in the affinity of this enzyme for its substrate.

III. HYPOKALEMIA

Hypokalemia occurs when the serum potassium concentration falls below 3.5 mEq/liter. A decrease in the serum potassium concentration may reflect a decrease in the total body stores of this cation but may also occur in the face of normal or even elevated levels of intracellular potassium (cf. Figure

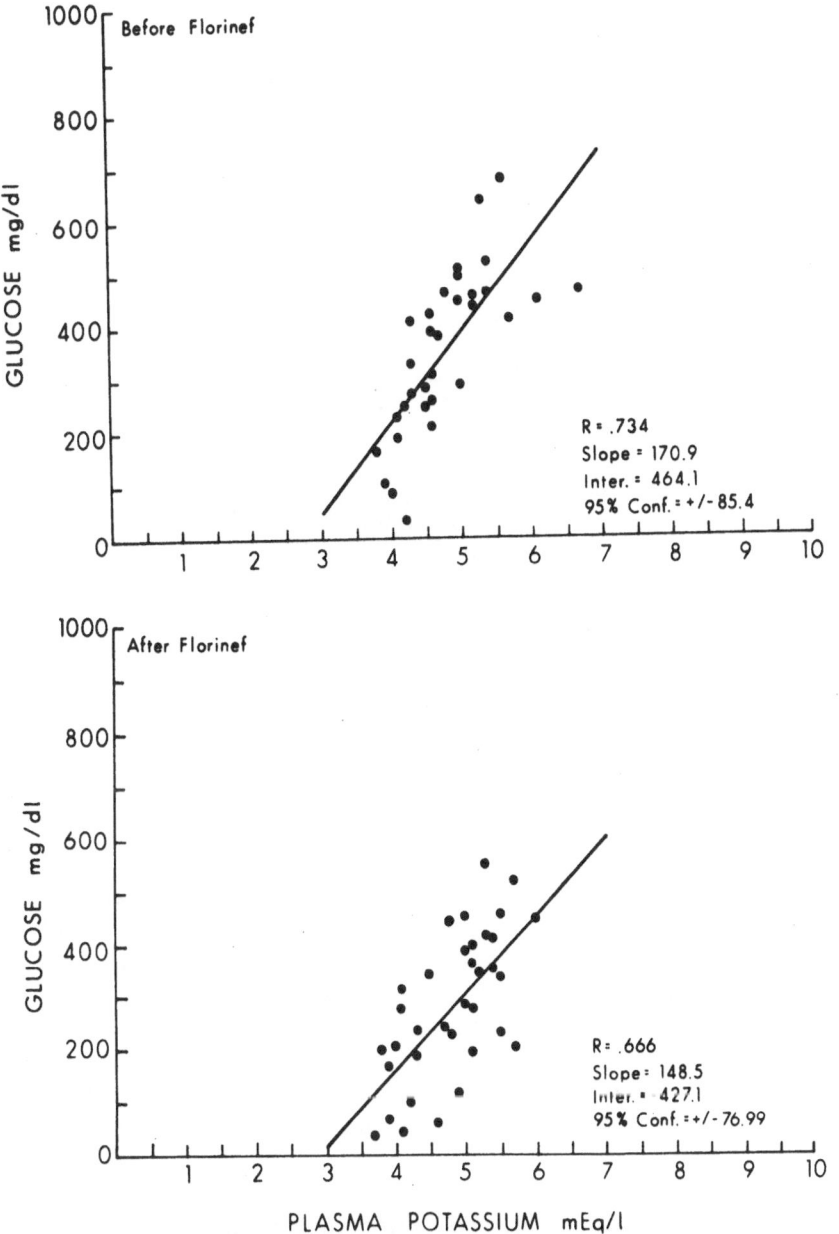

Figure 6. Relationship between levels of blood glucose and K in an insulin-dependent diabetic patient with a living related kidney transplant. The patient had a serum creatinine of 2 mg/dl and normal activities of renin and aldosterone. Hyperglycemia (insulin deficiency) was invariably associated with hyperkalemia. The relationship of hyperglycemia (insulinopenia) to hyperkalemia was similar in the absence (upper panel) or presence (lower panel) of therapy with fluorocortisone acetate (Florinef®). (Reprinted with permission from Rosenbaum, R., Hoffsten, P. E., Cryer, P., and Klahr, S.: *Arch. Intern. Med.* 138:1270, 1978.)

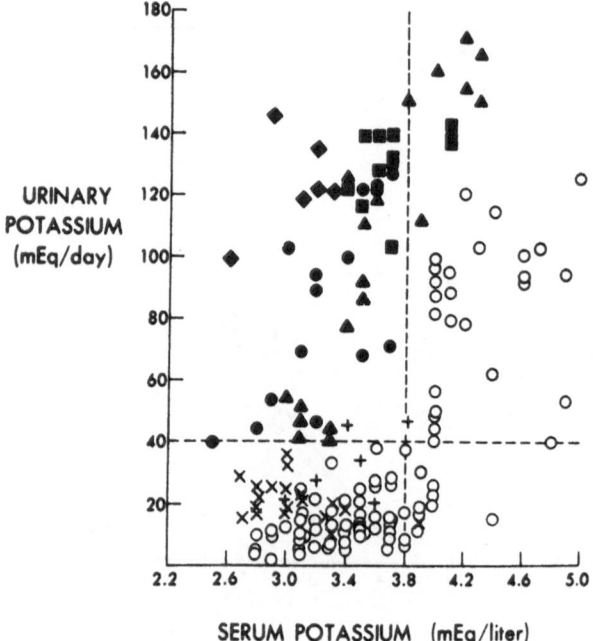

Figure 7. Relationship between urinary potassium excretion ($U_K V$) and plasma potassium concentration in subjects with normal renal function (open symbols, crosses) and in patients with renal tubular acidosis (closed symbols) in whom correction of the acidosis was sustained. Notice that in normal subjects with serum K < 3.8 mEq/liter the urine contains variable amounts of K, but the urinary excretion does not exceed 40 mEq/day. Patients with RTA and urinary K wasting excrete greater than 40 mEq of K even in the presence of severe hypokalemia. (Reprinted with permission from Sebastian, A., McSherry, E., and Morris, R. C.: *J. Clin. Invest.* 50:667, 1971.)

4). This stems from the fact that large shifts of potassium between cells and ECF space may occur in response to changes in hormonal levels (insulin) and acid–base status. The kidney has a limited ability to reduce the urinary excretion of potassium below 10–20 mEq/day and potassium depletion may occur when the dietary intake of this cation is reduced for prolonged periods. For practical purposes, the excretion of more than 40 mEq of potassium per day in the presence of hypokalemia and in the absence of diuretic therapy can be taken as evidence of renal potassium wasting (Figure 7).

A. Clinical Manifestation of Hypokalemia

Reduction of the body stores of potassium may occur with relatively few clinical manifestations or may be attended by a syndrome which affects (1) skeletal muscles (weakness, fatigue, flaccid paralysis, rhabdomyolysis), (2) smooth muscles (decrease in gastric and small intestinal motility, paralytic ileus), (3) cardiac muscle (decreased amplitude of the T wave, prolonged QT intervals, prominent U waves, widening of the QRS complex, and second- or

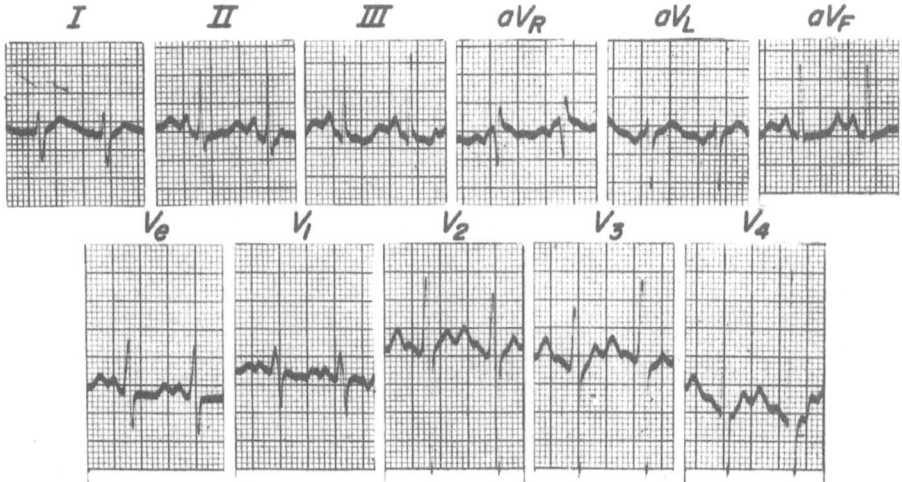

Figure 8. Electrocardiographic changes associated with hypokalemia. The patient had meningitis, metabolic alkalosis (iatrogenic), and a serum potassium of 2.6 mEq/liter. Serum calcium was normal. Notice the prolonged QT interval (0.37 sec; upper limit of normal for this ventricular rate is 0.3 sec) and prominent U waves in precordial leads (V1–V4) (Reprinted with permission from Roesler, H., and Fletcher, E.: *An Atlas of Electrocardiography*. The Williams & Wilkins Co., Baltimore, 1963, p. 28.

even third-degree AV block) (Figure 8), and (4) peripheral nerves (paresthesias and clumsiness of the extremities).

These clinical manifestations are essentially a consequence of changes in the resting membrane potential of muscle and nerves and decreased excitability associated with hypokalemia (cf. Figure 3). In addition, prolonged potassium deficiency may impair the concentrating ability of the kidney with marked increases in urine output (polyuria, nocturia) (Figure 9). The

Figure 9. Effect of K depletion and subsequent repletion on urinary concentrating ability during hydropenia in man. U_{osm} is the maximal urine osmolality after overnight dehydration. Vasopressin (ADH) does not correct the hyposthenuria. The concentrating defect is corrected by K repletion. *C*, control period. (Reprinted with permission from Rubini, M. E.: *J. Clin. Invest.* 40:2215, 1961.)

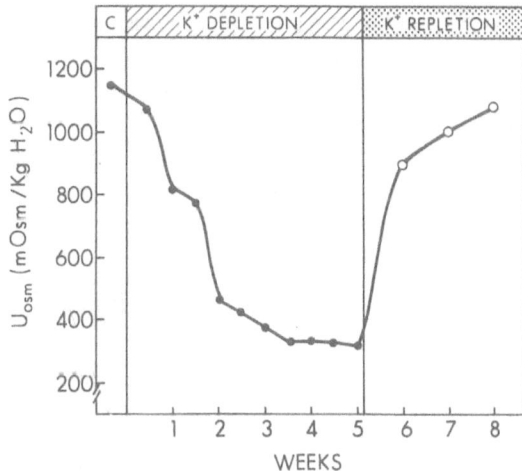

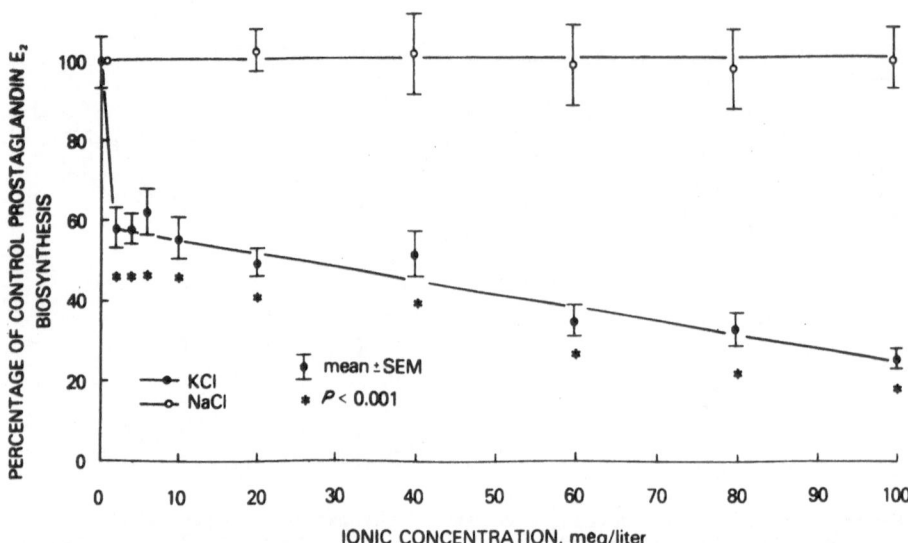

Figure 10. Effect of ionic concentration on prostaglandin biosynthesis (PGE_2) by rabbit reno-medullary interstitial cells in tissue culture. PGE_2 biosynthesis is markedly inhibited by increasing K concentration (closed circles) in the culture medium. The inhibitory effect of K is not due to changes in ionic strength because similar concentrations of Na (open circles) have no effect on PGE_2 synthesis. (Reprinted with permission from Zusman, R. M., and Keiser, H. R.: *J. Clin. Invest.* 60:215, 1977.)

pathogenesis of the renal concentrating defect is poorly understood. It has been ascribed to an increase in the renal synthesis of prostaglandins (PGE_1, PGE_2) (Figure 10) which are known to antagonize the cellular effects of antidiuretic hormone (ADH) on the collecting tubule (Figure 11). This inference is strengthened by the observation that *in vitro* stimulation of renal medullary adenylate cyclase by vasopressin is markedly blunted in experimental K^+ deficiency. However, inhibition of prostaglandin synthesis with indomethacin does not improve the renal concentrating defect observed in hypokalemic rats. This raises serious doubts as to the role of prostaglandins in the renal concentrating defect of hypokalemia. It has also been suggested that potassium deficiency stimulates thirst and that this may aggravate the polyuria. Although the extent of potassium depletion is usually reflected in a reduction of the serum level of potassium, this may be misleading in the presence of significant ECF acidosis due to the shifting of potassium previously discussed (cf. Figure 4).

B. Differential Diagnosis of Hypokalemia

The main causes of hypokalemia are outlined in Table III and will be briefly discussed.

When dietary potassium intake is markedly restricted, hypokalemia may result because of the limited ability of the kidney to reduce renal potassium excretion.

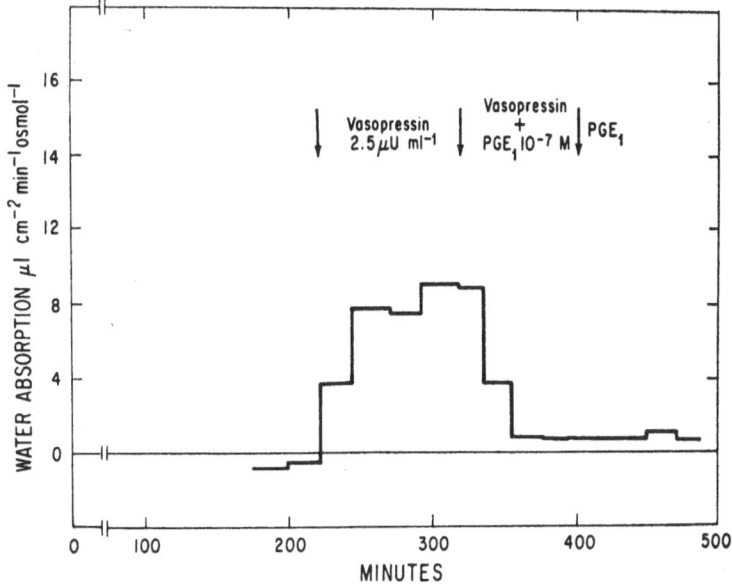

Figure 11. Effect of vasopressin (ADH) and prostaglandin (PGE$_1$), on water permeability of the isolated perfused cortical collecting tubule of rabbit kidney. Water absorption is negligible in the absence of vasopressin in spite of a large osmotic gradient (luminal solution: 125 mOsm/kg H$_2$O; outside bathing medium: 290 mOsm/kg H$_2$O). Low concentrations of vasopressin added to the outside bathing medium produce a large and sustained increase in water reabsorption and the effect is completely abolished by PGE$_1$. (Reprinted from Grantham, J. J., and Orloff, J.: *J. Clin. Invest.* 47:1154, 1968.)

Table III. Causes of Hypokalemia

I. Dietary deficiency
II. Primary hypermineralocorticism (↓ plasma renin activity)
    A. Primary aldosteronism (adenoma, hyperplasia carcinoma)
    B. Increased ACTH production
        1. Ectopic ACTH syndrome
        2. Cushing's disease
        3. Enzymatic deficiencies in corticol synthesis (11-hydroxylase, 17 hydroxylase)
    C. Licorice ingestion
III. Secondary hypermineralocorticism (↑ plasma renin activity)
    A. Accelerated or malignant hypertension
    B. Renovascular hypertension
    C. Edema-forming states (heart failure, cirrhosis, nephrotic syndrome)
    D. Renin-secreting tumor
IV. Renal tubular disorders
    A. Renal tubular acidosis (proximal, distal, Fanconi's syndrome)
    B. Bartter's syndrome
V. Miscellaneous
    A. Gastrointestinal losses (vomiting, diarrhea, laxative abuse)
    B. Diuretics
    C. Acute leukemia (monoblastic)
    D. Alkalosis
    E. Insulin therapy of diabetic ketoacidosis

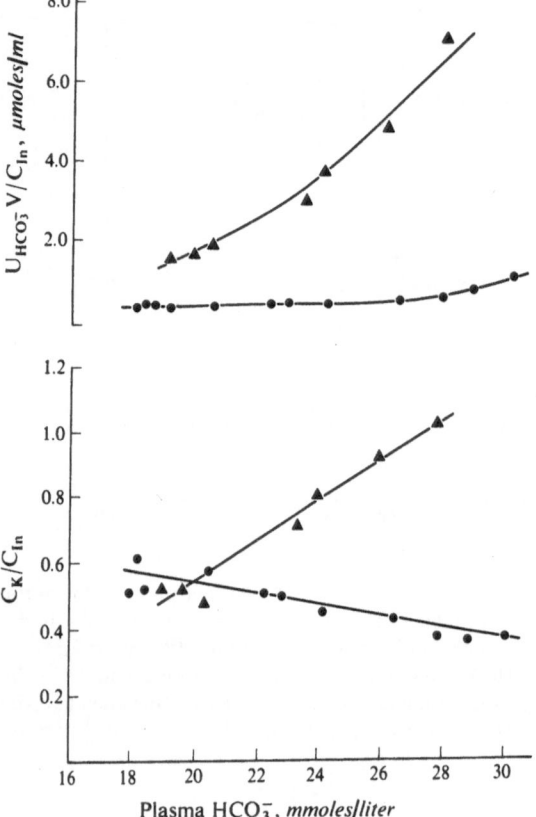

Figure 12. Effect of increases in plasma bicarbonate concentration on the urinary excretion of bicarbonate (upper panel) and K (lower panel) in a patient with proximal RTA (▲) and in a patient with distal RTA (●). In proximal RTA (▲) infusion of $NaHCO_3$ results in bicarbonaturia (upper panel) and marked kaliuresis (lower panel). No changes in bicarbonate or K excretion occur in distal RTA (●). (Reprinted with permission from Morris, R. C., Sebastian, A., and McSherry, E.: *Kidney Int.* 1:322, 1972.)

Excessive production of mineralocorticoid hormones (aldosterone) is an important cause of hypokalemia in clinical medicine. Hyperaldosteronism may be primary, if due to adenoma, hyperplasia or carcinoma of the zona glomerulosa of the adrenal cortex, or secondary, if associated with edema-forming states (congestive heart failure, cirrhosis of the liver, nephrotic syndrome), renovascular hypertension, and malignant hypertension. In all the states associated with secondary aldosteronism, the high circulating levels of aldosterone are due to a primary increase in plasma renin activity; by contrast, primary aldosteronism is typically accompanied by a decrease (suppression) of plasma renin activity. Increased ACTH secretion stimulates the production of glucocorticoid hormones (cortisol, corticosterone) and to a lesser extent of mineralocorticoids (aldosterone, deoxycorticosterone) and hypokalemia results. Ingestion of large quantities of licorice may result in hypokalemia because of the mineralocorticoidlike effect of glycirrhizic acid. In proximal RTA, the increased delivery of sodium and the relatively impermeant anion bicarbonate to distal nephron segments increase the transtubular electrical potential and produce kaliuresis (Figure 12). In addition, secondary aldosteronism is almost invariably present, which worsens the renal wasting of potassium. The mechanisms responsible for kaliuresis in distal RTA are poorly understood. The tendency to urinary potassium wasting in distal RTA is not dependent on the acidosis per se because significant kaliuresis occurs in these patients even after sustained correction of the systemic acidosis (cf. Figure 7). Experimental evidence suggests that the inability of distal nephron segments to maintain a hydrogen ion gradient in cases of distal RTA is not due to impairment of the hydrogen secretory capacity of the tubular cells but rather to a change in the conductance of the luminal membrane to protons which results in rapid dissipation of transmembrane proton gradients. Hence it is possible that changes in membrane conductance to potassium may account for the kaliuresis associated with distal RTA (see Section II, Chapter 8).

Bartter's syndrome is a condition in which hyperplasia of the juxtaglomerular apparatus results in increased renin levels and secondary aldosteronism. Clinically the syndrome is characterized by profound renal potassium wasting, hypokalemia, metabolic alkalosis, and normal or low blood pressure. Owing to the high levels of renin and angiotensin the patients manifest resistance to the pressor effects of infused angiotensin II. Renal potassium wasting is only partly explained by excessive aldosterone secretion because of the failure of bilateral adrenalectomy to completely correct potassium wasting. It is possible that the features of Bartter's syndrome are the result of several pathogenetic mechanisms such as (1) a defect in sodium chloride reabsorption in the proximal nephron with increased delivery of sodium to distal nephron segments and potassium wasting, which would be enhanced, but not entirely dependent on increased aldosterone levels, or (2) as recent studies have shown, patients with Bartter's syndrome have a marked increase in the renal production of prostaglandins and that renal potassium wasting can be reduced substantially by treatment with inhibitors of prostaglandin biosynthesis (e.g., indomethacin). However, the relationship of increased prostaglandin synthesis to renal potassium wasting is not clear. There is evidence that experimental potassium depletion in dogs is accompanied by marked increases in the urinary excretion of prostaglandins. Further, hypokalemia stimulates prostaglandin biosynthesis (PGE_2) in cultures of renomedullary interstitial cells (cf. Figure 10). Thus, it is possible that the increased renal synthesis of prostaglandins in Bartter's syndrome is the consequence rather than the cause of kaliuresis.

The gastrointestinal tract may be a major source of potassium loss leading to significant hypokalemia. Excessive use of laxatives or repeated enemas is perhaps the most common cause of hypokalemia encountered in medical practice. Likewise, any conditions associated with severe diarrhea (Zollinger–Ellison syndrome, inflammatory bowel disease, malabsorption) may produce severe hypokalemia. Villous adenomas of the rectum and colon may be associated with excessive potassium secretion and may quite rapidly lead to potassium depletion and hypokalemia. Some patients with acute monoblastic leukemia have a tendency to renal potassium wasting; this has been associated with the presence in the urine of large quantities of lysozyme

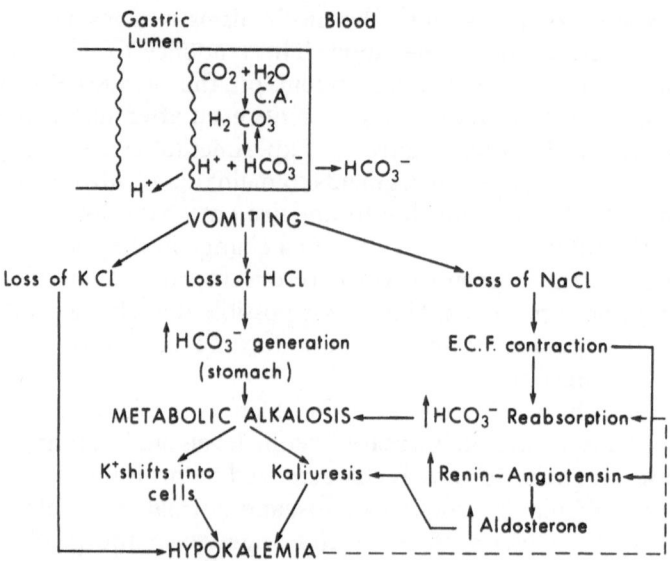

Figure 13. Pathogenesis of hypokalemia and metabolic alkalosis associated with vomiting. C.A., carbonic anhydrase.

(muramidase), but the mechanism of this effect has not been ascertained. Alkalosis is invariably accompanied by renal potassium wasting by mechanisms previously alluded to. It should also be remembered that hypokalemia in turn may lead to alkalosis by a direct effect related to increased ammonia production and increased bicarbonate reabsorption by the renal tubule (see Chapter 8). Finally, one of the most common causes of hypokalemia in clinical practice is vomiting. The pathogenetic events responsible for hypokalemia associated with vomiting are outlined in Figure 13. The concentration of potassium in gastric fluid is approximately 15–20 mEq/liter. Thus even in protracted vomiting the amount of potassium lost with the gastric fluid is relatively small and cannot account for the severe hypokalemia observed in these patients. There are two important pathogenetic mechanisms responsible for the hypokalemia of vomiting: metabolic alkalosis (a consequence of the loss of fixed acid HCl in the vomitus) and volume contraction. As hypokalemia develops, the kidney is further stimulated to reabsorb bicarbonate and the urinary pH may be acid in spite of very high levels of plasma bicarbonate. This explains the so-called "paradoxical acid-urea" (acid urinary pH in the presence of metabolic alkalosis) associated with protracted vomiting.

C. Management of Hypokalemia

Prevention. Recognize situations in which potassium intake must be supplied or increased (Table III). Do not supplement dietary potassium unless it is clear that the patient can handle extra potassium without becoming hyperkalemic. Since potassium is well absorbed from the intestinal tract, the only protection against hyperkalemia is adequate renal excretion. If urine flow is at least 1 ml/min (1400 ml/day), it is safe to supplement dietary potassium.

Specific Treatment of Cause of Hypokalemia. See Table III.

Potassium Replacement. (a) Orally, if possible. Normal potassium intake in an adult is about 100 mEq/day. To correct a deficit, intake should exceed the continuing potassium loss by no less than 100 mEq/day. (b) Intravenous potassium. Do not give potassium intravenously without first determining that serum potassium concentration is low.

The unequivocal electrocardiographic evidence of hypokalemia is the only acceptable substitute for direct measurement of serum potassium in an emergency. Emergency indications for intravenous potassium: rapidly progressive weakness or paralysis of limb muscles, any involvement of muscles of respiration (sucking inspiration), ECG changes consistent with hypokalemia. Potassium concentration in intravenous fluids should be less than 100 mEq/liter (6 g KCl = 81 mEq K). Infuse at constant rate; take no less than 2 hr to give 1 liter. Maintain constant medical attention. Monitor ECG at least every 15 min.

IV. HYPERKALEMIA

Hyperkalemia (a rise in serum potassium concentration above 5 mEq/liter) can occur with relatively few clinical signs prior to the appearance of major cardiac conduction abnormalities. An increase in the serum concentration of potassium lowers (depolarizes) the resting membrane potential of nerve and muscle cells. The immediate consequence of this is that impinging stimuli can rapidly depolarize the resting membrane potential to the threshold level and hyperexcitability of the cells results (cf. Figure 3). With greater elevations of serum potassium, the resting potential may approach the threshold potential and excitability may be lost. The major manifestations of hyperkalemia are disturbances of the cardiac rhythm: with progressive increases in serum potassium level the electrocardiogram will show peaking of the T waves, widening of the QRS complex, prolongation of the PR interval, and subsequent appearance of a smooth, biphasic QRS-T wave. In addition, there may be supra ventricular tachycardia, sinus arrest, AV dissociation, ventricular fibrillation, and/or cardiac standstill (Figure 14).

A. Differential Diagnosis of Hyperkalemia

The most common causes of hyperkalemia are listed in Table IV. These will be discussed here briefly.

In normal man, substantial increases in potassium intake are rarely attended by significant increases in serum potassium level, thus attesting to

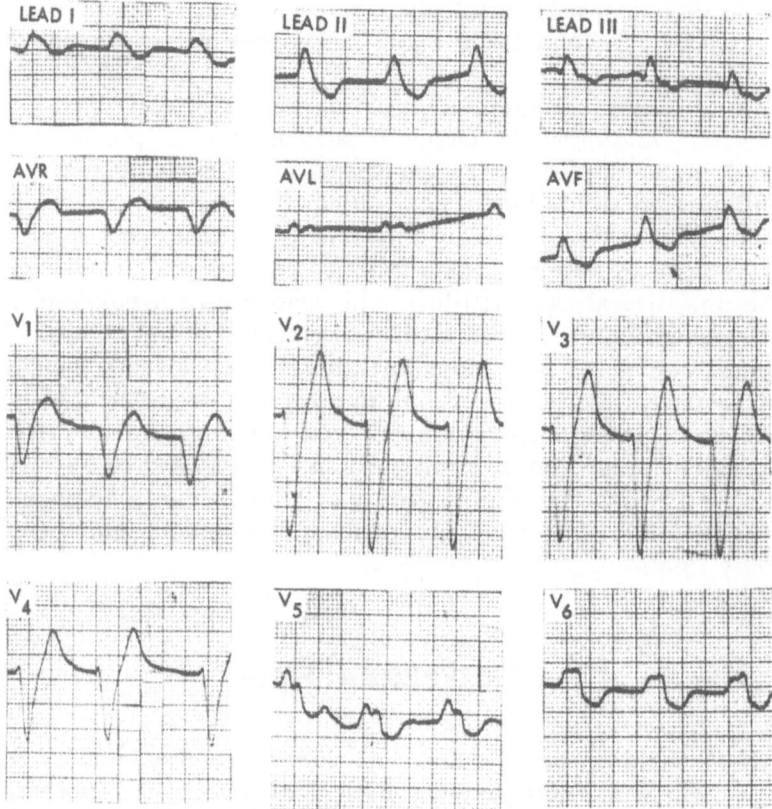

Figure 14. Electrocardiographic changes associated with hyperkalemia. The patient had oliguric acute renal failure with a blood pH of 7.19 and a plasma potassium of 7.2 mEq/liter. Notice the tall, peaked T waves (V_2, V_3, V_4), widening of the QRS complex, and the presence of a smooth-bifasic QRS-T wave (I, II, III, V_5, V_6).

the ability of the kidney to excrete potassium loads. However, in acute oliguric states (acute renal failure) serum potassium levels may increase rapidly in the absence of significant external potassium loads. By contrast, hyperkalemia is a relatively uncommon occurrence in chronic stable renal failure despite decreases in glomerular filtration rate to less than 15 ml/min. Since urinary potassium excretion is basically a secretory function of the distal nephron and is minimally dependent on glomerular filtration, it then follows that as long as urine output is maintained renal potassium excretion is essentially adequate to handle dietary loads. Hyperkalemia may occur in chronic stable renal failure when (1) the dietary intake is substantially increased, (2) mineralocorticoid levels are decreased (see below), or (3) following the administration of certain drugs (spironolactone, triamterene, amiloride).

Patients with Addison's disease (adrenal cortical insufficiency) present with hyperkalemia but more often manifest salt wasting and generalized debility. Adrenocortical insufficiency is by far the most common cause of hyperkalemia in patients with normal renal function. Recently, it has become apparent that a significant group of patients with chronic renal disease may present with hyperkalemia and hyperchloremic metabolic acidosis out of proportion to the decrease in renal function (as estimated by glomerular filtration rate). Studies in these patients have revealed a selective defect in aldosterone secretion (hypoaldosteronism) that appears to be secondary to a defect in renal renin secretion (hyporeninism). These defects have been commonly associated with diabetic nephropathy, and tubulo-interstitial diseases and they may be due to vascular damage to the cells of the juxtaglomerular apparatus and/or the tubular cells engaged in distal potassium secretion. In diabetic patients, insulin deficiency may be a contributing factor to hyperkalemia (cf. Figure 6). Patients with hyporenin hypoaldosteronism may be distinguished from those with Addison's disease by the presence in the former of normal glucocorticoid function.

Spironolactone acts as an antagonist to aldosterone by binding to the mineralocorticoid receptor protein in the cytosol of target cells and forming a complex spironolactone receptor which does not activate gene transcription.

Table IV. Causes of Hyperkalemia

   I. Due to decreased renal excretion
      A. Oliguric renal failure
         1. Acute
         2. Chronic
      B. Mineralocorticoid deficiency
         1. Addison's disease
         2. Hyporeninemic hypoaldosteronism
      C. Drugs that impair renal potassium excretion
         1. Spironolactones (aldosterone antagonist)
         2. Triamterene
         3. Amiloride
      D. Tubular defects in renal potassium excretion
  II. As a result of redistribution of K from cells to extracellular fluid
      A. Acidosis
         1. Metabolic
         2. Respiratory
      B. Rapid release of cell K^+
         1. Crush injury
         2. Chemotherapy of lymphomas, leukemia, multiple myeloma
         3. Arginine infusion
         4. Familial hyperkalemic episodic paralysis
 III. As a result of a high K intake
      A. Oral K supplementation
      B. Salt substitutes
      C. Intravenous K administration
  IV. Pseudohyperkalemia
      A. Hemolysis of blood
      B. Thrombocytosis

This results in inhibition of the aldosterone-dependent sodium reabsorption in the distal nephron (cortical collecting tubule) and a decrease in the electrical gradients with a correspondent inhibition of distal tubular secretion of potassium. In addition, spironolactone appears to change the permeability of the luminal membrane to sodium and markedly reduces the transmembrane potential which, as previously mentioned, is a major driving force for potassium secretion. It should be emphasized that drug-related hyperkalemia is rarely severe except in the presence of renal disease.

The term *pseudohyperkalemia* refers to spurious elevations of serum potassium. It may occur (1) when blood is hemolyzed during collection and/or processing, or (2) in patients with marked elevations of platelet or white blood cell counts. Hyperkalemia in the latter case appears to be due to potassium release from platelets or leukocytes during blood clotting. Determination of potassium in plasma rather than serum will show a normal potassium level. Needless to say, patients with pseudohyperkalemia do not show any clinical sign of potassium excess.

B. Management of Hyperkalemia

The effect of acute increases in the ECF concentration of potassium can be reversed by several maneuvers.

1. Physiologic Antagonists (Most Rapid Therapy in an Emergency)

Calcium Gluconate. Two grams of a 10% solution of calcium gluconate may be given intravenously every 2–4 hr. As previously discussed, a rise in ionized calcium decreases the threshold potential and increases the difference between the resting membrane potential and the threshold potential. This decreases tissue excitability and thus antagonizes the effects of hyperkalemia on the heart (cf. Figure 3). Calcium should be used if the electrocardiogram suggests imminent disaster or if serum potassium is greater than 8 mEq/liter. (Be careful not to produce hypercalcemia in digitalized patients.)

2. Reduction of Serum Potassium Concentration

One or more of these measures must be taken, even if a physiologic antagonist is used.

a. Promote the Shift of K^+ from Serum into Cells

(1) Correct severe acidosis. Administer IV sodium bicarbonate to raise serum HCO_3^- to at least 15 mEq/liter. This effect is transient and dependent on the changes in hydrogen ion activity (pH) that follow administration of bicarbonate.

(2) Insulin, IV, 15–30 units, crystalline zinc insulin every 3 hr, indefi-

nitely. To prevent hypoglycemia, add 2–5 g of glucose per unit of insulin to the intravenous infusion flask. The mechanism of action of insulin appears to be a direct stimulation of the activity of the sodium–potassium pump with a corresponding increase in the active uptake of potassium by muscle cells.

b. Remove Potassium from the Body

(1) Oral or rectal administration of an ion-exchange resin, such as sodium-cyclic sulfonic polystyrene (Kayexelate®), 40–80 g/day in divided doses. This is a slow measure. Serum potassium is reduced by only 0.5–1 mEq/liter in 24 hr by the resin. Resin therapy is, therefore, ideally prophylactic; begin it early in the course of acute renal failure. Watch carefully for signs of intestinal obstruction occasionally produced by the resin mass. Can be combined with production of osmotic diarrhea by sorbitol, 10–20 ml of 70% sorbitol, every 2 hr until diarrhea is produced. Adjust sorbitol dose to yield one or two watery stools a day.

(2) Peritoneal dialysis. Convenient but slow.

(3) Hemodialysis. If serum potassium rises rapidly and exceeds 7 mEq/liter, hemodialysis may be the only effective measure.

SUGGESTED READINGS

Ammon, R. A., May, W. S., and Nightingale, S. D.: Glucose-induced hyperkalemia with normal aldosterone levels. *Ann. Intern. Med.* 89:349, 1978.

Berl, T., Linas, S. L., Aisenbrey, G. A., *et al.*: On the mechanism of polyuria in potassium depletion: The role of polydipsia. *J. Clin. Invest.* 60:620, 1977.

Berl, T., Aisenbrey, G. A., and Linas, S. L.: Renal concentrating defect in the hypokalemic rat is prostaglandin independent. *Am. J. Physiol.* 238:F37–F41, 1980.

Brenner, B. M., and Stein, J. H.: *Contemporary Issues in Nephrology. Acid–Base and Potassium Homeostasis*, Vol. 2. Churchill Livingstone, New York, 1978.

Doucet, A., and Katz, A. I.: Renal potassium adaptation: Na-K-ATPase activity along the nephron after chronic potassium loading. *Am. J. Physiol.* 238:F380–F386, 1980.

Hayslett, J. P., Myketey, N., Binder, H. J., and Aronson, P. S.: Mechanism of increased potassium secretion in potassium loading and sodium deprivation. *Am. J. Physiol.* 239:F378–F382, 1980.

Knochel, J. P.: The syndrome of hyporeninemic hypoaldosteronism. *Annu. Rev. Med.* 30:145–153, 1979.

Kunau, R. T., and Stein, J. H.: Disorders of hypo- and hyperkalemia. *Clin. Nephrol.* 7:173–190, 1977.

Muggia, F. M.: Hyperkalemia and chemotherapy. *Lancet* 1:602, 1973.

Rodriguez, H. J., Hogan, W. C., Hellman, R. N., and Klahr, S.: Mechanism of activation of renal Na^+-K^+-ATPase in the rat: effects of potassium loading. *Am. J. Physiol.* 238:F315–F323, 1980.

Sachs, G.: Ion pumps in the renal tubule. *Am. J. Physiol.* 233(5):F359–F365, 1977.

Sopko, J. A., and Freeman, R. M.: Salt substitutes as a source of potassium. *J. Am. Med. Assoc.* 238:608, 1977.

Tannen, R. L.: Symposium on potassium homeostasis. *Kidney Int.* 11:389–505, 1977.

Wright, F. S., and Giebisch, G.: Renal potassium transport: contributions of individual nephron segments and populations. *Am. J. Physiol.* 235(6):F515–F527, 1978.

Pathophysiology of Acid–Base Metabolism

KEITH HRUSKA

I. INTRODUCTION

The hydrogen ion (H^+) concentration of the extracellular fluid (ECF) is regulated within narrow limits. The normal blood pH of 7.4 is the negative log of 40 nEq/liter (40×10^{-9} moles/liter) of H^+. By contrast, sodium and potassium are present in the ECF in mEq/liter (10^{-3} moles/liter) concentrations. Thus, the concentration of H^+ is about one millionth the concentration of sodium and potassium in the ECF, and the regulation of the H^+ concentration is two orders of magnitude more precise than the regulation of these two cations which exhibit changes in concentration in terms of mEq/liter instead of nEq/liter. This close regulation of H^+ concentration is essential for normal cell function because of the high reactivity of H^+. Small changes in H^+ concentration have dramatic effects on body functions. The process through which H^+ concentration remains nearly constant, even in the presence of continual addition of organic acids to the extracellular fluid, involves three basic steps. The first is chemical buffering by extracellular and intracellular buffers; secondly the carbon dioxide (CO_2) level of the blood is controlled by alveolar ventilation; and thirdly, the bicarbonate

KEITH HRUSKA • Department of Medicine, Washington University School of Medicine and The Jewish Hospital of St. Louis, St. Louis, Missouri 63110.

(HCO_3^-) concentration in the blood is controlled by regulation of renal H^+ excretion. This chapter will review the basic principles of acid–base physiology and discuss the clinical disorders of acid–base homeostasis.

II. CHEMISTRY OF ACIDS AND BASES

Acids are substances which donate H^+ and bases are substances which accept H^+. The function of a substance as an acid or a base may be independent of charge. For instance, some of the physiologically important acids and bases are as follows:

Acids		Bases
H_2CO_3	$\rightleftharpoons$	$H^+ + HCO_3^-$
$H_2PO_4^-$	$\rightleftharpoons$	$H^+ + HPO_4^{2-}$
H_2SO_4	$\rightleftharpoons$	$2H^+ + SO_4$
NH_4^+	$\rightleftharpoons$	$H^+ + NH_3$
HCl	$\rightleftharpoons$	$H^+ + Cl^-$

Physiologically important acids fall into two general categories: (1) Carbonic acid, which is produced through the action of carbon dioxide combining with water. Since 15,000 mmoles of CO_2 are produced by the metabolism of carbohydrates and fats each day, progressive accumulation of carbonic acid would occur if the lungs failed to excrete CO_2. (2) Noncarbonic acids, which are produced primarily from the metabolism of proteins. Only 50–100 mEq of H^+ are produced from these sources each day. These H^+ ions are buffered and are then excreted by the kidney.

The dissociation of all acids and bases conforms to the law of mass action:

$$K_a = \frac{[H^+][A^-]}{[HA]} \tag{1}$$

An acid (HA) dissociates into H^+ and A^- and K_a is the apparent ionization or dissociation constant for this acid. Each acid has its own dissociation constant. Acids or bases may be classified as strong or weak, according to their dissociation constant. A strong acid has a high dissocation constant and exists predominantly as H^+ and A^-. HCl is a strong acid and exists completely dissociated. In comparison, $H_2PO_4^-$ is only 80% dissociated at the normal extracellular H^+ concentration and is a weak acid. In general, the salts of weak acids (A^-) are the principal buffers in the body.

The normal ECF H^+ concentration is approximately 40 nmoles/liter. H^+ concentration is most commonly expressed as the negative logarithm of the H^+ concentration, the pH. In the measurement of pH, it is assumed that the H^+ concentration in plasma is the same as the H^+ activity of blood. The latter can be measured by a glass membrane electrode permeable only to H^+.

The equation for the law of mass action for the dissociation of acids [equation (1)] can be rewritten $[H^+] = K_a [HA]/[A^-]$. By converting to negative logarithms both sides of this formula and by substituting pH for $-\log H^+$ and defining minus log of the K_a as pK:

$$pH = pK_a + \log \frac{[A^-]}{[HA]} \tag{2}$$

This is the Henderson–Hasselbalch equation. It is used to describe the dissociation of acids and to calculate the H^+ concentration of fluids. The A^- represents the base and the HA represents the acid.

III. EXTRACELLULAR BUFFERS AND FUNCTION OF THE BICARBONATE–CO₂ SYSTEM AS A PHYSIOLOGIC BUFFER

Substances which prevent large changes in H^+ concentration are called buffers. These are primarily salts of weak acids capable of binding or releasing H^+ so that changes in the H^+ concentration are minimized. The most important buffers in the ECF are bicarbonate and secondary phosphates. In the presence of free H^+, the basic forms of these substances accept the H^+ and prevent large changes in the pH of the solution that would occur in the presence of H^+ release. The titration curves of phosphate ions and the bicarbonate ion are shown in Figure 1. The shape of these curves is sigmoidal. Each curve has a relatively straight region in which large amounts of strong acid can be added without much change in the pH. The straight portion of these titration curves extend approximately $\pm$ 1.0 pH unit from the pK, the pH at which the weak acid is 50% dissociated, of the buffer pair. In this pH range, 90% of the acid neutralizing capacity of a buffer will be expended. Additional acid equal to 9% of that neutralized within one pH unit

Figure 1. Titration curve of HPO_4^{2-} and HCO_3^- by addition of strong acid. The alkaline pH of the dissociated buffer pairs (HPO_4^{2-} and HCO_3^-) becomes increasingly acid as they accept H^+ when a strong acid is added. The pK of the ion pair is the point at which they exist as 50% dissociated and undissociated. The strength of a buffer in preventing large changes of pH as H^+ is added or withdrawn from solution lies within the straight portion of the titration curve which is about 1.0 pH unit on either side of the pK.

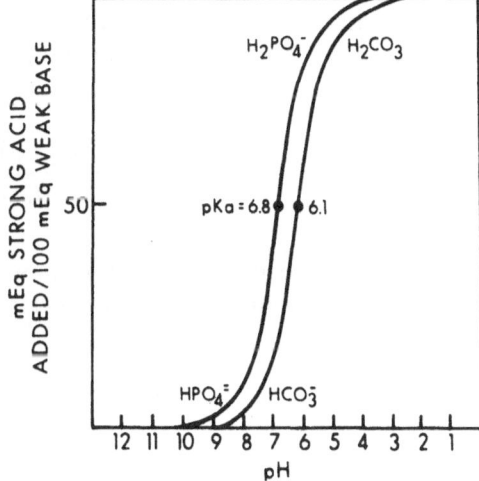

of the pK will lower the pH another whole pH unit. Thus, an ideal ECF buffer would be expected to have a p$K \pm 1.0$ pH unit from 7.4, the normal blood pH.

The principal buffer in the ECF is the bicarbonate ion. Its pK is 6.1 (Figure 1) which is further removed than optimal for functioning as the major buffer for blood with a pH of 7.4. Bicarbonate ion is formed from the dissociation of carbonic acid into H^+ and bicarbonate. Carbonic acid in turn is formed from the hydration of CO_2. The reactions of CO_2, carbonic acid, and bicarbonate can be written as

$$CO_2 + H_2O \rightleftharpoons H_2CO_3 \rightleftharpoons H^+ + HCO_3^- \qquad (3)$$
$$\text{(Aqueous)}$$

The ability of the lungs to remove tremendous amounts of CO_2 from the blood and the ability of the kidney to regenerate bicarbonate ion allows the bicarbonate ion–carbonic acid pair to function well as the major ECF buffer despite its lower-than-optimal pK.

Since all gases dissolve in water to some extent, the degree to which this occurs is proportional to the partial pressure of the gas in the solution. In humans, the partial pressure of CO_2 (P_{CO_2}) in the arterial blood is in equilibrium with that in the alveolar air. This is approximately 40 mm Hg at 37°C. Thus, the amount of CO_2 dissolved in the plasma is

$$[CO_2] \text{ dis} = 0.03 P_{CO_2}$$

$$= 0.03 \times 40 = 1\ 2 \text{ mmoles/liter}$$

where 0.03 is the solubility constant for CO_2 in the plasma. The equilibrium of the reaction ($[CO_2]$ dis $+ H_2O \rightleftharpoons H_2CO_3$) is normally far to the left and there are approximately 500 molecules of CO_2 in solution for each molecule of carbonic acid. Despite this, an increase in P_{CO_2} increases the dissolved CO_2 and therefore the carbonic acid concentration. Thus CO_2, which is not an acid, increases the acidity of the solutions through the formation of carbonic acid. The law of mass action for the above reaction of the hydration of CO_2 and dissociation of carbonic acid can be written

$$K_a = \frac{[H^+][HCO_3^-]}{[CO_2] \text{ dis}}$$

The pK of this reaction is 6.1; if we now solve this equation for hydrogen ion concentration using the Henderson–Hasselbalch equation, the

$$pH = 6.1 + \log \frac{[HCO_3^-]}{0.03 P_{CO_2}} \qquad (4)$$

The normal blood pH can then be calculated from the plasma HCO_3^- and the CO_2 dissolved in plasma (carbonic acid):

$$7.4 = 6.1 + \log\frac{[24]}{[1.2]}$$

where the ratio of bicarbonate/$[CO_2]$ dis is 20, and the log of 20 is 1.3.

In clinical practice, the plasma bicarbonate concentration can be calculated by measuring pH and P_{CO_2} by specific electrodes and solving the Henderson–Hasselbalch equation [equation (4)] for bicarbonate concentration.

$$7.4 = 6.1 + \log\frac{[HCO_3^-]}{0.03P_{CO_2}}$$

$$\log[HCO_3^-] = 7.4 - 6.1 + \log(0.03 \times P_{CO_2})$$

where $\log 1.2 = 0.08$ and the antilog of 1.38 is 24. Plasma bicarbonate can be measured by adding a strong acid to plasma and measuring the amount of CO_2 generated, e.g., as the added hydrogen combines with the plasma bicarbonate and H_2CO_3 then CO_2 is formed. This method measures total CO_2 content which is equal to all the forms by which CO_2 is carried in the blood:

$$\text{Total } CO_2 \text{ content} = [HCO_3^-] + [CO_2]\text{ dis}$$

Since H_2CO_3 exists in blood essentially as dissolved CO_2, it is omitted. If 0.03 of the P_{CO_2} is substituted for CO_2 dissolved, then

$$[HCO_3^-] = \text{total } CO_2 - 0.03P_{CO_2} \tag{5}$$

The ventilatory response to acidemia produces a reduction in P_{CO_2} of approximately 1.1 mm Hg for each 1.0 mmole/liter fall in plasma bicarbonate. Hyperventilation is much more effective in maintaining the pH than hypoventilation, which occurs in response to alkalosis, since needs for oxygenation limit the degree of hypoventilation. Both of these compensatory mechanisms of ventilation are temporary and their driving force is such that they very rarely, if ever, return the pH of blood completely to normal.

Beside the bicarbonate–CO_2 system there are other quantitatively less important buffers in the ECF, including inorganic phosphates (plasma phosphate concentration is 1.0 vs 24.0 mM bicarbonate), hemoglobin, and the plasma proteins. In the blood, the total noncarbonate buffering capacity amounts to 47% of all available buffer. Of this, hemoglobin and oxyhemoglobin contribute the greatest fraction, about 34%. The plasma bicarbonate contributes 35% and an additional 18% comes from the bicarbonate in the erythrocytes. Thus 53% of the total buffering capacity of whole blood is through the bicarbonate–CO_2 system.

IV. INTRACELLULAR BUFFERING

Besides the extracellular buffer mechanisms discussed above, acids are also buffered within the cells. Acidosis also decreases the normal intracellular H^+ production from metabolism and organic acid production and this indirectly serves to enhance the intracellular buffering capacity. Buffering of H^+ in the cells has important effects on the plasma potassium concentration. In order to maintain electroneutrality, the movement of H^+ into the cells is associated with movement of sodium and potassium out of the cells. This may result in a potentially serious increase of 1–4 mEq/liter in the plasma potassium concentration. Conversely, if the extracellular H^+ concentration is reduced because of hydrogen loss, H^+ are released from the intracellular buffers and enter the ECF. In this setting, sodium and potassium move into the cells, resulting in a fall in the plasma potassium concentration (see Chapter 7).

A. Bone as a Buffer Source

Bone carbonate represents a large store of buffer which contributes to the buffering of acid and base loads. Under some circumstances, the bone may contribute as much as 40% of the buffering of an acute acid load. Buffering of H^+ by bone carbonate results in release of calcium from bone into the ECF. In the presence of a chronic acid load, the bone buffering may be even greater than 40%. This is seen in patients with chronic renal failure.

V. PHYSIOLOGY OF ACID–BASE REGULATION

Daily, almost 15,000 mmoles of CO_2 are liberated from the metabolism of carbohydrates and fats. Since CO_2 combines with water to form carbonic acid, severe acidosis would ensue if the CO_2 produced were not excreted via the lungs. In addition, approximately 50–100 mEq of H^+ are produced each day from the metabolism of proteins and the hydrolysis of phosphoester acids:

$$\text{Methionine} + O_2 \rightarrow \text{Urea} + CO_2 + SO_4^{2-} + 2H^+$$

$$R\text{---}H_2PO_4 + H_2O \rightarrow ROH + 0.8HPO_4^{2-}/0.2H_2PO_4^- + 1.8H^+$$

Table I. Normal Arterial and Venous Blood Values

	pH	H^+ (nEq/liter)	P_{CO_2} (mm Hg)	HCO_3^- (mEq/liter)
Arterial	7.37–7.43	37–43	36–44	22–26
Venous	7.32–7.39	42–48	42–50	23–27

The response of the body to the production of CO_2 and H^+ occurs in three stages: (1) chemical buffering by extracellular and intracellular buffers, (2) changes in alveolar ventilation to control the P_{CO_2}, and (3) alteration in renal H^+ excretion to maintain the bicarbonate concentration. These adjustments are adequate under normal conditions to maintain a steady state of H^+ and CO_2 excretion equal to their rates of production. As a result, the H^+ concentration is maintained within narrow limits. Normal values for arterial and venous pH, H^+ concentrations, P_{CO_2}, and bicarbonate levels are shown in Table I.

A. Renal Excretion of Hydrogen

The kidney contributes to the maintenance of normal H^+ concentration in plasma by (1) reabsorbing the filtered bicarbonate thus, preventing loss of base in the urine, and (2) excreting the 50–100 mEq of H^+ produced per day in the form of nonvolatile acids. Since the urine pH is never less than 4.5 in man (a value which cannot account for the amount of H^+ excreted daily), it is apparent that H^+ in the urine is buffered. The main urinary buffers are ammonia (NH_3), which combines with H^+ to form ammonium ion (NH_4^+), and other urinary buffers referred to as titratable acidity (which are largely $H_2PO_4^-$ and HPO_4^{2-}). However, H^+ excretion cannot take place until the filtered bicarbonate is reabsorbed since loss of bicarbonate in the urine would be equivalent to the addition of H^+ to the body. In a normal subject with a GFR of 180 liters/day and plasma bicarbonate of 24 mEq/liter, the reabsorption of 4300 mEq of bicarbonate is required before the excretion of 50–100 mEq of H^+ can be accomplished.

The reabsorption of bicarbonate, and the excretion of titratable acidity and NH_4^+ all occur by active H^+ secretion from the tubular cell into the lumen (Figures 2 and 3). Secretion of H^+ appears to be coupled to passive sodium movement across the luminal membrane of the tubular cells (Figure 2). The secreted H^+ ions are generated within the tubular cells by the action of carbonic anhydrase. This enzyme catalyzes the hydration of CO_2 to H_2CO_3, which immediately dissociates into H^+ and bicarbonate ion. The H^+ is secreted into the tubular fluid and the bicarbonate ion formed is returned to the plasma. Thus, H^+ secretion represents generation of bicarbonate in the plasma. If the H^+ secreted into the tubular fluid combines with filtered bicarbonate then the net effect is bicarbonate reabsorption (Figure 2). This

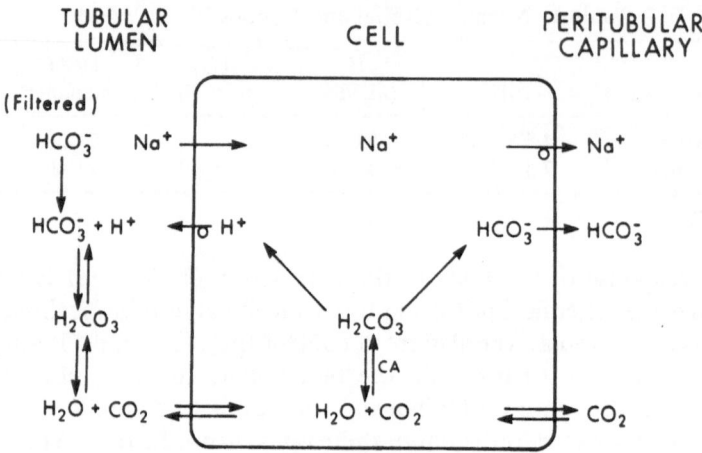

Figure 2. Conceptual treatment of the luminal and cellular events involved in renal tubular HCO_3^- reabsorption. CA indicates the action of carbonic anhydrase.

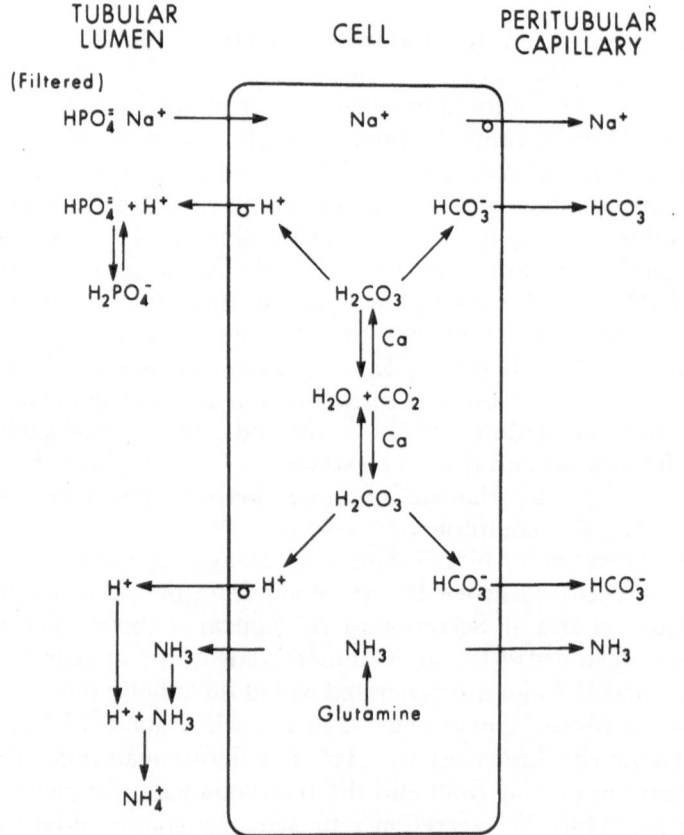

Figure 3. Formation of titratable acidity and NH_4^+ in the tubule. Each H^+ secreted results in the generation of a HCO_3^- in the peritubular capillary.

maintains the plasma bicarbonate concentration normal by reclaiming all of the bicarbonate filtered. If the secreted H^+ combines with buffers, such as HPO_4^{2-} or NH_3, a new bicarbonate ion is added to the peritubular capillary blood (Figure 3). This results in an increase in the plasma bicarbonate concentration to replace the bicarbonate which was lost in buffering the daily H^+ load from nonvolatile acids. Thus, the quantity of H^+ excreted in the urine, the net H^+ excretion, can be written as follows:

$$\text{Net } H^+ \text{ excretion} = NH_4 + \text{titratable acidity} - \text{urinary } HCO_3 \quad (6)$$

In the steady state, the net amount of H^+ excreted is equal to the hydrogen load, about 50–100 mEq/day. At times, net H^+ excretion is absent or has a negative value. This occurs after ingestion of bicarbonate load such as drinking a citrate-containing fruit juice. As the citrate is metabolized to bicarbonate, the urine will become alkaline as bicarbonaturia appears and titratable acid and ammonia excretion will be zero.

1. Bicarbonate Reabsorption

Bicarbonate ion in the blood is freely filtered by the renal glomerulus. It is removed from the glomerular filtrate by combining with secreted H^+ to form H_2CO_3. The latter rapidly dissociates into H_2O and CO_2, which are then reabsorbed. Within the cell, the dehydration of carbonic acid to produce the H^+ that is secreted also results in the formation of a bicarbonate ion. This is returned to the peritubular blood. The net effect of the luminal and intracellular processes can be viewed as an indirect reabsorption of the bicarbonate ion. The bulk of bicarbonate reabsorption (about 80%–84%) occurs in the proximal portion of the nephron. The distal tubule and the collecting ducts reabsorb the remaining 15%–20% of the filtered bicarbonate, again by active H^+ secretion as in the proximal nephron.

2. Titratable Acidity

Several weak acids present in plasma are filtered and serve as buffers in the urine. Their buffering capacity, referred to as "titratable acidity" (Figure 3), is measured by the amount of sodium hydroxide that must be added to a 24-hr urine specimen to titrate the urine pH back to 7.4. Under normal conditions, "titratable acidity" is 10–40 mEq/day of H^+. The buffering capacity of these weak acids in the urine is related to their quantity in the urine and their pK. Remember that the pK is important since maximum buffering capacity occurs at ± 1.0 pH unit from the pK of the buffer. Because of its relatively high urinary concentration and its favorable pK (6.8), the bulk of the urinary buffering is accomplished by HPO_4^{2-} according to the equation $H^+ + HPO_4^{2-} \rightleftharpoons H_2PO_4^-$. Other weak acids such as uric acid, creatinine, and sulfates make lesser contributions to urine buffering. The ability of phosphate to buffer H^+ is illustrated by the following example. From the Henderson–Hasselbalch equation for the $HPO_4^{2-}/H_2PO_4^-$ system ($pK = 6.8$),

$$pH = 6.8 + \log \frac{HPO_4^{2-}}{H_2PO_4^-}$$

At the pH of plasma (7.4) the log of the ratio $HPO_4^{2-}/H_2PO_4^-$ is 0.6 and the antilog of this is 4.0. Thus, the normal ratio of $HPO_4^{2-}/H_2PO_4^-$ buffer pair is 4:1. If 50 mM of phosphate is excreted in the urine and the rest reabsorbed, then 40 mM will exist as HPO_4^{2-} and 10 mM as $H_2PO_4^-$ at pH 7.4 as in the glomerular filtrate. In the proximal tubule, as H^+ is secreted, the tubular fluid pH is lowered to approximately 6.8. From the above equation for $HPO_4^{2-}/H_2PO_4^-$, the ratio of $HPO_4^{2-}/H_2PO_4^-$ will fall to 1:1. As a result there will now be 25 mM of both HPO_4^{2-} and $H_2PO_4^-$ in the tubule. This represents the buffering of 15 mM of H^+ by HPO_4^{2-} with an increase in the free H^+ concentration from 40 nmoles/liter (pH of 7.4) to only 160 nmoles/liter (pH of 6.8). Thus, over 99.9% of the secreted H^+ has been buffered. If the tubular fluid pH is lowered to 4.8 (H^+ concentration of 0.016 nmoles/liter), essentially all the HPO_4^{2-} will have been converted to $H_2PO_4^-$ and a total of 40 mM of H^+ will have been buffered by $H_2PO_4^-$.

The amount of H^+ buffered by HPO_4^{2-} increases as the tubular fluid pH is reduced. When the urine pH reaches its minimum of 4.5–5.0, further buffering by HPO_4^{2-} cannot occur unless there is an increase in phosphate excretion. However, phosphate excretion is relatively constant in the presence of an acid load, and the ability to enhance net H^+ excretion by increased formation of titratable acidity is limited. An exception to this is in ketoacidosis where large amounts of β-hydroxybutyrate ($pK = 4.8$) is excreted in the urine. This ketoacid can act as a urinary buffer augmenting titratable acid excretion by as much as 150 mEq/day.

3. Ammonia

Ammonia is a base which can combine with H^+ to form ammonium ion (NH_4^+):

$$NH_3 + H^+ \rightleftharpoons NH_4^+$$

the pK of the NH_3/NH_4^+ system is 9.3. Therefore, at a normal arterial pH the ratio of NH_3/NH_4^+ is almost 1:100. Thus, NH_3 is an ineffective buffer. However, as NH_3 enters the tubular lumen, by a passive nonionic diffusion, it will bind with H^+ forming NH_4^+. This process depends on the solubility characteristics of NH_3 and NH_4^+. NH_3 is lipid soluble and crosses cell membranes passively in a manner similar to CO_2. In contrast, the NH_4^+ ion is polar and water soluble, thus crossing lipid membranes poorly. Once

NH_4^+ is formed in the tubular lumen, it cannot diffuse out. Thus, as NH_3 binds with secreted hydrogen, the H^+ is trapped in the lumen as NH_4^+ (Figure 3).

Ammonia is formed in the tubular cells from the metabolism of amino acids, particularly glutamine, according to the following reaction:

$$\text{Glutamine} \rightleftharpoons \text{Glutamine acid } + NH_3$$

$$\Updownarrow$$

$$\alpha\text{-Ketoglutarate } + NH_3$$

The enzyme glutaminase-1 catalyzes the reaction of glutamine to glutamic acid with the release of ammonia. A second NH_3 is released when glutamic acid is metabolized to α-KG. The glutaminase-1 reaction is pH dependent and increases with acidosis and decreases with alkalosis. The effect of acidosis on glutamine metabolism takes several days to reach its maximum. The effect may be due to increased glutamine entry into the mitochondria, the site of glutaminase-1 activity, or an increase in the activity of the glutaminase-1 enzyme. Whichever mechanism is operative, the pH dependence of glutamine metabolism may be mediated by changes in intracellular pH. Although only 30–50 mEq of H^+ is excreted as NH_4^+ per day under normal conditions, NH_4^+ excretion can increase to more than 250 mEq/day in the presence of metabolic acidosis. The ability to augment NH_3 production and NH_4^+ excretion is the main adaptive response of the kidney to an acid load. In addition to the pH of the urine and the blood and the availability of glutamine, NH_4^+ excretion is dependent upon two other factors. The first is the functioning renal mass. In patients with chronic renal failure, there is a reduction in NH_4^+ excretion that is proportional to the reduction in glomerular filtration rate (GFR). This decrease in net H^+ excretion accounts in a large part for the metabolic acidosis observed in chronic renal failure (see Section V, Chapter 14). Second, ammonium (NH_4^+) excretion is affected by changes in effective circulating volume. In patients who are volume depleted and avidly reabsorbing sodium, NH_4^+ excretion may be increased independent of acid–base balance.

4. Urine pH

As shown in Figure 4, the urine pH falls in the terminal portion of the nephron, probably the collecting ducts, because of H^+ secretion and to some extent continued fluid readsorption. In humans, a pH minimum of 4.5–5.0 is reached in the collecting ducts. This represents a plasma to tubular fluid H^+ gradient of almost 1 to 1000. The inability to lower the pH further may reflect a limitation in the electromotive force of the H^+ secretory process or backflux of H^+ from the tubular fluid into the cell. The low values of urine pH are important because the formation of titratable acidity and NH_4^+ are pH dependent. They both increase as the urine is made more acid. If the

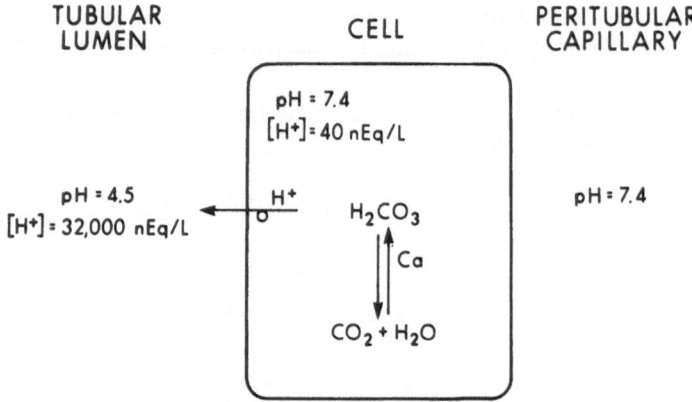

Figure 4. In the terminal nephron, continued H^+ secretion results in a reduction of the tubular fluid pH to a minimum of 4.5. The pH differential between the cell and the urine represents secretion of H^+ against a concentration gradient of nearly 1000:1.

urine pH does not fall below 5.5 or 6.0, titratable acid and NH_4^+ excretion are significantly reduced. Thus, the excretion of the daily H^+ load may be prevented. This appears to be the mechanism responsible for acidosis in patients with distal renal tubular acidosis (distal RTA), as discussed below.

B. Regulation of Renal Hydrogen Ion Excretion

The preceding sections have discussed the mechanism by which the kidney excretes H^+. This section will review factors that regulate H^+ excretion by the kidney. The major factors that influence H^+ secretion are (1) effective circulating volume, (2) reabsorbability of the anions in the tubular fluid, (3) arterial pH, (4) plasma potassium concentration, and (5) aldosterone.

1. Effective Circulating Volume

As reviewed in the chapter on sodium (Chapter 4), the renal response to hypovolemia is conservation of sodium. In this situation, the urinary sodium is reduced to very low levels. Since chloride is the only quantitatively important, reabsorbable anion in the glomerular filtrate, electrical neutrality is maintained in the face of sodium reabsorption according to the following concept:

$$Na^+ \text{ reabsorption} \cong Cl^- \text{ reabsorption} + (H^+ + K^+) \text{ secretion}$$

Of these factors, potassium secretion is the least important quantitatively, representing only 40–100 mEq/day as opposed to 20,000 mEq of chloride ion and 4300 mEq of bicarbonate reabsorbed (bicarbonate reabsorption is representative of H^+ secretion). If the glomerular filtrate Na^+ concentration if 140 mEq/liter, the filtrate HCO_3^- is 24 mEq/liter and the filtrate chloride is 105 mEq/liter, then only 130 mEq/liter of Na^+ can be reabsorbed with the existing HCO_3^- and chloride concentrations. In order to maintain electro-neutrality, further sodium reabsorption must be accompanied by either H^+ or potassium secretion. Hydrogen accounts for most of the sodium reab-sorption in this case. Thus, when sodium is conserved maximally as in volume depletion, H^+ secretion is increased. This results in increased HCO_3^- generation in the peritubular capillary and systemic alkalosis may develop. Conversely, volume expansion which diminishes fractional Na^+ reabsorption also decreases H^+ secretion and bicarbonate reabsorption.

2. Reabsorbability of the Anions in the Tubular Fluid

If significant amounts of Na^+ in the glomerular filtrate exist in associ-ation with nonreabsorbable anions, i.e., sulfate ions, then complete Na^+ reabsorption requires H^+ secretion in excess of the amount needed to reabsorb the filtered HCO_3^- just as in hypovolemic states. Thus, the state of the effective circulating ECF volume and the reabsorbability of the anion accompanying sodium to the distal nephron are important determinants of renal H^+ secretion.

3. Arterial pH

Net acid excretion [equation (6)] varies inversely with the arterial pH, increasing in acidosis and decreasing in alkalosis. This relationship plays an important role in the maintenance of acid–base homeostasis. Production of acidosis either by a decrease in the plasma bicarbonate concentration or an elevation in P_{CO_2} will augment H^+ excretion and raise the plasma bicarbonate concentration, thus returning the pH toward normal [equation (3)]. The role of arterial pH in the control of net acid excretion may be mediated by changes in renal tubular cell pH. In general, alterations in extracellular pH

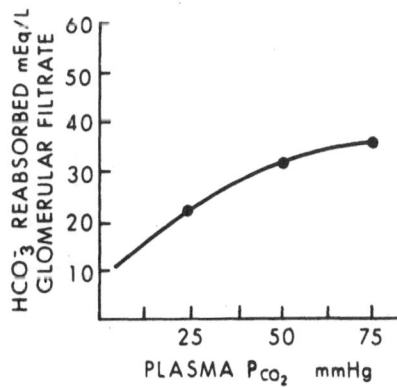

Figure 5. As the P_{CO_2} rises, increased H^+ secre-tion (HCO_3^- reabsorption) results. Conversely, during hyperventilation the lowering of the P_{CO_2} will decrease HCO_3^- reabsorption. (Adapted from data of Rector, F. C., et al.: *J. Clin. Invest.* 39:1706, 1960.)

result in parallel, although not equal, changes in intracellular pH. Thus, acidosis increases intracellular H^+ concentration thereby favoring H^+ secretion into the lumen. Intracellular acidosis also stimulates NH_3 formation, permitting secreted H^+ to be trapped in the lumen as NH_4^+. In alkalotic states, as H^+ concentrations decrease, the kidney excretes increasing amounts of bicarbonate in the urine. However, in clinical states of metabolic alkalosis, this adaptive response is frequently blunted. If the alkalosis is associated with volume depletion then the sodium-mediated stimulation of H^+ secretion and bicarbonate reabsorption becomes predominant and can prevent the excretion of bicarbonate. If alveolar ventilation induces changes in CO_2 elimination and the P_{CO_2} increases or decreases, respiratory alkalosis or acidosis results. The kidney minimizes the change in arterial pH in these states by varying H^+ excretion and bicarbonate reabsorption. The adaptive response of the kidney to an increase in P_{CO_2} or decrease in P_{CO_2} is directly related to a change in H^+ secretion (bicarbonate reabsorption) (Figure 5). As the plasma P_{CO_2} increases, there is an increase in H^+ secretion as NH_4^+, resulting in

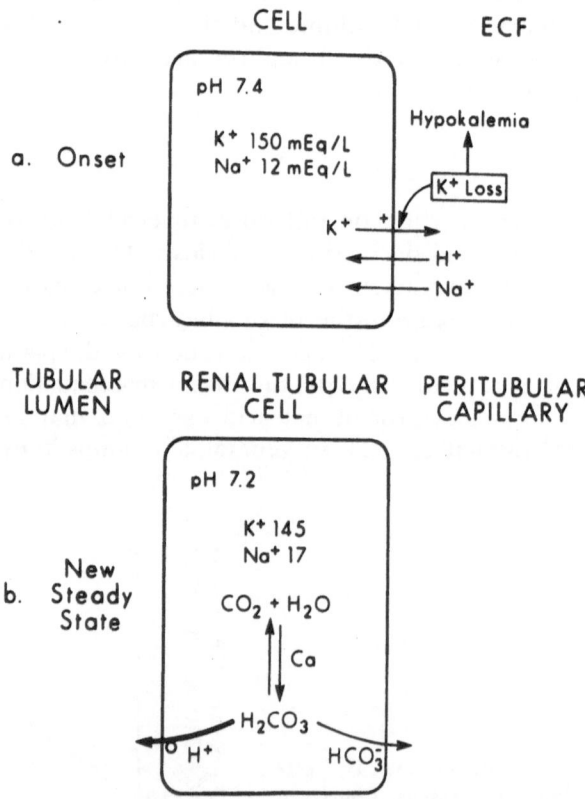

Figure 6. (a) Potassium loss from the ECF results in hypokalemia and potassium exit from the cellular compartments in exchange for increased intracellular H^+ and Na^+ concentrations. (b) In the new steady state the intracellular acidosis increases HCO_3^- reabsorption in renal tubular cells.

increased bicarbonate generation in the plasma. This adaptive response is relatively slow (it begins in 8–10 hr) but does not reach completion for 4–5 days.

4. Plasma Potassium Concentration

An inverse relationship between the plasma potassium concentration and bicarbonate reabsorption has been demonstrated. This effect appears to be related to changes in cell H^+ concentration induced by cation shifts between the cell and the ECF (Figure 6). If hypokalemia develops, potassium leaves the cell down a concentration gradient. In order to maintain electrical neutrality, H^+ and sodium enter the cell, resulting in intracellular acidosis. The increase in cell H^+ concentration (intracellular acidosis) accounts for the enhanced H^+ secretion and bicarbonate reabsorption observed with potassium depletion.

5. Aldosterone

Aldosterone stimulates both potassium secretion and H^+ secretion in the distal nephron. Aldosterone is thus a factor in the increased bicarbonate reabsorption associated with volume depletion and secondary hyperaldosteronism and hypokalemia. Aldosterone excess is associated with a metabolic alkalosis, and aldosterone deficiency is associated with decreased H^+ excretion and metabolic acidosis.

VI. CONTROL OF VENTILATION

Alveolar ventilation is controlled by changes in P_{CO_2}. The stimulus appears to be sensed by changes in arterial pH. Thus, increases in P_{CO_2} lower the pH, resulting in hyperventilation and the elimination of excess CO_2. This is extremely important in the maintenance of arterial pH since 15,000 mmoles of CO_2 are produced daily from endogenous metabolism. The pH stimulus to ventilation is sensed by chemoreceptors in the medulla oblongata which respond to changes in cerebral interstitial pH and by peripheral chemoreceptors in the carotid bodies and the aortic arch, which respond to changes in arterial pH.

Alveolar ventilation is also affected by alterations in pH produced by changes in the plasma bicarbonate concentration. In metabolic acidosis, the volume of ventilation may increase from the normal of 5.0 liters/min to greater than 30 liters/min as the arterial pH falls from 7.4 toward 7.0. The reduction in P_{CO_2} is induced by the increased ventilation. Conversely, when the plasma bicarbonate concentration is increased in a patient with metabolic alkalosis hypoventilation with consequent elevation in the P_{CO_2} reduces the pH toward normal. These respiratory compensations for metabolic acidosis and alkalosis are extremely important and can turn a life-threatening change in pH into one that is much less dangerous. In contrast to the renal compensation for respiratory acid–base disorders, which takes three to five days for complete response, the respiratory adaptation to metabolic disorders of pH is rapid, beginning within minutes and reaching its maximum effect within 12–24 hr.

VII. CHARACTERISTICS OF ACID–BASE DISORDERS

In a variety of clinical conditions to be discussed below, the arterial H^+ concentration becomes abnormal. An increase in H^+ concentration lowers the blood pH and is referred to as acidosis. From equation (4), it is apparent that acidosis can be produced by either a reduction in the blood HCO_3^- concentration or by an elevation in the P_{CO_2}. This fact is illustrated graphically in Figure 7, which shows the relationship between blood pH, the HCO_3^- concentration, and the P_{CO_2}. The H^+ concentration is depicted by a series of isobars radiating from the origin of the figure. A pH in the range of the acidosis isobars can be produced by either a primary elevation in the P_{CO_2} or a reduction in the plasma HCO_3^-. Conversely, a decrease in H^+ concentration will elevate the blood pH and is referred to as alkalosis. Again from equation (4), a decrease in the P_{CO_2} or an increase in the plasma HCO_3^- will result in an elevation of the blood pH. In Figure 7, the situation is again portrayed graphically. The blood pH in the range of the alkalosis isobars can be produced by either a primary elevation in the plasma HCO_3^- or a reduction in the P_{CO_2}. Changes in pH result from abnormal renal or respiratory

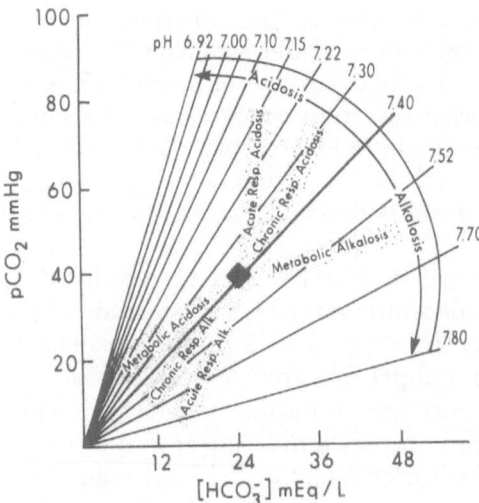

Figure 7. The relationships between P_{CO_2}, HCO_3^-, and pH. The normal status of the blood pH and the CO_2/HCO_3^- ion buffer is shown as the darkened area in the figure. As can be seen, alkalosis or acidosis may result from a change in either the P_{CO_2} or the HCO_3^- as the primary disturbance. (This nomogram and subsequent ones in this chapter have been adapted from Cohen, J. J., *et al.*, in Maxwell, M. H., and Kleeman, C. R. (eds.): *Clinical Disorders of Fluid and Electrolyte Metabolism*, Third edition. McGraw-Hill, New York, 1980.)

Table II. Primary Disturbances and Compensatory Responses in the Four Basic Acid–Base Disorders

Disorder	pH	$[H^+]$	Primary disturbance	Compensatory response
Metabolic acidosis	↓	↑	↓ $[HCO_3^-]$	↓ P_{CO_2}
Metabolic alkalosis	↑	↓	↑ $[HCO_3^-]$	↑ P_{CO_2}
Respiratory acidosis	↓	↑	↑ P_{CO_2}	↑ $[HCO_3^-]$
Respiratory alkalosis	↑	↓	↓ P_{CO_2}	↓ $[HCO_3^-]$

function or an acid or base load sufficient to overwhelm the body's defense mechanisms. There are four basic acid–base disorders: metabolic and respiratory acidosis and alkalosis. Their characteristics are shown in Table II.

A. Metabolic Acidosis

Metabolic acidosis is characterized by a low pH (high H^+ concentration) and a low bicarbonate concentration. This can either be due to bicarbonate loss or to the buffering of nonvolatile acid by bicarbonate ion. The reduction in pH stimulates ventilation within minutes, resulting in a compensatory decrease in P_{CO_2}. Ultimate correction of the pH depends upon the renal excretion of the acid load, a process which takes several days.

B. Metabolic Alkalosis

Metabolic alkalosis is characterized by high pH (low H^+ concentration) and an increased plasma bicarbonate concentration. It can be produced by bicarbonate administration, H^+ loss, or infrequently by the movement of H^+ from the extracellular fluid into the cells. The respiratory compensation consists of hypoventilation and an increase in bicarbonate reabsorption (see the description of metabolic alkalosis below).

C. Respiratory Acidosis

Respiratory acidosis is due to impaired pulmonary excretion of CO_2, resulting in an increase in the P_{CO_2}. The kidney compensates by an enhanced H^+ secretion raising the plasma bicarbonate concentration, a response taking several days to reach completion. The restoration of normal acid–base balance requires correction of the underlying ventilatory abnormality.

D. Respiratory Alkalosis

The primary disturbance in respiratory alkalosis is hyperventilation, resulting in a decrease in the P_{CO_2} and an increase in the pH (reduction in

H^+ concentration). The compensatory response consists of diminished renal H^+ excretion producing bicarbonate loss in the urine and reduction in the plasma bicarbonate concentration. Again, as in respiratory acidosis, correction of the acid–base abnormality requires correction of the underlying ventilatory abnormality.

E. Mixed Acid–Base Disorders

Not uncommonly, a patient may have a combination of the above disorders. Suppose a patient has a high arterial pH, then, as shown in Table II, an increased plasma bicarbonate concentration and a low P_{CO_2} will lead to the diagnosis of combined metabolic and respiratory alkalosis. In addition, renal and respiratory compensations to acidosis or alkalosis are incomplete, returning the pH toward but not actually to normal. Therefore, a normal pH in the face of marked changes in the plasma bicarbonate concentration and P_{CO_2} should alert one to the presence of a mixed disorder. This fact stresses an obvious point that is often forgotten in the clinical setting. That is, an acid–base disorder cannot be diagnosed with certainty from the plasma bicarbonate concentration. Although a reduction in the plasma bicarbonate concentration may be due to metabolic acidosis, it can also reflect the renal compensation to respiratory alkalosis. Similarly, a high plasma bicarbonate may represent either a metabolic alkalosis or the compensatory response to respiratory acidosis. The aim of treating an acid–base disorder is correction of acid–base imbalance not the plasma bicarbonate concentration. For this reason, it is important to establish the correct diagnosis which requires the measurement of the pH.

The use of an acid–base nomogram may provide a useful additional aid in the correct diagnosis of acid–base disorders. There are several different forms of these available. One example is shown in Figure 7. The shaded areas portray the changes in the P_{CO_2} and plasma $[HCO_3^-]$ seen during the development of simple acid–base disturbances of graded severity. Acid–base parameters falling outside of the shaded areas represent mixed acid–base disorders. Values that fall within the shaded areas do not rule out a mixed acid–base disorder.

VIII. METABOLIC ACIDOSIS

Metabolic acidosis may occur due to the addition of H^+ or the loss of bicarbonate from the ECF. Whether H^+ is added to the ECF or bicarbonate lost, metabolic acidosis produces a lowering of the pH and the bicarbonate buffer concentration of the ECF (Figure 8). The lowered pH stimulates the CNS respiratory control centers to increase the rate and depth of respiration, which in turn lowers the ECF P_{CO_2} This decreases the fall in the pH. As shown in Figure 8, the relationship between bicarbonate ion and P_{CO_2} in metabolic acidosis is predictable. Generally, each mEq/liter reduction in

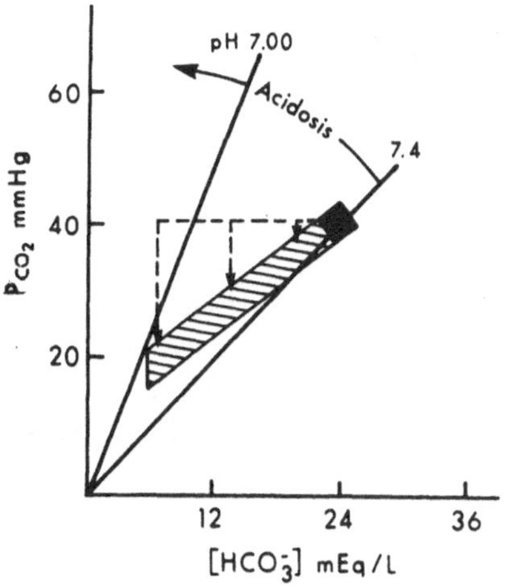

Figure 8. Effect of metabolic acidosis on acid–base equilibrium. As H^+ lowers blood pH, the HCO_3 buffer is consumed (–). The lowered pH stimulates the CNS respiratory control centers to cause increased respiration, lowering the P_{CO_2} (|). Shaded area indicates the relationship between HCO_3^- and P_{CO_2} at blood pH's below 7.4. Each mEq/liter reduction in HCO_3^- produces a 1.2-mm Hg fall in the P_{CO_2}.

bicarbonate ion produces a 1.2-mm Hg fall in the P_{CO_2}. Thus, the response of the body to an increase in H^+ concentration involves several processes: (1) extracellular buffering, (2) intracellular buffering, (3) respiratory compensation, and (4) renal excretion of the H^+ load. The first three processes act to minimize the increase in H^+ concentration until the kidneys restore acid–base balance by eliminating the excess H^+ in the urine.

A. Extracellular Buffering

As described above, a buffer system is most efficient within 1.0 pH unit of its pK_a. Although the pK_a of the bicarbonate–CO_2 system is 1.3 pH units below the normal ECF pH of 7.4, this system is a very effective buffer in body fluids. This is because the P_{CO_2} is regulated by changes in alveolar ventilation. As ventilation increases, CO_2 excretion is augmented, the P_{CO_2}

Table III. Relationship between the pH and H^+ Concentration in the Physiologic Range

pH	$[H^+]$ (nmole/liter)
7.80	16
7.70	20
7.60	26
7.50	32
7.40	40
7.30	50
7.20	63
7.10	80
7.00	100
6.90	125
6.80	160

is lowered, and dissolved CO_2 is decreased. A reduction in ventilation decreases the CO_2 excretion, resulting in an increase in P_{CO_2}. As H^+ is buffered by bicarbonate [equation (3)], an increase in the P_{CO_2} can be prevented by an increase in alveolar ventilation. This prevents an accumulation of dissolved CO_2 (carbonic acid).

The ability of bicarbonate ion as the most important buffer in the ECF to prevent large changes in arterial pH can be appreciated from the Henderson–Hasselbalch equation [equation (4)] and the data in Table III relating pH to H^+ concentrations. If we add 12 mEq/liter of H^+ to each liter of ECF, the concentration of the ECF bicarbonate will fall from 24 to 12 mEq/liter. If the P_{CO_2} remains constant,

$$pH = 6.1 + \log \frac{12}{0.03(40)} \qquad [P_{CO_2} = 40 \text{ mm Hg}]$$

$$= 6.1 + \log \frac{12}{1.2} \qquad [\text{since the log of 10 is 1}]$$

$$= 7.1$$

Even though 12 mEq/liter (12 million nEq) of H^+ has been added to each liter, the pH of 7.4 ($[H^+]$ of 40 nEq/liter) is only reduced to 7.1 ($[H^+]$ of 80 nEq/liter). Thus, more than 99% of the extra H^+ has been taken up by bicarbonate thereby preventing the H^+ concentration from exceeding 160 nEq/liter (pH 6.8), the highest H^+ concentration compatible with life.

B. Intracellular Buffering and the Plasma Potassium Concentration

H^+ is also buffered in cells. The intracellular buffers are mainly proteins and phosphates. Intracellular buffers will eventually account for about 60% of an acid load including the buffering of H^+ by bone carbonate. The ability of H^+ to enter the cell has an important effect on the plasma potassium (K^+) concentration. To maintain electrical neutrality the entry of H^+ into the cells is accompanied by diffusion of K^+ out of cells. In general, for every 0.1-unit change in pH there is roughly a reciprocal 0.6 mEq/liter change in the plasma K^+ concentration. In the above example, where the pH fell from 7.4 to 7.1, a 1.8-mEq/liter increase in the plasma K^+ concentration might be expected. Hyperkalemia in the presence of metabolic acidosis is very common. Hyperkalemia may even be seen in the presence of total body K^+ depletion. When an acidotic patient manifests normokalemia or hypokalemia this represents a severe degree of potassium depletion. As the acidosis is corrected these patients may develop hypokalemia of a life-threatening degree. In this setting, potassium repletion must be started at the same time as the correction of acidosis.

C. Respiratory Compensation

Acidosis stimulates chemoreceptors controlling respiration resulting in the increase in alveolar ventilation. As a result, P_{CO_2} will fall, and this will return the pH toward normal [equation (4)]. The increase in ventilation is characterized more by an increase in tidal volume than in respiratory rate, when hyperventilation reaches a severe degree it is called Kussmaul's respiration. This is apparent on physical examination and should alert the physician to the possible presence of metabolic acidosis. In general, the P_{CO_2} will fall 1.2 mm Hg for every 1.0-mEq/liter reduction in the plasma bicarbonate concentration down to a minimum P_{CO_2} of 10–15 mm Hg. From the example used before, a reduction of plasma bicarbonate from 24 to 12 mEq/liter, a fall of 12 mEq/liter, should be associated with a 14 mm Hg fall in the P_{CO_2} to 26 mm Hg (pH = 7.23). Thus, in metabolic acidosis when the plasma bicarbonate concentration is 12 mEq/liter, the normal P_{CO_2} is 26 mm Hg not 40 mm Hg. Values markedly different from this P_{CO_2} would suggest a mixed acid–base disorder. If the P_{CO_2} remained at 40 mm Hg when the plasma bicarbonate concentration fell to 12 mEq/liter this would represent a combined metabolic and respiratory acidosis. This fact is portrayed graphically in an acid–base nomogram such as Figure 7. This might occur in a patient with chronic lung disease who develops metabolic acidosis. Conversely, if the P_{CO_2} is 15 mm Hg when the plasma bicarbonate concentration was 12 mEq/liter this would reflect a combined metabolic acidosis and respiratory alkalosis since the fall in the P_{CO_2} is greater than the normal respiratory compensation for the metabolic acidosis. This is often seen in salicylate intoxication (see Section VIII.E, page 248).

D. Renal Hydrogen Excretion

In the absence of therapy with sodium bicarbonate, the kidney must eventually excrete the H^+ load to correct the metabolic acidosis. It does so by reclaiming all the filtered bicarbonate and secreting H^+, which combines with urinary buffers (phosphoric acid, titratable acidity, and NH_4^+). In response to an increased H^+ load, the kidney augments cellular NH_3 production and consequently NH_4^+ excretion. In patients with metabolic acidosis, NH_4^+ excretion can exceed 250 mEq/day. Generally, there is usually only a limited ability to enhance titratable acid excretion.

E. Causes of Metabolic Acidosis

Metabolic acidosis results from an inability to excrete the daily H^+ load or from an acute increase in the H^+ load either because of the addition of H^+ or loss of bicarbonate (Table IV).

Table IV. Causes of Metabolic Acidosis and the Anion Gap in Each Type

Cause	Anion gap
I. Inability to excrete endogenous H^+ loads	
A. Diminished NH_3 production	
Renal failure	Usually increased; may be normal
B. Diminished H^+ secretion	
1. Renal tubular acidosis (distal)	Normal
2. Hypoaldosteronism	Normal
II. Increased H^+ load	
A. Ketoacidosis	Elevated
B. Lactic acidosis	
C. Ingestions	
1. Salicylates	
2. Ethylene glycol	
3. Methanol	
4. Paraldehyde	
5. Ammonium chloride	Normal
6. Hyperalimentation fluids	
III. Increased HCO_3^- loss	
A. Gastrointestinal	
1. Diarrhea and fistulas	Normal
2. Cholestyramine	
3. Ureterosigmoidostomy	
B. Renal	
1. Renal failure	
2. Renal tubular acidosis (proximal)	

1. Anion Gap

Sodium, chloride, and bicarbonate are the electrolytes present in highest concentration in the ECF. The sodium concentration normally exceeds the sum of the chloride concentration plus bicarbonate by 9–13 mEq/liter. The negative charges of the plasma proteins account for most of the differences between the cation charges and the anion charges. This is referred to as the anion gap. The causes of metabolic acidosis listed in Table IV can be divided into those which increase the anion gap and those that do not. Determining the anion gap is very helpful as an initial step in the differential diagnosis of metabolic acidosis. Gastrointestinal or renal loss of sodium bicarbonate results in milliequivalent for milliequivalent replacement of extracellular bicarbonate by chloride since the kidney retains sodium chloride in an effort to preserve the volume of the extracellular fluid. This type of acidosis will result in an elevation in the plasma chloride concentration and is referred to as hyperchloremic acidosis. Conversely, if H^+ accumulates with any ion other than chloride, extracellular bicarbonate will be replaced by an unmeasured anion (A^-): $HA + NaHCO_3 \rightarrow NaA + H_2CO_3 \rightarrow CO_2 + H_2O$. As a result there will be a decrease in the sum of chloride plus bicarbonate ion concentration as an increase in the anion gap due to A^- accumulation. In acidosis with an increased anion gap identification of the specific disease process is often obtained by measuring serum concentrations of BUN, creatinine, glucose, lactate, pyruvate, and by checking the serum for the presence of ketones and intoxicants (salicylates and occasionally methanol or ethylene glycol). Occasionally, an increase in the anion gap is also seen in respiratory alkalosis where lactic acid production is increased (see discussion on respiratory alkalosis).

2. Ketoacidosis

Ketoacidosis results from incomplete oxidation of free fatty acids to CO_2 and water (Figure 9). This leads to increased production of beta hydroxybutyric and acetoacetic acids. Ketoacid overproduction appears to be dependent on two factors: (1) enhanced lipolysis, which increases the supply of free fatty acids, and (2) preferential conversion of free fatty acids in the liver to ketoacids rather than triglycerides. This latter step appears to be dependent upon the activity of the enzyme acylcarnitine transferase (ACTase) which

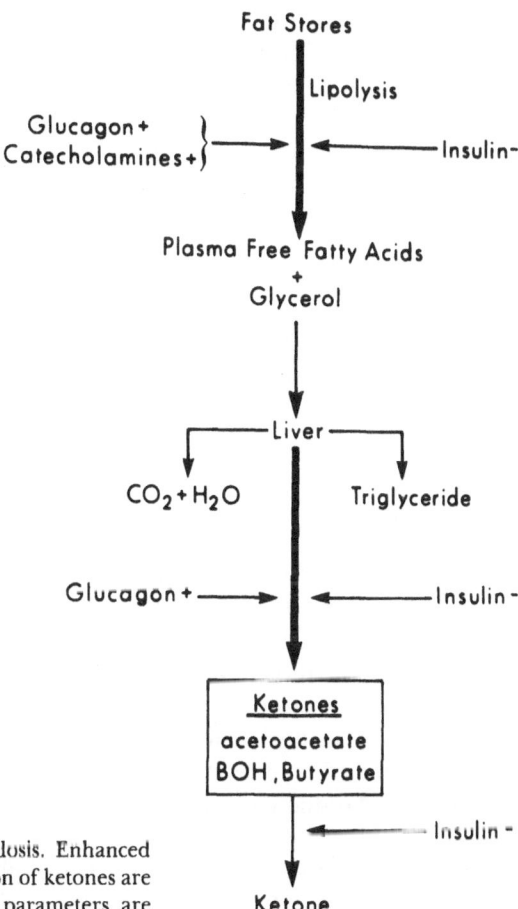

Figure 9. Lipid metabolism in ketoacidosis. Enhanced lipolysis and increased hepatic production of ketones are the major aberrations. Both of these parameters are produced by insulin deficiency and stimulated by glucagon.

facilitates the entry of free fatty acids into the mitochondria of hepatocytes where the conversion takes place. Normally, insulin is a potent inhibitor of ketone production reducing both lipolysis and ACTase activity. In the absence of insulin, or in fasting, lipolysis and ACTase activity are enhanced, resulting in ketone acid accumulation in the ECF and metabolic acidosis. Glucagon may also directly promote ketone synthesis by enhancing lipolysis and ACTase activity. In conjunction with insulin deficiency, endogenous hypersecretion of glucagon and catecholamines can contribute to the development of hyperglycemia and ketoacidosis in uncontrolled diabetes mellitus.

Diabetes mellitus is the most common cause of ketoacidosis. Fasting can also cause a mild self-limited ketosis as blood sugar falls and insulin secretion also decreases. With continued fasting, ketones replace glucose as the principal metabolic fuel of the body. Rarely, the combination of alcohol ingestion and poor dietary intake produces ketoacidosis. Poor carbohydrate intake plus the effects of alcohol on inhibiting gluconeogenesis are necessary to produce this clinical state. In addition, ethanol directly enhances lipolysis.

The diagnosis of ketoacidosis requires a demonstration of ketones in the blood. This is usually done with nitroprusside (Acetest) tablets. In a patient with metabolic acidosis, a 4^+ nitroprusside reaction in serum diluted $1:1$ and a high anion gap is strongly suggestive of ketoacidosis. Nitroprusside reacts with acetoacetate and acetone but not with β-hydroxybutyrate. Since β-hydroxybutyrate comprises about 75% of the circulating ketones in diabetic ketoacidosis and 90% of the ketones with concurrent lactic acidosis or alcoholic ketoacidosis, the nitroprusside test is insensitive and underestimates the severity of ketoacidosis.

Insulin is the keystone of therapy in diabetic ketoacidosis, but it is dangerous in the nondiabetic forms of ketoacidosis since the blood sugar is not high in these. In the nondiabetic forms of ketoacidosis, provision of glucose will increase endogenous insulin secretion and normalize ketone production.

3. Lactic Acidosis

Lactic acid is produced in the liver from anaerobic metabolism of pyruvic acid originating from the metabolism of glucose and amino acids (Figure 10). Normally, 45% of the glucose metabolized yields lactic acid. This lactic acid is rapidly buffered by the extracellular bicarbonate. In the liver 80% of the lactate is converted to CO_2 and water and 20% into glucose. Either of these reactions results in the regeneration of the bicarbonate lost in buffering the lactic acid and maintenance of acid–base balance. However, if production of lactic acid is enhanced, the capacity of the liver may be overwhelmed with resultant lactic acidosis.

The normal plasma lactate is 1.0 mEq/liter and that of pyruvate is 0.1 mEq/liter. Any condition which enhances glycolysis increases pyruvate and lactate formation. In these states, lactate/pyruvate ratio remains normal ($10:1$). Acidosis is not a problem since most of the pyruvate is converted to

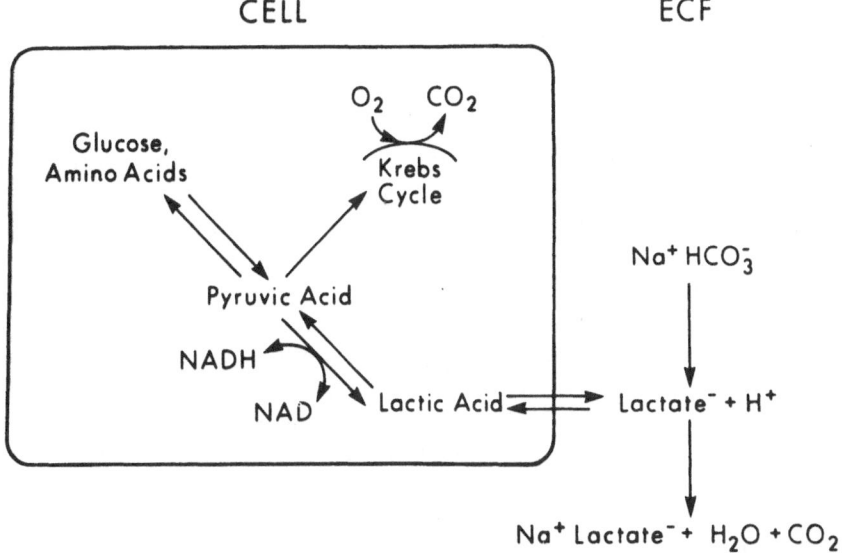

Figure 10. Schematic diagram of lactic acid production. Glycolytic metabolism of glucose and to a lesser extent amino acids results in production of pyruvic acid. This normally is further metabolized by entering the Krebs cycle. The equilibrium between pyruvic and lactic acids is governed by the ratio NADH:NAD. In anaerobic conditions, the NADH:NAD ratio is increased favoring production of lactic acid by the enzymatic activity of lactic dehydrogenase. Upon release from cells, lactic acid immediately dissociates and is buffered by ECF bicarbonate. In the liver, lactate uptake and utilization proceed by reversal of these steps.

CO_2 and water. In clinical disorders of lactic acidosis, the overproduction of lactate results in an elevation of the lactate/pyruvate ratio, separating the elevated lactate of acidosis from normal states of enhanced glycolysis.

The most commmon cause of lactic acidosis is shock. Shock may be caused by sepsis, hemorrhage, pulmonary edema, or cardiac failure. The common denominator in these conditions is decreased tissue delivery of oxygen which favors the anaerobic formation of lactate from pyruvate.

Acute pancreatitis, diabetes mellitus, leukemia, and other disorders may also be associated with increased production of lactic acid. Occasionally, no underlying cause for the lactic acidosis can be ascertained. In this instance, lactic acidosis is termed *idiopathic*. There is marked overproduction of lactate and despite treatment with massive amounts of bicarbonate, mortality is quite high. The underlying defect in this disorder is unknown.

A mild form of lactic acidosis is seen in chronic alcoholism. In this condition, lactate production may be normal but lactate utilization is diminished. As a result, there is no regeneration of the bicarbonate consumed in the initial buffering of lactic acid.

A diagnosis of lactic acidosis can be made with certainty only by the demonstration of an elevated plasma lactate concentration and a lactate/pyruvate ratio greater than 10:1. In patients with severe metabolic acidosis, a high anion gap and shock, or one of the other disorders known to produce lactic acidosis, the diagnosis may be suspected.

4. Acidosis Due to Ingestions

a. Salicylates

Aspirin (acetylsalicylic acid) is present in most analgesic tablets. It is rapidly converted to salicylic acid in the body. In addition to the direct effect of salicylic acid on the pH, salicylate interferes with carbohydrate metabolism and causes the accumulation of organic acids. Salicylate also directly stimulates the respiratory center, resulting in an increase in ventilation and a fall in the P_{CO_2}. Therefore, the primary acid–base disorder is usually respiratory alkalosis but may be either metabolic acidosis and/or combined metabolic acidosis–respiratory alkalosis. Often times respiratory alkalosis precedes the development of a severe metabolic acidosis following large ingestions. The diagnosis can be made with certainty by the measurement of the plasma salicylate concentration. The presence of a severe metabolic acidosis with a large anion gap and the history of ingestion strongly suggests the diagnosis. Fatal overdose may occur after the ingestion of 10–30 g by adults and as little as 3 g by children. There is no absolute correlation between plasma salicylate levels and intoxication. However, most patients show signs of intoxication when the plasma levels exceed 40–50 mg/dl. The therapeutic range of salicylate for conditions such as arthritis is 20–35 mg/dl. The symptoms of early salicylate intoxication include tinnitus, vertigo, nausea, vomiting, and diarrhea. Later, mental abberations which may progress to hallucinations and death develop.

b. Others

Other intoxications can also produce metabolic acidosis. Ethylene glycol, a component of antifreeze, produces a toxic metabolite, oxalic acid. Antifreeze is occasionally ingested during attempted suicide. Methanol ingestion by alcoholics is occasionally seen. Methanol is metabolized to formaldehyde and formic acid. A lethal dose is as little as 70–100 ml. Ingestion frequently causes permanent blindness. Ingestion of paraldehyde and ammonium chloride are other uncommon causes of metabolic acidosis.

Hyperalimentation fluids containing cationic amino acids such as arginine, lysine, and histidine are metabolized to H^+:

$$R—NH_3{}^+ + O_2 \rightarrow Urea + Co_2 + H_2O + H^+$$

Some hyperalimentation fluids, especially neoaminosol, contain 40–50 mEq/liter of cationic amino acids. Administration of these solutions can produce a metabolic acidosis.

5. Gastrointestinal Loss of Bicarbonate

Intestinal secretions below the stomach which include pancreatic and biliary secretions are alkaline. Therefore, diarrhea or removal of pancreatic, biliary, or intestinal secretions, either by tube drainage or fistulas to the skin, may result in bicarbonate loss and metabolic acidosis. In addition, the intestine (ileum and colon) has an anion exchange pump which produces chloride absorption and bicarbonate secretion. Patients who suffer loss of bladder function due to neurologic abnormalities are treated with implantation of the ureters into the sigmoid colon or the ileum. In this setting, a hyperchloremic acidosis may occur if the contact time between the urine and the intestine is sufficient for reabsorption of urinary chloride and bicarbonate secretion. An additional factor in this metabolic acidosis is reabsorption of NH_4^+ by the colonic mucosa and bacterial metabolism of urea in the colon, producing resorbable H^+. Implantation of the ureters into a short loop of ileum has made the development of metabolic acidosis from ureteral diversion less common by decreasing the contact time between intestinal mucosa and urine.

F. Acidosis of Chronic Renal Failure

Metabolic acidosis is a common finding in patients in the later stages of chronic renal failure (CRF). It is due to a decrease in net acid excretion [equation (6)].

The decrease in net acid excretion is mainly due to a decrease in NH_4^+ excretion. Titratable acidity excretion and bicarbonate reclamation are better maintained throughout the course of renal failure than is NH_4^+ excretion.

1. Ammonium (NH_4^+)

Normal NH_4^+ excretion in the presence of decreased functional renal mass requires an increase in NH_3 production per unit of mass. However, in CRF the quantity of NH_3 excreted, although increased somewhat per unit of excretory mass, is decreased below the level needed to excrete the daily endogenous H^+ production. Because of the inability of the diseased kidney to adequately increase NH_3 production, an amount of organic acid production must be buffered elsewhere each day.

2. Titratable Acidity

Titratable acidity is maintained close to normal throughout the course of CRF until phosphate restriction or decreased dietary phosphate intake occurs. When phosphate retention is prevented, titratable acid excretion decreases. Under normal conditions the decrease in titratable acid excretion would be countered by an increase in NH_3 synthesis and net acid excretion would not be changed. In CRF, the biosynthesis of NH_3 is not substantially increased and a fall in titratable acid excretion results in a greater decrease in net acid excretion.

3. Bicarbonate

Bicarbonate reabsorption studies in patients with CRF demonstrate a decreased capacity for H^+ secretion by the diseased nephron. Thus, a larger portion of the nephron is required for bicarbonate reclamation to be complete. In fact, at normal plasma levels of bicarbonate the urinary pH is alkaline in patients with CRF indicating the reclamation is not complete. However at plasma levels of bicarbonate in the range seen in the presence of established acidosis (usually 12–20 mEq/liter) the urinary pH is acid and bicarbonate reclamation is complete. Thus, the diseased kidney of patients with CRF can maintain the steep H^+ gradient necessary to acidify the urine, but the total H^+ secretory capacity is significantly reduced. The ability to acidify the urine at low plasma levels of bicarbonate and the inability to reclaim bicarbonate completely at normal plasma levels of bicarbonate are characteristics of the acidification defect seen in patients with proximal renal tubular acidosis. In this sense, patients with CRF have a proximal renal tubular acidosis (RTA).

The acidosis of CRF usually develops late (GFR = 25 ml/min) in the course of the disease. In this setting, the retention of organic acid anions such as phosphate and sulfate contribute to an increased anion gap as discussed above. Thus, the acidosis of renal failure is more often characterized by increased anion gap.

In some patients with CRF due to diseases that affect mainly the renal interstitium such as hypercalcemia, medullary cystic diseases or interstitial nephritis, an acidosis develops due to a loss of NH_3 production at an earlier stage of the disease (a higher GFR) than is seen in other forms of CRF. This appears to be due to preponderant destruction of tubular functions while the GFR is better maintained. When this occurs, the GFR is sufficient to prevent significant retention of organic acid anions. In this situation, a hyperchloremic acidosis develops.

In some patients with CRF who develop a hyperchloremic metabolic acidosis relatively early in the course of their disease, hyperkalemia is also observed. The cause of the hyperkalemia is due to decreased potassium secretion by the diseased kidney. These patients frequently have hyporeninemic, hypoaldosteronism, or impaired renal response to aldosterone stimulation. The abnormality in aldosterone metabolism or response produces a decrease in potassium secretion by the kidney and hyperkalemia. Hyperkalemia further impairs acid excretion by inhibiting ammonia production from glutamine. The hypoaldosteronism may also decrease H^+ secretion and can contribute to the metabolic acidosis. Whether hypoaldosteronism or decreased NH_3 production, due to tubular damage, is the predominant factor in the pathogenesis of the metabolic acidosis in these patients is not clear. However, the urinary pH in these patients is usually 5.5 or less, which indicates a pathogenesis of the acidosis which is characterized by a decrease in H^+ secretory capacity but maintenance of the ability to acidify the urine.

In summary, three clinically distinguishable types of metabolic acidosis are associated with CRF: an increased anion gap acidosis, a hyperchloremic normokalemic acidosis, and a hyperchloremic hyperkalemic acidosis.

The metabolic acidosis of CRF is usually mild to moderate and emergency treatment is rarely needed. The contribution of the metabolic acidosis of CRF to other complications of the uremic state such as encephalopathy or osteodystrophy remains unclear. Thus, the need for therapy of the acidosis is not apparent until it becomes severe (pH < 7.2, $[HCO_3^-] < 15$ mEq/liter). Then sufficient HCO_3^- should be provided to raise the $[HCO_3^-$ to >15 mEq/ liter and correct the pH to > 7.25. Avoidance of worsening ECF volume overload and increasing congestive heart failure by $NaHCO_3$ treatment of the acidosis are important cautions to keep in mind.

G. Renal Tubular Acidosis

The diagnosis of the metabolic acidosis in patients who present with a normal anion gap (hyperchloremic metabolic acidosis) is easily established in most instances. Elimination of causes such as gastrointestinal loss of bicarbonate, ingestions such as ammonium chloride, or hyperalimentation fluids and renal insufficiency is not difficult. Thus, patients with hyperchloremic acidosis due to impaired urinary acidification are usually suspected clinically before the diagnostic tests are performed to confirm the diagnosis. There are three major types of renal tubular acidosis (RTA). The first results from impaired bicarbonate reclamation (proximal RTA). The second results from impaired acidification of the urine (distal RTA), and it is usually associated with hypokalemia. The third type may share pathophysiologic properties of both of the former, but is associated with hyperkalemia. Renal function in these patients is otherwise normal.

1. Proximal RTA

Under normal conditions all of the filtered bicarbonate is reabsorbed unless the bicarbonate concentration in the glomerular filtrate exceeds 26 mEq/liter. Above this level of plasma bicarbonate, bicarbonate begins to appear in the urine (Figure 11). Approximately 85% of bicarbonate reabsorption occurs in the proximal tubule. In patients with proximal RTA, there is a reduction in proximal bicarbonate reabsorption resulting in elevated bicarbonate delivery to the distal nephron and bicarbonate loss in the urine and resultant metabolic acidosis. This can be viewed as a decrease in the reabsorptive capacity for bicarbonate such that the maximal reabsorptive capacity is reduced from the normal of 26 mEq/liter to a new value of a smaller quantity. For example, if the new reabsorptive capacity for bicarbonate was 18 mEq/liter of glomerular filtrate, then bicarbonate would be lost in the urine at a level of 26 mEq/liter until the plasma bicarbonate concentration reached 18 mEq/liter. At this point, a new steady state would be achieved and all the filtered bicarbonate would now be reabsorbed. Thus, proximal RTA is a self-limiting disorder in which the plasma bicarbonate concentration is set at a value lower than normal. At this new level of plasma bicarbonate, bicarbonate reabsorption is complete, the kidney is capable of regenerating the bicarbonate titrated each day by organic acid production, and the urinary pH will be acid. Therefore, these patients are not in a continual positive H^+ balance.

When bicarbonate is administered to patients with proximal RTA, their urinary pH becomes alkaline. Large quantities of bicarbonate are required to raise the plasma bicarbonate to normal levels. This is because all of the administered bicarbonate is excreted in the urine since the reabsorptive capacity of the proximal tubule has been exceeded as bicarbonate is administered. This response is diagnostic of proximal RTA. It also makes the correction of metabolic acidosis in patients with proximal RTA difficult since the quantity of bicarbonate required to maintain a normal plasma bicarbonate will be very large.

In addition to the defect in bicarbonate reabsorption, patients with proximal RTA often exhibit other impairments in proximal tubular function. Thus defects in phosphate, uric acid, amino acids, and glucose reabsorption are often associated with proximal RTA. As shown in Table V, proximal

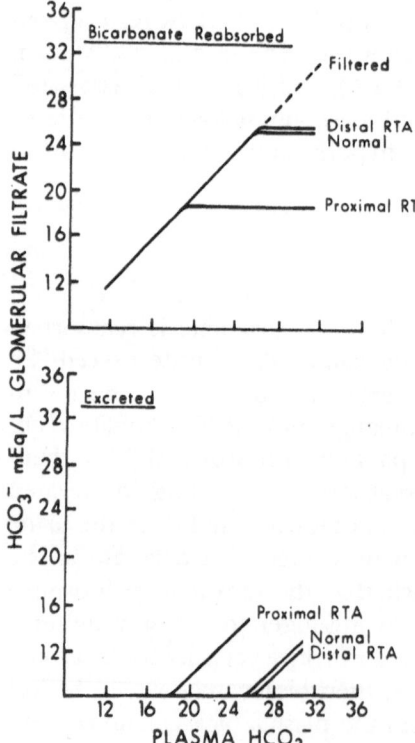

Figure 11. Reabsorption and excretion of filtered bicarbonate during bicarbonate infusions in normals, and subjects with distal and proximal RTA. In normals and patients with distal RTA, bicarbonate reabsorption is complete up to a plasma bicarbonate of 26 mEq/liter. As bicarbonate is elevated above 26 mEq/liter, bicarbonaturia develops. In patients with proximal RTA, the maximal reabsorption of bicarbonate and the urinary bicarbonate threshold are reduced. (Data from Morris, R. C.: *N. Engl. J. Med.* 281:1405, 1969.)

Table V. Causes of Proximal RTA

I. Primary—hereditary or sporadic
II. Cystinosis
III. Wilson's disease
IV. Hyperparathyroidism
V. Disorders of protein metabolism
    A. Nephrotic syndrome
    B. Multiple myeloma
    C. Sjögren's syndrome
    D. Amyloidosis
VI. Medullary cystic disease
VII. Renal transplantation
VIII. Acetazolamide

RTA can be produced by a wide variety of disorders. In many of these conditions, particularly those due to toxins or metabolic disorders, the tubular defect may be reversed by treatment of the primary disorder. The explanation for the tubular dysfunction in these patients is not understood.

2. Distal RTA

In patients with distal RTA, bicarbonate reabsorptive capacity is normal (Figure 11) as compared to proximal RTA. However, there is decreased distal H^+ secretion manifested by an inability to lower the urine pH below 5.3 (normal minimal urine pH is 4.5–5.0). This inability to lower urine pH could be produced in one of two ways. First, there may be a defect in H^+ secretion itself in the distal nephron. Second, and probably more commonly, there may be an increase in the permeability of the distal nephron to H^+. As H^+ secretion makes the tubular fluid more acid than the cells and the ECF, there is a tendency for the secreted H^+ to diffuse back out of the lumen into the cell or into the ECF space. Thus, there is an inability to keep secreted H^+ in the tubular fluid despite a normal capacity for H^+ secretion. Regardless of the mechanism of the defect in lowering urine pH, the net effect is a decrease in net H^+ excretion and HCO_3^- regeneration resulting in a bicarbonate deficit whenever nonvolatile H^+ generated from metabolism is added to the body. Thus, patients with distal RTA are unable to excrete completely the dietary H^+ load and are in a state of chronic positive H^+ balance. The limitation to H^+ secretion may be viewed as an inability to maintain the steep gradient necessary to acidify the urine. This gradient limitation to H^+ secretion results in positive H^+ balance, which is easily reversed by sodium bicarbonate administration. The dose of bicarbonate required is modest, and it is equal to the daily unexcreted load of nonvolatile acids. This is a small requirement compared to that needed to correct a proximal RTA.

In patients with distal RTA, several complications are observed. There is impaired growth and these patients usually develop nephrolithiasis, nephrocalcinosis, and renal insufficiency due to precipitation of calcium phosphate salts in the medullary portions of the kidney. The pathogenesis of the nephrocalcinosis is twofold. First, as a result of the high urinary pH, urinary citrate excretion is decreased. Citrate is a major inhibitor of calcium precipitation in the urine since it chelates calcium ions in a molar ratio of 4:1. Secondly, because of the daily net positive H^+ balance, patients with distal forms of RTA utilized bone carbonate as a major buffer of the daily organic acid load. This results in hypercalciuria in patients with distal RTA, and further promotes nephrocalcinosis.

The diagnosis of distal RTA should be suspected in any patient with metabolic acidosis and urinary pH greater than 5.5. In the absence of an infection with a urea-splitting organism which can elevate the urinary pH, the only other disorder that can produce this combination is proximal RTA when the plasma bicarbonate concentration is above the tubular reabsorptive capacity. Proximal and distal RTA can be differentiated from each other by response to a bicarbonate load. In a patient with proximal RTA, who is given bicarbonate, the urine pH will increase, but it will not be affected in a patient with distal RTA (Figure 12). Alternatively, if the acidosis is mild, an acid load can be given as ammonium chloride in a dose of 0.1 g/kg. Within 4–6 hours the plasma bicarbonate concentration will fall 4–5 mEq/liter. In patients

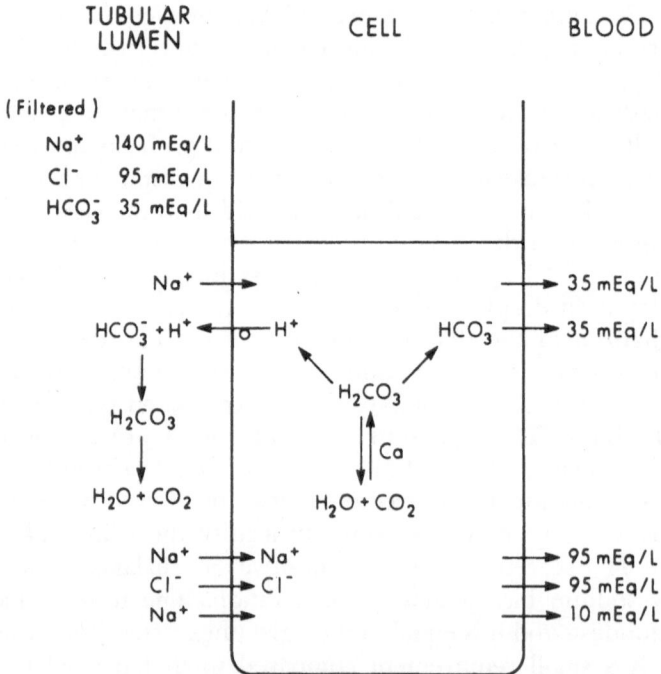

Figure 12. Fluid and solute reabsorption in hypovolemic metabolic alkalosis. The hypochloremia induced by the alkalotic state lessens the fraction of sodium reabsorbed with chloride. Avid sodium reabsorption thus induces accelerated H^+ secretion and reclaims all of the filtered HCO_3^-, maintaining the alkalotic state.

with distal RTA, the urinary pH will remain above 5.5 despite the fall in plasma bicarbonate. However, in proximal RTA (and in normal subjects) the urine pH will fall to less than 5.5 and usually below 5.0. This is the short NH$_4$Cl loading test originally described by Wrong and Davies.

It should be noted that the acidifying defect seen in distal RTA does not always lead to metabolic acidosis. Patients with an acidification defect of the distal variety but a normal plasma bicarbonate are referred to as having incomplete RTA. These patients exhibit a persistently elevated urinary pH but an absence of metabolic acidosis. Apparently these patients are able to increase NH$_3$ production by the tubular cell to increase net acid excretion sufficiently to prevent an acidosis despite an elevated urinary pH. Why these patients are able to augment NH$_3$ production in contrast to those with a complete form of distal RTA is not known. It is also of interest that these patients, with the incomplete form of distal RTA, may manifest the complications of hypercalciuria, nephrocalcinosis, nephrolithiasis, and low urinary citrate excretion seen in distal RTA.

Patients with either distal or proximal RTA are natriuretic, kaluretic, and often hypokalemic. However, the mechanisms for these associated defects of solute transport differ between the two types. In patients with distal RTA, the urinary excretion rates of potassium, sodium, and aldosterone decrease when the acidosis is corrected with alkali therapy. This observation has led to the hypothesis that the renal sodium and potassium wasting in patients with distal RTA result from a reduction in net rate of sodium–hydrogen exchange in the distal nephron which is imposed by a limitation on the attainable lumen to peritubular H$^+$ concentration gradient. This reduction in the rate of sodium–hydrogen exchange results in a reciprocal, not fully compensatory increase in the rate of sodium–potassium exchange. As a consequence, renal wasting of both sodium and potassium develops. Hyperaldosteronism resulting from sodium depletion augments the rate of sodium–potassium exchange. When acidosis is corrected with alkali therapy increasing the filtered load of bicarbonate, the attendant increase in the intraluminal bicarbonate concentration is presumed to remove the gradient restriction on sodium–hydrogen exchange in the distal nephron, and thereby reduce the urinary excretion rate of sodium. As sodium wasting disappears, so does the stimulus for aldosterone secretion, accelerated sodium–potassium exchange, and urinary potassium excretion. However, as natriuresis has been reported to persist following correction of the acidosis, the mechanisms of sodium and potassium wasting in distal RTA are not totally clarified as yet.

In patients with proximal RTA, the renal potassium wasting becomes more severe when acidosis is corrected with alkali therapy. These findings are attributed to excessive sodium bicarbonate delivery to the distal nephron accelerating sodium–potassium exchange. In these patients, a direct relationship between the excretion of bicarbonate and the excretion of potassium is observed during administration of bicarbonate therapy. In patients with distal RTA, bicarbonaturia does not develop with bicarbonate therapy and urinary excretion of bicarbonate and the excretion of potassium tends to diminish. Thus, the natriuresis and kaliuresis of proximal RTA appear to be directly linked to decreased H^+ secretory capacity.

3. RTA Associated with Hyperkalemia

Hyperchloremic metabolic acidosis with hyperkalemia instead of hypokalemia is a common clinical syndrome. As discussed under the section of acidosis due to renal failure, most of these patients also have mild-to-moderate chronic renal insufficiency. However, hypoaldosteronism in the absence of CRF may produce a metabolic acidosis with hyperkalemia. Aldosterone increases both potassium and H^+ secretion in the distal nephron. Its deficiency will result in a decrease in H^+ secretion in the distal nephron and impaired acidification. In the setting of hypoaldosteronism with a normal GRF, patients will exhibit an elevated urine pH, an impaired response to ammonium chloride, like patients with distal RTA. In the presence of both chronic renal insufficiency and hypoaldosteronism, most patients exhibit an acid urinary pH of 5.0, indicating the role of the renal failure and the hyperkalemia (decreased NH_3 production) as the major factors in the pathogenesis of the acidosis.

Patients with RTA and hyperkalemia respond to mineralocorticoid replacement with correction of the hyperkalemia (the most important factor) first and an improvement in the metabolic acidosis more slowly.

H. Principles of Treatment for Metabolic Acidosis

Repair of the altered body composition produced by metabolic acidosis centers on the provision of adequate amounts of HCO_3^-. If the cause of acidosis is self-limited, bicarbonate therapy may not be necessary because the normal kidney can replete body bicarbonate stores over a period of several days. Also, if the plasma bicarbonate concentration is only mildly to moderately depressed, therapy is not indicated in all cases. If, however, the cause of acidosis cannot be eliminated (e.g., chronic renal failure) long-term alkali therapy may be necessary. Bicarbonate, or an organic anion that can be converted to bicarbonate (e.g., citrate), may be administered orally for this purpose in a dose adjusted empirically to maintain the desired plasma bicarbonate concentration.

If bicarbonate concentration is markedly depressed, rapid therapeutic intervention may be required even if the underlying cause can be removed quickly (diabetic acidosis). Rapid correction of metabolic acidosis is accomplished most reliably by the intravenous administration of sodium bicarbonate. Generally, therapy should be designed to replace only about one half the total bicarbonate deficit over the initial 12 hr of treatment in order to avoid the consequences of abrupt changes in extracellular acid–base equilibrium. When this precaution is observed, complications that have been observed with too rapid a correction of metabolic acidosis occur rarely (i.e., altered mental status, convulsions, and tetany).

In determining the amount of bicarbonate required to produce a desired increase in the plasma bicarbonate concentration, the effect of nonbicarbonate buffers on the fate of administered bicarbonate must be considered. Since up to 50% of the excess H^+ concentration in metabolic acidosis is buffered by nonbicarbonate buffers, no less than 50% of an administered bicarbonate load is dissipated immediately by H^+ relinquished from these buffers. To determine the appropriate dose of bicarbonate for administration, the desired increment in plasma concentration must be multiplied by an apparent space of distribution at least twice as large as the normal extracellular fluid volume (approximately 40% of the body weight). This space of bicarbonate distribution takes into account the role of nonbicarbonate buffers in the response to an acid load. The apparent space of bicarbonate distribution may be even larger in patients with severe metabolic acidosis ($HCO_3^- < 5$ mEq/liter). Estimates of bicarbonate requirements serve only as rough guidelines and must be adjusted to suite individual circumstances. This is particularly true when increased acid production (especially lactic acidosis) or bicarbonate losses continue during the period of therapy.

Other alkalinizing agents (lactate, citrate) offer no advantage over bicarbonate in the urgent treatment of metabolic acidosis. This is because their net effect on acid-base equilibrium is achieved only through their capacity to increase bicarbonate concentrations. If cardiac or renal failure precludes administration of adequate amounts of bicarbonate (sodium load), it may be necessary to institute peritoneal or hemodialysis.

IX. METABOLIC ALKALOSIS

Metabolic alkalosis can be produced by the retention of bicarbonate or the loss of H^+ from the gastrointestinal tract or in the urine. Understanding the pathophysiology of metabolic alkalosis requires a knowledge of the factors that lead to the *generation* of the alkalotic state and the factors that prevent its correction or, in effect, *maintain* the alkalosis. For example, H^+ lost through removal of gastric secretions are derived from the intracellular dissociation of carbonic acid in gastric mucosa cells [equation (3)]. For each milliequivalent of H^+ lost, there will be an equimolar generation of bicarbonate in the plasma. Additionally, as gastric secretions are removed, plasma volume is decreased and aldosterone secretion is stimulated, resulting in hypokalemia. Subsequently, K^+ moves from the cells due to the hypokalemia and H^+ moves in, representing an additional loss of plasma H^+. The effect on H^+ concentrations is dramatic because of the small concentration of H^+ in the ECF. Thus, the *generation* of metabolic alkalosis from loss of gastric secretions involves both H^+ loss and movement of H^+ into intracellular space due to hypokalemia.

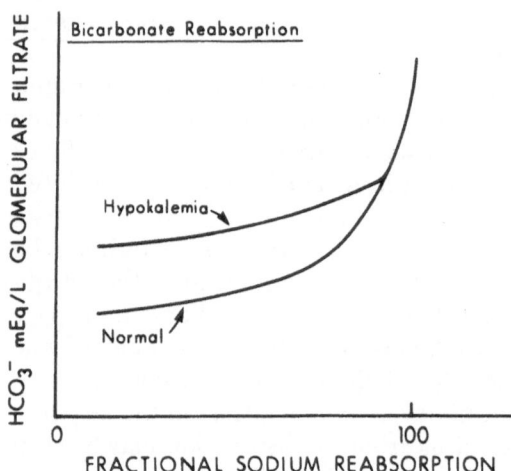

Figure 13. The relationships between volume depletion (reflected here as fractional sodium reabsorption) and HCO_3^- reabsorption in the presence of hypokalemia. At any state of ECF fluid volume hypokalemia stimulates HCO_3^- reabsorption. Hypovolemia itself also directly stimulates HCO_3^- reabsorption and if severe can sustain extremely high plasma bicarbonate levels. (Data from Kurtzman, N. A.: *Arch. Intern. Med.* 131:702, 1973.)

Maintenance of metabolic alkalosis, once generated, requires retention of the elevated bicarbonate levels. The kidney possesses the capacity to excrete all the filtered bicarbonate. Thus, the perpetuation of metabolic alkalosis requires an impairment in renal bicarbonate excretion. In most instances, this results from an enhanced bicarbonate reabsorption. Renal bicarbonate reabsorption by H^+ secretion from the tubular cell into the lumen is stimulated by three major control factors: intracellular acidosis (metabolic or respiratory), hypovolemia, and potassium depletion. In acidotic states, the increase in hydrogen secretion represents an attempt to excrete H^+ and return the pH to normal. In metabolic alkalosis from loss of gastric secretions, hypovolemia and potassium depletion augment H^+ secretion and bicarbonate reabsorption. They thereby *maintain* the alkalosis. The increase in H^+ secretion also accounts for the paradoxical finding of acid urine pHs (H^+ excretion) in the presence of extracellular alkalosis.

How volume depletion maintains an alkalotic state through augmenting H^+ secretion and, consequently, bicarbonate reabsorption, is illustrated in Figure 12. In the presence of hypovolemia, fractional sodium reabsorption is enhanced in an attempt to restore normovolemia and can be considered essentially complete. To maintain electrical neutrality, sodium reabsorption must either be accompanied by reabsorption of chloride, the only important reabsorbable anion, or balanced by the secretion of H^+ or potassium. Of the 140 mEq/liter of sodium in the glomerular filtrate, normally only 25 mEq/liter is reabsorbed in association with H^+ secretion. In metabolic alkalosis, the increase in the plasma bicarbonate concentration to 35 mEq/liter is associated with a decrease in the plasma chloride concentration. Now 35 mEq/liter of sodium reabsorption is associated with H^+ secretion. The remaining Na^+ is reabsorbed in association with undetermined anions or K^+ secretion. Thus, avid Na^+ reabsorption increases H^+ secretion and therefore bicarbonate reabsorption. The net effect of maintaining extracellular volume at the expense of pH homeostasis is the *maintenance* of a metabolic alkalosis.

The mechanisms whereby hypokalemia augments H^+ secretion are shown in Figure 6. In hypokalemic states, intracellular acidosis results from the shift of H^+ into the cell and is responsible for the increase in H^+ secretion. The combined effects of volume depletion and hypokalemia on bicarbonate reabsorption are portrayed graphically in Figure 13. The relationship between $[K^+]$, ECF fluid volume, and HCO_3^- reabsorption have important therapeutic implications. Removal of the stimuli to increased bicarbonate reabsorption by either volume expansion or potassium chloride administration will allow bicarbonate to be lost in the urine. This alleviates the alkalosis.

A. Respiratory Compensation to Metabolic Alkalosis

In Figure 14, the relationship between blood HCO_3^-, pH, and P_{CO_2} in metabolic alkalosis is portrayed. As metabolic alkalosis is generated by an increase in the bicarbonate concentration of the ECF, the development of alkalosis is sensed by chemoreceptors controlling ventilation. This results in hypoventilation and an increase in the P_{CO_2}, which reduces the pH toward normal. On the average, the P_{CO_2} increases 0.6–0.7 mm Hg for every 1 mEq/liter increment in the plasma bicarbonate concentration. For example, if the plasma bicarbonate concentration is 10 mEq/liter greater than normal, there should be a 6- to 7-mm Hg increase in the P_{CO_2} from the normal of 40 to 46–47 mm Hg. In the clinical setting observation of P_{CO_2} values significantly different from those predicted would indicate a superimposed respiratory acidosis or alkalosis.

The respiratory compensation for metabolic alkalosis is limited by hypoxemia. Since hypoxemia is a potent stimulus to ventilation itself, its development as the P_{CO_2} rises will limit the hypoventilatory response to metabolic alkalosis. In a patient with metabolic alkalosis who is breathing room air, the maximum P_{CO_2} usually achieved is 60 mm Hg. This limitation is due to significant hypoxemia at this rate of respiration. In a patient with

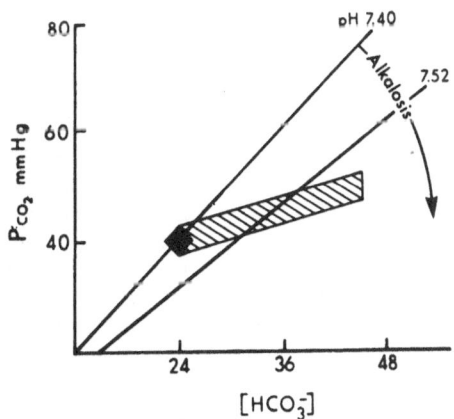

Figure 14. Effect of metabolic alkalosis on acid–base equilibrium. As plasma bicarbonate is increased, lowering H^+ concentration (elevating pH), ventilation decreases. The P_{CO_2} is elevated 0.6 mm Hg for every 1-mEq/liter increment in HCO_3^-. The shaded area indicates the relationship between P_{CO_2}, HCO_3^-, and pH at varying degrees of metabolic alkalosis.

underlying pulmonary disease and resting hypoxemia, the limitation to respiratory compensation for metabolic alkalosis occurs even sooner.

B. Etiology of Metabolic Alkalosis

Metabolic alkalosis is caused by three general mechanisms: (1) H^+ loss, (2) bicarbonate retention, and (3) contraction alkalosis. These are listed in Table VI according to their responsiveness to ECF volume replenishment.

1. Gastrointestinal H^+ Loss

Gastric juice contains high concentrations of saline, hydrochloric acid, and lesser concentrations of potassium chloride. Each milliequivalent of H^+ secreted generates 1 mEq of bicarbonate in the ECF. Under normal conditions, the increase in plasma bicarbonate concentration is only transient since the entry of H^+ to the duodenum stimulates an equal amount of bicarbonate secretion from the pancreas into the intestinal lumen. However, if the gastric juice is removed either by vomiting or nasogastric suction, there is no stimulus

Table VI. Causes (Generation) of Metabolic Alkalosis Listed According to Their Responsiveness to Increases in ECF Volume

I. ECF volume responsive
  A. H^+ loss
    1. Gastrointestinal loss
      Removal of gastric secretions (vomiting, suction)
    2. Renal H^+ loss
      Diuretics (late)
    3. H^+ movement into cells
      Hypokalemia
      Diuretic induced
  B. Contraction alkalosis
    Diuretics
II. ECF volume unresponsive
  A. H^+ loss
    1. Renal H^+ loss
      a. Mineralocorticoid excess
        i. Primary hyperaldosteronism
        ii. Hyperreninemia
        iii. Licorice ingestion
        iv. Glucocorticoid excess (Cushing's syndrome)
        v. Congenital adrenal hyperplasia
      b. Posthypercapnic alkalosis
    2. H^+ movement into cells
      Hypokalemia
      Mineralocorticoids
  B. Bicarbonate retention
    Administration of $NaHCO_3$ or Na citrate

to bicarbonate secretion. The result is an increase in the plasma bicarbonate concentration and metabolic alkalosis. The tendency toward alkalosis is enhanced and maintained by the concomitant volume depletion.

2. Diuretic-Induced Alkalosis

The potent diuretics in common use (thiazides, furosemide, ethacrynic acid) promote excretion of sodium and potassium almost exclusively in association with chloride. Net acid excretion is also augmented at times during the diuresis. Metabolic alkalosis is generated by the combination of the direct loss of acid and disproportionate chloride loss causing extracellular bicarbonate concentrations to rise. The alkalosis is maintained by volume contraction and hypokalemia. This is especially the case in patients adhering to low-salt diets during diuretic therapy.

During the generation phase of metabolic alkalosis due to diuretic administration, the urinary chloride concentrations are high as sodium and potassium losses develop. With continued diuretic administration, a new steady state develops at a lower ECF volume. In this situation, a reduced ECF volume, sodium and chloride retention is avid and the urinary chloride and sodium concentration will decrease. Thus, the maintenance stage of metabolic alkalosis due to diuretic administration is characterized by a low urinary chloride concentration.

The urinary sodium or chloride concentration may be helpful in differentiating between the two general types of metabolic alkalosis (volume responsive and volume independent). In states of metabolic alkalosis associated with hypovolemia and hypochloremia, the renal conservation of sodium and chloride will result in maximal lowering of the urinary sodium and chloride concentration to less than 10 mEq/liter. In patients with mineralocorticoid excess who are volume expanded, as discussed below, the urinary sodium and chloride concentration should exceed 20 mEq/liter. In Table VI, the causes of metabolic alkalosis are divided by the expected response to ECF volume replenishment. The volume responsive causes of metabolic alkalosis will be associated with urinary sodium or chloride concentration of less than 20 mEq/liter and often less than 10 mEq/liter, while the ECF volume independent causes of metabolic alkalosis usually exhibit concentration of greater than 20 mEq/liter.

3. Contraction Alkalosis

In situations where sodium chloride and water are lost from the ECF without concomitant bicarbonate loss, the ECF volume contracts around a constant amount of extracellular bicarbonate, resulting in an increase in the bicarbonate concentration and a rise in the pH. This syndrome is referred to as contraction alkalosis. It is rarely the sole cause of metabolic alkalosis, but it is a common contributing factor, especially in the case of diuretic ingestion.

4. Mineralocorticoid Excess

Since aldosterone stimulates hydrogen and potassium secretion and sodium reabsorption in the distal nephron, the excessive ·production of aldosterone can lead to H^+ loss and metabolic alkalosis. The effect of aldosterone on H^+ secretion is enhanced in the presence of hypokalemia. Thus, the generation of metabolic alkalosis in states of mineralocorticoid excess is probably due to the direct effect of mineralocorticoids on H^+ secretion. However, this mechanism has not been fully established since attempts to produce experimental metabolic alkalosis in man by long-term administration of mineralocorticoids have been unsuccessful. The mainte-nance of the alkalotic state is, at least in part, due to hypokalemia induced by the mineralocorticoids.

The action of aldosterone in the distal nephron on H^+ and potassium secretion requires the presence of sodium in the tubular fluid. When delivery of sodium out of the proximal tubule is reduced, as in secondary hyperal-dosteronism due to volume depletion, hydrogen and potassium secretion is only slightly enhanced by aldosterone. Thus, in patients with congestive heart failure who have a decreased effective circulating volume and secondary hyperaldosteronism, the tendency toward generation and maintenance of a metabolic alkalosis is blunted by decreased delivery of sodium to the distal nephron. The degree of metabolic alkalosis seen in patients with congestive heart failure, not treated by diuretics, is only mild. However, secondary hyperaldosteronism may lead to significant increases in H^+ and potassium secretion if loop diuretics, which enhance distal delivery of sodium, are administered. Also, the administration of impermanent anions such as sodium carbenicillin or penicillin would increase sodium delivery to the distal tubule in a volume-depleted subject. In this setting, the sodium in the distal tubular fluid will be reabsorbed in exchange for H^+ and potassium, resulting in hypokalemia and metabolic alkalosis.

The combination of primary mineralocorticoid excess, hypokalemia, high distal sodium delivery, and metabolic alkalosis can be seen in a variety of conditions listed in Table VI. In these settings, aldosterone augments sodium reabsorption and secretion of potassium and hydrogen. The sodium retention seen in these disease states does not result in edema since as sodium is retained the ensuing volume expansion activates natriuretic mechanisms which result in renal excretion of most of the excess sodium. This phenom-enon is called aldosterone escape and is discussed in greater detail in the chapter on sodium (Chapter 4). It is important to note that the metabolic alkalosis in these patients will not respond to sodium chloride since their ECF volume is already expanded. Correction of the hypokalemia or aldos-terone antagonists will serve to treat the alkalosis.

5. Posthypercapnic Alkalosis

Chronic respiratory acidosis is associated with a compensatory increase in renal bicarbonate reabsorption. If a patient with this disorder is treated with mechanical ventilation, P_{CO_2} can be rapidly returned to normal. However, the plasma bicarbonate concentration will remain elevated, resulting in metabolic alkalosis. Since this acute increase in arterial pH can produce serious neurologic abnormalities and death, the P_{CO_2} should be lowered slowly and carefully in patients with chronic hypercapnia.

6. Retention of Bicarbonate

Because of the ability of the kidney to excrete bicarbonate, it is difficult to produce more than a small increment in the plasma bicarbonate concentration by chronic administration of sodium bicarbonate. However, a significant alkalosis can be produced by the acute infusion of base or administration of alkali in a patient in whom renal bicarbonate excretion is impaired.

X. RESPIRATORY ACIDOSIS

Ventilation is controlled by chemoreceptors in the respiratory center of the medulla oblongata sensitive to CO_2. This results in adjustments of alveolar ventilation and the respiratory excretion of the daily CO_2 load and the maintenance of a normal P_{CO_2} of 40 mm Hg. Interference with any step in the process of ventilation, from the respiratory center in the medulla to the chest wall and respiratory muscles, to gas exchange across the alveolar capillary, can produce a decrease in alveolar ventilation resulting in CO_2 retention. If CO_2 retention occurs and the ventilatory function is not restored, the decrease in the pH produced by CO_2 retention is minimized first by cellular buffers and later by increased renal hydrogen secretion. The renal response occurs over several days and the compensation to acute respiratory acidosis is thus less effective than that in chronic respiratory acidosis.

A. Acute Respiratory Acidosis

Acute elevations in P_{CO_2} result in large changes in pH since very little extracellular buffering is available. This is because bicarbonate cannot buffer CO_2. Thus, the only buffering for an acute increase in P_{CO_2} are the intracellular buffers, hemoglobin and proteins. These constitute the only defense against acute hypercapnia:

$$CO_2 + H_2O \rightleftharpoons H_2CO_3 + Hb^- \rightleftharpoons HHB + HCO_3$$

The bicarbonate formed from these reactions diffuses out of the red cell into the extracellular fluid in exchange for chloride. As a result of the cell buffers, there is an increase in plasma bicarbonate concentration of 1 mEq/liter for every 10-mm Hg rise in the P_{CO_2}, but as shown in Figure 15, this is an

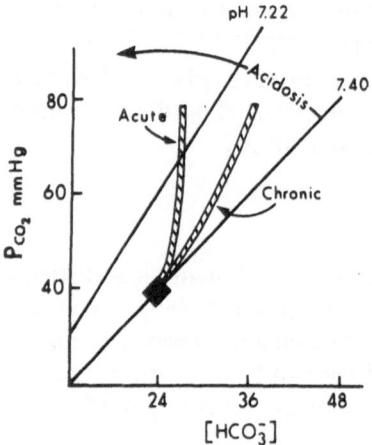

Figure 15. Effects of acute and chronic respiratory acidosis on acid–base equilibrium. Decreased alveolar gas exchange elevates the P_{CO_2} of the ECF. Acutely, since HCO_3^- cannot buffer H^+ from CO_2, the increase in H^+ from CO_2 is buffered by intracellular release of HCO_3^- from hemoglobin and nonbicarbonate buffers. This buffer capacity is minimal and large changes in pH result. Chronically, the intracellular acidosis increases renal H^+ secretion, elevating the plasma HCO_3^-. The enhanced renal H^+ excretion minimizes the change in pH.

ineffective defense of the ECF pH. Treatment of acute respiratory acidosis must be directed at prompt improvement of alveolar ventilation. The use of bicarbonate might blunt developing acidemia but it is only a temporizing maneuver at best.

B. Chronic Respiratory Acidosis

The renal response to hypercapnia appears more slowly than cell buffering, taking 3–4 days to reach completion. The reduction in the arterial pH from the increased P_{CO_2} stimulates renal hydrogen secretion, resulting in an addition of bicarbonate to the extracellular fluid. Because of the effects of cell buffers and the renal compensation, patients with chronic respiratory acidosis have roughly a 3.5 mEq/liter increase in the plasma bicarbonate for every 10-mm Hg increment in the P_{CO_2}. This is more efficient in preventing a change in ECF pH than the compensation seen in acute respiratory acidosis (Figure 15). In the untreated chronic respiratory acidosis, the plasma bicarbonate level represents the renal threshold for bicarbonate. Thus, sodium bicarbonate administration would be ineffective in producing a further increase in the plasma bicarbonate and a correction of the acidosis since the administered bicarbonate would simply be excreted. Chronic respiratory acidosis is a relatively common disturbance, most often due to chronic obstructive pulmonary disease (bronchitis and emphysema in smokers). Therapy is aimed at improving alveolar ventilation. The specifics of this are beyond the scope of this chapter. Infrequently, extrapulmonary disorders such as extreme obesity and the Pickwickian syndrome can produce chronic alveolar hypoventilation and CO_2 retention. The Pickwickian syndrome is the term used to refer to chronic hypocapnia seen in extremely obese patients in whom the increased weight of the chest wall increases the work of breathing. Weight loss in these patients has been effective in producing a normal ventilatory pattern.

XI. RESPIRATORY ALKALOSIS

If effective alveolar ventilation is increased beyond the level needed to eliminate the daily CO_2 load because of an increase in respiratory rate or the effect of tidal volume, the result will be a reduction in P_{CO_2} and an increase in the systemic pH [equation (3)]. Hypocapnia (the reduction in P_{CO_2}) can result either from a physiologic or nonphysiologic stimulus to respiration. Since ventilation results in the uptake of O_2 and the excretion of CO_2, which increases the pH, it is appropriate that hypoxemia and acidosis are the principle stimuli to ventilation.

The pH stimulus to ventilation is sensed centrally in the medullary respiratory centers and to a lesser degree peripherally in the carotid and aortic bodies. Since the pH of the CSF and the cerebral interstitium tends to change in the same direction as the pH of the ECF, the hyperventilation seen with acidosis is primarily due to a reduction in the pH of the fluid bathing the medullary respiratory centers. In certain conditions, an isolated CSF acidosis has been thought to be responsible for the primary increase in ventilation and respiratory alkalosis. For example, this occurs in patients with metabolic acidosis who have hyperventilation and hypocapnia as the normal respiratory compensation. However, if the ECF acidosis is corrected by bicarbonate administration, the reduction in P_{CO_2} may persist for hours to days resulting in respiratory alkalosis. This may be mediated by a persistent CSF acidosis due to two factors. First, bicarbonate crosses the blood–brain barrier slowly and so the medulla does not initially sense the increase in the bicarbonate concentration. Secondly, there may be a moderate increase in the P_{CO_2} toward normal since ventilation is slowed as the peripheral chemoreceptor senses the increase in ECF pH. Since the CO_2 enters the brain rapidly, this causes an elevation in the CSF P_{CO_2}, resulting in a paradoxical fall in the CFS pH, which tends to perpetuate the hyperventilatory state. Another situation in which a primary CSF acidosis may be responsible for respiratory alkalosis occurs in patients with subarchnoid hemorrhage where blood products of hemolysis may directly stimulate the respiratory center.

In many patients with respiratory alkalosis, the P_{O_2} is normal and the CSF pH reflects the systemic pH and is increased. Presumably, the hypocapnia in these situations is due mainly to emotional stress or salicylate intoxication, which directly stimulates respiratory centers. Other direct stimuli to the respiratory centers appear to be cirrhosis, sepsis, and exercise, all of which augment ventilation by poorly understood mechanisms.

If normal ventilation is not restored, the increase in the systemic pH induced by a fall in P_{CO_2} is minimized by a reduction in the plasma bicarbonate concentration. Both the cell buffers and an increase in renal bicarbonate excretion contribute to this response. Since the latter occurs relatively slowly over several days, the pH is less well maintained in acute respiratory alkalosis than in chronic respiratory alkalosis (Figure 16). The initial response to hyperventilation and respiratory alkalosis is movement of H^+ from the cells into the ECF where they combine with bicarbonate,

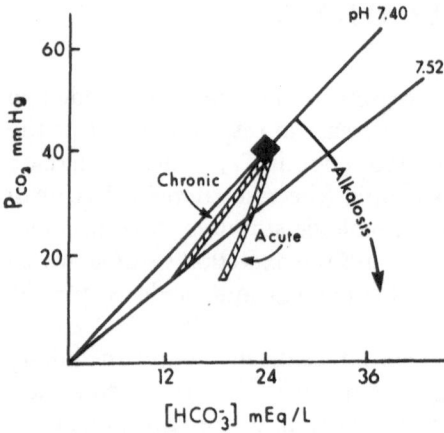

Figure 16. Effects of acute and chronic metabolic alkalosis on acid–base equilibrium. Acutely, the increased alveolar gas exchange lowers P_{CO_2} [H^+]. H^+ movement from cells is not efficient in preventing large falls in blood pH. Chronically, reduction in intracellular H^+ decreases renal H^+ secretion causing a loss of base in the urine and preventing large elevation in pH during hypocapnia.

resulting in a fall of the plasma bicarbonate concentration. These H^+ are derived from cell buffers and from increased lactic acid production produced in the cells by the alkalosis. In general, enough H^+ enters the ECF to lower the plasma bicarbonate concentration by 1 mEq/liter for each 10-mm Hg decrease in the P_{CO_2}. This is not a very efficient defense of the ECF pH and relatively large changes in pH result from acute respiratory alkalosis.

A. Chronic Respiratory Alkalosis

In the presence of persistent hypocapnia, there is a decrease in renal H^+ secretion resulting in bicarbonate loss in the urine (Figure 16). On the average, the combined effects of the cell buffers releasing bicarbonate and this renal compensation will lower the plasma bicarbonate concentration 5 mEq/liter for each 10-mm Hg reduction in the P_{CO_2}. If the P_{CO_2} were chronically reduced to 20 mm Hg the plasma bicarbonate concentration would fall by 10 mEq/liter to 14 mEq/liter. This is a very effective response since the pH would only be increased to 7.47.

SUGGESTED READINGS

General

Cogan, M. G., Rector, F. C., Jr., and Seldin, D. W.: Acid–base disorders, in Brenner, B. M., and Rector, F. C., Jr. (eds.): *The Kidney*. W. B. Saunders, Philadelphia, 1981.

Kassirer, J. P.: Serious acid–base disorders. *N. Engl. J. Med.* 291:773, 1974.

Maxwell, M. H., and Kleeman, C. R.: *Clinical Disorders of Fluid and Electrolyte Metabolism*, Third edition. McGraw-Hill, New York, 1980.

Rose, B. D. (ed.): *Clinical Physiology of Acid–Base and Electrolyte Disorders*. McGraw-Hill, New York, 1977.

Metabolic Acidosis

Felig, P.: Diabetic ketoacidosis. *N. Engl. J. Med.* 290:1360, 1974.

Kreisberg, R. A.: Lactate homeostasis and lactic acidosis. *Ann. Intern. Med.* 92:227, 1980.

Narins, R. G.: The renal acidoses, in Brenner, B. M., and Stein, J. H. (eds.): *Contemporary Issues in Nephrology. Acid–Base and Potassium Homeostasis 2.* Churchill Livingstone, New York, 1978.

Oh, M. S., and Carroll, H. J.: The anion gap. *N. Engl. J. Med.* 297:814, 1977.

Relman, A. S.: Lactic acidosis, in Brenner, B. M., and Stein, J. H. (eds.): *Contemporary Issues in Nephrology. Acid–Base and Potassium Homeostasis 2.* Churchill Livingstone, New York, 1978.

Renal Tubular Acidosis

Battle, D., and Arruda, J. A. L.: The renal tubular acidosis syndromes. *Miner. Electrolyte Metab.* 5:83, 1981.

Kurtzman, N. A., and Arruda, J. A. L.: Physiologic significance of urinary carbon dioxide tension. *Miner. Electrolyte Metab.* 1:241, 1978.

Sebastin, A., McSherry, E., and Morris, R. C., Jr.: Impaired renal conservation of sodium and chloride during sustained correction of systemic acidosis in patients with Type 1, classic renal tubular acidosis. *J. Clin. Invest.* 48:454, 1976.

Metabolic Alkalosis

Sebastian, A., Hulter, H. N., and Rector, F. C., Jr.: Metabolic alkalosis, in Brenner, B. M., and Stein, J. H. (eds.): *Contemporary Issues in Nephrology. Acid–Base and Potassium Homeostasis 2.* Churchill Livingstone, New York, 1978.

Seldin, D. W., and Rector, F. C., Jr.: The generation and maintenance of metabolic alkalosis. *Kidney Int.* 1:306, 1972.

Shear, L., and Brandman, I. S.: Hypoxia and hypercapnia caused by respiratory compensation for metabolic alkalosis. *Am. Rev. Respir. Dis.* 107:836, 1973.

Respiratory Acid–Base Disorders

Cohen, J. J., and Madias, N. E.: Acid–base disorders of respiratory origin, in Brenner, B. M., and Stein, J. H. (eds.): *Contemporary Issues in Nephrology, Acid–Base and Potassium Homeostasis 2.* Churchill Livingstone, New York, 1978.

Respiratory Acidosis

Cohen, J. J., Madias, N. E., Wolf, C. J., and Schwartz, W. B.: Regulation of acid–base equilibrium in chronic hypocapnia: evidence that the response of the kidney is not geared to the defense of extracellular [H^+]. *J. Clin. Invest.* 57:1483, 1976.

Madias, N. E., Schwartz, W. B., and Cohen, J. J.: The maladaptive renal response to secondary hypocapnia during chronic HCl acidosis in the dog. *J. Clin. Invest.* 60:1393, 1977.

9

Pathophysiology of Calcium, Magnesium, and Phosphorus Metabolism

EDUARDO SLATOPOLSKY

I. CALCIUM

A. Introduction

1. General Considerations

Calcium, the principal mineral of the human skeleton and the most abundant cation of the body, is essential to the integrity and function of cell membranes, neuromuscular excitability, transmission of nerve impulses, multiple enzymatic reactions, and regulation of parathyroid hormone secretion. The primary factor in the regulation of extracellular calcium is parathyroid hormone. It acts on the skeleton, small intestine, and kidney and interrelates with vitamin D and calcitonin to maintain the extracellular calcium concentration within narrow limits. Parathyroid hormone increases serum calcium by (1) increasing the activity and number of osteoclasts, inducing bone resorption, and consequently mobilizing calcium from bone; (2) augmenting

EDUARDO SLATOPOLSKY • Department of Medicine, Washington University School of Medicine, St. Louis, Missouri 63110.

calcium reabsorption by the kidney; and (3) increasing calcium absorption by the small intestine, indirectly, due to greater production of 1,25(OH)$_2$ vitamin D$_3$ (see Chapter 3). Since more than 99% of the body calcium resides in the skeleton, and some of it is in dynamic equilibrium with soluble forms of circulating calcium, bone plays a key role in calcium metabolism. Thus, factors affecting calcium metabolism may lead to skeletal derangements. In order to understand the pathophysiological mechanisms underlying a given clinical disorder of calcium metabolism, it is necessary to review calcium balance in health.

2. Distribution of Calcium

The total amount of calcium in the human body ranges from 1000 to 1200 g or 20–25 g/kg of fat-free body tissue. Approximately 99% of the body calcium resides in the skeleton, the other 1% is present in the ECF and ICF spaces. About 1% of the calcium in the skeleton is freely exchangeable with calcium in the ECF. Together, these two fractions are known as the miscible pool of calcium and account for 2% of the total body calcium. Calcium in bone is found primarily in the form of small crystals similar to hydroxy-apatite although some calcium exists as amorphous crystals in combination with phosphate. The normal calcium to phosphate ratio in bone is 1.5:1. In humans, the serum calcium concentration is kept remarkably constant between 9 and 10 mg/100 ml or 4.5–5 mEq/liter or 2.25–2.5 mM/liter. About 50% of serum calcium is ionized and 10% is complexed with citrate, phosphate, bicarbonate, and lactate. These two fractions, ionized plus complexed calcium ("ultrafiltrable calcium"), comprise approximately 60% of the total serum calcium. The rest, 40% is protein bound, mainly to albumin (Figure 1). The relationship between ionized calcium (Ca^{2+}) and the concentration of proteins in blood can be expressed as follows:

$$\frac{(Ca^{2+}) \, (proteinate)}{Calcium \; proteinate} = K$$

where proteinate equals the concentration of plasma protein. Since K is a constant the numerator and the denominator must change proportionally. In hypoproteinemic states, such as the nephrotic syndrome or cirrhosis, although total serum calcium may be low, the ionized fraction may be within the normal range. Five to ten percent of the calcium is bound to globulins. It is unusual for total serum calcium concentrations to change because of alterations in the levels of serum globulins. However, in cases of severe hyperglobulinemia such as in multiple myeloma or other dysproteinemias, elevations of total serum calcium concentrations may be observed.

One gram of albumin binds approximately 0.7 mg of calcium. The normal plasma albumin concentration is 4.0–4.5 g/100 ml, and only about 10%–15% of the binding sites for calcium are occupied. Consequently, when excess calcium is added to blood either *in vitro* or *in vivo,* all the fractions increase in the same proportion and the ultrafiltrable fraction as a percentage

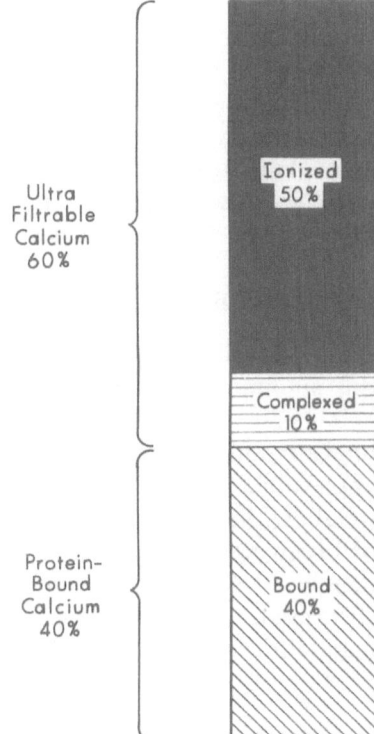

Figure 1. Relative amounts of the different forms of calcium in human serum.

of the total calcium does not change. The binding of calcium by albumin, therefore, acts as a buffer which reduces by about half the potential changes in ionized calcium which may result from acute gains or losses of calcium by the blood. The most important factor modifying the binding of calcium to albumin is the pH of plasma. Alkalosis increases the binding of free calcium resulting in a fall in ionized calcium concentration and acidosis has the opposite effect. This is due not only to competition between H^+ and Ca^{2+} for binding sites in albumin but also to changes in the conformation of the albumin molecule. Changes in P_{CO_2} do not affect calcium binding other than via changes in pH. In the past, ionized calcium was difficult to measure. This difficulty has been overcome in the past five years by the use of very sensitive flow-through electrodes, some of which can measure changes in ionized calcium as small as 0.1 mg/100 ml.

The intracellular concentration of calcium is extremely small. Most cells apparently have an active "calcium pump" which extrudes calcium and can maintain a 1000-fold concentration gradient between the cytosolic and ECF calcium. Intracellular calcium may be complexed with ions such as ortho-phosphate or pyrophosphate or bound to organic molecules such as ATP; however, a large amount of intracellular calcium may be sequestered within organelles such as mitochondria or cytoplasmic reticulum. In general, cell membranes are less permeable to calcium than to sodium. The permeability of cell membranes to calcium may change dramatically in response to several influences such as the action of hormones on target cells (i.e., PTH). In cardiac muscle and nerve, calcium extrusion is directly coupled to sodium transport. The cytosolic calcium concentration is also maintained by an active transport into mitochondria and microsomes. It has been shown that mitochondria accumulate calcium and phosphate ions to form insoluble amorphous tricalcium phosphate, a reaction which releases hydrogen ions into the cytosol. Cell injury may lead to a rise in intracellular calcium because of its release from organelles.

3. Calcium Balance

Approximately 1 g of calcium is ingested daily in the diet. However, this amount may vary depending on the amount of milk consumed. Milk and cheese are the major sources of calcium and contribute 50%–70% of the total amount ingested in the diet. In the United States, 1 liter of milk contains approximately 800–900 mg of calcium. About 10–15 mg calcium/kg body weight is the recommended daily intake. However, during the last trimester of pregnancy, there is an increased requirement for calcium since approximately 20–30 g of calcium enter the fetus. With age, intestinal calcium absorption declines, thus, an increase in calcium intake may be necessary to maintain calcium homeostasis. When 1 g of calcium is ingested in the diet,

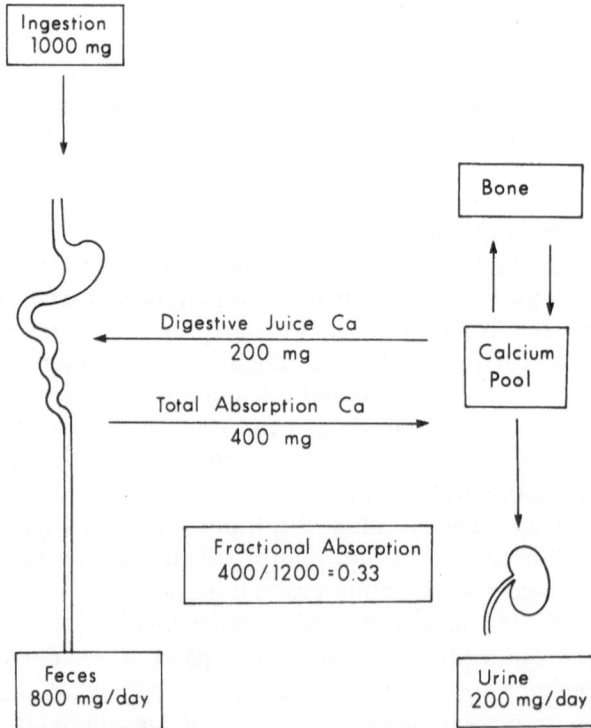

Figure 2. Diagrammatic representation of calcium metabolism in man showing the contribution of the gastrointestinal tract, the kidney, and bone to the maintenance of the calcium pool.

approximately 800 mg are excreted in the feces and 200 mg in the urine (Figure 2). With a normal calcium intake (700–1000 mg), approximately 30%–40% of the ingested calcium is absorbed in the intestine; however, on a low-calcium diet (less than 400 mg/day) the percent absorbed increases. On the other hand, the percent of calcium absorbed decreases when the diet has a high calcium content (greater than 1500 mg/day). The mechanisms responsible for this adaptation have been partially characterized and require the participation of parathyroid hormone, vitamin D, and perhaps, calcitonin. When a patient or an experimental animal is fed a low-calcium diet, the development of mild and transient hypocalcemia triggers the release of parathyroid hormone which increases the conversion of 25-hydroxycholecalciferol [25(OH)D_3] to 1,25-dihydroxycholecalciferol [1,25(OH)$_2D_3$] in the renal cortex (see Chapter 3). This metabolite of vitamin D [1,25(OH)$_2D_3$], increases the intestinal absorption of calcium and also mobilizes calcium from bone, in a synergistic way with PTH. Thus, serum calcium returns to normal. On the other hand, if the patient is fed a high-calcium diet, the mild hypercalcemia that may be produced suppresses the release of parathyroid hormone and stimulates the release of calcitonin. In the absence of parathyroid hormone, the activity of the 1,α-hydroxylase is diminished and the 24-hydroxylase is activated, thus, the kidney makes preferentially 24,25-dihydroxycholecalciferol [24,25(OH)$_2D_3$], which is less efficient than 1,25(OH)$_2D_3$ in promoting calcium absorption from the gastrointestinal (GI) tract and mobilizing calcium from the skeleton.

4. Intestinal Calcium Absorption

The mechanisms of calcium transport across the intestinal mucosa are complex and not fully understood. This process involves three steps: (1) the transport of calcium from the lumen into the cell, (2) the movement of calcium within the cell, and (3) the movement of calcium from the cell into the interstitial fluid. Many factors regulate intestinal calcium absorption including (1) dietary calcium intake, (2) vitamin D intake, (3) age of the patient, (4) the general state of calcium balance, and (5) circulating levels of PTH. The fecal calcium consists of the fraction of calcium ingested that is not absorbed plus 100–200 mg of calcium secreted by the intestine daily. This secreted calcium is known as "endogenous fecal calcium." The amount of calcium secreted by the intestine seems to be fairly constant and not greatly influenced by hypercalcemia.

Intestinal calcium absorption occurs by two general mechanisms: active and passive transport. Calcium movement from the mucosa to the serosal surface of the intestine occurs against a concentration gradient. This suggests that the intestinal cells contain a "pump" capable of moving calcium against an electrochemical gradient. There is evidence to suggest that a passive process plays an important role in calcium absorption. When the intestine is perfused in vitro with increasing calcium concentrations, the rate of movement of calcium from mucosa to serosa increases without evidence of saturation or a maximum transport rate. It would be expected that an active transport process would be saturable. It has been estimated that at luminal calcium concentrations above 7.0 mM, calcium is transported primarily by a diffusional process. This would suggest that in regions of the intestine, such as the ileum, where the calcium concentration is high, the passive transport process predominates. In the duodenum and jejunum, where the luminal calcium concentration is lower than 6 mM, the active transport process assumes a predominant role.

The transfer of calcium across the intestinal brush border surface seems to be rate limited by vitamin D deficiency. This suggests that a brush border component is instrumental in the transfer of calcium into the epithelial cell (Figure 3). Intestinal brush border preparations have a calcium-dependent ATPase whose activity is increased by vitamin D. The increase in calcium ATPase parallels the change in calcium transport after vitamin D repletion. Also an alkaline phosphatase is present in the brush border of the small intestine. Both calcium ATPase and alkaline phosphatase may play a role in the movement of calcium into the mucosal cell. A calcium-binding protein has been demonstrated in the mucosal cells of the intestine of many species. Its molecular weight ranges from 8000 in rats to 25,000 in chickens. Calcium-binding protein has some of these characteristics: its concentration increases in response to vitamin D, it is present in intestinal mucosal cells, but not in bone, the time course of its appearance after vitamin D treatment is similar to the time course of changes in calcium transport, and it is localized in the glycocalyx surface of the brush border of the mucosal intestinal cells. However, the exact role of this protein in calcium transport by mucosal cells is still controversial. Recently it has been demonstrated that the early effects of $1,25(OH)_2D_3$ on calcium transport are mediated by changes in the structure of the luminal membrane of the intestine. Glucocorticoids block the effect of vitamin D on calcium transport without altering the synthesis of calcium-binding protein. Increased intestinal calcium absorption is accompanied by an increase in the amount of calcium-binding protein without changes in the intrinsic binding affinity (K_m) of the protein for calcium. In addition to parathyroid hormone and vitamin D, other factors such as phosphate influence calcium absorption. High phosphate diets decrease calcium absorption. This may be due to decreased $1,25(OH)_2D_3$ synthesis secondary to hyperphosphatemia and to the formation of relatively insoluble calcium–phosphate complexes which decrease the availability of calcium for transepithelial uptake. Experimentally, large concentrations of lactose or other sugars (mannose, xylose) or certain amino acids (lysine, arginine) inhibit intestinal calcium absorption. The physiological significance of these observations is unknown. The decreased calcium absorption produced by glucocorticoids has therapeutic implications in the management of hypercalcemic disorders associated with excessive intake or increased sensitivity to vitamin D.

Less is known about the movement of calcium within the cell. When calcium enters the cell it either diffuses or is carried across the cell to the basolateral membrane where it is pumped out into the serosal medium. This

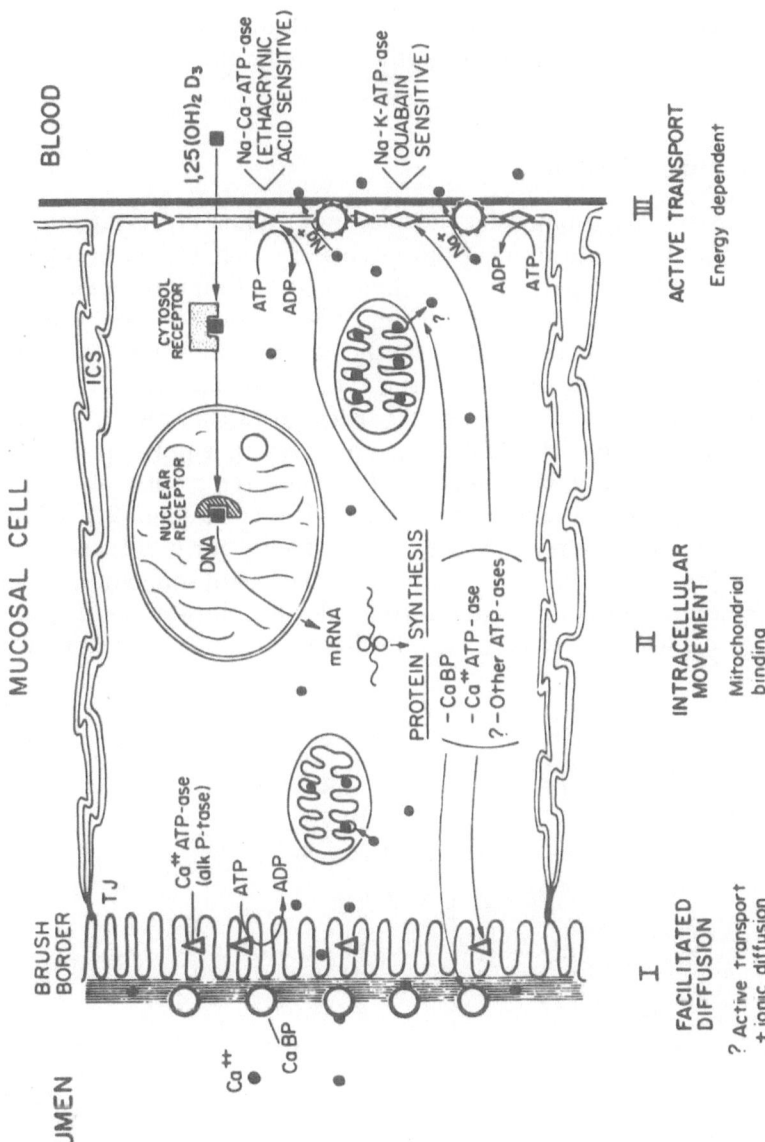

Figure 3. Diagrammatic representation of the mechanisms involved in the transport of calcium across the intestinal cell. Abbreviations: CaBP, calcium-binding protein; TJ, tight junction; ICS, intercellular space. (Reprinted with permission from Coburn, J. W., et al.: Kidney Int. 4:96, 1973.)

extrusion of calcium into the ECF may be dependent on external sodium. Apparently, the exit of calcium from the cells is driven by the inward (downhill) transport of sodium into the cells. Thus, the energy necessary to translocate calcium is not used to activate a specific calcium pump but to maintain the activity of a sodium pump which maintains a sodium gradient across the cell surface. This sodium gradient may be the driving force for calcium extrusion.

5. Renal Handling of Calcium

In humans at GFR (glomerular filtration rate) values of 170 liters/24 hr and serum ultrafiltrable calcium concentrations of 6 mg/100 ml, roughly 10 g of calcium are filtered per day. The amount of calcium excreted in the urine usually ranges from 100 to 200 mg/24 hr; hence 98%–99% of the filtered load of calcium is reabsorbed by the renal tubules. Micropuncture studies of the kidney in the Munich–Wistar rat (with surface glomeruli) have demonstrated that the fluid (in Bowman's space) to plasma ratio of calcium (TF/PCa) is approximately 0.6, indicating that only that portion of serum calcium not bound to protein is filtrable. There are remarkable similarities in the handling of calcium and sodium by the kidney: less than 2% of their filtered load is excreted normally; there is no evidence for tubular secretion of either calcium or sodium in the mammalian nephron, and urinary excretion of either sodium or calcium is controlled by adjustments in tubular reabsorption. Approximately 60% of the filtered calcium is reabsorbed in

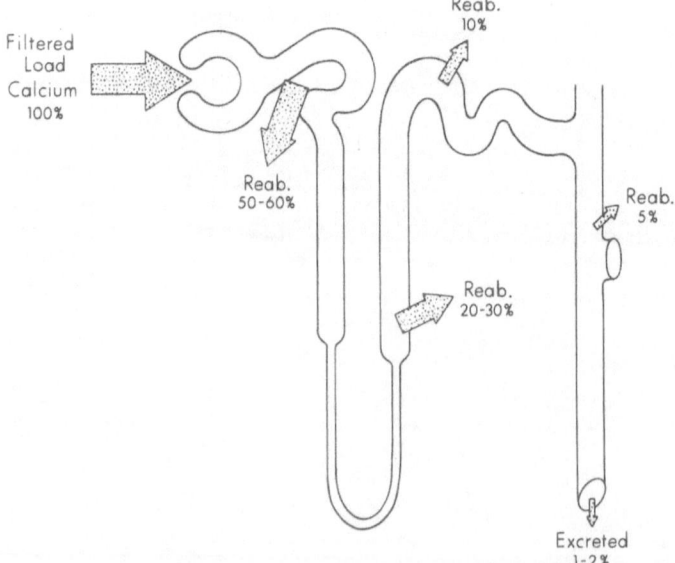

Figure 4. Schematic illustration of the reabsorption of calcium by different segments of the nephron. Only ultrafiltrable calcium contributes to the filtered load. The arrows show the relative amounts of calcium reabsorbed in the different nephron segments.

the proximal convoluted tubule, 20%–25% in the loop of Henle, 10% by the distal convoluted tubule, and 5% by the collecting system (Figure 4). The terminal nephron, (late distal tubule and collecting system), while responsible for the reabsorption of only 5%–8% of the filtered calcium load, seems to be the major site for the final regulation of calcium excretion. The distal nephron appears to be the major site of parathyroid hormone action on calcium reabsorption. PTH enhances calcium reabsorption in the thick ascending limb of Henle's loop and in the collecting duct. The reabsorption of calcium in the proximal convoluted tubule parallels sodium and water reabsorption with the ratio of tubular fluid to plasma ultrafiltrable calcium being 1.0 : 1.1. This would be compatible with passive calcium reabsorption secondary to sodium and water reabsorption. If calcium is reabsorbed transcellularly, rather than through intercellular channels, it must be extruded at the peritubular surface of cells by active transport since its intracellular concentration, as mentioned above, is probably 1000-fold lower than in the lumen or the peritubular capillaries. A calcium ATPase present in the basolateral membrane could provide the energy for calcium extrusion from cells. Alternatively, a calcium sodium exchange has been suggested. Calcium is transported in the pars recta by a process which is not inhibited by ouabain. Neither the thin descending limb or thin ascending limbs of Henle's loop plays an important role in calcium reabsorption. In contrast, however, the isolated thick ascending limb of Henle's loop *in vitro* reabsorbs calcium from lumen to bath in the absence of water movement. About 20%–30% of the filtered calcium is reabsorbed in this segment. Although the movement of calcium may be due to the potential gradient generated by active chloride transport (see Chapter 2), studies on the thick ascending limb of Henle suggest that the flux ratio for calcium may be greater than can be accounted for by the positive intraluminal potential; thus an additional active transport process for calcium may be present in this segment. Furosemide or ethacrynic acid, which block sodium transport in the thick ascending limb of Henle's loop (see Chapter 17), also block calcium transport. Parathyroid hormone, on the other hand, increases calcium absorption in this portion of the nephron. In the distal convoluted tubule, calcium reabsorption seems to be independent of sodium transport or electrical potential gradients. A progressive fall in the tubular fluid to plasma ultrafiltrable calcium and the rise in the TF/P inulin between early and distal sites of distal convoluted tubule have been observed, indicating that an active absorption of calcium occurs in this segment. Thiazides (see Chapter 17) block sodium reabsorption and enhance calcium reabsorption in the distal tubule.

Maneuvers such as administration of parathyroid hormone, cyclic AMP, ECF volume expansion, insulin administration, and phosphate depletion have all been shown to inhibit proximal tubule reabsorption of calcium and to increase the delivery of calcium to the more distal nephron segments. The effect of these maneuvers on urinary calcium excretion, however, may be a decrease, no change, or an increase in calcium excretion, emphasizing again the critical role of the distal tubule in the final regulation of calcium excretion. Both metabolic acidosis and phosphate depletion are accompanied by increased calcium excretion in the urine. Studies in experimental animals suggest that the "defect" in calcium reabsorption of metabolic acidosis and phosphate depletion is located in the distal tubule, although phosphate depletion may also affect calcium transport in the proximal tubule. The administration of sodium bicarbonate, with a rapid correction of acidosis, increases calcium reabsorption in the late distal tubule. Similar results are found when phosphate is given to an animal which has been previously phosphate depleted.

6. The Skeleton as a Calcium Reservoir

More than 99% of the total body calcium is found in the skeleton. Bone consists of approximately 40% mineral, 30% organic matrix, and 30% water. Bone mineral exists in two physical forms, the amorphous and the crystalline. The amorphous form consists mainly of brushite and tricalcium phosphate; the crytstalline form is composed mainly by hydroxy-apatite. Greater than 90% of the organic material of the bone matrix is in the form of collagen fibers which are arranged in bundles. The remaining of the organic intra-cellular substance of bones is composed by carbohydrate protein complexes, lipids, and peptides. From the architectural point of view, the skeleton is composed of two types of bone: (1) compact cortical bone, which surrounds the marrow cavity and forms the shaft of the long bones, and (2) cancellous or trabecular bone, which is the main component of flat bone and vertebra.

A differentiation between two other general types of bone is critical in the diagnosis of metabolic bone disease. The first, called woven bone (immature bone) is a loosely organized highly mineralized bone in which the collagen fibers are coarsely arranged and the osteocytes are large and irregular in size and shape. Woven bone is formed by simultaneous and unorganized actions of many cells. The calcification of the tissue is patchy, occurring in a speckled pattern and independent of the presence of vitamin D activity. Woven bone is present in the fetus but after age 14 is no longer in the human skeleton except in pathological conditions such as hyperpara-thyroidism and during rapid bone turnover, as in the presence of healing fractures. The second type is lamellar bone (mature bone), which is the major component of the normal adult skeleton. It is a highly organized bone in which the collagen bundles are arranged in successive extending layers between which are rows of cells called osteocytes. Lamellar bone is the product of a synchronized activity of the osteoblast depositing collagen materials at a specific call surface. Another difference between woven bone and lamellar bone is the relation of mineral to collagen. In lamellar bone, the relative amounts of collagen and minerals are closely related and make these bones difficult to hypermineralize. Mineralization of woven bone is disorderly and the degree of mineralization varies enormously; thus hypermineralization may occur in this type of bone.

The skeleton is under a constant process of resorption and formation. Although, this long-term process is responsible for bone turnover, it probably does not play a minute-to-minute role in the maintenance of serum calcium.

However, in pathological states where bone resorption is greatly increased, profound changes in calcium homeostasis may occur. The osteoclasts responsible for bone resorption are multinuclear giant cells lying in a regular indentation of the bone surface known as Howship's lacunae. The degree of bone resorption depends on the number and activity of osteoclasts. Resorption can also be produced by other cells such as mononuclear cells resembling monocytes and macrophages, which are believed to be precursors of the osteoclast. The process of resorption produced by the osteoclasts includes the production of lactic and citric acids, lyzosomal enzymes, and collagenase, which digest bone matrix. The osteoblasts, on the other hand, are the cells responsible for the repair process or bone formation. Usually, this process is initiated by the biosynthesis of collagen, which forms the bone matrix. Thereafter, the matrix is mineralized by the deposition of calcium and phosphate, with formation of amorphous material initially and then the development of hydroxy-apatite. The deposition of mineral occurs along a well-defined front ("calcification front") outside of which there is an osteoid border or seam. The osteoid begins to calcify about 10 days after deposition. Tetracycline when given to a patient is incorporated in the calcification front. By giving two doses of tetracycline separated by an interval of 14–21 days it is possible to calculate the linear rate of mineral deposition by measuring the distance between the two fluorescing bands of tetracycline, under the ultraviolet light. Parathyroid hormone in conjunction with vitamin D plays a key role in bone turnover. At physiological doses, parathyroid hormone has an anabolic effect, increasing bone formation. Thus, parathyroid hormone, by increasing calcium reabsorption by the kidney and gut and through stimulation of the osteoblast, affects the rate of bone formation. However, in pathological conditions, i.e., hyperparathyroidism, the concentration of PTH in serum may be increased 10 to 50-fold. At this high concentration, PTH increases the activity and number of osteoclasts; thus bone resorption predominates over bone formation, and minerals and organic matrix are removed from bone and enter the ECF. Not only parathyroid hormone, but other hormones like thyroxine or prostaglandins (PGE_2) also can produce severe hypercalcemia by increasing the activity of the osteoclast. Moreover, there are pathological processes such as multiple myeloma in which the malignant cells are known to produce an osteoclastic activating factor (OAF) which leads to an increase in bone resorption.

B. Hypercalcemia

Hypercalcemia is an elevation of total serum calcium above 11.0 mg/100 ml (when serum protein values are normal). The manifestations of hypercalcemia differ among patients. Mild hypercalcemia may be totally asymptomatic and may be detected during a routine blood chemistry determination; however, hypercalcemia may be so severe as to produce lethargy, disorientation, coma, and death. Pathologically, three general mechanisms may lead to the development of hypercalcemia (Table I): (1) increased mobilization of

Table I. Causes of Hypercalcemia

I. Hypercalcemia secondary to an increased Ca mobilization from bone
  A. Malignancy
    1. Metastatic
    2. Nonmetastic
      a. Osteoclastic activating factor (OAF)
      b. Prostaglandin (PGE_2)
      c. Ectopic hyperparathyroidism
  B. Hyperparathyroidism
    1. Primary
      a. Adenoma
      b. Hyperplasia
      c. Neoplastic
    2. Secondary
    3. Multiple endocrine neoplasias
      a. Type I with pituitary and pancreatic tumors
      b. Type II with medullary carcinoma of thyroid and pheochromocytoma
  C. Immobilization
  D. Hyperthyroidism
  E. Vitamin D intoxication
  F. Renal disease
    1. Chronic renal failure
    2. Postrenal transplantation
    3. Diuretic phase of acute renal failure
  G. Thiazide diuretics
  H. Vitamin A intoxication
II. Hypercalcemia secondary to an increase in calcium absorption from the gastrointestinal tract
  A. Sarcoidosis
  B. Vitamin D intoxication
  C. Milk-alkali syndrome
III. Hypercalcemia secondary to a decrease in urinary calcium excretion
  A. Thiazide diuretics
IV. Miscellaneous
  A. Adrenal insufficiency
  B. Tuberculosis
  C. Berylliosis
  D. Dysproteinemias
  E. Hemoconcentration
  F. Hyperalimentation regimens

---

calcium from bone, by far the most common and important mechanism, (2) increased absorption of calcium from the gastrointestinal tract, and (3) decreased urinary excretion of calcium (of minor importance). In some clinical disorders, although one or more of these mechanisms may be operative, compensatory adaptations develop and hypercalcemia may not occur. For example, in idiopathic hypercalciuria due to increased calcium absorption from the gastrointestinal tract, increased urinary excretion of calcium may prevent the development of hypercalcemia. On the other hand, in hyperparathyroidism, all three mechanisms (increased bone resorption, augmented GI absorption of calcium, and decreased urinary calcium excretion) lead to the development of hypercalcemia.

1. Hypercalcemia Secondary to Increased Calcium Mobilization from Bone

a. Hypercalcemia Secondary to Malignancies

Malignancy is the most common cause of hypercalcemia. Multiple mechanisms underlie the development of hypercalcemia of malignancy but, in general, it is due to increased mobilization of calcium from the skeleton, secondary to increased bone resorption by osteoclasts. The increased resorption could be due to the action of malignant cells that have metastasized to bone from tumors such as breast, prostate, kidney, lung, and thyroid. However, in certain types of tumors hypercalcemia occurs with no evidence of bone metastasis. In certain occasions, the removal of the tumor results in correction of the hypercalcemia. In these cases, humoral agents may be involved. Increased levels of an immunoreactive parathyroid hormone-like material which may be responsible for the hypercalcemia have been described. Other mechanisms of hypercalcemia due to tumors include the secretion of prostaglandins (PGE_2), especially by solid tumors, or the production of proteins, capable of increasing the activity of the osteoclast (osteoclast activating factor—OAF) as in patients with multiple myeloma. In metastatic bone disease there are usually two effects: (1) increased bone resorption and (2) an increase in woven bone formation. If the osteoblastic process (bone formation) predominates, hypercalcemia may not develop. However, if the osteolytic process predominates, the patients develop severe hypercalciuria and hypercalcemia. In contrast to tumors that produce a "parathyroidlike material," the serum phosphorus or the tubular reabsorption of phosphate usually is not decreased in metastatic bone disease. However, the patient may develop hypophosphatemia when the disease progresses and malnutrition becomes evident. It should be emphasized, however, that the osteolysis produced by tumors may be chemically mediated by substances such as PGE_2 which increase bone resorption. In other malignancies, such as multiple myeloma, Burkitt's lymphoma, or other malignant lymphomas, a factor has been found in the supernatant of cultured lymphoid cells obtained from these patients. This peptide material (OAF) appears to be present in two interconvertible forms, with molecular weights of 14,000 and 2000 daltons, respectively. Ectopic hyperparathyroidism is characterized by the presence of PTH-like material in blood and the development of severe hypercalcemia. Although many tumors may secrete PTH-like material, by far the two most important ones are the epidermoid squamous cell carcinoma of the lung and the renal cell carcinoma. Disagreement exists in the literature as to the percentage of patients with hypercalcemia of malignancy that have elevated levels of circulating immunoreactive PTH. This discrepancy is mainly related to the type of antibody used in a given assay for PTH. In general, patients with ectopic hyperparathyroidism have a greater degree of hypercalcemia and lower levels of immunoreactive PTH than patients with primary hyperparathyroidism. Moreover, patients with ectopic hyperparathyroidism are sicker, have a greater weight loss and the history of hypercalcemia is shorter and more dramatic. As mentioned above, prostaglandins may be involved in the production of localized osteolysis around the metastasis, but they also may have a systemic effect. There are two experimental situations in which the transplant of a tumor may produce hypercalcemia (the fibrosarcoma in the mouse and the VX2 carcinoma in the rabbit). Both tumors secrete PGE_2 and produce bone resorption. The hypercalcemia can be corrected by the administration of inhibitors of prostaglandin synthesis such as indomethacin (see Chapter 3). Currently, it is not known if circulating prostaglandins per se are responsible for the hypercalcemia since the administration of prostaglandins to experimental animals does not produce hypercalcemia. The hypercalcemia observed in patients with prostaglandin-producing tumors has occurred in the presence of bone metastasis. Thus, the hypercalcemia may be due to a local effect of prostaglandins produced by the malignant cells that have metastasized to bone.

b. Primary Hyperparathyroidism

Primary hyperparathyroidism is the most common endocrine disorder causing hypercalcemia. It is probably the major cause of asymptomatic hypercalcemia in young people. A single adenoma of the parathyroid gland is the most common cause of primary hyperparathyroidism. In contrast, chief-cell hyperplasia is the lesion seen in practically all patients with secondary hyperparathyroidism due to renal insufficiency. The mechanism of hypercalcemia relates to the effects of parathyroid hormone. The levels of radioimmunoassayable PTH (i-PTH) are elevated in primary hyperparathyroidism. The percentage of positive results, to confirm the diagnosis, depend on the type of antibody used and the sensitivity of each particular radioimmunoassay for PTH. Sensitive assays, utilizing a carboxy-terminal antibody, demonstrate elevated levels of PTH in 90%–95% of the patients with primary hyperparathyroidism. Since parathyroid hormone increases the activity and number of osteoclasts, bone resorption is seen on bone histology. X-rays of the phalanges show subperiosteal bone resorption. The increased calcium mobilization from bone raises the filtered load of calcium and leads to the development of hypercalciuria, despite the effect of PTH in increasing the reabsorption of calcium in the distal nephron. Moreover, the hypercalcemia is aggravated by increased calcium absorption from the gut secondary to high levels of $1,25(OH)_2D_3$ in response to high levels of PTH in blood. Parathyroid hormone decreases the renal reabsorption of phosphorus in the proximal and distal tubule, resulting in hypophosphatemia. Patients with primary hyperparathyroidism have a high incidence of peptic ulcer, renal stones, and psychiatric disorders. Since hypercalcemia interferes with the renal countercurrent mechanism responsible for the concentration of the urine, the patient develops polyuria and polydipsia. By measuring ionized calcium and i-PTH some laboratories have been able to establish the diagnosis of primary hyperparathyroidism in greater than 95% of the cases. The treatment of this condition is surgery (parathyroidectomy).

c. Immobilization

Patients who are immobilized for several days develop some degree of hypercalciuria. However, some of these patients may develop hypercalcemia. This is seen in patients with increased bone turnover such as Paget's disease. Hypercalcemia is seen frequently in immobilized patients secondary to multiple fractures. It would seem that prolonged periods of immobilization disrupt the balance between bone resorption and formation. The resorptive process predominates due to depression of osteoblastic activity and calcium mobilization occurs. In a few patients, the circulating levels of parathyroid hormone are elevated.

d. Hyperthyroidism

Serum calcium concentration may increase in thyrotoxicosis. Usually, the increment is mild and does not produce severe symptoms. Bone histology reveals an increase in osteoclastic bone resorption and fibroblastic proliferation resembling osteitis fibrosa cystica. Moreover, patients with thyrotoxicosis who present with hypercalcemia usually have low or undetectable levels of parathyroid hormone in blood. There is evidence for a direct stimulation of bone resorption by thyroxine (T4) and triiodothyronine (T3) *in vitro*.

e. Vitamin D Intoxication

Vitamin D increases both calcium absorption from the gastrointestinal tract and bone resorption. Metabolites of vitamin D have been shown to increase the efflux of calcium from bone *in vitro*. Moreover, the administration of $1,25(OH)_2D_3$ to dogs fed a low-calcium diet leads to hypercalcemia suggesting that the effect on bone was responsible for the rise in ECF calcium. The manifestations of vitamin D intoxication are probably secondary to high levels of 25-hydroxycholecalciferol in blood. The circulating levels of $1,25(OH)_2D_3$ remain within the normal range. Of course, if a patient receives pharmacological doses of $1,25(OH)_2D_3$ this metabolite of vitamin D may produce toxic effects and the characteristic hypercalcemia.

f. Renal Disease

i. Chronic Renal Failure. Hypercalcemia is rare in patients with chronic renal failure. In fact, the majority of patients with renal disease have hypocalcemia which leads to the development of secondary hyperparathyroidism. However, hypercalcemia has been described in a few patients with chronic renal failure. The mechanism is not fully understood. Potentially, the extreme hyperplasia of the parathyroid glands that may develop in these patients progresses to a point that they no longer respond to normal feedback mechanisms. Thus, a greater degree of hypercalcemia may be necessary to suppress PTH secretion by such enlarged glands. In some patients, hypercalcemia may be seen after significant reduction of serum phosphorus or after the ingestion of large amounts of calcium carbonate.

ii. Post-Renal Transplantation. Hypercalcemia occurs more frequently after a successful renal transplant than in patients with chronic renal insufficiency. Since patients receiving kidney transplants usually have severe secondary hyperparathyroidism, the amount of $1,25(OH)_2D_3$ produced by the new kidney, if the graft is successful, is greatly increased as a result of both high levels of PTH and decreased serum phosphate levels due to the marked phosphaturia posttransplant. Synergistically, $1,25(OH)_2D_3$ and parathyroid hormone would increase calcium mobilization from bone leading to hyper-calcemia. Obviously, $1,25(OH)_2D_3$ also increases calcium absorption from the gastrointestinal tract. In most patients, the hypercalcemia does not require specific treatment and subsides after 3–4 weeks. However, in some patients specific measures should be taken to prevent nephrocalcinosis, and if the hypercalcemia is severe and persists for several months or years, the patients may require surgical parathyroidectomy.

iii. Diuretic Phase of Acute Renal Failure. Occasionally hypercalcemia may be seen in patients entering the diuretic phase of acute renal failure. Many of these patients' renal failure is secondary to severe rhabdomyolysis. Usually, the patients have severe hyperphosphatemia and hypocalcemia during the short period of renal insufficiency. During the diuretic phase, calcium is rapidly mobilized from different tissues in which it had precipitated previously due to the pronounced hyperphosphatemia.

g. Thiazide Diuretics

Patients taking thiazide diuretics may develop moderate hypercalcemia. The mechanism for the hypercalcemia is not fully understood and a series of factors are involved. Thiazides decrease urinary excretion of calcium by increasing calcium reabsorption in the distal tubule. This reduction in urinary calcium seems to require some degree of ECF volume contraction and the presence of parathyroid hormone, since patients with hypoparathyroidism do not greatly reduce the amount of calcium in the urine after the admin-istration of thiazides. Thus, in patients with increased calcium mobilization from bone, the administration of thiazides may blunt the expected hyper-calciuria and potentially raise serum calcium. However, thiazides per se may also have a direct effect on the skeleton. Administration of thiazides intra-venously produces a mild change in ionized calcium. This effect is apparently potentiated by parathyroid hormone since the effect is greater in patients with hyperparathyroidism than in normals. Finally, there is controversy as to whether or not thiazides per se increase the release of parathyroid hormone. Most of the evidence indicates that this is not the case.

h. Vitamin A Intoxication

This is a very rare cause of hypercalcemia, seen more frequently in children than adults. Vitamin A has been shown to increase bone resorption *in vitro.*

2. Hypercalcemia Secondary to Increased Calcium Absorption from the Gastrointestinal Tract

There are several clinical entities, such as sarcoidosis, vitamin D intoxication, and milk alkali syndrome, which are characterized by increased calcium absorption from the gut and positive calcium balance. Some patients also have widespread soft tissue calcification and nephrocalcinosis. Most of these patients have low or undetectable levels of parathyroid hormone.

a. Sarcoidosis

About 10%–25% of patients with sarcoidosis have mild hypercalcemia. Although this abnormality is secondary to an increase in calcium absorption, controversy still exists as to the mechanism responsible for the increased calcium absorption. The serum levels of $1,25(OH)_2D_3$ may be elevated in sarcoidosis, but this is not uniform. In general, patients with sarcoidosis are sensitive to small doses of vitamin D and exposure to ultraviolet radiation of the skin. It is possible that not only is the concentration of vitamin D metabolites, especially $1,25(OH)_2D_3$, increased but also the target cells in the intestine responsible for calcium transport may have an increased sensitivity to vitamin D or an increased rate of calcium transport independent of vitamin D. The administration of corticosteroids in these patients decreases intestinal calcium absorption and corrects the hypercalcemia.

b. Vitamin D Intoxication

Vitamin D and its metabolites, especially $1,25(OH)_2D_3$, increase intestinal calcium absorption. Thus, high concentrations of D metabolites in blood are responsible for the hypercalcemia observed in vitamin D intoxication. As described above, vitamin D also has a direct effect on bone resorption which contributes to the development of hypercalcemia.

c. Milk Alkali Syndrome

This syndrome was seen frequently in the past in patients with peptic ulcer disease who ingested large amounts of calcium carbonate. Calcium carbonate contains 40% of elemental calcium. Some patients who ingested up to 20 g of calcium carbonate in 24 hr developed severe hypercalcemia. Moreover, alkalosis increases renal calcium reabsorption in the distal tubule and also reduces bone turnover thus decreasing calcium uptake by bone.

3. Hypercalcemia Secondary to Decreased Urinary Calcium Excretion

The decrease in urinary excretion of calcium may be secondary to a fall in the filtered load of calcium or to an increase in the tubular reabsorption of calcium. The fall in the filtered load of calcium may be secondary to a decrease in serum calcium or GFR. By definition, if the patient has a disorder which produces hypocalcemia with a decrease in urinary calcium excretion, the patient cannot be at the same time hypercalcemic, thus, such disorders can be excluded. A fall in GFR may decrease calcium delivery to the distal tubule and less calcium may be excreted in the urine. This situation which may occur in profound dehydration is self-limited and the hypercalcemia does not persist for a prolonged period of time. Moreover, dehydration or other conditions which decrease GFR may also modify the transport of sodium and water and affect the reabsorption of calcium by the nephron.

4. Clinical Symptoms of Hypercalcemia

Patients with mild hypercalcemia may be totally asymptomatic, however, as serum calcium increases, usually above 11 mg/100 ml numerous symptoms may be present and practically every organ of the body is affected. The most common symptoms are nausea, vomiting, polyuria, polydipsia, lack of concentration, fatigue, somnolence, mental confusion, and even death (see Table II).

5. Renal Effects of Hypercalcemia

Hypercalcemia may cause both an acute and reversible decrement in GFR or a chronic nephropathy. The mechanisms by which hypercalcemia decreases GFR are multifactorial. Hypercalcemia may lead to vasoconstriction of the afferent arteries and decreased renal blood flow. It can decrease ultrafiltration across glomerular capillaries. In addition, acute hypercalcemia may produce natriuresis and ECF volume contraction. In chronic hypercalcemic nephropathy, there is a fall in GFR, a decrease in the maximum concentrating capacity, and the urine is free of cells or casts, although mild proteinuria may be observed. The findings are similar to those seen in

Table II. Clinical Manifestations of Hypercalcemia

I. General
   Apathy, lethargy, weakness
II. Cardiovascular
   Cardiac arrhythmias, hypertension, vascular calcification
III. Renal
   Polyuria, hypercalciuria, stones, nephrocalcinosis, impaired concentration of urine, renal insufficiency
IV. Gastrointestinal
   Anorexia, nausea, vomiting, polydypsia, constipation, abdominal pain, gastric ulcer, pancreatitis
V. Neuropsychiatric and muscular
   Headache, impaired concentration, loss of memory, confusion, hallucination, coma, myalgia, muscle weakness, arthralgia
VI. Metastatic calcification
   Band keratopathy, conjunctival irritation, vascular calcification, periarticular calcification

---

patients with interstitial nephritis. The characteristic abnormality of hypercalcemic nephropathy is the inability to concentrate the urine. This abnormality persists even after the administration of ADH. The mechanisms by which hypercalcemia impairs the concentration of the urine are multiple. First, the osmotic gradient of the medulla is decreased, in part, due to decreased sodium transport in the thick ascending portion of the loop of Henle (see Chapter 6). Moreover, hypercalcemia decreases the permeability of the collecting duct to water by inhibiting the adenylate cyclase activity and generation of cyclic AMP in response to ADH. There is some evidence to suggest that increased prostaglandin synthesis may mediate part of this effect. PGE_2 enhances medullary blood flow, inhibits NaCl transport in the loop of Henle and antagonizes the effect of ADH on the collecting duct. It is possible that several of the effects of hypercalcemia on the concentrating mechanism could be related to increased prostaglandin synthesis in the medulla. Chronic persistent hypercalcemia eventually leads to the development of nephrocalcinosis most commonly localized to the medulla of the kidney. Thus, a salt-wasting nephropathy and the inability to concentrate the urine may explain part of the symptoms such as polyuria and polydipsia seen in patients with hypercalcemia.

6. Cardiovascular Effects

Calcium has an inotropic effect on the cardiovascular system. Calcium increases peripheral resistance and hypertension occurs in 20%–30% of patients with chronic hypercalcemia. Renal parenchymal damage with elevated levels of renin, increased cardiac output, and severe vasoconstriction may all participate in the development of hypertension. The most significant change in the electrocardiogram is a shortening of the QT interval. The positive inotropic effect of digitalis is enhanced by calcium, thus digitalis toxicity may be aggravated by hypercalcemia.

7. Gastrointestinal Manifestations

Anorexia, nausea, and vomiting are frequently seen in patients with hypercalcemia. Occasionally, abdominal pain, distension, and ileus may be present. There is an increased incidence of peptic ulcer in patients with primary hyperparathyroidism and it has been shown that calcium increases the release of gastrin and hydrochloric acid in the stomach. Moreover, the incidence of pancreatitis is also greatly increased. Several mechanisms have been implicated in the development of pancreatitis. Usually, hypercalcemia increases pancreatic enzyme secretion and intraductal proteins may cause obstruction of the pancreatic duct. Enhanced conversion of trypsinogen to trypsin due to elevated calcium levels may contribute to the inflammatory process.

8. Neurological and Psychiatric Effects of Hypercalcemia

Patients with hypercalcemia are frequently admitted to psychiatric wards because of nonspecific complaints characterized by lethargy, apathy, depression, and decreased memory. Patients with hypercalcemia secondary to increased parathyroid levels have electroencephalographic changes which are reversible after removal of the parathyroid adenoma. Moreover, the administration of large doses of parathyroid hormone to dogs results in increased brain calcium and changes in the electroencephalogram.

9. Metastatic Calcification

Patients with hypercalcemia may develop band keratopathy, which is the appearance of corneal calcification. The changes in the cornea are usually permanent. However, conjunctival irritation disappears after the correction of the hypercalcemia. Arterial and periarticular calcification are observed more frequently in patients who have also some degree of renal insufficiency, especially those who also have hyperphosphatemia.

C. Hypocalcemia

The clinical manifestations of hypocalcemia vary greatly among patients. Patients with chronic renal insufficiency adjust well to low levels of serum calcium and seldom become symptomatic. On the other hand, patients who suddenly become hypocalcemic, such as those with postsurgical hypoparathyroidism, may develop profound symptomatology, including tetany, even after a moderate decrease in serum calcium. Before one can correlate the pathophysiological mechanisms responsible for the hypocalcemia with the clinical symptomatology, it is critical to determine whether both total and ionized calcium are low. In conditions such as the nephrotic syndrome and cirrhosis with severe hypoalbuminemia, total serum calcium may be decreased, but ionized calcium levels may be normal or only slightly decreased and the patients remain asymptomatic.

In most patients, six general mechanisms may be responsible for the development of hypocalcemia (Table III): (1) absence of parathyroid hormone, (2) abnormalities of vitamin D metabolism or decreased magnesium levels that may make the bones resistant to the action of parathyroid hormone, (3) a genetic disorder known by the name of "pseudohypoparathyroidism" in which the target organs do not respond to the action of parathyroid hormone, (4) a decreased absorption of calcium from the GI tract, (5) translocation of calcium between different compartments of the body, and (6) increased urinary excretion of calcium.

Table III. Causes of Hypocalcemia

I. Hypocalcemia secondary to low or absent levels of PTH in blood
  A. Hypoparathyroidism
    1. Congenital
    2. Idiopathic
    3. Di-George syndrome
    4. Postsurgical
    5. Infiltration of parathyroid glands by malignancy or amyloidosis
  B. Transient hypoparathyroidism
    1. Neonatal
    2. Postsurgery for parathyroid adenoma
  C. Magnesium deficiency
II. Hypocalcemia secondary to a decrease in calcium mobilization from bone
  A. Vitamin D deficiency
    1. Decreased ingestion
    2. Decreased absorption (GI disorders)
      a. Partial gastrectomy
      b. Intestinal bypass
      c. Sprue
      d. Pancreatic insufficiency
  B. $25(OH)D_3$ deficiency
    1. Severe liver disease
      a. Biliary cirrhosis
      b. Amyloidosis
    2. Ingestion of anticonvulsant medication
    3. Nephrotic syndrome
  C. $1,25(OH)_2D_3$ deficiency
    1. Advanced renal failure
    2. Severe hyperphosphatemia
    3. Hypopathyroidism
  D. Pseudohypoparathyroidism Types I and II
  E. Magnesium deficiency
III. Hypocalcemia secondary to reduced calcium absorption in the gastrointestinal tract
  A. Deficiency in vitamin D or its metabolites
IV. Hypocalcemia secondary to translocation of calcium into different compartments
  A. Hyperphosphatemia
  B. Administration of citrate
  C. Administration of EDTA
V. Miscellaneous conditions
  A. Pancreatitis
  B. Colchicine intoxication
  C. Pharmacological dose of calcitonin
  D. Administration of mithramycin

---

1. Hypocalcemia Secondary to Low or Absent Levels of Parathyroid Hormone in Blood

A decrease or absence of parathyroid hormone will have significant effects on calcium metabolism. Since parathyroid hormone plays a key role in the regulation of osteoclasts, the cells responsible for bone resorption, the decrease in the activity or number of these cells will eventually decrease the efflux of calcium from bone. In the absence of parathyroid hormone, the capacity of the ascending portion of the loop of Henle and distal nephron to transport calcium is decreased; thus at any filtered load of calcium a greater amount of calcium will be excreted in the urine. Moreover, the absence of PTH decreases the activity of the 1α-hydroxylase in the kidney and leads to decreased formation of $1,25(OH)_2D_3$ and a fall in calcium absorption from the gastrointestinal tract. Thus, decreased mobilization of calcium from bone, excretion of larger amounts of calcium in the urine, and decreased absorption of calcium from the GI tract lead to profound hypocalcemia. The most common cause of hypoparathyroidism is excision or damage to the parathyroid glands at surgery. This may be secondary to thyroid or parathyroid surgery or to radical neck dissection performed for the treatment of cancer. It should be emphasized, however, that some patients may develop transient hypocalcemia. This phenomenon is observed in patients who have one adenoma of the parathyroid gland. The hypercalcemia produced by the excessive secretion of PTH by the adenoma usually suppresses the other glands and the removal of the adenoma may produce a transient period of hypoparathyroidism and hypocalcemia. However, the remaining glands, if they are intact, will respond to the hypocalcemia and this abnormality will be reversible in a relatively short period of time. Idiopathic hypoparathyroidism is a rare disease and tetany may occur soon after birth. Idiopathic hypoparathyroidism may be associated with the congenital absence of the thymus (Di-George syndrome). These patients have depressed cell immunity and many other malformations; they frequently have mucosal candidiasis and usually die in early childhood of severe hypocalcemia and/or severe infections. The parathyroid gland may be suppressed at birth due to maternal hypercalcemia, thus, neonatal tetany should be looked for in the presence of hypercalcemia of any cause in the mother. The fetal parathyroid glands are suppressed by maternal hypercalcemia and when the infant is stressed, for example, with a phosphate load (cow's milk), tetany may result. Another factor which plays a key role in the secretion of parathyroid hormone is magnesium. As will be discussed in a subsequent section, profound hypomagnesemia may decrease the release of parathyroid hormone. In this syndrome, the administration of magnesium with a correction of the hypomagnesemia increases the release of parathyroid hormone within minutes.

2. Hypocalcemia Secondary to Decreased Calcium Mobilization from Bone

Vitamin D has a synergistic effect with parathyroid hormone increasing the mobilization of calcium from bone. The mechanism by which vitamin D and its metabolites increase bone resorption is not fully understood. Many disorders can alter the metabolism of vitamin D and different D metabolites could be responsible for decreased mobilization of calcium from bone. In vitamin-D-deficient rickets, a nutritional condition observed in children, the lack of vitamin D is responsible for hypocalcemia, hypophosphatemia, and mild secondary hyperparathyroidism. Disorders of the gastrointestinal tract such as partial gastrectomy, intestinal bypass, tropical and nontropical sprue, and Crohn's disease may impair the absorption of vitamin D from the diet. Pathological processes which involve the liver, such as hepatobiliary cirrhosis, may decrease the production of $25(OH)D_3$. The lack of this metabolite greatly diminishes the calcification front and adults with low levels of $25(OH)D_3$ may develop osteomalacia. Although there may be an increase in the level of parathyroid hormone, the osteoclasts are unable to remove calcium since the osteoid material lacks minerals; therefore there is a decrease in the mobilization of calcium from bone. The administration of anticonvulsant medication is also characterized by low levels of $25(OH)D_3$ in serum. This may be due to an increase in microsomal activity in the liver and increased catabolism of $25(OH)D_3$. Moreover, in situations characterized by decreased renal mass (advanced renal insufficiency) or severe hyperphosphatemia, the serum levels of $1,25(OH)_2D_3$ may decrease, rendering the bone insensitive to the action of parathyroid hormone.

In patients with profound hypomagnesemia the skeleton becomes resistant to the action of parathyroid hormone and there is decreased calcium mobilization from bone. Another important condition is pseudohypoparathyroidism, which is a genetic disorder characterized by symptoms and signs of hypoparathyroidism associated with distinctive skeletal and somatic defects. The secretion of parathyroid hormone is increased as assessed by elevated levels of i-PTH; thus the hypocalcemia in pseudohypoparathyroidism is felt to represent a bone resistance to the effects of parathyroid hormone. Many patients also have renal resistance to the action of the hormone since administration of exogenous PTH does not lead to increased urinary excretion of cyclic AMP and phosphate. Recently, the syndrome has been subclassified as pseudohypoparathyroidism Type I, in which there is neither cyclic AMP nor phosphaturic response to exogenous PTH, and Type II, where there is no phosphaturic effect despite a normal response in cyclic AMP excretion to PTH. Some of these patients have low levels of $1,25(OH)_2D_3$, perhaps representing the renal resistance to PTH stimulated 1α-hydroxylase activity. Thus, the high levels of PTH and the lack of response to the exogenous administration of PTH differentiates this syndrome from true hypoparathyroidism. The hyperphosphatemia that is present in this syndrome also may be, in part, responsible for the low levels of $1,25(OH)_2D_3$. It should be emphasized that this is a heterogenous disorder. Some patients have resistance to PTH at the renal level only, others at the skeletal level, and still others exhibit resistance to PTH in both organs.

3. Hypocalcemia Secondary to Reduced Intestinal Calcium Absorption

A normal individual who ingests a low calcium diet usually does not develop hypocalcemia, or its degree is minimal since compensatory secondary hyperparathyroidism will correct the mild hypocalcemia. Usually, hypocalcemis is associated with pathological processes of the GI tract which affect the absorption of vitamin D. Under these circumstances, the low absorption of calcium plus abnormalities in vitamin D metabolism greatly affect calcium homeostasis and the patients may develop profound hypocalcemia.

4. Hypocalcemia Secondary to Translocation of Calcium into Different Compartments

Precipitation of ionized calcium is seen in disorders in which there is retention of phosphorus. Patients with advanced renal insufficiency, malignancies, or severe rhabdomyolisis and hyperphosphatemia can precipitate calcium rapidly and develop symptoms characterized by tremors, muscular irritability, and tetany. In the neonate, administration of cow's milk, which is high in phosphorus content when compared to human milk, can produce severe hyperphosphatemia and hypocalcemia. Neonatal parathyroid function is not adequate to cope with this challenge and the neonate may develop severe symptoms secondary to hypocalcemia. When large amounts of blood containing citrate are given to patients (open heart surgery, exchange transfusions for neonatal hyperbilirubinemia) the ionized calcium is complexed by citrate and hypocalcemia leading to tetany may develop.

5. Hypocalcemia Secondary to Increased Urinary Excretion of Calcium

This condition is rare and self-limited. The expansion of the extracellular fluid compartment produces a remarkable decrease in the reabsorption of sodium and calcium and large amounts of these cations can be excreted in the urine. However, these are transitory mechanisms which are rapidly corrected by the release of parathyroid hormone. Thus, if the PTH, vitamin D, and skeletal axis are intact, an increase in urinary calcium excretion should not result in significant hypocalcemia. Diuretics such as furosemide or ethacrynic acid which block the reabsorption of calcium in the thick ascending portion of the loop of Henle are effective drugs in the treatment of hypercalcemia. However, very seldom do patients ingesting these drugs develop hypocalcemia.

6. Miscellaneous Conditions

Approximately 10%–20% of patients with acute pancreatitis develop some degree of hypocalcemia. The hypocalcemia is related to deposition of calcium salts in areas of lypolysis and tissue necrosis. Some investigators have postulated that proteolytic digestion of PTH may explain the lack of elevated levels of PTH in the serum of patients with acute pancreatitis. Some drugs such as calcitonin, mithramycin (used for testicular carcinoma), and colchicine (used in gout) can produce profound hypocalcemia by decreasing bone resorption. There are a series of disorders characterized by increased bone formation in which the uptake of calcium by the skeleton is greatly increased. Such patients may develop profound hypocalcemia. A disorder known as "hungry bone syndrome" is seen in patients with chronic renal insufficiency and severe secondary hyperparathyroidism. The removal of the parathyroid glands produces profound hypocalcemia, which sometimes is difficult to correct even with pharmacological doses of $1,25(OH)_2D_3$. Under these conditions, when the factors producing bone resorption have been removed and the osteoblastic activity is greatly increased there is a remarkable increase in bone formation and the greater uptake of minerals by the skeleton may produce profound hypocalcemia.

7. Clinical Symptoms of Hypocalcemia

Patients with significant hypocalcemia have increased neuromuscular irritability. The hallmark of hypocalcemia is tetany. Latent tetany may be detected by tapping over the facial nerves resulting in a contraction of the facial muscles (Chvostek's sign) or by producing carpal spasm following occlusion of arterial blood supply to the forearm (Trousseau's sign). The symtomatology depends on the rapidity of onset of hypocalcemia. Patients with chronic renal failure occasionally have marked hypocalcemia; however, tetany is extremely rare. In part, this may be due to the presence of metabolic acidosis. However, the changes in ionized calcium produced by metabolic acidosis in the majority of patients with profound hypocalcemia is not sufficient to correct the ionized calcium back to normal. On the other hand, respiratory alkalosis due to hyperventilation (see Chapter 8) can precipitate tetany. Clinically, the patients may complain of tingling in the tips of the fingers, stiff muscles, and cramps. They may also develop convulsions or impaired mental function. Children may develop mental retardation and dementia may occur in adults. Extrapyramidal disorders also have been found in some patients. Psychiatric manifestations are characterized by confusion and hallucinations. Proximal muscle weakness is more frequently seen when the hypocalcemia is secondary to vitamin D deficiency.

Severe complications include the development of cataracts, papilledema, and rarely optic neuritis. In general, the skin may be dry and puffy and the patients may develop dermatitis. Hypocalcemia may produce hypotension and a delay in ventricular repolarization, thus increasing the QT interval and ST segment. Ventricular arrhythmias and refractoriness to digoxin in patients with atrial fibrillation have been seen in patients with hypocalcemia. As mentioned before, since calcium has an inotropic effect, hypocalcemia, can be responsible in part for a decrease in cardiac output.

II. MAGNESIUM

A. Introduction

1. General Considerations

Magnesium is the fourth most abundant cation of the body, and, after potassium, the second most abundant intracellular cation. It plays an essential role as a cofactor for a variety of enzymes, most of which utilize ATP. Magnesium increases the stimulus threshold in nerve fibers and in pharmacological doses has a curarelike action on neuromuscular function, likely inhibiting the release of acetylcholine at the neuromuscular junction. Magnesium decreases peripheral resistance and lowers blood pressure. Magnesium like calcium, plays a role in the regulation of parathyroid hormone secretion. Hypermagnesemia suppresses the release of parathyroid hormone. Acute hypomagnesemia has the opposite effect; however, profound magnesium depletion decreases the release of parathyroid hormone. *In vitro*, magnesium increases the solubility of both calcium and phosphorus.

2. Body Stores of Magnesium

Total body magnesium is approximately 2000 mEq or 25 g. Similarly to calcium, only a small fraction (about 1%) of the body magnesium is present in the ECF compartment. Approximately 60% of total body magnesium is found in bone. Most of the magnesium in bone is associated with apatite crystals. A significant amount of the magnesium in bone is present as a surface-limited ion on the bone crystal and is freely exchangeable. Approximately 20% of the total body magnesium is localized in the muscle. The remaining 20% is localized in other tissues of the body. The liver has a high magnesium content. The concentration of magnesium in blood is maintained within narrow limits and ranges between 1.5 and 1.9 mEq/liter. Approximately 75%–80% of the magnesium in serum is ultrafiltrable, the rest is protein bound. Most of the ultrafiltrable magnesium is present in the ionized form. As indicated above, magnesium is the second most abundant intracellular cation, after potassium, and its concentration in muscle is in the order of 70–80 mEq/kg of fat-free solids. Red cell magnesium concentration is approximately 5 mEq/liter.

3. Magnesium Balance

Approximately 300 mg or 25 mEq of magnesium are ingested daily in the diet. A large proportion of the magnesium in the diet is provided by the ingestion of green vegetables. A minimal magnesium intake of 0.3 mEq/kg body weight is apparently necessary to maintain magnesium balance in the average person. Of the total amount of magnesium ingested in the diet, about one third is eliminated in urine and the rest in feces. Thus, on a normal diet containing approximately 300 mg of magnesium, 30%–40% of the ingested magnesium is absorbed (Figure 5). Small amounts of magnesium, on the order of 15–30 mg/day, are secreted by the gastrointestinal tract. Many studies have shown that animals fed low magnesium diets can excrete urine that is very low in magnesium. However, the gastrointestinal tract continues to secrete small amounts of magnesium, and the animal becomes magnesium depleted. Most of the magnesium is absorbed in the upper gastrointestinal tract. Magnesium shares with calcium similar pathways for absorption in the intestine, but while most of the evidence suggests that calcium is actively absorbed from the GI tract, magnesium is absorbed mainly by ionic diffusion and "solvent drag" resulting from the bulk flow of water. There is no good evidence to indicate that magnesium is actively transported. The factors controlling the absorption of magnesium from the GI tract are not fully understood. Although there is some evidence to suggest that vitamin D may influence the absorption of magnesium, this role seems to be less important than the one played by the vitamin in the absorption of calcium. It is known that patients with severe renal insufficiency and low levels of $1,25(OH)D_3$ can develop profound hypermagnesemia by slightly increasing the amount of magnesium in the diet and without modifying the metabolites of vitamin D in serum. The sigmoid colon has the capability to absorb magnesium and there are several reports in the literature of patients who developed magnesium toxicity after receiving enemas containing magnesium; most of these patients also had renal insufficiency. The role of parathyroid hormone on magnesium absorption is not fully understood. There is evidence to suggest that PTH increases the absorption of magnesium from the gastrointestinal tract. Studies performed in everted gut sacs of the rat demonstrated that magnesium transport from the mucosal to the serosal side was a linear function of the mucosal magnesium concentration over the range of 0–30 mM. Experimental evidence in different species suggests an

Figure 5. Diagrammatic representation of magnesium metabolism in man showing the contribution of the gastrointestinal tract, the kidney, bone, and soft tissues to the magnesium pool. (Reprinted with permission from Slatopolsky, E., *et al.*, in Massry, S., Ritz, E., and Rapado A. (eds.): *Homeostasis of Phosphate and Other Minerals.* Plenum Press, New York, 1978.)

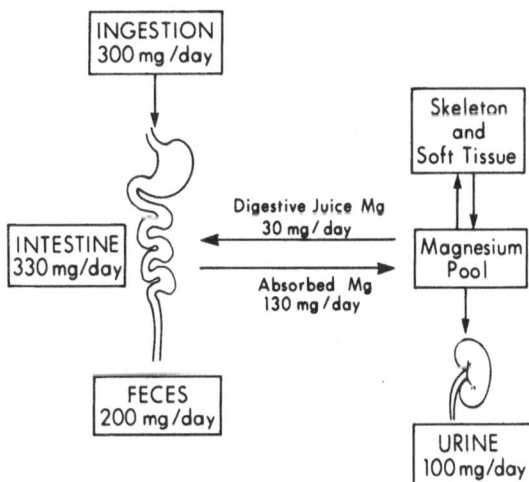

interrelationship between magnesium and calcium absorption from the GI tract. Diets high in calcium decrease the absorption of magnesium, and diets containing low magnesium increase the absorption of calcium.

4. Renal Handling of Magnesium

Approximately 2 g of magnesium are filtered daily by the kidney and about 100 mg appear in the urine. Thus, 95% of the filtered load of magnesium is reabsorbed and 5% is excreted in the urine (Figure 6). In states of magnesium deficiency the kidney can reduce the amount of magnesium excreted in the urine to less than 0.5% of the filtered load. On the other hand, during magnesium infusion or as is commonly seen in patients with far advanced renal insufficiency, the kidney can excrete 40%–70% of the filtered load of magnesium. Moreover, in some species like the rat, secretion of magnesium by the nephron has been demonstrated during the infusion of magnesium. The proximal tubule is poorly permeable to magnesium. There are some differences in the renal handling of magnesium between dogs and rats. In the dog, about 50% of the filtered magnesium is reabsorbed in the proximal tubules; in rats, probably no more than 30% is reabsorbed in this segment. In the descending limb of the loop

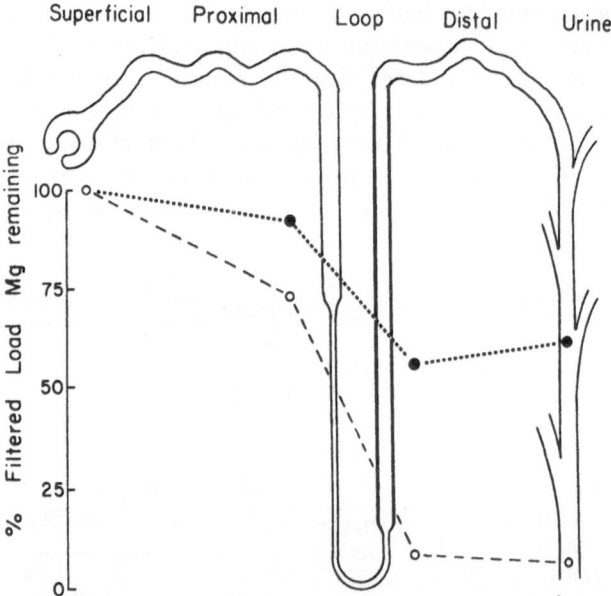

Figure 6. Schematic illustration of the fraction of ultrafiltrable magnesium remaining in different segments of the nephron in normal, hydropenic conditions (O···O) and following acute $MgCl_2$ loading (●- - -●). The results observed emphasize the importance of the thick ascending loop of Henle on Mg reabsorption. (Reprinted with permission from Dirks, J. H., and Quamme, G. A., in Massry, S., Ritz, E., and Rapado A. (eds.): *Homeostasis of Phosphate and Other Minerals.* Plenum Press, New York, 1978.)

of Henle, the magnesium concentration raises severalfold over the ultrafiltrable serum concentration owing to water removal. The thick ascending limb of the loop of Henle seems to play a critical role in the reabsorption of magnesium. The ascending limb reabsorbs 60% of the filtered load of magnesium. The permeability of the ascending limb to magnesium is quite different from that of the proximal tubule. Two mechanisms have been proposed to explain magnesium transport in the thick ascending limb of Henle's loop: (1) passive, secondary to the potential difference generated by the active transport of chloride which facilitates the entry of magnesium into the cell; and (2) active, since the chemical concentration of magnesium in the cells is higher than in the lumen and the potential gradient may not be great enough to explain the entry of magnesium into cells. Diets deficient in magnesium or the administration of parathyroid hormone enhance the reabsorption of magnesium in the thick ascending limb of Henle's loop. On the other hand, diets containing large amounts of magnesium or factors that decrease the reabsorption of sodium chloride in this portion of the nephron (ECF volume expansion, administration of diuretics such as furosemide or ethacrynic acid) also decrease the reabsorption of magnesium in this portion of the nephron. The terminal segment of the nephron (late distal tubule and collecting duct) appear to play a minor role in the reabsorption of magnesium under normal conditions. Chronic administration of mineralocorticoids increases magnesium excretion. Several interrelationships between calcium and magnesium reabsorption have been demonstrated. The administration of one of these two elements decreases the reabsorption of the other. When large amounts of magnesium are given intravenously, there is a remarkable decrease in the renal reabsorption of calcium and vice versa. Alcohol also affects the handling of magnesium by the kidney. A remarkable short-lived hypermagnesuria is seen after alcohol is given to experimental animals or humans. The intravenous administration of glucose has a similar effect.

In summary, and in contrast to calcium it seems that the thick ascending portion of Henle's loop is the most important portion of the nephron in the regulation of magnesium reabsorption. Moreover, the reabsorption of magnesium in contrast to sodium, calcium and phosphate is rather limited in the proximal tubule.

B. Hypomagnesemia

Hypomagnesemia is defined as a decrease in serum magnesium to levels below 1.5 mg/100 ml. Diseases involving the small intestine may decrease magnesium absorption and are the most common cause of hypomagnesemia (Table IV). It is difficult to predict the degree of total body magnesium deficiency by determining only serum magnesium. Since only 1% of magnesium is present in the ECF compartment, changes in intracellular magnesium and skeletal magnesium can modify the concentration of serum magnesium and one may not be able to precisely assess the degree of

Table IV. Causes of Hypomagnesemia

I. Decreased intestinal absorption
   A. Severe diarrhea
   B. Intestinal bypass
   C. Surgical resection
   D. Tropical and nontropical sprue
   E. Celiac disease
   F. Invasive and infiltrative process: lymphomas
   G. Prolonged gastrointestinal suction
II. Decreased intake
   A. Starvation
   B. Protein–calorie malnutrition
   C. Chronic alcoholism
   D. Prolonged therapy with IV fluids lacking magnesium
III. Excessive urinary losses
   A. Diuretic phase of ATN
   B. Postobstructive diuresis
   C. Diuretic therapy
   D. Diabetic ketoacidosis (during treatment)
   E. Chronic alcoholism
   F. Hypercalcemic states
   G. Primary aldosteronism
   H. Inappropriate antidiuretic hormone secretion
   I. Gentamicin toxicity
   J. Idiopathic renal magnesium wasting

---

magnesium deficiency by determining serum magnesium. Probably the determination of skeletal or muscle magnesium may provide a better index of magnesium deficiency. However, the determinations are not practical in clinical medicine. In patients with magnesium deficiency, the administration of 50–100 mEq magnesium per day usually corrects the hypomagnesemia after a short period of time. Magnesium depletion can also produce changes in other electrolytes. Usually, there is an increase in potassium excretion in the urine and patients may develop hypokalemia. However, the most important manifestation of hypomagnesemia is the development of hypo-calcemia and tetany. Experimental animals fed a low magnesium diet develop profound hypocalcemia. Patients with hypomagnesemia also develop hypo-calcemia. The pathogenesis of hypocalcemia in magnesium depletion is multifactorial. Hypomagnesemia has profound effects on parathyroid hor-mone metabolism and bone physiology. It would seem that neither the biosynthesis nor the conversion of proparathyroid hormone to parathyroid hormone is greatly affected by the concentration of magnesium. However, the release of parathyroid hormone is influenced by the serum magnesium concentration. Several investigators have demonstrated that the administra-tion of magnesium, to patients with severe hypomagnesemia who have low levels of i-PTH in serum, increases the release of PTH a few minutes after magnesium administration. Also, there is evidence to indicate that during hypomagnesemia, the skeleton is resistant to the action of parathyroid hormone, and in general the administration of mildly pharmacological doses of parathyroid hormone does not elicit a normal calcemic response in patients with magnesium depletion. Recent studies have further clarified this abnormality. The uptake of parathyroid hormone by bones obtained from dogs with experimental magnesium depletion was greatly diminished, and the release of cyclic AMP by bone was also blunted in hypomagnesemia. It seems that the ionic exchange from the hydration shell of bone between calcium and magnesium also is decreased; thus, on a physicochemical basis, less calcium is mobilized from bone in hypomagnesemia. Thus, the decrease in the release of parathyroid hormone, the low uptake of parathyroid hormone by bone, and the decreased heteroionic exchange of calcium for magnesium at the bone, are all pathogenetic factors responsible for the hypocalcemia observed in patients with profound magnesium depletion.

1. Clinical Manifestation of Hypomagnesemia

Patients with severe hypomagnesemia usually develop some degree of mental confusion, anorexia, and vomiting. In general, there is increased neuromuscular irritability; thus tremors and seizures are signs usually observed in these patients. Muscle fasciculation and positive Trousseau's and Chvostek's signs can be observed. Most of these patients also have profound hypocalcemia and sometimes it is difficult to determine if the symptoms are due to magnesium deficiency per se or the concommitant hypocalcemia. Other neurological manifestations may include vertigo, ataxia, nystagmus, and dysarthria. Changes in personality, depression, and sometimes hallucinations and psychosis also have been observed. Nodal or sinus tachycardia and premature atrial or ventricular contractions may occur. The electrocardiogram may show prolongation of the QT interval and broadening and flattening or even inversion of the T waves. Magnesium deficiency potentiates the action of digoxin and there is an enhanced sensitivity in magnesium deficiency to the toxic effects of digitalis. Since magnesium plays a key role in regulating the activity of Na–K-ATPase, the enzyme responsible for the maintenance of intracellular potassium concentration, severe alterations in skeletal muscle and myocardium function are observed. Sometimes it is difficult to interpret if the changes in the electrocardiogram are related to magnesium or potassium depletion. Patients also may show some degree of hypophosphatemia. In the rat, it has been shown that magnesium deficiency promotes renal phosphate excretion.

2. Mechanisms Responsible for the Development of Hypomagnesemia

From the pathogenetic point of view, three main mechanisms are responsible for the development of hypomagnesemia (Table IV): (1) decreased intestinal absorption, (2) decreased intake, and (3) excessive urinary losses.

a. Hypomagnesemia Secondary to Decreased Intestinal Absorption of Magnesium

By far, the most common causes responsible for the development of hypomagnesemia are pathological entities affecting the small bowel. In these conditions, the kidney adapts to the hypomagnesemia and decreases the urinary excretion of magnesium. However, the amount of magnesium in the stools does not decrease appropriately (probably the secretion of magnesium is not greatly reduced) and the patient develops hypomagnesemia. Pathological processes such as celiac disease, tropical and nontropical sprue, malignancies (characteristically lymphoma), surgical resection, intestinal bypass, and profound diarrhea have all been described as being responsible for the development of hypomagnesemia. In the past ten years, when the number of surgical bypass procedures was greatly increased for the treatment of obesity, it was noted that many of these patients developed profound hypomagnesemia and tetany. Hypomagnesemia is especially prominant in patients with idiopathic steatorrhea and diseases affecting the terminal ileum.

b. Hypomagnesemia Secondary to Decreased Magnesium Intake

Magnesium depletion has been described in children with protein-calorie malnutrition. The hypomagnesemia results from a combination of decreased intake and gastrointestinal losses due to diarrhea, often times severe vomiting. In a hospital setting, perhaps, the most common reason for the development of hypomagnesemia is prolonged therapy with intravenous fluids lacking magnesium. Often, if surgical patients require intestinal suction, they are fed with intravenous fluid, sometimes for several weeks, and seldom is magnesium given to these patients. The chronic administration of alcohol produces hypomagnesemia. The mechanisms are multifactorial. Usually chronic alcoholics ingest diets poor in magnesium, but there is also an increase in the urinary excretion of magnesium. From the point of view of differential diagnosis, the clinical history, evidence of malnutrition, the presence of diarrhea and vomiting, or a history of surgery may help to differentiate individuals with decreased absorption of magnesium due either to a primary gastrointestinal disease or decreased intake from individuals with increased urinary excretion of magnesium. As mentioned above, when there is decreased intake or absorption of magnesium from the gastrointestinal tract, the amount of magnesium excreted in the urine is greatly reduced, on the order of 10–15 mg/day.

c. Hypomagnesemia Secondary to Increased Urinary Losses of Magnesium

Since 60%–70% of the magnesium is absorbed in the thick ascending limb of Henle's loop, any factor that blocks the reabsorption of sodium chloride in this part of the nephron will also promote the urinary excretion of magnesium. In conditions in which the ECF volume is increased, or entities characterized by profound diuresis (diuretic phase of acute tubular necrosis, postobstructive diuresis), the patients may excrete 20%–30% of the filtered load of magnesium and develop profound hypomagnesemia. The administration of large amounts of diuretics such as ethacrynic acid or furosemide has a significant effect on renal magnesium excretion. Patients with ketoacidosis may develop hypomagnesemia. Serum magnesium as well as phosphorus and potassium concentrations may be elevated during periods of ketoacidosis; however, the levels usually fall after the administration of insulin and fluid replacement. Increased excretion of magnesium has been seen after the treatment of ketoacidosis. Metabolic conditions characterized by an excess of mineralocorticoids such as primary aldosteronism, or an increase of ADH, such as entities characterized by inappropriate secretion of ADH (see Chapter 6), are also accompanied by hypomagnesemia secondary to increased excretion of magnesium in the urine. Recently, a specific defect has been described in a few patients receiving gentamycin or cis-platinum (an antitumoral agent). The usual lesion produced by gentamycin is acute tubular necrosis, renal insufficiency, and hypermagnesemia; however, several patients have developed a specific tubular defect characterized by profound hypermagnesuria and hypomagnesemia that may persist for several weeks after the drug is discontinued.

C. Hypermagnesemia

By far the most common cause of hypermagnesemia is chronic renal insufficiency (Table V). The kidney can excrete large amounts of magnesium in the urine. Thus, in patients with normal renal function hypermagnesemia develops very seldom, even if the patient ingests large amounts of magnesium such as drugs like antacids containing magnesium or laxatives such as milk of magnesia. It should be emphasized, however, that hypermagnesemia is a late manifestation of renal insufficiency and seldom does hypermagnesemia occur in patients with GFR values greater than 15 ml/min. Mild hypermagnesemia may be seen in patients with GFR values of approximately 10 ml/min. However, moderate hypermagnesemia is usually seen in patients with GFR values of less than 5 ml/min. As renal insufficiency progresses, there is a significant increase in the fractional excretion of magnesium in the urine. Patients with a GFR of 120 ml/min excrete approximately 5% of the filtered

Table V. Causes of Hypermagnesemia

I. Decreased renal excretion
   A. Acute renal failure
   B. Chronic renal disease
   C. Adrenocortical insufficiency
II. Increased entrance into ECF
   A. Laxatives containing magnesium ⎫
   B. Antacids containing magnesium ⎬ Usually seen in patients with renal failure
   C. Enemas containing magnesium ⎭
   D. Intravenous fluids containing magnesium
   E. Intramuscular administration of magnesium (eclampsia)

load of magnesium. However, patients with far advanced renal failure (GFR less than 10 ml/min) can excrete up to 40%–70% of the filtered load of magnesium. Thus, patients with chronic renal failure may not be able to further increase magnesium excretion after ingestion of large amounts of magnesium since they may already be excreting 40%–70% of the filtered load. Therefore, if magnesium ingestion is increased (administration of laxatives or antacids containing magnesium) in patients with advanced renal failure, profound hypermagnesemia and death may occur. In obstetric wards, magnesium is still being used for the treatment of eclampsia. Some of these patients have a decrease in GFR and the administration of large amounts of magnesium sulfate may result in hypermagnesemia. Moreover, some of the magnesium may enter the fetus, increasing the concentration of magnesium in the newborn. Although most of the magnesium is absorbed in the small intestine, the sigmoid colon can also absorb magnesium. Several reports have described cases of severe hypermagnesemia after administration of enemas containing magnesium.

1. Symptoms and Signs of Hypermagnesemia

Profound hypermagnesemia blocks neuromuscular transmission and depresses the conduction system of the heart. It would seem that the neuromuscular effects of magnesium are antagonized by the administration of calcium. Mild hypermagnesemia is well tolerated. However, if serum magnesium levels increase to 5–6 mg/100 ml, there may be a decrease in tendon reflexes and some degree of mental confusion. If the serum magnesium increases to 7–9 mg/100 ml, there is a decrease in the respiratory rate and a fall in blood pressure. If serum magnesium levels increase to about 10–13 mg/100 ml there is usually profound hypotension and severe mental depression. When the levels increase further to about 15 mg/100 ml, death may occur. In uremic patients, the adverse effect of hypermagnesemia may be worsened by the presence of hypocalcemia. Acute hypermagnesemia can also produce mild hypocalcemia. This may be due to (1) suppression of the release of parathyroid hormone and (2) competition for tubular reabsorption between calcium and magnesium leading to decreased calcium reabsorption and hypercalciuria which aggravates the hypocalcemia produced by decreased release of parathyroid hormone. In chronic renal insufficiency, there is probably an increase in red cell magnesium and muscle magnesium, but the results are controversial. The amount of magnesium in bone is apparently increased in both cortical and trabecular bone. If the patient develops hypermagnesemia at GFR values greater than 10 ml/min, ECF volume expansion with saline, the administration of furosemide, and the addition of calcium will promptly correct the symptoms of hypermagnesemia. On the other hand, if the GFR is very low, the only practical means of correcting the hypermagnesemia is hemodialysis.

III. PHOSPHATE

A. Introduction

1. General Considerations

The term *phosphate* in this section refers to inorganic phosphorus. Its concentration in serum is maintained between 3.5 and 4.5 mg/100 ml or 1.12 and 1.45 mmoles/liter. Serum phosphate concentrations may exhibit daily variations of as much as 50%. Serum phosphate has a diurnal variation of 0.6–1 mg/100 ml, with the nadir occurring between 8 AM and 11 AM. Carbohydrate ingestion decreases serum phosphate concentration as a result of internal redistribution. In the ECF, phosphate is present mainly in the inorganic form. In serum, phosphate exists mostly as the free ion and only a small fraction, less than 15%, is protein bound. Approximately 85% of the phosphate is present in the skeleton. The rest is widely distributed throughout the body in the form of organic phosphate compounds. Phosphate plays a key role in many aspects of cellular metabolism. It influences the oxygen-carrying capacity of hemoglobin through its regulation of 2,3 DPG synthesis. Phosphate is an important constituent of cell membrane phospholipids. It may influence many metabolic pathways such as ammoniagenesis, glycolysis, and the activation of the 25-hydroxy-vitamin D 1-hydroxylase. Inorganic phosphate can enter the organic phosphate pool by different mechanisms. During oxidative phosphorylation, mitochondrial inorganic phosphate is used directly to form ATP from ADP. During glycogenolysis, inorganic phosphate reacts directly with glycogen to form glucose 1-phosphate, and finally during glycolysis, glyceraldahyde 3-phosphate combines with cytoplasmic inorganic phosphate to form 1,3-diphosphoglycerate, which reacts with ADP to form ATP and 3-phosphoglycerate (see Chapter 3).

2. Phosphate Absorption

On an average diet, 1 g of phosphorus is ingested daily of which approximately 70% is absorbed and the remainder is excreted in the stool (Figure 7). Absorption of phosphate occurs throughout the small intestine but transport is greater in the jejunum than in the duodenum with minimal absorption occurring in the ileum. The movement of phosphate across the intestinal epithelium occurs by two mechanisms, active transport and diffusion between cells through the paracellular "shunt" pathway. Recent studies of phosphate accumulation by rat intestinal brush border vesicles demonstrated that, at physiological pH, phosphate uptake was dependent on luminal sodium but was unaffected by the transmembrane potential, a finding which is consistent with an electroneutral cotransport of sodium and monovalent phosphate (H_2PO_4); at lower pH values (6.0) the accelerated uptake was independent of intraluminal sodium concentration and appeared to involve

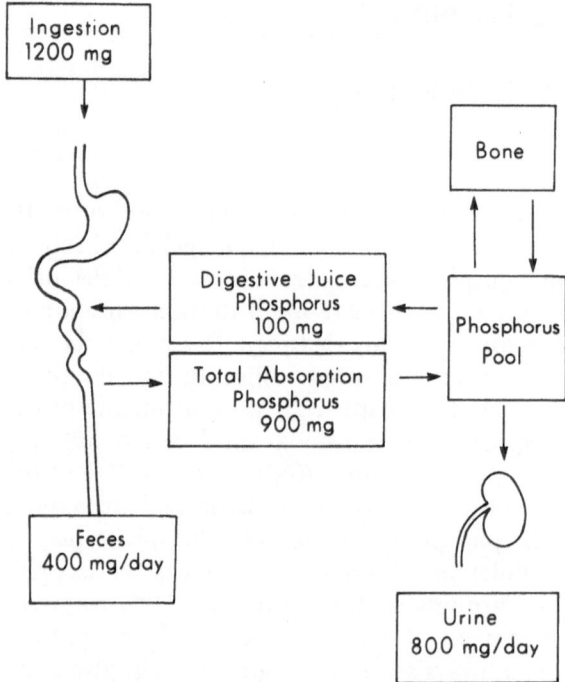

Figure 7. Diagrammatic representation of phosphorus metabolism in man, showing the contribution of the gastrointestinal tract, bone, and kidney to the maintenance of the phosphorus pool.

transfer of net negative charge. Vitamin D seems to stimulate phosphate absorption by two mechanisms: a calcium-dependent duodenal process and a calcium-independent jejunal system. The metabolite responsible for the stimulation of phosphate transport appears to be 1,25-dihydroxy D_3, which increases both calcium and phosphate transport in D-deficient rats within

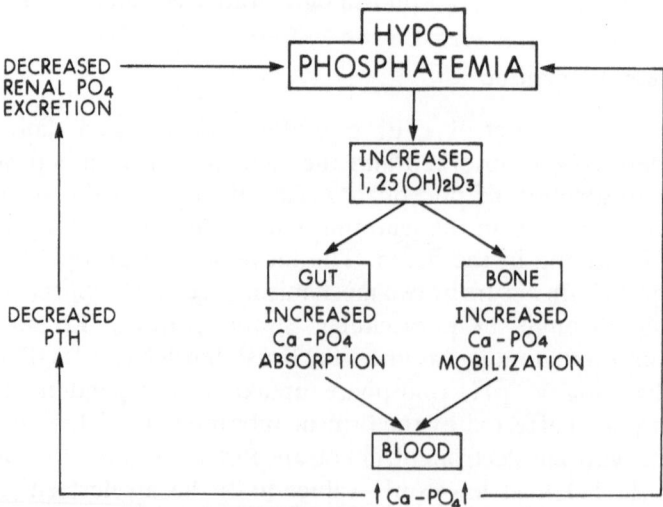

Figure 8. Illustration of the adaptative mechanisms observed during a low phosphate intake (hypophosphatemia). See text for a more detailed description.

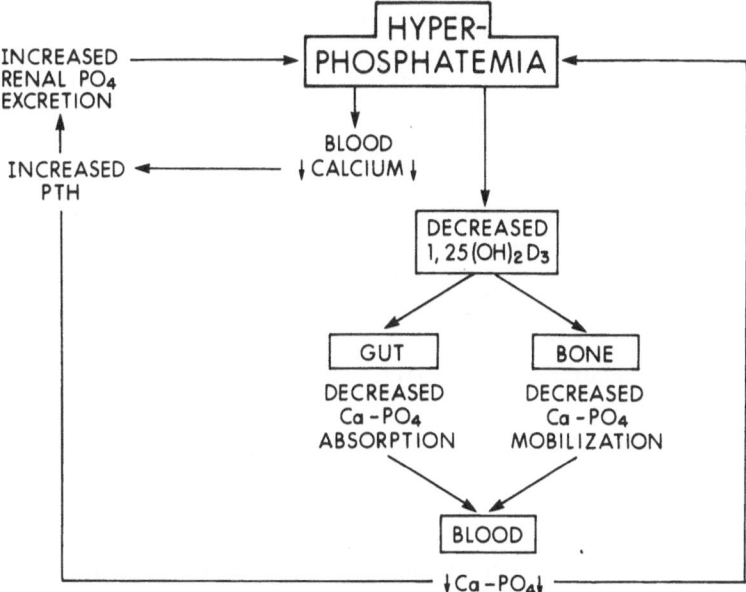

Figure 9. Illustration of the adaptative mechanisms observed during a high phosphate intake (hyperphosphatemia). See text for a more detailed description.

three to six hours of administration. In the rat, the major effect of $1,25(OH)_2D_3$ on phosphate absorption appears to involve increased active transport. The effects of parathyroid hormone and calcitonin on phosphate transport in the gut are controversial. Increased absorption of phosphate in response to PTH and calcitonin has been reported, but these results have not been confirmed by other investigators. The amount of phosphate ingested in the diet plays a key role in the overall phosphate balance. In animals fed a low phosphorus diet, the production of $1,25(OH)_2D_3$ increases and, the efficiency of the intestine to absorb calcium and phosphate is greatly enhanced. The mild hypercalcemia that develops suppresses the release of parathyroid hormone and renal conservation of phosphorus occurs (Figure 8). On the other hand, in animals fed a high phosphate diet, the production of $1,25(OH)_2D_3$ decreases resulting in a fall in calcium and phosphate absorption from the intestine and mobilization from bone. Moreover, the development of hypocalcemia (due to a decreased calcium absorption and hyperphosphatemia) will enhance the release of parathyroid hormone, which will promote urinary phosphate excretion and reestablish phosphate balance (Figure 9).

3. Renal Handling of Phosphate

Approximately 10%–15% of plasma phosphate is bound to proteins. However, when the Donnan factor for inorganic phosphorus across membranes (1.09) and the water content of plasma are considered, the ratio of ultrafiltrable phosphate to total plasma phosphate is not far from unity, approximately 95%–98%. Thus, virtually all the unbound inorganic phosphate in plasma water is ultrafiltrable at the glomerulus. Approximately 7 g, of phosphate are filtered daily by the kidney, of which 80%–90% is reabsorbed by the renal tubule and the remainder excreted in the urine (about 700 mg on a 1-g phosphorus diet). About 60%–70% of the filtered phosphate is reabsorbed in the proximal tubule. However, there is also evidence to indicate that significant amounts of phosphate are reabsorbed in the distal tubule (Figure 10). Although renal secretion of phosphate has been demonstrated in certain animals (amphibians, birds), the results obtained in mammals are controversial. Even if renal phosphate secretion occurs in mammals, this mechanism seems to play a minor role in the overall regulation of phosphate balance. As serum phosphate and the filtered load of phosphate increases, the capacity to reabsorb phosphate increases. However, a maximum rate of transport (T_m) for phosphate reabsorption is obtained usually at serum phosphate concentrations of 6 mg/100 ml. There is a direct correlation between T_m phosphate values and GFR even when the latter is varied over a broad range. Parathyroid hormone, volume expansion, or the administration of glucose all decrease phosphate reabsorption. Apparently, two independent mechanisms are responsible for the reabsorption of phosphate in the proximal tubule. In the early portion of the proximal tubule where only 10%–15% of filtered sodium and fluid is reabsorbed, the ratio of the tubular fluid phosphate to plasma ultrafiltrable phosphate has already fallen

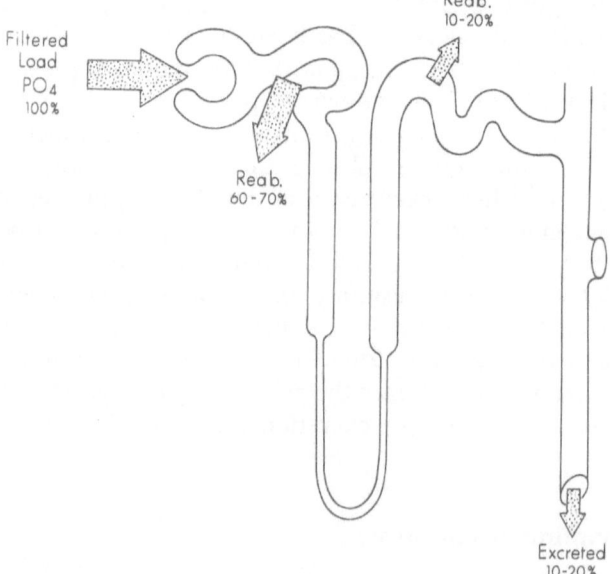

Figure 10. Schematic illustration of the relative amounts of phosphate reabsorbed by different segments of the nephron. Urinary excretion of phosphorus varies normally from 10% to 20%.

significantly to values of approximately 0.6. Thus, the early portion of the proximal tubule accounts for approximately 50% of the total amount of phosphate reabsorbed in this segment. In late segments of the proximal tubule, the reabsorption of phosphate is mainly dependent on the movement of salt and water. Thus, in the remaining 80% of the pars convoluta, the (TF/UF) phosphate ratio remains at a value of 0.6–0.7, while fluid reabsorption increases to approximately 60%–70% of the filtered load. Thus, in the last two thirds of the proximal tubule, phosphate reabsorption parallels and is directly proportional to sodium and fluid reabsorption. A significant amount of phosphate, perhaps on the order of 20%–30%, is reabsorbed beyond the portion of the proximal tubule accessible to micropuncture (in the pars recta, loop of Henle, and/or early distal tubule). Parathyroid hormone seems to play an important role in phosphate reabsorption in this segment of the nephron and several investigators have demonstrated the presence of parathyroid hormone stimulated adenylate cyclase activity. Controversy exists as to the role of the collecting duct in phosphate reabsorption and secretion. Studies performed in rats receiving intravenous phosphate have shown that the amount of phosphate appearing in the urine is greater than can be accounted for by the amount leaving the late distal tubule. Thus, phosphate may have been added at the level of the collecting duct, or alternatively, there may be differences in the transport of phosphate between superficial and deep nephrons. When a larger amount of phosphate appears in the urine than leaves the distal tubule of surface nephrons, it is difficult to ascertain if there is addition of phosphate by a secretory mechanism in the collecting duct or there is a greater delivery of phosphate into the collecting duct by the distal tubules of the deep nephrons. Numerous factors affect the reabsorption of phosphate by the nephron. Perhaps, the most important one is the amount of phosphate ingested in the diet. In individuals ingesting a very low phosphate diet, the tubular reabsorption of phosphate approaches 100% and a very small amount of phosphate appears in the urine. On the other hand, if a patient increases the amount of dietary phosphate to 2–3 g, 60%–70% of this amount will be excreted in the urine. By a series of complicated feedback mechanisms, when the amount of phosphate entering the body is increased, changes in ionized calcium increase the release of parathyroid hormone. Parathyroid hormone plays a key role in the regulation of phosphate in different segments of the nephron. This peptide binds to receptors at the contraluminal side of the proximal tubule and activates the adenylate cyclase system, cyclic AMP increases, and phosphate reabsorption is decreased. Moreover, this action is also seen in the distal portion of the nephron. Thus, in the presence of an excess of parathyroid hormone, phosphate excretion can increase from roughly 10% to 30%. The T_m for phosphate is also greatly diminished. On the other hand, in the absence of parathyroid hormone, the capacity of the nephron to reabsorb phosphate is greatly enhanced. Patients who lack parathyroid hormone, hypoparathyroidism, have an increased reabsorptive capacity for phosphate, therefore they develop hyperphosphatemia. Volume expansion of the ECF can decrease the reabsorption of phosphate. However, the phosphaturia of volume expansion is blunted by the previous removal of the parathyroid glands. During volume expansion, proximal phosphate reabsorption is greatly diminished independently of the presence or absence of parathyroid hormone. However, during volume expansion, in the presence of parathyroid hormone, the phosphate delivered from the proximal tubule is not reabsorbed in the distal tubule and is excreted in the urine; hence the marked phosphaturia. Volume expansion leads to a similar decrease in phosphate reabsorption in the proximal tubule in the absence of parathyroid glands. However, in the absence of the hormone, the excess phosphate delivered from the proximal tubule is reabsorbed in the distal tubule, and the phosphaturia is markedly blunted. Acidosis produces a remarkable phosphaturia. The mechanism is complex since profound acidosis mobilizes calcium and phosphate from bone, and decreases phosphate reabsorption by the nephron. Metabolic alkalosis also promotes phosphaturia. It was suggested initially that alkalinization of the urine decreases the reabsorption of phosphate. However, recent studies suggest that the phosphaturia observed after administration of sodium bicarbonate is due mainly to changes in serum pH with a decrease in ionized calcium and release of parathyroid hormone and to ECF volume expansion produced by the administration of sodium bicarbonate. Other hormones, besides PTH, also have been implicated in the regulation of phosphate reabsorption by the nephron. Calcitonin and glucocorticoids appear to decrease the amount of phosphate reabsorbed; on the other hand, growth hormone increases phosphate reabsorption. The exact role of these three hormones in the day-to-day regulation of phosphate is unknown. The role of vitamin D and its metabolites on phosphate reabsorption by the kidney is controversial, since different results have been obtained. It would seem that in general vitamin D tends to increase phosphate reabsorption. Further studies are needed to establish firmly such an effect. Another factor which may influence the reabsorption of phosphate is the concentration of calcium in the ECF. Again, the results reported are controversial. In normal animals or man, the administration of calcium increases phosphate reabsorption mainly by the suppression of parathyroid hormone. Different results, however, have been obtained in parathyroidectomized animals. In some circumstances, calcium administration has increased and in others decreased the renal reabsorption of phosphate. Also, the degree of hypercalcemia may be important. Mild hypercalcemia seems to increase phosphate reabsorption. However, profound severe hypercalcemia may not have the same effect since changes in GFR and renal plasma flow may complicate the interpretation of the results obtained. Glucose plays a role in the renal phosphate reabsorption. Luminal addition of increasing concentrations of glucose to the isolated perfused nephron decreases phosphate transport. Thus, patients with diabetes and severe hyperglycemia may excrete increased amounts of phosphate in the urine.

B. Hyperphosphatemia

Hyperphosphatemia (a serum phosphate concentration greater than 5 mg/100 ml in adults) is seen frequently in clinical medicine. By far, the most common cause of hyperphosphatemia is decreased phosphate excretion in the urine secondary to renal failure. However, hyperphosphatemia can be the consequence of increased intake of phosphate or increased entry of phosphate, from tissue breakdown, into the ECF. The causes of hyperphosphatemia are listed in Table VI.

1. Decreased Renal Excretion of Phosphate

a. Renal Insufficiency

In chronic renal insufficiency, phosphate balance is maintained by a progressive increase in phosphate excretion by the remaining nephrons. (see Chapter 14). The phosphaturia per nephron seen in renal insufficiency is part of an adaptive process responsible for the maintenance of phosphate homeostasis, and severe hyperphosphatemia is seen only in patients with advanced chronic renal failure, usually when the glomerular filtration rate is less than 25 ml/min. A normal person with a glomerular filtration rate of

Table VI. Causes of Hyperphosphatemia

I. Decreased renal excretion of phosphate
    A. Renal insufficiency
        1. Chronic
        2. Acute
    B. Hypothyroidism
    C. Pseudohypoparathyroidism
        1. Type I
        2. Type II
    D. Abnormal circulating PTH
    E. Acromegaly
    F. Tumoral calcinosis
    G. Diphosphonates
II. Increase in phosphate entrance to ECF
    A. Neoplastic diseases
        1. Leukemia
        2. Lymphoma
    B. Increased catabolism
    C. Respiratory acidosis
III. Administration of PO_4 Salts or vitamin D
    A. Pharmacological administration of vitamin D metabolites
    B. Ingestion and/or administration of phosphate salts
IV. Miscellaneous
    A. Cortical hyperostosis
    B. Intermittent hyperphosphatemia
    C. Artifacts

---

120 ml/min excretes 5%–15% of the filtered load of phosphate. However, as the number of nephrons decreases, fractional excretion of phosphate can increase to 60%–80% of the filtered load. This phosphaturia per nephron plays a key role in the maintenance of phosphate balance in renal insufficiency. However, when the number of nephrons is greatly diminished and if the intake of phosphate in the diet remains constant, phosphate balance can no longer be maintained and hyperphosphatemia develops. The filtered load of phosphate per nephron, therefore, will increase, phosphate excretion also will rise, and phosphate balance will be reestablished (Figure 11). Hyperphosphatemia is a usual finding in patients with acute renal insufficiency. The degree of hyperphosphatemia varies among patients; however, it is significant in those patients with renal insufficiency secondary to severe trauma or nontraumatic rhabdomyolysis (as in patients ingesting large amounts of alcohol or in heroin addicts). In patients with acute renal failure,

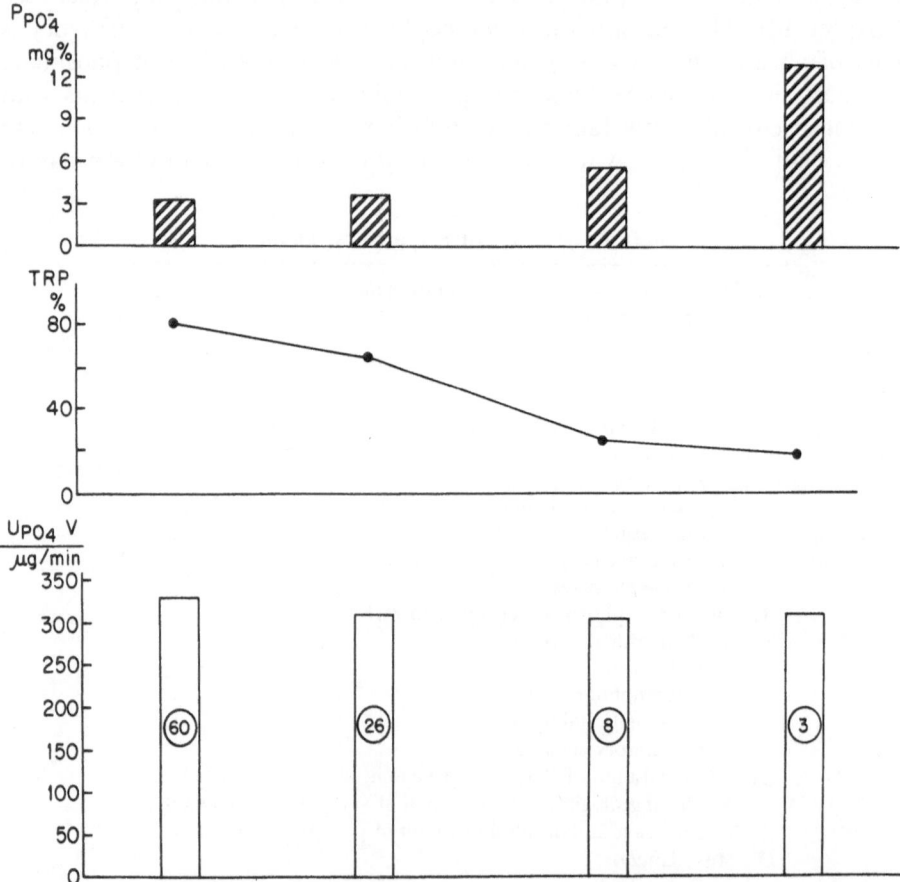

Figure 11. Plasma phosphate ($P_{PO_4^-}$), tubular reabsorption of phosphate (TRP) and phosphate excretion ($U_{PO_4}V$) in a group of four patients with a range of values for glomerular filtration rate from 60 to 3 ml/min while they were on a controlled phosphate intake (650 ± 50 mg/day). (Reprinted with permission from Slatopolsky, E., *et al.*, *J. Clin. Invest.* 47:1865, 1968.)

the hyperphosphatemia is transient, and in most patients serum phosphate returns to normal as the renal function recovers.

b. Hypoparathyroidism

Regardless of its etiology, hypoparathyroidism is characterized by low or absent levels of parathyroid hormone, low serum calcium, and hyperphosphatemia. Since parathyroid hormone normally inhibits the renal reabsorption of phosphate, the absence of this hormone leads to an elevation in the T_m for phosphate and the patients develop hyperphosphatemia (serum phosphate in the range of 6–8 mg/100 ml). Even in the absence of parathyroid hormone, when the serum phosphate is elevated to the levels mentioned above, the kidney can reestablish balance and phosphate homeostasis is maintained; however, the patients characteristically have hyperphosphatemia.

c. Pseudohypoparathyroidism

In this condition, there is organ resistance to the action of parathyroid hormone. Although the serum levels of parathyroid hormone may be elevated, the response of the renal epithelial cells to the phosphaturic effect of parathyroid hormone is abnormal; thus a greater amount of phosphate is reabsorbed, and the patients characteristically develop hyperphosphatemia. Other features of this syndrome are discussed in the section on calcium.

d. Abnormal Circulating Parathyroid Hormone

This syndrome, described recently, is characterized by hyperphosphatemia, hypocalcemia, chronic tetany, and cataracts. These manifestations are similar to those observed in patients with hypoparathyroidism. However, the patients have normal or high serum levels of parathyroid hormone, they do not have the features of pseudohypoparathyroidism, and the kidney responds to the administration of PTH with an increase in excretion of cyclic AMP and phosphate. The presence of an abnormal endogenous parathyroid hormone has been postulated, but this explanation has not been substantiated.

e. Acromegaly

Growth hormone decreases urinary phosphate excretion and increases the T_m for phosphate. The hypersecretion of growth hormone may lead to the development of gigantism if the increased secretion occurs prior to the closure of the epiphisis or to acromegaly if the excessive secretion occurs after puberty. Hyperphosphatemia has been observed in many patients with acromegaly. It is known that serum phosphate concentrations in children are higher (5–8 mg/100 ml) than in adults. This may be due, in part, to increased circulating levels of growth hormone in children. However, it is now known at present whether or not the hyperphosphatemia of childhood is related to increased levels of growth hormone alone or to other factors.

f. Tumoral Calcinosis

This condition, seen more frequently in young blacks, is usually characterized by hyperphosphatemia, ectopical calcification around large joints, normal levels of parathyroid hormone, and normal response to the administration of exogenous parathyroid hormone. Sometimes the masses of calcium are the size of an orange, overlying hips, elbows and shoulders. Likely, the extensive calcification of soft tissues seen in this condition is due to an elevated calcium–phosphate product. The pathogenesis of this disease is probably related to a primary increase in tubular phosphate reabsorption. Of interest is the fact that despite hyperphosphatemia, these patients do not develop high serum levels of parathyroid hormone. This may be due to the fact that the levels of 1,25-dihydroxy D_3 are normal in these patients, despite hyperphosphatemia, and to increased reabsorption of calcium by the kidney. The combination of a normal gastrointestinal calcium absorption and decreased urinary calcium excretion may serve to maintain a normal serum calcium and prevent the development of secondary hyperparathyroidism.

g. Diphosphonates

Hyperphosphatemia may occur during the administration of disodium etridronate (EHDP), a drug of the diphosphonate class, which reduces bone turnover and is used in the treatment of Paget's disease. The mechanism by which diphosphonate increases serum phosphorus is complex and may involve alterations in phosphate redistribution between different cellular compartments and a decrease in renal phosphate excretion. It seems that the levels of circulating PTH and the urinary excretion of cyclic AMP after PTH administration are normal during therapy with diphosphonates.

2. Redistribution of Phosphate between Intracellular and Extracellular Pools

a. Neoplastic Diseases

Hyperphosphatemia has been described in patients with malignant disorders. Patients receiving treatment for lymphoblastic leukemia may develop an increase in serum phosphate with a concomitant decrease in serum calcium. The phosphate load originates primarily from the destruction of lymphoblasts, which have four times the amount of organic and inorganic phosphorus present in mature lymphocytes. Similar findings have been described in Burkitt's lymphoma. This tumor is characterized by very rapid growth, which makes it very sensitive to chemotherapy. Thus, a remarkable lysis of malignant cells can occur during treatment. Other biochemical alterations include hyperuricemia, hyperkalemia, hyperphosphatemia, and hypocalcemia. Some of the patients have serum phosphate elevations in the range of 20–30 mg/100 ml which may contribute to the development of renal insufficiency due to calcium deposition in the kidney and other tissues.

b. Increased Catabolism

Several conditions characterized by increased protein breakdown (severe tissue of muscle damage, severe infections) are sometimes accompanied by hyperphosphatemia. Although the hyperphosphatemia may be due simply to a translocation of intracellular phosphate into the extracellular space other factors seem to play a role. Hyperphosphatemia has been described in patients with ketoacidosis prior to treatment. After IV fluids and insulin therapy the entrance of glucose into the cells is usually followed by movement of phosphate back into the intracellular space and some of the patients now may develop hypophosphatemia. Thus, the combination of dehydration, acidosis, and tissue breakdown in different catabolic states may lead to hyperphosphatemia.

c. Respiratory Acidosis

Acute rises in P_{CO_2} in experimental animals lead to an increase in serum phosphate. In chronic respiratory acidosis, the degree of hyperphosphatemia, if any, is extremely small since there is renal compensation and phosphate balance is maintained.

3. Administration of Phosphate Salts or Vitamin D

a. Pharmacological Administration of Vitamin D Metabolites

The active metabolite of vitamin D_3 1,25(OH)$_2$D$_3$ increases phosphate transport from the gastrointestinal tract. A rise in serum phosphate has been observed in uremic patients receiving metabolites of vitamin D. If these drugs are used in patients with reduced GFR, they may increase the concentration of both calcium and phosphate in blood and deposition of calcium in the kidney may lead to further deterioration of renal function. Physicians should be aware that D and its metabolites can produce hyperphosphatemia and obviously they should not be used in the presence of hypercalcemia because of the risks mentioned above.

b. Ingestion and/or Administration of Phosphate Salts

When the newborn is fed cow's milk (which is higher in phosphate content than human milk), hyperphosphatemia may develop. This may be an important factor in the genesis of neonatal tetany. Hyperphosphatemia has been observed in adults ingesting laxatives containing phosphate salts, or after administration of enemas containing large amounts of phosphate. Intravenous phosphate administration has been used in the treatment of hypercalcemia of malignancy. The administration of 1–2 g of phosphate intravenously decreases the concentration of serum calcium. Unfortunately, the severe hyperphosphatemia induced by the administration of large amounts of phosphate intravenously may lead to calcium precipitation in important organs such as the heart and kidney, and several deaths have been reported as a consequence of this form of therapy.

4. Clinical Manifestations of Hyperphosphatemia

Most of the clinical effects of hyperphosphatemia are related to secondary changes of calcium metabolism. Besides hypocalcemia, ectopic calcification is one of the most important manifestations of hyperphosphatemia. This association has been seen in several clinical settings including renal failure, hypoparathyroidism, and tumoral calcinosis. It seems that when the calcium–phosphate product exceeds 70, the chances for precipitation are greatly increased. In addition to the calcium–phosphate product, local tissue factors may play a role in calcium precipitation. For example, local alkalosis may favor calcification of the cornea and lungs. In patients with severe calcification (calcifilaxis) it appears that the presence of high levels of parathyroid hormone may also aggravate this condition. Hyperphosphatemia also plays a key role in the development of secondary hyperparathyroidism in renal insufficiency. When phosphate ingestion is decreased and hyperphosphatemia is avoided in animals with experimental renal insufficiency, the development of secondary hyperparathyroidism can be prevented. Hyperphosphatemia also affects vitamin D metabolism by decreasing the activity of the 1-hydroxylase enzyme in the renal cortex. In patients maintained on chronic hemodialysis, the concentrations of serum phosphorus correlated well with the severity of secondary hyperparathyroidism. Those patients who do not follow the therapeutic regimens and do not take phosphate binders seem to develop severe and persistent hyperphosphatemia and profound secondary hyperparathyroidism and bone disease. Vascular calcification observed in some of these patients may produce necrosis and gangrene of the extremities. Slit lamp examination may show ocular calcification and some patients may develop acute conjunctivitis, a syndrome called the "red eye" of uremia. Precipitation of calcium in the skin may be, in part, responsible for pruritus, a symptom that usually is seen in patients with far advanced uremia. From the therapeutic point of view, the most effective way to control hyperphosphatemia is to use phosphate binders that decrease the absorption of phosphate from the gastrointestinal tract. Obviously, if the patient is dehydrated, expansion of the ECF with saline will greatly increase the amount of phosphate excreted in the urine.

C. Hypophosphatemia

Hypophosphatemia (serum phosphate concentration below 2.5 mg/100 ml) usually results from an increase in urinary phosphate excretion, a decrease in the gastrointestinal absorption of phosphate, or a translocation of phosphate from the extracellular to the intracellular space. The causes of hypophosphatemia are listed in Table VII.

1. Increased Renal Excretion of Phosphate

a. Primary Hyperparathyroidism

Primary hyperparathyroidism is seen frequently in clinical medicine. (see Section I on calcium). The excess parathyroid hormone secreted into the circulation greatly influences phosphate balance. There is a remarkable decrease in renal phosphate reabsorption with consequent hypophosphatemia. The degree of hypophosphatemia varies among patients since mobilization of phosphate from bone will, in part, ameliorate the hypophosphatemia. Moreover, if the patient ingests large amounts of phosphate in the diet, the degree of hypophosphatemia may be mild. Since these patients also have elevated calcium, the diagnosis is rather easy in the majority of patients and the treatment of this condition is surgery.

Table VII. Causes of Hypophosphatemia

 I. Increased renal excretion of phosphorus
   A. Primary hyperparathyroidism
   B. Secondary hyperparathyroidism
   C. Renal tubular defects
   D. Diuretic phase of ATN
   E. Postrenal transplantation
   F. ECF volume expansion
 II. Decrease in gastrointestinal phosphate absorption
   A. Administration of PO_4 binders
   B. Malabsorption
   C. Starvation–malnutrition
 III. Abnormalities in vitamin D metabolism
   A. Vitamin-D-deficient rickets
   B. Vitamin-D-resistant rickets
   C. Vitamin-D-dependent rickets
 IV. Miscellaneous
   A. Diabetes mellitus: during treatment for ketoacidosis
   B. Severe respiratory alkalosis
   C. Recovery phase of malnutrition
   D. Alcohol withdrawal

---

b. Secondary Hyperparathyroidism

Hyperphosphatemia rather than hypophosphatemia occurs in chronic renal disease as a result of decreased phosphorus excretion by the kidney as GFR falls. However, certain conditions (diseases of the gastrointestinal tract with normal renal function) decrease calcium absorption from the GI tract and may produce secondary hyperparathyroidism and hypophosphatemia. In secondary hyperparathyroidism due to GI abnormalities usually both serum calcium and phosphorus are low. It is the hypocalcemia that is responsible for the increased release of parathyroid hormone. The levels of PTH may be extremely high, promoting phosphaturia. Thus, in these conditions the malabsorption of phosphate from the gastrointestinal tract is aggravated by an increased excretion of phosphate by the kidney.

c. Renal Tubular Defects

There are conditions in which, despite normal GFR, specific renal tubular defects result in decreased phosphate reabsorption. In the Fanconi syndrome, the patients excrete not only increased amounts of phosphate in the urine, but also increased quantities of amino acids, uric acid, and glucose, resulting in hypoglycemia, hypouricemia, and hypophosphatemia. There are other conditions in which an isolated defect in the renal tubular transport of phosphate is found (as in fructose intolerance, an autosomal recessive disorder).

d. Diuretic Phase of Acute Tubular Necrosis

During the oliguric phase of acute renal failure, patients develop secondary hyperparathyroidism and phosphate retention (see Chapter 13). During the diuretic phase, the presence of profound diuresis, secondary hyperparathyroidism, and the continued use of phosphate binders may lead to the development of severe hypophosphatemia. Usually, the hypophosphatemia is only temporary and serum phosphate levels return to normal in a relatively short period of time.

e. Post-Renal Transplantation

Patients frequently develop profound hypophosphatemia after renal transplantation. This is due to severe secondary hyperparathyroidism, and a GFR that is greatly increased after transplantation. The high serum levels of PTH will decrease the reabsorption of phosphate with the concommitant development of hypophosphatemia. However, some of these patients may also develop a renal tubular defect in phosphate transport and the hypophosphatemia may persist for several years, even in the absence of secondary hyperparathyroidism. Thus, the hypophosphatemia seen after transplantation may result from a combination of factors: (1) ingestion of phosphate binders, (2) secondary hyperparathyroidism, (3) improvement in renal function, and (4) tubular defects. When phosphate binders are decreased or discontinued and hyperparathyroidism subsides, phosphorus levels return to normal in most patients. However, in some cases, hypophosphatemia does not subside and this could be due to tubular defects. Prolonged periods of severe hypophosphatemia may lead to bone disease characterized by severe osteomalacia.

f. Extracellular Fluid Volume Expansion

Expansion of the extracellular space, by the administration of solutions containing sodium, increases the excretion of phosphate. An important mechanism by which ECF volume expansion produces phosphaturia is due to a fall in ionized calcium and subsequent release of PTH. If this condition occurs in clinical medicine, it is of minor importance, and will subside after the expansion of the ECF is discontinued.

2. Decrease in Gastrointestinal Phosphate Absorption

a. Administration of Phosphate Binders

Phosphate binders, mainly aluminum salts (aluminum hydroxide, aluminum carbonate gel), are drugs used in the treatment of hyperphosphatemia. However, when these drugs are given in excess they may produce profound hypophosphatemia. These gels trap phosphate in the small intestine and increase the amount of phosphate in the stool. Patients ingesting large amounts of phosphate binders and not followed closely may develop phosphate depletion. Over a period of time, these patients may develop severe weakness, bone pain, and osteomalacia.

b. Malabsorption

Since most of the phosphate is absorbed in the small intestine, gastrointestinal disorders such as celiac disease, tropical and nontropical sprue, regional enteritis, etc. may decrease the absorption of phosphate. The degree of hypophosphatemia varies among patients being extremely mild in some and severe in others. Recently, phosphate malabsorption has been described in patients who have undergone surgical bypass procedures for obesity.

c. Malnutrition

Most of the phosphorus ingested in the diet is present in protein especially milk, cheese, meat, eggs, and the like. In many parts of the world, where protein consumption is poor, hypophosphatemia occurs, predominantly in children. Overall growth is greatly diminished and a series of metabolic disorders are present.

3. Abnormalities in Vitamin D Metabolism

Vitamin D and its metabolites play a key role in phosphate metabolism. Physiological amounts of vitamin D in the diet are necessary to maintain the normal mineralization process in bone and to promote the intestinal absorption of calcium and phosphorus. Dietary deficiency of vitamin D increases the amount of osteoid tissue in the skeleton and decreases normal mineralization.

a. Vitamin-D-Deficient Rickets

Vitamin-D-deficient diets are responsible for the metabolic disorder known as rickets, when it occurs in children, or osteomalacia, when it occurs in adults. Vitamin D deficiency in childhood causes severe deformities because of the rapid growth of bone. These deformities are characterized by soft lucent areas in the skull known as craniotabes and costochondral swelling or bending (known as ricketic rosary), the chest usually becomes flattened, the sternum may be pushed to form the so-called "pigeon chest." The volume of the thorax may be greatly reduced with impairment of respiratory function. Kyphosis is frequently seen. There is a remarkable swelling of the joints, especially the wrists and ankles, with characteristic anterior bowing of the legs, and fractures of the "green stalk" variety may also be present. In the adult form of the disease the symptoms are not as striking and are usually characterized by vague bone pain, weakness, radiolucent area, and pseudofractures. The pseudofractures represent stretch fractures in which the normal process of healing is impaired by the mineralization defect. Mild hypocalcemia may be present; however, hypophosphatemia is by far the most frequent biochemical alteration. This pathological process responds well to small pharmalogical doses of vitamin D.

b. Vitamin-D-Resistant Rickets or Familial Hypophosphatemic Rickets

This condition is an X-linked dominant disorder characterized by hypophosphatemia, decreased renal tubular reabsorption of phosphate, decreased absorption of calcium and inorganic phosphate, and varying degrees of rickets or osteomalacia. Two key hypothesis have been postulated to explain this abnormality: (1) A defect in the conversion of vitamin D to 25-hydroxy D_3. However, it has been demonstrated recently that the levels of 25-hydroxy D_3 are normal in this condition, and that administration of 25-hydroxy D_3 or 1,25-dihydroxy D_3 does not correct the hypophosphatemia. (2) A defect in the reabsorption of inorganic phosphate by the kidney and intestine. There is evidence to suggest that the decreased tubular reabsorption of phosphate is not due to an increase in PTH levels. It seems that a component of the renal phosphate transport which may be PTH independent may be abnormal and responsible for the increased phosphaturia.

c. Vitamin-D-Dependent Rickets

This is a recessively inherent form of vitamin D refractory rickets. This condition is also characterized by hypophosphatemia, hypocalcemia, elevated levels of serum alkaline phosphatase, and sometimes generalized aminoaciduria and severe bone lesions. This condition usually responds to massive doses of vitamin D.

4. Miscellaneous Conditions

a. Diabetic Ketoacidosis

Hypophosphatemia is frequently seen during the treatment of diabetic ketoacidosis. When diabetic patients develop ketoacidosis, usually they have an increase in phosphate excretion in the urine; however serum phosphate may be slightly elevated due to acidosis. During the administration of insulin there is a rapid decrease in the levels of glucose with translocation of phosphate from the extracellular space to the intracellular space, resulting in hypophosphatemia.

b. Severe Respiratory Alkalosis

Acute respiratory alkalosis decreases urinary phosphate excretion but produces marked hypophosphatemia. In contrast, patients who receive sodium bicarbonate excrete large amounts of phosphate in the urine; however, the hypophosphatemia that may develop is only moderate in nature. It has been postulated that in respiratory alkalosis there is an increase in the intracellular pH with activation of glycolysis and increased formation of phosphorylated carbohydrate compounds leading to a precipitous fall in serum phosphate concentration. The mild hypophosphatemia that may be seen during administration of sodium bicarbonate is probably secondary to increased renal phosphate excretion due to a decrease in ionized calcium and release of parathyroid hormone.

c. Recovery Phase of Malnutrition

In malnourished patients, the administration of high caloric diets without an appropriate amount of phosphorus produces severe hypophosphatemia.

d. Alcohol Withdrawal

The pathogenesis of the hypophosphatemia observed in some patients during alcohol withdrawal is not fully understood. The previous state of nutrition plays an important role in the development of hypophosphatemia. Many alcoholics develop borderline hypophosphatemia as the result of a poor dietary intake or decreased phosphorus absorption. However, when

Table VIII. Clinical and Biochemical
Manifestations of Marked Hypophosphatemia

I. Hematological alterations
  A. Red blood cells
    1. Decreased ATP content
    2. Decreased 2,3 DPG
    3. Decreased P_{50}
    4. Increased oxygen affinity
    5. Decreased life span
    6. Hemolysis
    7. Spherocytosis
  B. Leukocytes
    1. Decreased phagocytosis
    2. Decreased chemotaxis
    3. Decreased bactericidal activity
  C. Platelets
    1. Impaired clot retraction
    2. Thrombocytopenia
    3. Decreased ATP content
    4. Megakaryocytosis
    5. Decreased life span
II. Skeletal abnormalities
    1. Bone pain
    2. Radiolucent areas (X-ray)
    3. Pseudofractures
    4. Rickets or osteomalacia
III. Central nervous system
    1. Anorexia
    2. Irritability
    3. Confusion
    4. Parasthesias
    5. Dysarthia
    6. Coma
IV. Cardiovascular
    1. Decreased cardiac output
    2. Increased left ventricular end diatolic pressure
V. Muscular
    1. Muscle weakness
    2. Rhabdomyolysis
    3. Decreased transmembrane resting potential
VI. Biochemical
    1. Low PTH levels
    2. Increased 1,25 $(OH)_2D_3$
    3. Hypercalcemia
    4. Hypomagnesemia
    5. Hypermagnesuria
    6. Hypophosphaturia
    7. Decreased GFR
    8. Decreased T_m for bicarbonate
    9. Decreased renal gluconeogenesis
    10. Decreased titrable acid excretion
    11. Increased creatine phosphokinase
    12. Increased aldolase

the patient is admitted to the hospital the hypophosphatemia may be aggravated by alcohol withdrawal. This, in part, may be due to respiratory alkalosis which will translocate phosphate into the intracellular space. Moreover, the administration of phosphate binders for the treatment of gastritis worsens the hypophosphatemia. It should be emphasized that hypophosphatemia is a common disorder in patients with chronic alcoholism.

5. Clinical and Biochemical Manifestations of Hypophosphatemia

Since phosphate plays a key role in the formation of ATP, the source of energy, practically every cell of the body and every organ is affected in patients who have chronic, profound hypophosphatemia. Patients can tolerate mild degrees of hyposphphatemia and are usually asymptomatic. However, if profound hypophosphatemia is present with serum phosphate levels lower than 1 mg/100 ml a series of hematological, neurological, and metabolic disorders may develop. In general, the patient becomes anorectic, develops weakness, and mild bone pain may be present if the hypophosphatemia persists for several months (Table VIII).

6. Hematologic Manifestations

Important biochemical abnormalities of the red cells include a decline in the levels of 2,3 DPG and ATP. Low levels of 2,3 DPG may depress P50 values so that the release of oxygen to peripheral tissue is decreased. Thus, severe hyposphphatemia may limit oxygen release at the cellular level. Severe hypophosphatemia in man and dog has been reported to produce hemolytic anemia with parallel reductions in hematocrit and ATP which reverse after phosphate administration. In dogs, it has been demonstrated that hypophosphatemia produces severe platelet dysfunction characterized by thrombocytopenia, reduced ATP levels, increased platelet size, impaired clot retraction, and hemorrhage in gut and skin. There is some evidence in dogs that hypophosphatemia also affects leukocyte function. Important functions like chemotaxis, phagocytosis, and intracellular bacterial killing seem to be impaired in severe hypophosphatemia.

7. Cardiovascular Manifestations

Severe cardiomyopathies, decreased cardiac function with lowering of cardiac output, have been described in patients with severe hypophosphatemia. Studies of the myocardium showed that the resting muscle membrane potential fell, sodium chloride and water content of the tissue increased, and potassium content decreased in severe hypophosphatemia. The values returned to normal after phosphate was administered.

8. Skeletal Manifestations

Phosphate, as well as calcium, plays a key role in the mineralization of osteoid tissue. After the osteoid is laid down by the osteoblast, deposition of minerals such as calcium amorphous phosphate is critical to mineralize collagen. In the presence of severe hypophosphatemia this process is impaired and there is a widening of the osteoid seam and a lack of uptake of tetracycline. These patients usually have mild microfractures difficult to detect on X-ray, and bone pain is a characteristic finding.

9. Central Nervous System

Many patients with profound hypophosphatemia have increased irritability and develop numerous parasthesias and mental confusion. It is possible that the decrease in the 2,3 DPG becomes important in tissues where oxygen is necessary for energy production. Some patients also may develop decreased nerve conduction velocity.

10. Muscular Manifestations

Muscle weakness and electromyographic abnormalities are associated with chronic hypophosphatemia and phosphate depletion. Dogs fed low phosphate diets for several months developed changes in muscle, rhabdomyolysis, and characteristic increases in the levels of CPK and aldolase in blood. The syndrome of rhabdomyolysis has been observed in alcoholic patients with hypophosphatemia.

11. Renal Effect of Hypophosphatemia

Numerous metabolic alterations are seen in patients with profound hypophosphatemia. A commonly observed alteration is the presence of hypercalciuria. Experimental evidence has shown that in phosphate depletion, there is a defect in proximal and distal tubule calcium reabsorption. Acute administration of phosphate to phosphate-depleted animals results in a rapid increase in the distal tubule reabsorption of calcium. Phosphate-depleted dogs demonstrate a decrease in hydrogen ion secretion and the T_m for bicarbonate is greatly reduced. At lower levels of serum bicarbonate the amount of bicarbonate in the urine is greatly increased. In severe phosphate depletion, the biological action of parathyroid hormone is greatly impaired. Although the administration of parathyroid hormone may increase the release of cyclic AMP, the phosphaturia is abolished.

IV. TREATMENT OF DISORDERS OF CALCIUM, PHOSPHATE, AND MAGNESIUM METABOLISM

Although the treatment of alterations in the metabolism of calcium, phosphorus, and magnesium should be geared toward the pathogenetic mechanisms responsible for its genesis, there are different practical and effective ways to increase or decrease the absorption of Ca, P, and Mg by the kidney, gastrointestinal tract, and their mobilization from bone.

Space constraints do not allow us to review the general medical guidelines that may take priority in the care of patients. Obviously, if a concomitant infection is present, the patient is hypotensive, or has decreased cardiac output or hypoxia, these alterations should be corrected immediately before any other therapeutic modalities are attempted.

A. Treatment of Disorders of Calcium Metabolism

1. Hypercalcemia

From the practical point of view, the easiest and most useful maneuver to correct hypercalcemia is to decrease the reabsorption of calcium by the kidney. As discussed previously, only 1%–2% of the filtered load of calcium is excreted by the kidney. This percentage can be greatly increased, and the kidney may thus become an excellent excretory organ for calcium. Since the majority of patients with hypercalcemia develop dehydration and volume contraction with a consequent decrease in glomerular filtration rate (GFR), one of the first therapeutic maneuvers will be the expansion of the extracellular fluid space. Since expansion with saline will require several liters per day it is mandatory that strict records be kept in order to maintain accurate determinations of the intake and output of fluids. In the majority of patients it is convenient to determine central venous pressure which will allow us to expand the patient and to prevent the potential risk of overexpansion and heart failure. Thus, after a CVP line is inserted, the patient should be expanded with saline until the venous pressure increases to 10–14 mm Hg. This maneuver alone will increase GFR and will decrease the reabsorption of calcium in the proximal tubule as well as in the ascending part of the loop of Henle. Thus, fractional excretion of calcium will be greatly increased. This effect can be enhanced by administration of diuretics such as furosemide or ethacrynic acid. The administration of 40–120 mg of furosemide every four hours is recommended in most patients. Using these maneuvers fractional excretion of calcium can be increased to 10% of the filtered load. Thus, 1 g of calcium can be easily excreted in the urine in 24 hr. The administration of large amounts of saline and diuretics usually increases the excretion of potassium. In order to prevent arrhythmias, serum potassium should be maintained between 3.5 and 5 mEq/liter. This can be achieved by adding 10–30 mEq of potassium to each liter of saline.

Although expansion of the ECF may control the hypercalcemia, this effect is temporary and since in most circumstances the hypercalcemia is secondary to increased mobilization of calcium from bone, we may be forced to add a second line of medication to decrease the efflux of calcium from bone.

Calcitonin produces hypocalcemia by decreasing the activity of the osteoclasts. It is a safe drug with few secondary effects. The dose commonly used ranges from 2 to 5 MRC units per kilogram of body weight every 6–12 hr. The degree of hypocalcemia produced by this drug is mild and the decrease is usually of 1–3 mg/100 ml. Calcitonin can be given either intramuscularly or intravenously in the concentration of 5 MRC units/kg dissolved in 500 ml of 5% dextrose in water to be given over a period of 6 hr. Unfortunately, in the majority of patients there is an escape from the hypocalcemic effect of calcitonin after 6–10 days of administration.

Mithramycin is an antibiotic originally introduced for the treatment of testicular tumors. Mithramycin blocks the activity of the osteoclasts and may result in severe hypocalcemia. It is usually given intravenously in the dose of 25 µg/kg of body weight dissolved in 500 ml of 5% dextrose in water or saline and given over a period of 3–4 hr. Mithramycin is an extremely effective drug. However, the effects may be seen only after 48–72 hr. One of the toxic effects of the drug is severe thrombocytopenia and bleeding. In general the drug should not be given more than once every 4 or 5 days.

Recently, a derivative of the diphosphonates, *disodium dichloromethylene diphosphonate* (Cl_2MDP), has been used on an experimental basis in patients with tumors and bone metastases and severe hypercalcemia. Although the results reported up to the present time are scanty, this experimental drug may be of great value in the treatment of hypercalcemia in these patients. Most of the investigators have used 300 mg four times daily for several months with remarkable results. More information is necessary before we can use this drug on a routine basis. There are several tumors which produce prostaglandins which have resulted in the development of hypercalcemia. Some of these patients have solid tumors such as lung or renal carcinoma. The use of aspirin in the dose of 1 g four times daily or indomethacin 75 mg twice daily has ameliorated the hypercalcemia.

If hypercalcemia is mainly due to increased absorption of calcium from the gastrointestinal tract, it is obviously important to decrease the amount of calcium in the diet and to administer *glucocorticosteroids* which will result in decreased absorption. Usually prednisone 20 mg twice daily has been effective in conditions like sarcoidosis which is characterized by increased calcium absorption from the intestinal tract.

Phosphate has been used in the treatment of hypercalcemia. However, the presence of a normal or slightly elevated serum phosphorus or decreased renal function will preclude the use of this medication. Phosphorus should be given *only in those circumstances in which serum phosphorus is low*. If a remarkable elevation of serum phosphorus is achieved and serum calcium decreases, the patient may deposit calcium phosphate in soft tissues. Thus, in the presence of hypophosphatemia 1–2 g of neutral phosphate can be given orally to the patients in order to increase serum phosphorus to a maximum of 4–5 mg/100 ml. It is not clear how phosphorus decreases serum calcium. Calcium, in general, is not increased in the urine or stools. The changes are rapidly observed and the effects may last for several days. In some circumstances there is precipitation of calcium in soft tissue, in others it is sequestered by bone.

EDTA, ethylenediaminetetraacetate, is an effective therapeutic agent in reducing the ionized calcium in hypercalcemic patients. The effect is very rapid and the changes are on the order of 1–2 mg/100 ml in ionized calcium. Usually 50 mg/kg of body weight of EDTA (disodium salt) is dissolved in 500 ml of saline and is given over a period of four hours. Although this is an effective way to correct hypercalcemia, the effect only lasts a few hours. This approach to treat hypercalcemia has been abandoned by most. On the other hand, EDTA infusion is an important tool to test the ability of the parathyroid glands to respond to an acute hypocalcemic stimulus.

There are a series of general measures which are important in the treatment of hypercalcemia. Immobilization should be avoided as much as possible especially in those patients with rapid bone turnover such as in Paget's disease. Since the great majority of patients with hypercalcemia have an underlying tumor as a cause for the hypercalcemia, physicians should be aware of this pathogenetic mechanism and join efforts with oncologists in the treatment of the malignancy. Finally, in situations in which the hypercalcemia is very severe and the patient has advanced renal insufficiency, acute hemodialysis is an effective way to correct the hypercalcemia (Table IX).

2. Hypocalcemia

The treatment of severe hypocalcemia and tetany is a medical emergency. The administration of calcium is mandatory to prevent severe complications and even death in these patients. If the patient has severe hypocalcemia and tetany in the absence of hypomagnesemia, these symptoms can be easily relieved by administration of one or two ampules of calcium gluconate given intravenously *over a period of 10 min* (1 amp of calcium gluconate has approximately 100 mg of elemental calcium). This initial treatment can be followed by administration of 1 g of elemental calcium dissolved in 500 ml of dextrose in water and given intravenously over a period of 4–6 hr. If the condition responsible for the hypocalcemia cannot be corrected, i.e., hypoparathyroidism, a program for the chronic treatment of hypocalcemia should be instituted. First, the amount of calcium in the diet should be supplemented by 1–3 g of elemental calcium. Calcium carbonate has roughly 40% of elemental calcium. Commercial preparations like Titralac® or Oscal® can be used in this situation. However, in many circumstances the administration of large amounts of calcium may not be sufficient to increase the absorption by the intestine; therefore, different metabolites of vitamin D should be used. In acute situations, 1,25-dihydroxycholecalciferol, known commercially by the name of Rocatrol®, could be used. The dose used ranges from 0.5 μg up to 2 μg/24 hr. Most of the patients eventually require 0.5 μg/day. If this metabolite of vitamin D is not available, vitamin D_2 or D_3 about 50,000 units three times a week could be given to the patient. The dose could be gradually increased up to 50,000 to 100,000 units daily. The serum calcium should be carefully monitored to prevent severe hypercalcemia.

Table IX. Treatment of Hypercalcemia

Agent	Dosage	Route of administration[a]	Effect	Mechanism of action	Side effects
I. Measurements directed to enhance renal excretion of calcium					
Saline	1–3 liters every 6 hr	IV	4–8	↑ GFR	Heart failure
				↓ Tubular reabsorption of Ca	Electrolyte imbalance
Furosemide	40–120 mg every 2–4 hr	IV	2–4 hr	↓ Tubular reabsorption of Ca	Hypokalemia
II. Measurements directed to decrease calcium efflux from bone					
Calcitonin	2–5 MRC/kg every 4–8 hr	IM	4–12 hr	Decrease bone resorption (DBR)	Allergic reaction, nausea, flushing
Mithramycin	25 µg/kg in 500 ml saline	IV	24–72 hr	DBR (marked)	Thrombocytopenia, bleeding
Indocin	75 mg every 12 hr	PO	2–4 days	DBR secondary to prostaglandins	GI disorders
Aspirin	1 g every 6 hr	PO	2–4 days	DBR secondary to prostaglandins	GI disorders, allergic reaction
*Disodium-dichloromethylene diphosphonate (Cl_2MDP)[b]	300 mg every 6–8 hr	PO	3–10 days	DBR to osteolytic metastases	Unknown
III. Measurements directed to decrease calcium absorption in the GI tract					
Prednisone	20–30 mg every 12 hr	PO	2–4 days	Decrease GI absorption	Acute toxic steroid effects
IV. Measurements directed to decrease serum calcium					
Disodium EDTA	50 mg/kg in 500 ml saline; 4 hr infusion	IV	1–4 hr	Chelation	Nephrotoxicity, nausea, vomiting, arrhythmias
Phosphate	0.5–1 g every 8 hr	PO	12–72 hr	Precipitation, bone sequestration	Metastatic calcification, decreased renal function
Hemodialysis	Low dialysate calcium				

[a] IV, intravenous; IM, intramuscular; PO, by mouth.
[b] Experimental drug.

B. Treatment of Disorders of Phosphate Metabolism

1. Hyperphosphatemia

The most effective way to treat hyperphosphatemia is to decrease phosphate absorption from the gastrointestinal tract by use of phosphate binders. Of course, if the diet contains high amounts of phosphate it should be changed. However, the administration of aluminum salts has been the traditional treatment to control hyperphosphatemia. Aluminum hydroxide and aluminum carbonate gel are the two most common forms (Alucap®, Dialume®, and Basaljel®). The liquid form of these preparations has a greater capacity to bind phosphorus in the gastrointestinal tract. However, many patients cannot tolerate large amounts of these liquid gels for prolonged periods of time because of nausea and vomiting. In general, patients' compliance for the liquid form is very poor. Because of this, the liquid gels have been dehydrated and incorporated into tablets or capsules. Most of these preparations require the administration of two to four tablets or capsules three to four times daily in order to correct the hyperphosphatemia. If the patient develops constipation, one of the complications of these medications, magnesium should be incorporated into these preparations. However, if the patient has hyperphosphatemia secondary to severe renal insufficiency, *magnesium should not be given* because of the likelihood of producing severe hypermagnesemia which may lead to magnesium intoxication and death. Although decreased absorption of phosphate is the most effective way to control hyperphosphatemia, the kidney is also an effective organ for phosphate excretion. Thus, expansion of the ECF with saline can result in significant phosphaturia. Parathyroid hormone has been used in the past especially in patients with primary hypoparathyroidism to increase phosphate excretion by the kidney. Although the administration of parathyroid hormone is an important tool in the differential diagnosis between hypoparathyroidism and pseudohypoparathyroidism, because in the latter condition the excretion of phosphate in the urine does not increase after PTH administration, from the practical point of view, parathyroid hormone is not effective in the treatment of chronic hyperphosphatemia.

2. Hypophosphatemia

Correction of hypophosphatemia is a relatively easy task in clinical medicine. The administration of a diet high in protein in general will correct hypophosphatemia. However, there are circumstances in which there is a need for a rapid increase in the levels of serum phosphate. Under these circumstances phosphate can be given intravenously. A solution containing 1–2 g of neutral phosphate, pH 7.4, dissolved in 500 ml of saline, can be given over a period of 6–8 hr. This procedure can be repeated the next day if the hypophosphatemia persists. On a chronic basis, hypophosphatemia can be corrected, as mentioned before, by improving the diet or by giving medications containing phosphorus. Approximately 1–2 g of neutral phosphate divided in three doses per day should be sufficient to correct the hypophosphatemia. There are conditions such as vitamin-D-resistant rickets (VDRR), a genetic disorder seen in children, in which it is very difficult to correct the hypophosphatemia. In this genetic disorder an elevation in serum phosphorus is usually followed by a significant increase in urinary phosphate. Thus, in patients with VDRR, it is critical that the patients receive phosphate four to six times daily in small amounts to produce an effect at the level of the bone. An easy way to give phosphorus to a patient is the use of Fleet's Phospho-soda®, which contains roughly 120 mg/ml. Thus, the administration of 5 ml four times daily will provide around 2 g of elemental phosphorus. If larger amounts are used patients may develop diarrhea.

C. Treatment of Alterations in Magnesium Metabolism

1. Hypermagnesemia

Hypermagnesemia very seldom is seen in clinical medicine. In general, it is observed in patients with far advanced renal insufficiency, usually with a GFR of less than 10 ml/min. The treatment is similar to the one for hypercalcemia, that is to say, expansion with saline and administration of furosemide. However, one should be careful since this therapeutic regimen will also increase the excretion of calcium in the urine and potentiate the toxic effects of hypermagnesemia. Thus, if expansion with saline and furosemide are used, calcium should be added to the solutions, approximately 1–3 ampules of calcium gluconate per liter of saline, to prevent hypocalcemia. If the patient's GFR is extremely low and expansion with saline and use of diuretics are not effective, dialysis with a zero magnesium dialysate should be instituted. The other circumstance in which hypermagnesemia is seen is when large amounts of magnesium are given intravenously to patients. A decrease in the dose administered will rapidly correct the hypermagnesemia.

2. Hypomagnesemia

Profound magnesium depletion may be accompanied by hypocalcemia and tetany. Thus the treatment of severe hypomagnesemia may constitute a medical emergency. Profound hypomagnesemia can be easily corrected by administration of magnesium intravenously provided that the patient has fairly normal renal function. Fifty to seventy-five mEq of magnesium sulfate or magnesium chloride should be mixed in 500 ml of dextrose in water and given intravenously over a period of 6–8 hr. The next morning serum magnesium should be measured and if the hypomagnesemia persists, the amount of magnesium should be increased to 100 mEq dissolved in the same type of solution and given over a period of eight hours. In some circumstances this procedure should be repeated two or three times until serum magnesium increases to 2.5 mg/100 ml. If the patient requires magnesium orally over a prolonged period of time, magnesium salts can be given to these patients. One gram of magnesium oxide has roughly 50 mEq or 600 mg of Mg. Thus, magnesium oxide in the dose of 250–500 mg can be given to patients two to four times daily. If larger doses are used, they are not well tolerated and most patients will develop diarrhea. It is important to emphasize that a normal diet provides approximately 25 mEq or 300 mg of magnesium.

SUGGESTED READINGS

Agus, Z. S.: Renal tubular transport of calcium: update, in Massry, S., Ritz, E., and Rapado, A. (eds.): *Homeostasis of Phosphate and Other Minerals.* Plenum Press, New York, 1978.

Anast, C. S., Winnacker, J. L., Forte, L. R., and Burns, T. W.: Impaired release of parathyroid hormone in magnesium deficiency. *J. Clin. Endocrinol. Metab.* 42:707, 1976.

Austin, L. A., and Heath III, H.: Calcitonin: physiology and pathophysiology. *N. Engl. J. Med.* 304:269, 1981.

Bikle, D. D., Morrissey, R. L., Zolock, D. T., and Rasmussen, H.: The intestinal response to vitamin D. *Rev. Physiol. Biochem.* 89:63, 1981.

Chapuy, M. C., Meunier, P. J., Alexandre, C. M., and Vignon, E. P.: Effects of disodium dichloromethylene diphosphonate on the hypercalcemia produced by bone metastases. *J. Clin. Invest.* 65:1243, 1980.

Chen, T. C., Costillo, L., Korycka-Dahl, M., and DeLuca, H.: Role of vitamin D metabolites in phosphate transport of rat intestine. *J. Nutr.* 104:1056, 1974.

Coburn, J., and Slatopolsky, E.: Vitamin D, PTH and renal osteodystrophy in the kidney, in Brenner, B. and Rector, F. C. (eds.): *The Kidney,* Second edition. W. B. Saunders, Philadelphia, 1981, pp. 2213–2305.

Dirks, J. H., and Quamme, G. A.: Renal handling of magnesium, in Massry, S., Ritz, E., and Rapado, A. (eds.): *Homeostasis of Phosphate and Other Minerals.* Plenum Press, New York, 1978.

Knochel, J.P.: The pathophysiology and clinical characteristics of severe hypophosphatemia. *Arch. Intern. Med.* 137:203, 1977.

Knox, F. G., Greger, R. P., Lang, F. C., and Marchand, G. R.: Renal handling of phosphate: update. in Massry, S., and Ritz, E. (eds.) *Phosphate Metabolism.* Plenum Press, New York, 1977.

Knox, F. G., Hoppe, A., Kempson, S. A., Shah, S. V., and Dousa, T. P.: Cellular mechanisms of phosphate transport, in Massry, S. G., and Fleisch, H. (eds.): *Renal Handling of Phosphate* Plenum Press, New York, 1980, p. 79.

Kumar, R., Cohen, W. R., Silva, P., and Epstein, F. H.: Elevated 1,25-dihydroxyvitamin D plasma levels in normal human pregnancy and lactation. *J. Clin. Invest.* 63.942, 1979.

Massry, S. G.: Pharmacology of magnesium. *Annu. Rev. Pharmacol. Toxicol.* 17:67, 1977.

Mundy, G. R., Raisz, L. G., Cooper, R. A., Schechter, G. P., and Salmon, S. E.: Evidence for the secretion of an osteoclast stimulating factor in myeloma. *N. Engl. J. Med.* 291:1041, 1974.

Norman, A. W.: Vitamin D metabolism and calcium absorption. *Am. J. Med.* 67:989, 1979.

Nusynowitz, M. L., Frame, B., and Kolb, F. O.: The spectrum of the hypoparathyroid states. *Medicine* 55:105, 1976.

Parfitt, A. M., and Kleerkoper, M.: The divalent ion homeostatic system. Physiology and metabolism of calcium, phosphorus, magnesium and bone, in Maxwell, M., and Kleeman, C. (eds.): *Clinical Disorders of Fluid and Electrolyte Metabolism.* McGraw-Hill, New York, 1980.

Rutherford, W. E., Bordier, P., Marie, P., Hruska, K., Harter, H., Greenwalt, A., Blondin, J., Haddad, J., Bricker, N., and Slatopolsky, E.: Phosphate control and 25-hydroxycholecalciferol administration in preventing experimental renal osteodystrophy in the dog. *J. Clin. Invest.* 60:332, 1977.

Seyberth, H. W., Segre, G. V., Morgan, J. L., Sweetman, B. J., Potts, J. T., Jr., and Oates, J. A.: Prostaglandins as mediators of hypercalcemia associated with certain neoplasia. *N. Engl. J. Med.* 293: 1278, 1975.

Slatopolsky, E., Rutherford, W. E., Hruska, K., Martin, K., and Klahr, S.: How important is phosphate in the pathogenesis of renal osteodystrophy? *Arch. Intern. Med.* 138:848, 1978.

Slatopolsky, E., Martin, K., and Hruska, K.: Parathyroid hormone metabolism and its potential as a uremic toxin. *Am. J. Physiol.* 239(8):F1, 1980.

Suki, W. N.: Calcium transport in the nephron. *Am. J. Physiol.* 237(1):F1, 1979.

Sutton, R. A. L., and Dirks, J. H.: Renal handling of calcium: overview, in Massry, S., and Ritz, E. (eds.): *Phosphate Metabolism.* Plenum Press, New York, 1977.

III

Pathophysiology of Hypertension

This section comprises a single chapter which discusses the pathophysiology of hyper-tension. Both essential hypertension and secondary causes of hypertension are consid-ered. Special emphasis is given to the role of the kidney in the genesis of both essential hypertension and secondary hypertension. The role of the renin—angiotensin system and that of extracellular fluid volume in the pathophysiology of hypertension are considered in detail.

10

Pathophysiology of Hypertension

HERSCHEL R. HARTER

I. INTRODUCTION

Hypertension is diagnosed if a blood pressure greater than 150/95 mm Hg is obtained in both upper extremities in individuals less than 50 years of age on at least three office visits. It is an extremely common syndrome affecting over 23,000,000 people in the United States. The complications of hypertension are reversible if the syndrome is recognized early and treated adequately. Probably the single most significant study illustrating the effects of antihypertensive therapy in controlling the morbid events caused by hypertension was the V.A. Cooperative Study initiated in 1963. If individuals with diastolic blood pressures between 115 and 129 mm Hg were vigorously treated, morbid events (cerebrovascular accidents, coronary artery disease, congestive heart failure, or renal damage) were significantly reduced within 18 months of followup. For those individuals with diastolic blood pressures between 90 and 114 mm Hg, 36 months of followup were required to document a reduction in these morbid events. The results of the V.A. Cooperative Study clearly defined the beneficial effects of therapy in patients with severe (diastolic blood pressure greater than 115 mm Hg) hypertension. Patients receiving antihypertensive therapy for diastolic blood pressure between 90

HERSCHEL R. HARTER • Department of Medicine, Washington University School of Medicine, St. Louis, Missouri 63110.

Table I. Primary and Secondary Causes of Hypertension

I. Essential hypertension
   A. Alterations in plasma volume
   B. Alterations in cardiac output
   C. Alterations in renal function
   D. Alterations in neurogenic activity
   E. Alterations in vascular resistance
II. Secondary causes of hypertension
   A. Renal insufficiency
      1. Volume-dependent hypertension
      2. Volume-independent hypertension
      3. High-renin hypertension
   B. Renal artery stenosis
      1. Stage one
      2. Stage two
      3. Stage three
   C. Hypertension associated with endocrine abnormalities
      1. Primary hyperaldosteronism and its variants
      2. Pheochromocytoma
      3. Hyper- and hypothyroidism
      4. Acromegaly
III. Low-renin hypertension
IV. High-renin hypertension

Table II. Potential Mechanisms Responsible
for Essential Hypertension

I. Increased plasma volume
   A. Role of increased salt intake
   B. Defect in renal sodium excretion
II. Increased cardiac output
   A. Neurogenic factors
   B. Effects of hormones
   C. Stress
   D. Hyperkinetic hypertension
III. Renal mechanisms
   A. Defect in renal sodium excretion
   B. Alterations in renin–angiotensin system
   C. Alterations in prostaglandin production
   D. Alterations in kallikrein production
IV. Neurogenic factors
   A. Cardiac effects
   B. Renal effects
   C. Vascular effects
V. Increased vascular resistance
   A. "Autoregulation"
   B. Neurogenic factors
   C. Role of sodium and water

and 114 mm Hg showed a significant reduction in some morbid events (cerebrovascular accidents, congestive heart failure) but no improvement in coronary artery disease events (myocardial infarction). The more current Oslo study confirms these results. It is not clear if hypertension accelerates atherosclerotic processes (coronary vessel disease and the like) especially in patients with less severe forms of hypertension. It is clear, however, that hypertension, especially with diastolic blood pressures over 115 mm Hg, is associated with significant increases in the incidence of cerebrovascular accidents, dissecting aortic aneurysms, renal impairment, and congestive heart failure. Thus, recognition and treatment of hypertension is critical to the long-term survival of these patients. Antihypertensive therapy is not the primary subject of this chapter but will be commented upon later in this text. A rational approach toward the diagnosis and therapy of the hypertensive patient requires a good understanding of the pathophysiology of this syndrome. The purpose of this chapter will be to acquaint the reader with the different types of hypertension and their causes. Owing to the complex nature of this topic, the discussion cannot be all inclusive. Rather general pathophysiologic concepts will be stressed. The general causes of hypertension are outlined in Table I.

II. ESSENTIAL HYPERTENSION

Approximately 80%–90% of all hypertensive patients have primary or essential hypertension. The exact etiology of this syndrome is unclear but certain general mechanisms have been defined. A specific blood pressure is generated by the cardiac output dissipated into the vascular tree at a given resistance. Thus, blood pressure = CO × TPR, where CO refers to cardiac output and TPR to total peripheral vascular resistance. An elevated blood pressure may be caused by an increased cardiac output with a normal or even low peripheral vascular resistance or by a high peripheral resistance with normal or even decreased cardiac output.

Essential hypertension may be due to changes in cardiac output or blood volume, alterations of renal function especially of the renin–angiotensin system or the prostaglandin or kallikrein systems, neurogenic factors, or alterations in vascular resistance (see Table II). We will review each of these independently.

A. Alterations in Plasma Volume (Figure 1)

Increased salt intake is associated with higher blood pressure. Thus, Japanese living at sea level ingest large quantities of salt and have a high incidence of hypertension (40% over the age of 40), while those living at higher elevations ingest much less salt and have a low incidence of hyper-

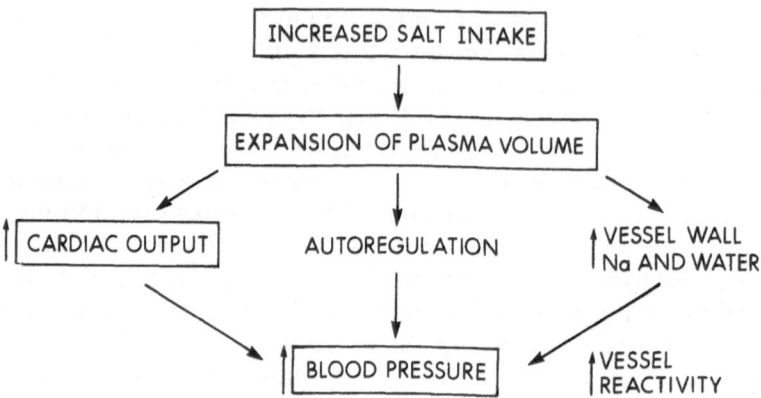

Figure 1. The potential effects of increased salt intake in the genesis of the hypertensive state.

tension (1%–2% of the population). Furthermore, a change from a low to high dietary salt intake is associated with increasing rates of hypertension. Salt intake in the United States has risen progressively over the past 30–40 years. Associated with this increased salt intake there has been an increased incidence of hypertension.

Augmented salt intake predisposes to an expanded extracellular fluid (ECF) volume. Blood flow to different organs is kept constant during expansion of the ECF volume by increased peripheral vascular resistance, which causes a rise in blood pressure. Sodium also has a direct vascular effect. Vessel wall sodium and water may be increased in the hypertensive patient. This may increase vessel reactivity and also augment vascular response to various pressor agents. Thus, the vasoconstrictive effect of angiotensin II may be greater in vessels with higher sodium content. In response to increased salt intake and changes in blood pressure, the vessel walls thicken and become more reactive to various stimuli. These changes in vessel wall reactivity may maintain the hypertensive state and also increase renal vascular resistance, which may limit the excretion of sodium necessary to reduce the intravascular blood volume and decrease the blood pressure to normal.

B. Alterations in Cardiac Output (Figure 2)

Increased plasma volume may lead to a reflex increase in cardiac output. Experimentally, volume expansion results in transient increases in cardiac output. After a period of time, however, cardiac output returns to normal but the increase in blood pressure persists owing to augmented peripheral vascular resistance. Increased cardiac output in the hypertensive population has been difficult to document. One syndrome, hyperkinetic hypertension, is associated with increased adrenergic activity, tachycardia, increased cardiac output, anxiety, diaphoresis, and sustained systolic hypertension. This relatively rare syndrome usually occurs in young males, is often self-limited, and

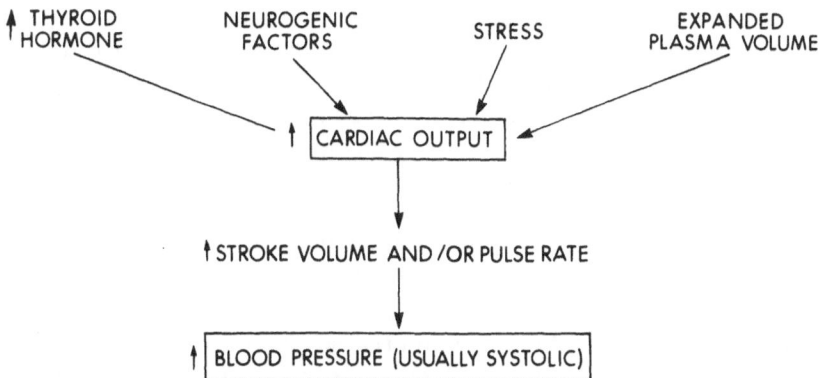

Figure 2. The potential causes of an increased cardiac output and its role in the genesis of the hypertensive state.

is reversed by treatment with B-blocking agents (propranolol). Thyrotoxicosis is also associated with an increased cardiac output and systolic hypertension. (See Section III.C on endocrine etiologies of hypertension for a more complete discussion.) Finally, as discussed later, stress may play a role in the maintenance of hypertension.

C. Alterations in Renal Function in Essential Hypertension (Figure 3)

1. Defect in Renal Sodium Excretion

Under normal circumstances, increases in plasma volume, cardiac output, or blood pressure lead to increased urinary excretion of sodium. An augmented sodium excretion is seen in hypertensive patients as compared

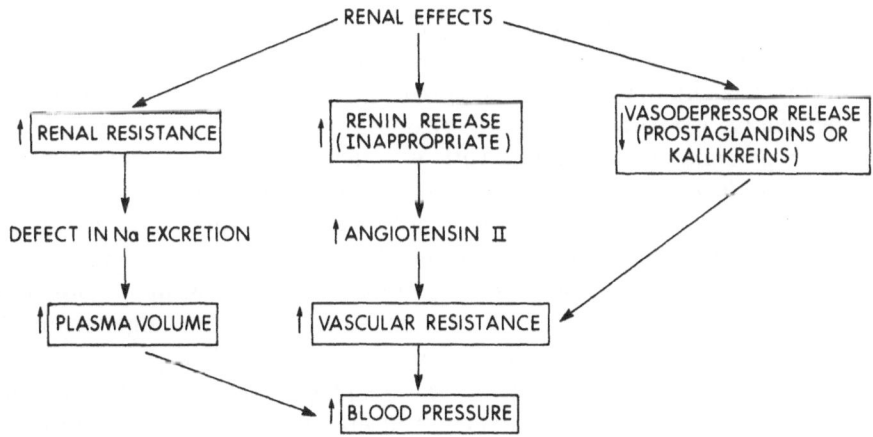

Figure 3. Potential renal defects leading to the hypertensive state.

to normals in response to a salt challenge. Normally, increases in blood perfusion pressure lead to an augmented sodium excretion. If a defect in this response exists, sodium excretion may not rise despite an increase in blood pressure leading to a further increase in blood pressure.

A defect in renal sodium handling in hypertensive patients has been difficult to document. Sodium retention may be so insidious and mild that present techniques may not allow demonstration of such changes. Renal vascular resistance is usually increased in most hypertensive animal models. This would decrease renal blood flow (RBF) and increase the filtration fraction (GFR/RBF), causing a rise in peritubular oncotic pressure which would increase proximal tubular sodium reabsorption with expansion of ECF volume, and a further increase in blood pressure (see Chapter 4).

Although a primary renal event as the initiating cause for essential hypertension has been difficult to demonstrate, there is inferential information to implicate the kidney as the primary factor in some forms of hypertension. Studies in experimental models suggest that the kidney may be responsible for the persistence of hypertension regardless of what stimulus was used to initiate the change in blood pressure. Furthermore, morphologic and physiologic renal changes have been documented in animal models and humans with hypertension. Renal tubular mass may be decreased, renal blood flow may fall, filtration fraction may rise, and/or redistribution of renal blood flow to juxta medullary (sodium-retaining) nephrons may occur. Such findings suggest that renal changes may be responsible for the persistence of the hypertension. Regardless of whether or not renal resistance is a primary or secondary event in essential hypertension, an increased efferent arteriolar tone must be present. This has been demonstrated in hypertensive rats that respond to increased salt intake with a further rise in blood pressure. Rat species which are not salt sensitive do not have increased tone and will not become hypertensive with a salt challenge.

2. Role of the Renin–Angiotensin System

While sodium retention and thus a modest increase in total body sodium may initiate the hypertensive state, renin and angiotensin may also play a role. Normally, increases in renal perfusion pressure due to increases in systemic blood pressure lead to decreased renin release (see Chapter 3). Sixty-five percent of all patients with essential hypertension have normal plasma renin levels. This would seem inappropriate since renin release falls in the normal kidney exposed to increased blood pressure. Also, as shown in experimental animals, increased vessel wall sodium and water increase the affinity of the vascular receptors for angiotensin II. Thus, owing to enhanced tissue binding or mildly increased or even normal levels of angiotensin II, hypertension may be maintained. This may explain the therapeutic benefits of drugs that block renin release, such as propranolol (a β blocker), or Captopril (which inhibits the conversion of angiotensin I to angiotensin II) in patients with essential hypertension.

Increased plasma levels of renin are seen in a small group of patients with essential hypertension. These increased levels presumably reflect renal ischemia due to sustained hypertension and concomitant vessel damage. High levels of renin cannot be incriminated as an initiating event in essential hypertension, but they play a role in its maintenance and in the genesis of malignant hypertension.

Low levels of renin are seen in approximately 20% of the patients with essential hypertension. This may reflect decreased renin due to increased mineralocorticoid activity (see Section IV on low renin hypertension).

3. Decreased Production of Vasodepressor Substances

The kidney produces large quantities of prostaglandin E_2, a known vasodilator. Unfortunately, documentation of decreased plasma levels of specific prostaglandins is difficult although reduced levels of urinary PGE have been documented in some hypertensives. Whether this is a consequence of hypertension or a cause of hypertension is not clear. Hypertension unrelated to volume can occur after total nephrectomy. This so-called "reno-prival hypertension" has been thought to be due to the absence of a vasodepressor substance (see Chapter 3 for a complete discussion). While prostaglandins are a most interesting possibility, other vasodepressor substances may also be involved. The kidney plays an important role in the kallikrein system. Plasma bradykinin which is generated from kininogen via kallikrein responds to stimuli in a fashion similar to renin. Plasma bradykinin produces arterial vasodilatation, venoconstriction, natriuresis, and activates prostaglandin synthesis. Urinary excretion rates of kallikrein are lower in some patients with essential hypertension and rise to a lesser degree during conditions of sodium depletion in these patients. Thus, there is a defect in the kallikrein–kinin system in some patients with essential hypertension but what role it plays in the genesis of the hypertension is unclear. For a more complete discussion of the prostaglandin and kallikrein systems the reader is referred to Chapter 3.

D. Neurogenic Factors (Figure 4)

Increased activity of the autonomic nervous system may be one of the factors responsible for essential hypertension. The increased autonomic activity could be due to increased sympathetic or decreased parasympathetic drive. This would have effects on specific target organs, particularly the heart, the vascular tree, and the kidney. Increased autonomic stimulation increases cardiac output, heart rate, stroke volume, and causes an increase in venous tone. These changes, however, can be documented only in a small percentage of hypertensive patients.

Overactivity of the autonomic nervous system increases total peripheral vascular resistance due to direct stimulation of the arterioles. It also increases

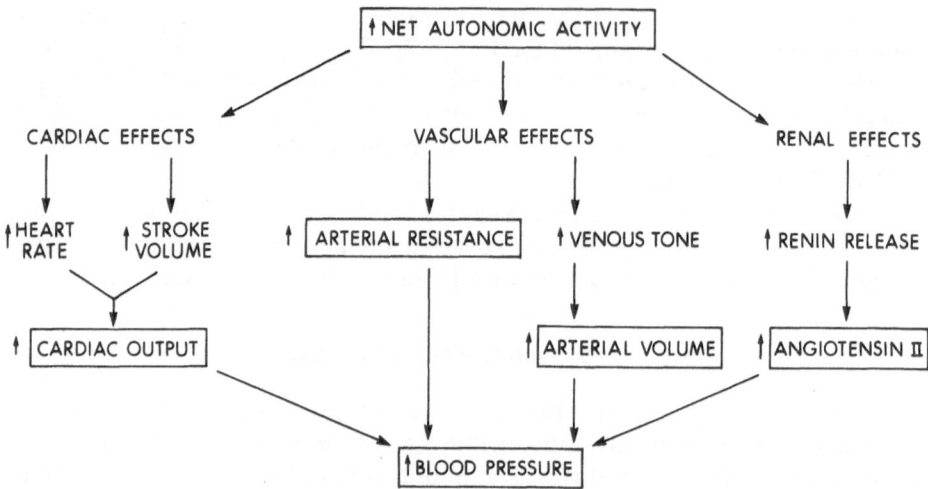

Figure 4. The effects of increased autonomic activity in the genesis of the hypertensive state.

venous tone leading to a decrease in total plasma volume and causes redistribution of this volume from the venous to the arterial tree. The net effect would be to increase the amount of blood circulating in an arterial system which already has increased resistance, and thus increase the blood pressure. Although the total plasma volume may be normal or even decreased in hypertensive patients, the distribution from the venous to the arterial system augments the hypertension. As hypertension progresses the net vascular volume actually decreases. Under these circumstances the resistance of the arterial tree may be so high that arterial and venous volume are actually decreased. Thus, while plasma volume may be increased early in hypertension, redistribution to the arterial tree with a reduction in venous volume may occur causing normalization of the total plasma volume. Ultimately, plasma volume may fall below normal in the late stages of hypertension. Another organ uniquely susceptible to autonomic overactivity is the kidney. As discussed in Chapter 3, the afferent arteriole is innervated by sympathetic nerve endings and stimulation of these nerves leads to renin release, which generates angiotensin II, which in turn raises the blood pressure. It is also possible, although not proven, that a low level of increased autonomic activity may lead to increased responsiveness of the renin–angiotensin system. Thus for any stimulus leading to increased renin release there will be augmented release and inappropriate elevations in blood pressure.

Increased sympathetic activity in certain hypertensives has been documented by the following: (1) increased circulating levels of catecholamines; (2) increased dopamine β-hydroxylase levels in some hypertensives; (3) blockage of the sympathetic nervous system is occasionally associated with a decrease in blood pressure; and (4) altered baroreceptor function, which usually lowers blood pressure, may allow for the maintenance of an elevated blood pressure. Unfortunately, documentation of these changes is scanty.

However, increased autonomic activity would affect neural end-plate activity more than circulating levels of epinephrine or norepinephrine.

E. Increased Vascular Resistance

The final common pathway leading to an increase in blood pressure is a rise in vascular resistance. If cardiac output increases and vascular resistance falls, blood pressure will be maintained within the normal range. If cardiac output remains constant but vascular resistance increases, hypertension will develop. Regardless of the initiating event, increased peripheral resistance is almost always present in the hypertensive patient (Figure 5). The mechanisms responsible for the increased resistance are not entirely clear. As discussed above, neurogenic factors may play a central role even though catecholamine levels are normal under most circumstances. When plasma volume is expanded peripheral vascular autoregulation will increase vascular resistance and thus increase blood pressure. The autoregulation is a normal control mechanism but when sustained it may lead to increased vascular resistance and hypertension. Another factor is vessel reactivity. Increased salt intake may lead to higher sodium and water content of the vessel wall. This may increase the binding to receptors of angiotensin II or neural hormones, leading to a greater increase in resistance for any given change in angiotensin II production. All of these factors probably play a role in the genesis of increased vascular resistance, which is the final common pathway responsible for the sustained increase in blood pressure in hypertension.

F. Other Factors

Other contributing factors in the development of hypertension include a genetic predisposition, race, and sex. It has been suggested that 50%–60% of the patients with essential hypertension have a genetic predisposition. If a patient is to become hypertensive he is more likely to reflect this trend by his fiftieth year. Furthermore, if a strong family history of hypertension is present, the individual is more likely to develop hypertension at an earlier age and at an incidence three- to fourfold greater than in the general population. While this information defines the risk it does not define the mechanism. Finally, blacks are more likely to develop hypertension and greater end-organ damage than whites. Males develop hypertension more frequently than premenopausal women. It is likely that environmental factors also play a role. Stress, if moderate to severe, may be an important contributing factor. Individuals with stressful jobs have a high incidence of hypertension. On the other hand, individuals living in isolated, nonstressful communities have a low incidence of hypertension. It is likely that increased sympathetic nervous activity induced by stress leads to hypertension. Thus,

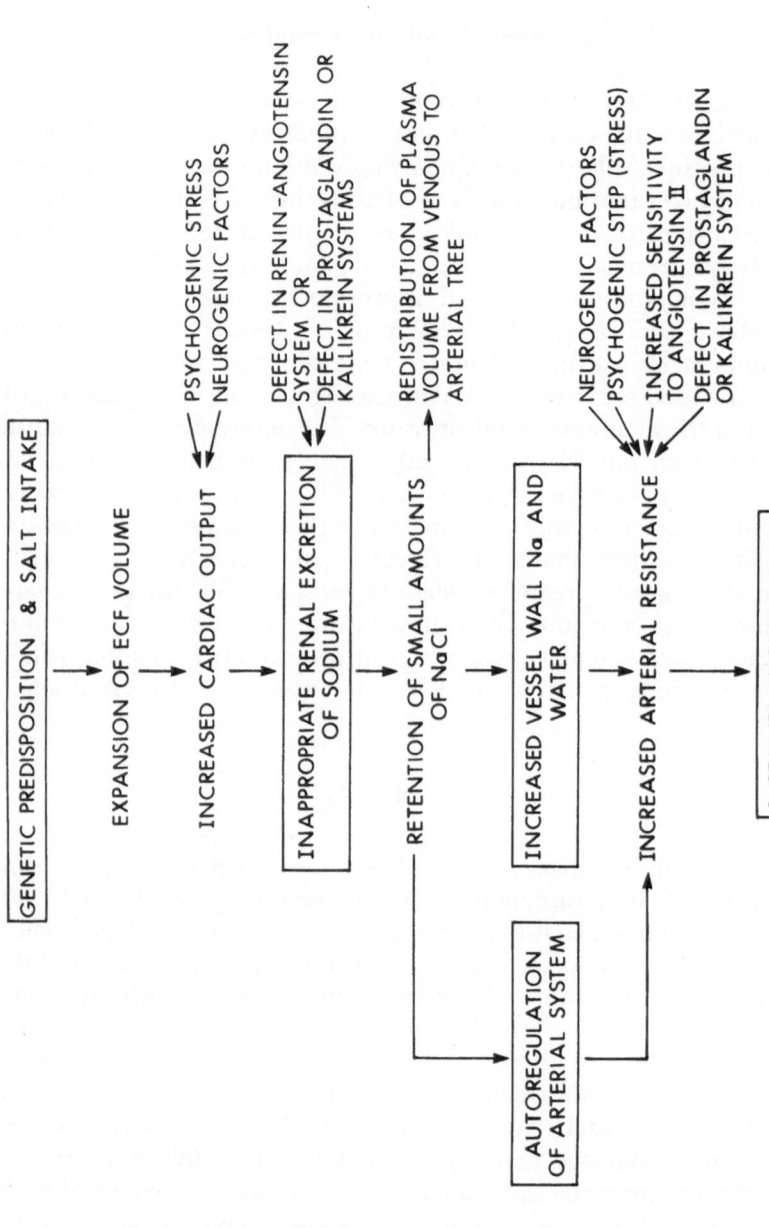

Figure 5. A composite sequence of events leading to the hypertensive state.

the incidence of essential hypertension may increase simply due to emotional and environmental factors.

In summary, essential hypertension is a common syndrome without a documented specific cause. Most certainly genetic predisposition, environmental factors, and dietary sodium intake play a role in its development. Sodium and water retention occurs, which expands the extracellular fluid volume, thus increasing cardiac output. Under normal circumstances increased renal excretion of salt and water should follow. The fact that this does not occur may reflect a defect in the renin–angiotensin system. At any rate, vascular autoregulation occurs which increases peripheral resistance. The retained salt and water and presumed increased vessel wall sodium enhances angiotensin II effects, further augmenting the hypertensive response. This enhanced vascular sensitivity may also sustain the hypertension under conditions of stress where catecholamine levels are elevated. The net effect of these changes is an elevation in blood pressure, which will continue to rise as vascular damage, especially to the kidney, progresses. Figure 5 outlines a possible sequence of pathogenetic mechanisms responsible for the development of essential hypertension. It must be remembered that part of this sequence of events has not been definitely established.

III. SECONDARY CAUSES OF HYPERTENSION

A. Hypertension Associated with Renal Insufficiency

Although renal disease (nephrosclerosis) is often the consequence of hypertension and not the cause of it, renal impairment is the most common cause of secondary hypertension. Furthermore, the kidney is also one of the target organs of hypertension, which may accelerate the rate of decrease in renal function produced by the original renal lesion. The pathogenetic mechanisms responsible for hypertension in patients with renal insufficiency are difficult to ascertain. It is known that patients with certain renal diseases, and some forms of chronic glomerulonephritis, are more prone to develop hypertension. Other renal diseases (certain forms of hereditary nephritis such as Alport's syndrome, pyelonephritis, and interstitial nephritis such as that induced by analgesic abuse) are less likely to lead to hypertension or if it occurs, it is mild. This separation, however, does not help to define the pathogenetic mechanisms responsible for the hypertension in patients with chronic renal insufficiency. With the advent of hemodialysis for the treatment of uremia, the types of hypertension in renal insufficiency have been clarified. Three general types exist: (1) volume-dependent hypertension, (2) volume-independent hypertension, and (3) high renin hypertension. Although careful studies have not been performed in a uremic population prior to dialysis, it is likely that these same three types of hypertension also exist in this population.

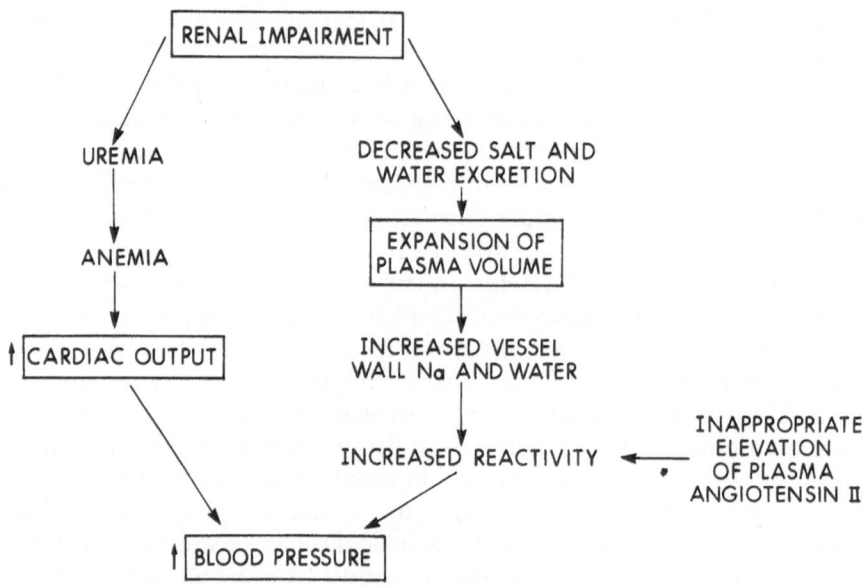

Figure 6. Volume-dependent hypertension in renal failure.

1. Volume-Dependent Hypertension (Figure 6)

The major factor responsible for hypertension in chronic renal insufficiency is an expanded ECF volume. About 80%–90% of the patients demonstrate this finding. Regardless of the etiology, as renal disease progresses and nephron mass decreases, the amount of salt excreted by each surviving nephron must increase in order to maintain salt balance (see Chapter 14). As the disease progresses there is a further decrease in the amount of salt that a patient with renal impairment can excrete. Thus, if a patient with modest renal impairment has an excessive salt intake, a transient increase in ECF volume may occur. Cardiac output will increase, leading to arterial autoregulation and hypertension. This type of hypertension would require plasma volume to be increased, and plasma renin levels to be normal or low. Reduction of salt intake and the use of diuretics should cause a return of blood pressure to normal levels. These findings have been documented in hypertensive subjects with mild to moderate renal insufficiency, severe renal insufficiency, and in hemodialysis patients.

Several other factors may play a role. In uremia, vessel wall sodium and water content may increase, leading to increased reactivity of the arterial tree. Also plasma renin levels are often normal in these patients. Theoretically, with ECF volume expansion renin levels should be low. Thus, despite being within normal limits, the renin levels may be inappropriately elevated for the degree of ECF volume expansion. A final factor which may contribute to the hypertension of uremia is an increased cardiac output which may be due to anemia, uremia itself, and/or the arteriovenous fistula created before hemodialysis is started.

2. Volume-Independent Hypertension (Figure 7)

A second form, volume-independent hypertension, affects approximately 5%–10% of hypertensive patients with renal impairment. In these patients, reduction of ECF volume does not return blood pressure to normal. Plasma renin levels are normal, although slightly higher than those described in the volume responsive group of patients. The pathogenetic mechanisms responsible for hypertension in these patients remain speculative. A defect in autonomic regulation has been suggested. An augmented sympathetic activity may exist, causing an increase in cardiac output and in total peripheral resistance. Use of β blockade (propranolol) may return the blood pressure to normal in these patients, suggesting that the renin–angiotensin system may play a critical role in the genesis of this form of hypertension. On the other hand, deficiency of vasodepressor substances such as prostaglandins or kinins has not been excluded.

3. High-Renin Hypertension

The third type seen in about 5%–10% of hypertensive patients with chronic renal impairment is high-renin hypertension. It appears more frequently in individuals with nephrosclerosis or vasculitis. The presumed mechanism relates to chronic renal ischemia, augmented renin release, elevated angiotensin II levels, and sustained, often refractory, hypertension. These patients do not respond to a reduction in plasma volume and occasionally are actually volume depleted when initially seen. Also, they may become more hypertensive as plasma volume is reduced by diuresis or dialysis. This presumably reflects a further decrease in plasma volume with reduced renal perfusion, further ischemia, and markedly increased renin release. These patients have also been shown to have severe secondary hyperaldosteronism. In many respects these patients are similar to those with malignant hypertension and normal renal function, which will be discussed

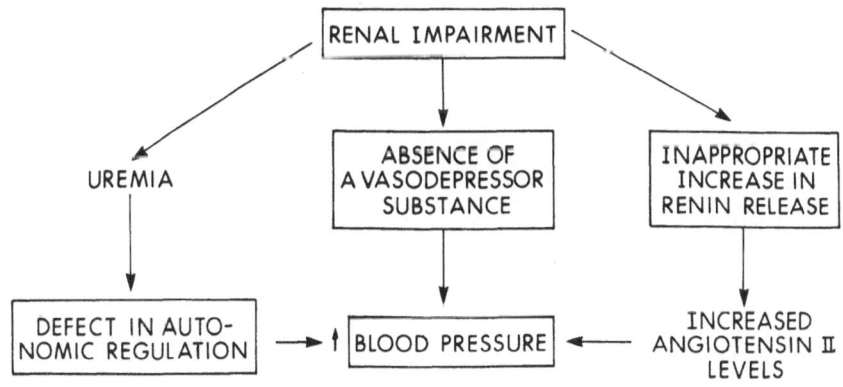

Figure 7. Volume-independent hypertension in renal failure.

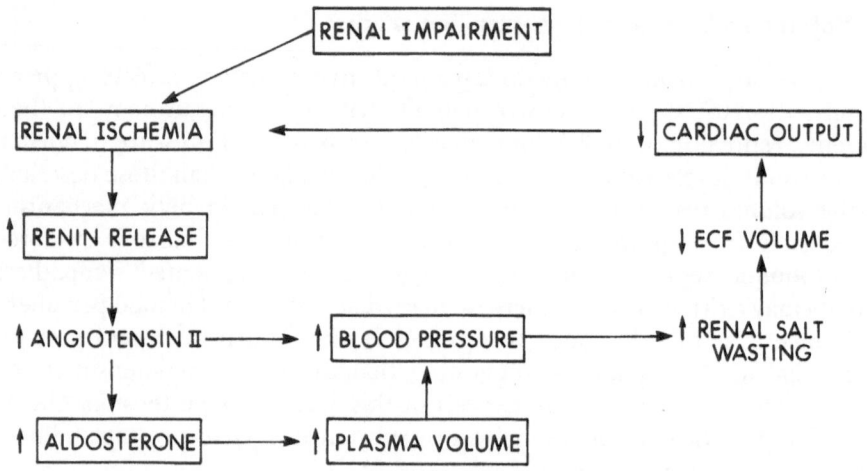

Figure 8. High-renin hypertension in renal failure.

later in this chapter. Figure 8 outlines the presumed sequence of events leading to hypertension in these patients.

It must be remembered that hypertension in patients with renal impairment is multifactorial. To break the causes down into three groups is probably artificial, but at the present time this scheme reflects the extent of our knowledge in this area.

4. Renal Artery Stenosis

Renal artery stenosis is the cause of hypertension in 1% of hypertensive patients. Renal artery stenosis itself is a common finding, especially in the aged and in diabetics as many of these patients have some form of renal artery stenosis. Usually, however, the stenosis is associated with but is not the cause of the hypertension, and surgical correction is rarely associated with reduction in blood pressure. The usual lesions causing renal artery stenosis

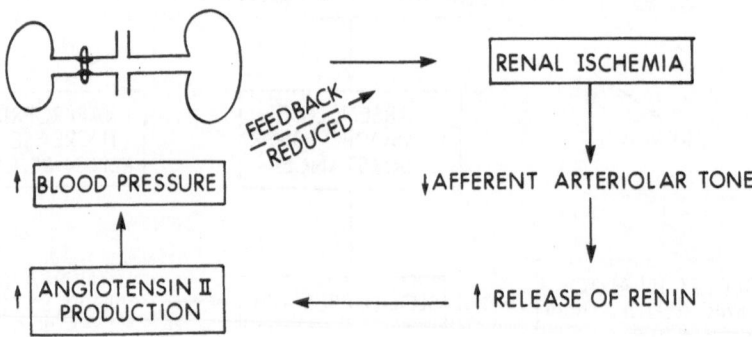

Figure 9. The first stage of hypertension in renal artery stenosis.

significant enough to induce hypertension are atherosclerotic plaques and fibromuscular hyperplasia. Atherosclerotic plaques, which account for 70%–80% of the stenoses, usually involve the proximal one third of the renal artery and are frequently unilateral. The majority of stenoses caused by fibromuscular hyperplasia involve the middle one third of the renal artery are frequently bilateral and most commonly occur in women. The hyperplasia may be intimal, medial, or adventitial. Other conditions, such as arteritis or extrinsic compression, may be associated with arterial stenosis and hypertension.

The mechanisms responsible for the hypertension in this condition are reasonably well understood. If a stenosis of the renal artery greater than 70% is induced by a ligature, immediate hypertension occurs. This initial response is due to augmented renin release as a consequence of renal ischemia. The potential mechanisms are outlined in Figure 9. Once the blood pressure rises, the ischemia is alleviated, renin release falls, but hypertension persists. This so-called "second phase" is characterized by increased angiotensin II vascular sensitivity. Thus, for any angiotensin II level, an augmented hypertensive response is seen. However, the steady state levels of renin remain higher than expected for the degree of blood pressure elevation. Also, plasma volume may be modestly increased. Figure 10 outlines the possible sequence of events. Sustained hypertension with inappropriately elevated plasma levels of renin (and presumably angiotensin II production) and a modestly expanded blood volume leads to vascular damage (nephrosclerosis) and impairment of renal function on the contralateral side. As vascular damage progresses in the contralateral (unprotected) kidney, renin no longer plays the major role. At this point, sodium retention and volume expansion are the main events responsible for sustained hypertension ("third stage") (Figure 11). At this stage, surgical correction of the stenotic lesion is usually not associated with amelioration of the hypertension.

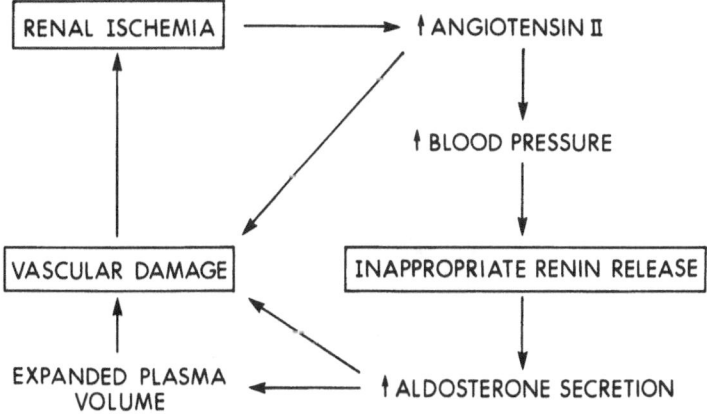

Figure 10. The second stage of hypertension in renal artery stenosis.

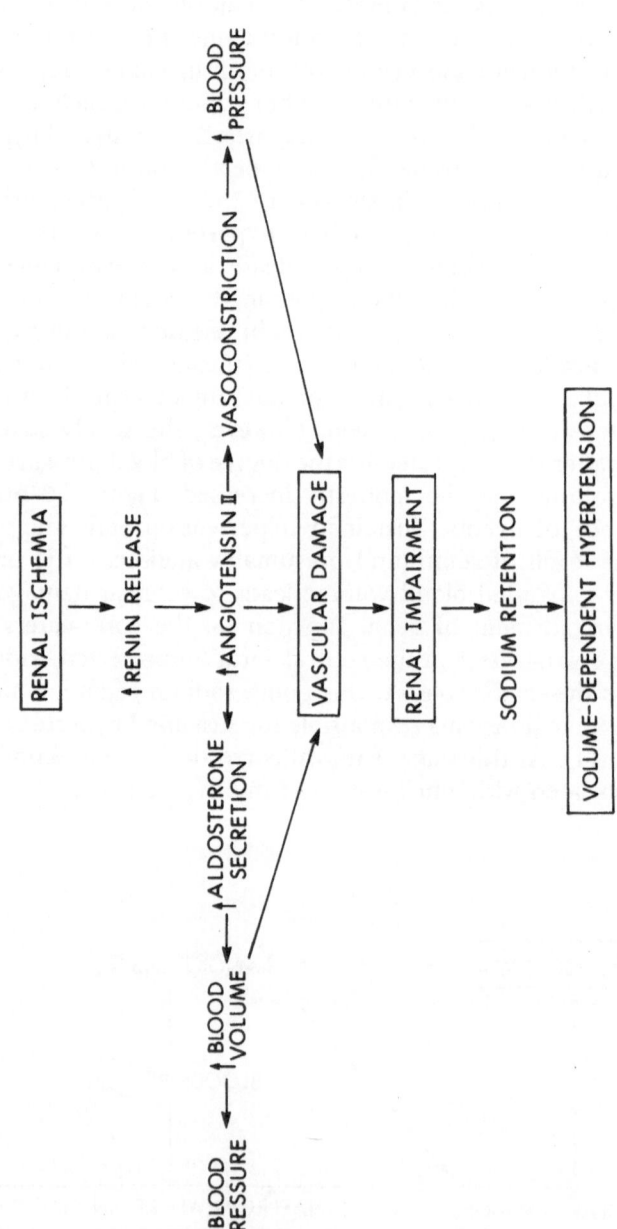

Figure 11. The third stage of hypertension in renal artery stenosis.

B. Hypertension Associated with Endocrine Abnormalities

1. Abnormalities in Secretion of Aldosterone or Other Mineralocorticoid Hormones

Primary hyperaldosteronism is a syndrome caused by excessive (not under normal feedback control) release of aldosterone. This syndrome probably is the cause of hypertension in less than 1% of all hypertensives and may be due to an adrenal adenoma involving the zona glomerulosa or to diffuse bilateral adrenal hyperplasia. Adenomas are from two- to sixfold more common than hyperplasia and are frequently unilateral. The exact cause for the increased release of aldosterone and the etiology of the adenomas or hyperplasia are unknown. Usually, the patient with bilateral adrenal hyperplasia has less severe hypertension, less severe hypokalemic alkalosis, and does not respond as well to adrenalectomy as the patient with an adenoma. Unfortunately, this is not a hard and fast rule and variable presentations can be seen with both adenomas and hyperplasia.

The initial event is an excess production of aldosterone which will lead to renal sodium retention and expansion of the ECF volume. Expansion will progress to a given level and then stabilize at which point sodium balance is maintained at an expanded ECF volume level. This "escape" phenomenon is due to natriuretic factors which cause the enhanced sodium excretion. Volume expansion is associated with arterial autoregulation, increased reactivity of the vessel wall, and increased blood pressure. The hypertension of primary hyperaldosteronism may be severe but usually diastolic blood pressures over 120 mm Hg are uncommon. As outlined previously, increased ECF volume and the rise in blood pressure suppress renin release.

The other effect of excessive aldosterone production is the development of hypokalemia due to increased renal tubular secretion of potassium. Thus plasma levels of potassium will fall. A secondary effect of this hypokalemia is the generation of a metabolic alkalosis. As potassium is lost in the urine, the total body potassium falls. To maintain electroneutrality, hydrogen and sodium ions will move into the intracellular space, leaving unbuffered bicarbonate in the plasma (alkalosis). More importantly, aldosterone will continue to promote sodium reabsorption from tubular fluid. As cellular levels of potassium fall, hydrogen will preferentially be lost into the urine to maintain electroneutrality as sodium is reabsorbed. Furthermore, aldosterone directly stimulates hydrogen secretion into the tubular fluid. As this hydrogen is lost and is buffered by ammonia or phosphate, new bicarbonate is generated, leading to the metabolic alkalosis.

Thus patients with primary hyperaldosteronism will have increased plasma levels of aldosterone, an expanded ECF volume, low or undetectable levels of plasma renin, metabolic alkalosis, and hypertension (see Figure 12). It should be noted that not all patients with primary hyperaldosteronism, elevated plasma aldosterone levels, and hypertension are hypokalemic. This may be due to somewhat lower plasma aldosterone levels, greater potassium

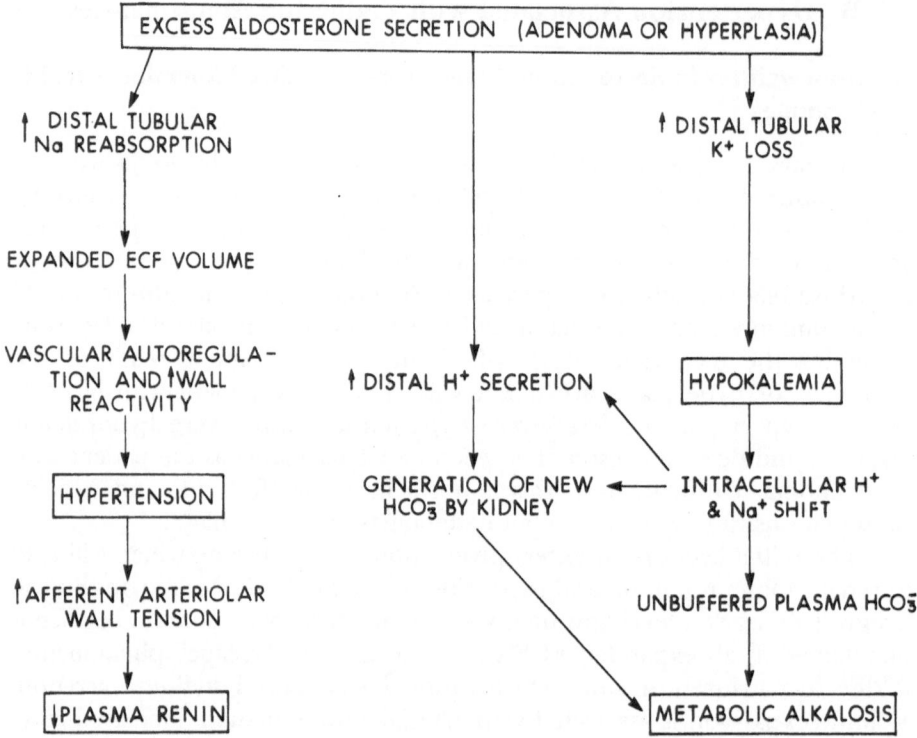

Figure 12. The systemic effects of excess mineralocorticoid activity.

intake, or decreased salt intake. Also, some patients with hypokalemic metabolic alkalosis and hypertension may have normal aldosterone levels owing to the effect of hypokalemia on aldosterone secretion. Some of these patients may secrete a mineralocorticoid different from aldosterone such as corticosterone or 18-hydroxy-deoxycorticosterone (18-OH-DOC) which may be responsible for the syndrome (consult a textbook on endocrinology— e.g., Williams—for a more detailed discussion).

2. Pheochromocytoma

The pheochromocytoma is a tumor, usually benign, of the chromaffin cells of the adrenal medulla or sympathetic chain. The chromaffin cells synthesize catecholamines (usually epinephrine) from tyrosine as depicted in Figure 13. Under conditions of stress, anesthesia, or the like, excessive amounts of norepinephrine and occasionally epinephrine are released into the plasma, causing severe elevations of blood pressure. This syndrome accounts for less than 1% of all hypertensive patients.

If epinephrine is released, which usually reflects an adrenal tumor, tachycardia with an increased cardiac output will lead to predominantly systolic hypertension. Sweating, flushing, and tremulousness also reflect epinephrine excess. When norepinephrine is predominantly secreted (usually from the adrenal medulla but occasionally from extra-adrenal sites such as the sympathetic chain), both diastolic and systolic hypertension occur. Intermittent release of the catecholamines due to stress, trauma, or anesthesia, causes paroxysmal hypertension, but sustained hypertension is seen in 50% of the cases. A syndrome resembling pheochromocytoma may also be induced in patients ingesting excess tyramine (from certain cheeses and imported chianti wine) and receiving monoamine oxidase inhibitors.

3. Disturbances in Thyroid Function

Thyrotoxicosis is frequently associated with systolic hypertension. The mechanism of hypertension is most likely due to the effects of thyroid hormone on cardiac function. Thyroxine and free T_3 both increase pulse rate (chronotropic effect) and force of ventricular contraction (ionotropic effect). This leads to increased cardiac output and hence systolic hypertension. Total peripheral vascular resistance is normal or low and blood volume usually is normal or slightly decreased. Hypothyroidism has the opposite effect. Lower thyroxine or T_3 levels decrease pulse rate and force of contraction, leading to a fall in systolic blood pressure. Total peripheral resistance rises by unknown mechanisms, causing an increase in diastolic blood pressure. Plasma volume may be normal or increased. The net effect is a narrow pulse pressure with diastolic hypertension.

4. Acromegaly

Excess growth hormone production in the adult leads to acromegaly. Organomegaly occurs with increased kidney and cardiac size. Cardiac output increases because of an increased stroke volume. Plasma volume is moderately expanded. The hypertension is mild but both systolic and diastolic hypertension are present.

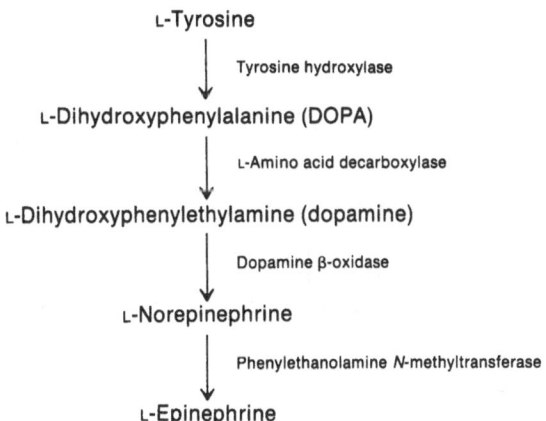

Figure 13. The enzymatic steps in the production of epinephrine.

IV. LOW-RENIN HYPERTENSION

Somewhere between 17% and 45% of all hypertensive patients will have low plasma renin activity (PRA). This may be an appropriate response by a kidney subjected to increased perfusion pressure. Several other factors must be considered when interpreting renin values. Renin levels decrease with age and thus hypertension in a 60-year-old male is most often related to increased volume. Nephrosclerosis may reduce afferent arteriolar responsiveness leading to low PRA. Blacks have lower PRA values than whites, and premenopausal women lower values than men. Diabetics may have low values owing to decreased autonomic activity and altered afferent arteriolar responsiveness. Patients with pyelonephritis may also have low PRA owing presumably to altered renal responsiveness.

Most of the patients with hypertension and low PRA do not have one of the above contributing factors. The most likely explanation for reduced PRA in hypertension is an expanded plasma volume (see above). The causes responsible for an expanded volume may be many. The most plausible mechanism would be increased mineralocorticoid activity. Thus patients with primary hyperaldosteronism would fit this picture. Many patients do not have increased aldosterone levels, and other metabolites such as deoxycorticosterone or 18-OH-DOC have been implicated. Unfortunately these

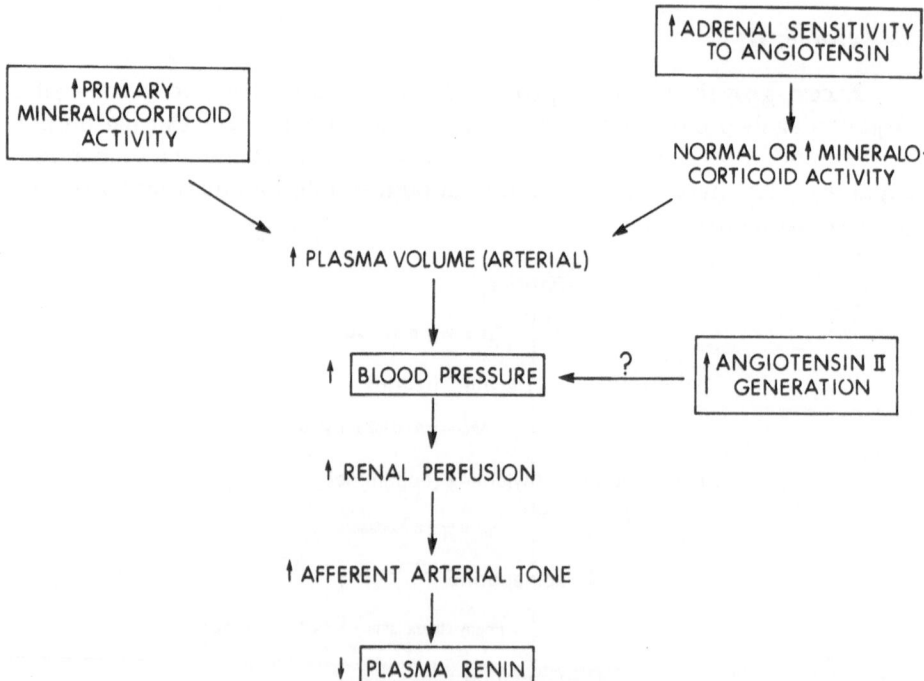

Figure 14. The possible mechanisms responsible for the production of low-renin hypertension.

compounds have weak mineralocorticoid activity and invoking them as a cause for low PRA is still debatable.

Furthermore, plasma volume measurements in patients with low PRA have been normal. This of course does not exclude a shift in the volume distribution of the ECF from the venous to the arterial system. While plasma volumes may be normal in these patients, they respond to a salt load with an exaggerated natriuresis, suggesting an expanded arterial system. Also, they often respond to aldosterone antagonists with a natriuresis and a drop in blood pressure. One of the reasons for implicating aldosterone is the fact that the levels are normal despite low PRA. One would expect the aldosterone values to be low. Recent data suggest that increased adrenal sensitivity to angiotensin II exists in at least some of these patients. Thus more aldosterone is secreted for any angiotensin II stimulus, leading to mild volume expansion (arterial) with low PRA and normal aldosterone levels. Also, increased angiotensin II generation for a given renin stimulus may be a potential mechanism responsible for low PRA but data are lacking to confirm this hypothesis. The relative contribution of each of these factors is still not resolved. The possible sequence of events leading to low levels of plasma renin is outlined in Figure 14.

V. HIGH-RENIN HYPERTENSION

A variable percentage of patients will have hypertension associated with elevated levels of plasma renin. Usually these patients have progressive hypertension with renal impairment, excluding, of course, renal artery stenosis. Pathologic studies have demonstrated that most patients with high-renin hypertension have changes on renal biopsy, including nephrosclerosis, interstitial nephritis, glomerulonephritis, or pyelonephritis. Over 40% of the patients have nephrosclerosis. As few as 1% and as many as 5% of the hypertensive population will have an accelerated course typified by high-renin hypertension.

From a pathophysiologic point of view, high-renin hypertension occurs because of vascular damage and renal ischemia. If hypertension is poorly controlled it may progress into an "accelerated phase." This is defined as a diastolic blood pressure of 120 mm Hg or greater with hemorrhage and exudates on funduscopic examination. This accelerated phase rapidly progresses into a malignant phase with diastolic blood pressures over 120 mm Hg, papilledema on funduscopic examination, and, usually, proteinuria (see Figure 8).

As hypertension progresses, vascular damage occurs with renal ischemia and increased renin release. Renin stimulates angiotensin II production, which increases blood pressure and promotes aldosterone secretion. This secondary hyperaldosteronism leads to sodium retention, expansion of the ECF volume, and a further rise in blood pressure. Under normal circumstances as perfusion pressure to the kidney increases, renin release decreases. However, because of vascular damage the plasma renin levels remain modestly elevated and rise progressively as vascular damage and renal ischemia progress. Ultimately, the patient presents with severe malignant hypertension. Several important facts are known. First, plasma renin levels are very high in these patients. Second, aldosterone levels are extremely elevated, indicating severe secondary hyperaldosteonism. Third, angiotensin II infusion in these patients is associated with a minimal or absent pressor response, indicating saturation of angiotensin II binding sites in these patients. Also, therapy with angiotensin II blockers (saralasin) induces a prompt reduction in blood pressure. Since the kidney is the target organ in malignant hypertension, early detection and treatment are critical to prevent further renal impairment.

VI. MECHANISMS OF VASCULAR DAMAGE SECONDARY TO HYPERTENSION

One of the most important aspects of accelerated hypertension is the associated vascular damage that occurs in this disease state. While the kidney is the primary target organ and its damage leads to progressive azotemia, the microvasculature in general is affected, including the retinal vessels, pancreas, spleen, and so forth. The events responsible for vascular damage have been well characterized and two main mechanisms postulated. Figure 15 outlines a scheme where renin and more probably angiotensin II is a vascular toxin that is potentiated if aldosterone is present. This toxic effect significantly damages the intima of vessels, allowing for exudation of plasma proteins as

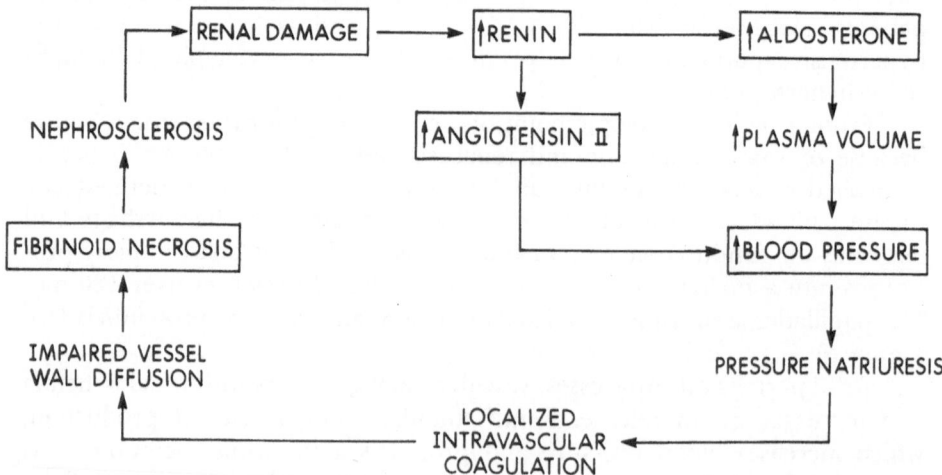

Figure 15. The proposed sequence of events leading to vascular damage secondary to elevated anigotensin II levels.

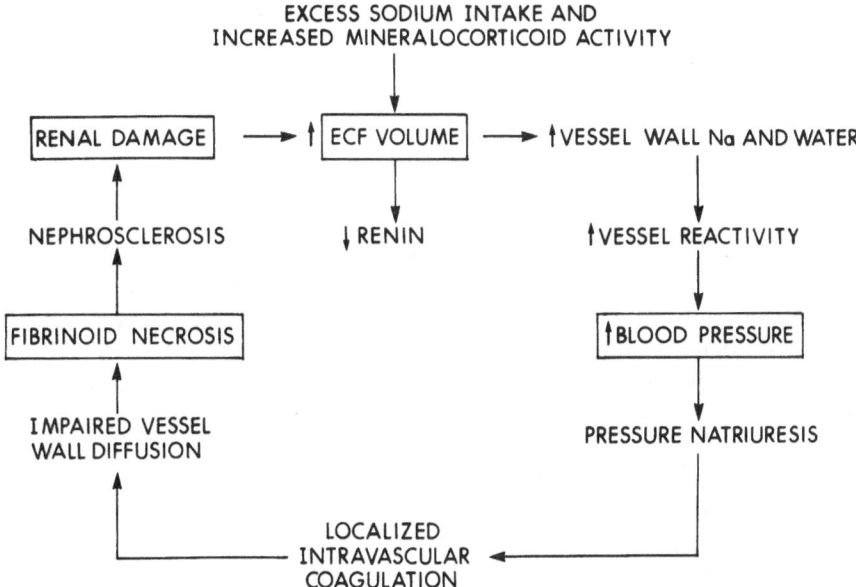

Figure 16. The proposed sequence of events leading to vascular damage secondary to an increase in blood pressure.

well as red cells, and may explain the funduscopic changes seen in these patients (hemorrhage, exudates, and papilledema). While there is little doubt that angiotensin and aldosterone may be vascular toxins, at least in experimental animals, the exact mechanism responsible for the damage is unclear. Localized intravascular coagulation induced by angiotensin, changes in plasma viscosity, or the pressure itself may trigger the process. It is likely that localized intravascular coagulation plays some role since experimentally it has been shown that heparinization will prevent the pathologic change induced by hypertension within the rat kidney. At any rate, fibrinoid necrosis occurs which leads to nephrosclerosis and further renal damage. A vicious cycle is started which will rapidly lead to renal failure unless antihypertensive therapy is instituted.

A second mechanism (Figure 16) has also been proposed. This theory states that the pressure itself is enough to cause the vascular damage. In this model, hypertension is induced in rats by excessive salt intake along with the administration of deoxycorticosterone acetate (a mineralocorticoid). Volume expansion occurs, which leads to hypertension and a pressure natriuresis. Localized intravascular coagulation is again felt to occur, which leads to fibrinoid necrosis, nephrosclerosis, and renal damage, initiating the cycle which ultimately culminates in malignant hypertension. Note that at least early in the course, angiotensin II and renin levels are suppressed. In this model the major vascular toxins appear to be the blood pressure, sodium, and possibly aldosterone. While either one of these two mechanisms may be involved, it is likely that both play some role in all patients during their course to malignant hypertension.

VII. THERAPEUTIC CONSIDERATIONS IN THE HYPERTENSIVE PATIENT

The treatment of hypertension depends, at least in part, on the type of hypertension the patient manifests. Since this chapter emphasizes general pathophysiologic mechanisms, only brief diagnostic information is included. The reader is referred to several texts which outline the diagnostic considerations in the hypertensive patient. The purpose of this section is to acquaint the reader with the general classification of antihypertensive drugs, their proposed modes of action, and their potential therapeutic application to the hypertensive patient. As stated earlier in this chapter, several studies have clearly defined the benefits of therapy in the hypertensive population. In general, strict blood pressure control is the ultimate goal of therapy, and blood pressures between 120/80 and 140/90 mm Hg should be achieved. The number of agents available today is large and is outlined in Table III. We will review each group separately.

Table III. Classification of Antihypertensive Drugs

I. Diuretics
   A. Thiazides and related compounds
   B. Furosemide and ethacrynic acid
   C. Spironolactone and triamterene
II. Drugs affecting the sympathetic nervous system
   A. Peripheral adrenergic blockers
      1. Reserpine
      2. Quanethidine
   B. Central adrenergic blockers
      1. Methyldopa
      2. Clonidine
   C. Peripheral β-adrenergic blockers
      1. Propranolol
      2. New β-blocking agents
   D. Peripheral α-adrenergic blockers
      1. Phentolamine
      2. Phenoxybenzamine
      3. Prazosin
III. Peripheral direct vasodilators
   A. Hydralazine
   B. Diazoxide
   C. Minoxidil
   D. Nitroprusside

A. Diuretics

In general, *thiazides* are the diuretics most commonly used to treat hypertension. These drugs include short-acting agents such as chlorothiazide or hydrochlorothiazide and long-acting agents such as chlorothalidone or polythiazide. Their mechanism of action as antihypertensive agents is still controversial.

As diuretics, thiazides exert their effects in the cortical diluting segment of the distal nephron (see Chapter 17). A moderate diuresis can be produced by maximal dosages of the selected agent. Their antihypertensive effects are probably related to (1) reduction of extracellular fluid and plasma volume, (2) reduction of vessel wall sodium and calcium, leading to a reduction in receptor binding for vasoactive substances, (3) direct arteriolar dilatation, and (4) reduction in renal vascular resistance.

The indications for the use of a diuretic as a primary or adjunctive therapeutic agent are listed below:

1. As a primary antihypertensive agent in mild hypertension.
2. As a combination with other agents to enhance their antihypertensive effects.
3. To reduce the sodium retention produced by vasodilator antihypertensive agents.
4. To reduce edema in patients who have the nephrotic syndrome, cirrhosis, or heart failure as well as hypertension.

Thiazide diuretics should not be used if the patient is allergic to sulfanimide derivatives or if severe oliguria is present. Thiazides are the drug of choice in mild hypertension (140/90–160/100 mm Hg on repeated examinations). Patients with more severe hypertension will usually require adjunctive therapy as outlined below.

Complications of the use of thiazide diuretics include (1) hypokalemia, (2) hyperuricemia, (3) progressive azotemia, (4) hyperglycemia, (5) hyponatremia, and (6) hypercalcemia.

The incidence of the above complications vary and relate in part to ancillary medical conditions present in the hypertensive patient, the duration of therapy and the dosage of the agent used.

There are other diuretic agents which can be used in hypertension. *Furosemide* is a diuretic chemically similar to the thiazides but considerably more potent. It acts primarily on the thick ascending limb of Henle's loop. The efficacy of furosemide alone as an antihypertensive agent is less than that of thiazides. As such it probably should not be used as a sole therapy in mild essential hypertension. The use of potent diuretics such as furosemide or ethacrynic acid should be considered (1) to reduce the sodium retention produced by potent vasodilator agents, (2) to induce natriuresis in patients with severe hypertension requiring the use of parenteral vasodilator agents (i.e., diazoxide in the therapy of malignant hypertension), or (3) as adjunctive therapy in patients with renal impairment if sodium retention has occurred secondary to the therapy of hypertension or due to the renal disease itself.

Complications of furosemide therapy include (1) hyponatremia, (2) hypokalemia and metabolic alkalosis, (3) hyperuricemia, (4) hyperglycemia, and (5) volume depletion with transient azotemia and hypotension.

Because diuretic therapy frequently leads to kaliuresis and hypokalemia, potassium-retaining drugs may be useful. In this country, two agents are available: triamterene and spironolactone. Since these agents are mild diuretics at best, they are usually used in conjunction with other diuretics rather than as the sole therapy.

Triamterene prevents potassium wasting by inhibiting sodium–potassium exchange in the distal tubule (see Chapter 7). It is a weak diuretic which can prevent potassium wasting during diuretic therapy in patients most prone to potassium wasting i.e., secondary hyperaldosteronism (patients with nephrotic syndrome, cirrhosis with ascites, and with severe right-sided heart failure). Caution should be used when administering this drug since fatal hyperkalemia may occur. Triamterene should not be used in patients with diabetes mellitus and signs of renal impairment since they are prone to hyporeninemic hypoaldosteronism and hyperkalemia, or in patients with progressive renal or hepatic disease.

Side effects of triamterene therapy include (1) hyperkalemia, (2) hyperuricemia, (3) hyperglycemia, and (4) elevations in blood urea nitrogen.

The other potassium-sparing agent is a competitive inhibitor of aldosterone and thus inhibits sodium–potassium exchange in the distal tubule. It is most effective in patients with primary or secondary hyperaldosteronism. *Spironolactone* may reduce blood pressure in these patients but is most effective in minimizing potassium wasting induced by other diuretics. Its side effects include (1) hyperkalemia, (2) gastrointestinal symptoms (nausea, vomiting, diarrhea), (3) gynecomastia, (4) amenorrhea, and (5) impotence.

The most common complication is hyperkalemia. While fatal hyperkalemia is rare, careful clinical evaluation is necessary. The risk of severe hyperkalemia in patients with hyporeninemic hypoaldosteronism (diabetes mellitus or interstitial nephritis with azotemia) does not exist with this agent as it does with triamterene.

B. Drugs Affecting the Sympathetic Nervous System

1. Peripheral Adrenergic Blockers

Reserpine is the most frequently utilized peripheral sympathetic blocker. It depletes stores of catecholamines and 5-hydroxytryptamine in many organs including the brain, smooth muscle, and adrenergic nerve endings. It inhibits the uptake of dopamine by chromaffin granules which may be its major effect as an antihypertensive agent. Reserpine is indicated in the treatment of mild hypertension or in combination with other agents such as a diuretic or vasodilator in more severe hypertension. It may also be utilized parenterally for the treatment of hypertensive emergencies especially malignant hypertension or in patients with hypertension associated with a dissecting aortic aneurysm.

Side effects occur frequently when this agent is used and include depression, sedation, weakness, nasal congestion, increased appetite, nightmares, palpitations and arrhythmias, diarrhea, dyspnea, and bronchospasm. While this agent may be effective in the treatment of many forms of hypertension, the frequency of side effects has reduced its effectiveness because of noncompliance.

Guanethidine, a guanidine derivative, produces hypotension by blockade of the adrenergic neuron. It has a selective effect on the peripheral sympathetic neurons depleting nerve endings and the myocardium of catecholamines. The adrenal medulla is not affected by this agent. Depletion of catecholamines results in decreased arterial vasoconstriction and a reduction in blood pressure. The drug is indicated in patients with severe hypertension and is usually used in association with a diuretic. Guanethidine is contraindicated in patients with a pheochromocytoma or in those patients with a known hypersensitivity to this agent. It should not be used in patients with congestive failure who are not hypertensive or in those patients receiving monoamine oxidase inhibitors since a malignant phase of hypertension may develop. Guanethidine is contraindicated in patients with moderate to severe renal damage since it reduces the glomerular filtration rate and renal blood flow. The side effects of this agent include dizziness, congestive heart failure, bradycardia with or without atrioventricular block, hypotension and shock, occasional diarrhea, lethargy and somnolence with a dry mouth, urinary retention, sexual dysfunction including impotence and decreased libido, and sodium retention with edema.

In general, guanethidine is utilized on a one time per day dosage and is reserved for those patients who are not responsive to other agents. It is most often used in conjunction with a diuretic because of its sodium-retaining characteristics. The side effects of guanethidine are frequent, thus reducing its effectiveness because of noncompliance.

2. Central Adrenergic Blockers

Methyldopa is a frequently used antihypertensive agent. It is a synthetic phenylalanine derivative of methyldopa which produces its effect most likely through central mechanisms. Initially the drug was felt to produce a false neurotransmitter (L-methyl norepinephrine) thus blocking the peripheral effects of norepinephrine. It has recently been demonstrated that the metabolic by-product of methyldopa metabolism, L-methyl norepinephrine in fact, stimulates central adrenergic receptors, but produces peripheral α-adrenergic blockade thus reducing peripheral resistance. Other potential antihypertensive effects of methyldopa include a reduction in cardiac output and renin release.

Methyldopa is indicated for all classes of hypertension. In low doses it can be very effective in the treatment of mild-to-moderate hypertension. Higher doses can be used for moderate-to-severe hypertension in conjunction with other agents. Because it reduces peripheral vascular resistance, sodium retention may occur and the antihypertensive effect may be potentiated with the use of a diuretic. Methyldopa is indicated in patients with renal impairment and hypertension since renal blood flow and GFR are not decreased by the drug and may be increased in some cases.

Methyldopa should not be given to patients with hepatitis or cirrhosis or to patients with known hypersensitivity to the drug. Side effects of methyldopa include sedation, somnolence, fatigue, dizziness, dry mouth, headache, and sometimes depression. Impotence may be a frequent problem and is seen in as many as 10% of the patients receiving this agent. As many as 20% of patients receiving methyldopa will develop a positive direct Coombs test but hemolytic anemia is uncommon.

Clonidine is an imidazoline derivative which can be utilized to treat many hypertensive patients who are refractory to other agents. It is a central α-adrenergic stimulator presumably acting at the level of the medulla oblongata, thus decreasing sympathetic activity in this area. The net effect is to decrease the sympathetic outflow to the peripheral vasculature. The drug also significantly lowers plasma renin and aldosterone levels, which may contribute to its antihypertensive effects. Occasionally a decrease in cardiac output has also been described with this agent, but no change in exercise tolerance is seen.

Clonidine can be used as a single agent or in combination with a thiazide to treat all stages of hypertension. It may be also added to the regimen of patients previously treated with a vasodilator and a diuretic. The dosages for clonidine are quite wide and it can be given on a two time per day basis with effective control of blood pressure in most patients. Several side effects may occur with the use of clonidine. Sudden withdrawal of clonidine therapy has been associated with an acute elevation in blood pressure. This sudden increase in blood pressure is usually to the pretreatment levels although blood pressures significantly higher than pretreatment levels have been described. The incidence of this complication is probably less than 1%. It may be related to the unique mechanism of the drug through central α stimulation and thus peripheral α blockade. Sudden withdrawl of the agent leads to increased α outflow and thus a sudden increase in blood pressure. This so-called "withdrawal syndrome" is not unique to clonidine and has been described with methyldopa and propranolol. Other adverse reactions include drowsiness, sedation, and fatigue, which may be quite common. Also, dry mouth is seen in most patients initially but decreases with time. Constipation, dizziness, and vertigo have also been described. The patient may rarely develop congestive heart failure, angina pectoris, or a positive Coombs test.

3. Peripheral β-Adrenergic Blockers

The most commonly used β-adrenergic blocker is *propranolol*, which will be described as a prototype of these agents. Propranolol is chemically similar to isoproterenol except for a double (penthrene) ring and therefore competes with the β-adrenergic receptor stimulating agents for available β-receptor sites. As such, propranolol will reduce the chronotropic, ionotropic, and vasodilator responses to β-adrenergic stimulation. Its mechanism of action in hypertension is still debatable. Propranolol is a potent inhibitor of renin release and as such may reduce blood pressure in patients with high-renin hypertension by reducing renin release and therefore angiotensin II production. However, modest decreases in blood pressure may occur even in patients without significantly elevated plasma renin levels. The reduction in blood pressure in these patients may relate to a decrease in cardiac output, owing to suppressed ionotropic and chronotropic stimulation on myocardial function. It is probable that each of these effects plays a role in the antihypertensive action of propranolol.

Indications for use of these agents include the treatment of hyperkinetic hypertension especially in young adults who frequently present with tachycardia and increase in cardiac output. Propranolol may be added to a therapeutic regimen including a vasodilator and a diuretic as part of the so-called triple therapy in moderate or severe hypertension. Propranolol is particularly beneficial when used with a peripheral vasodilator like hydralazine since it blocks the reflex sympathetic activity of direct vasodilatation. Propranolol may be combined with a thiazide in patients who are unresponsive to thiazides alone, and finally it is specifically indicated in hyperreninemic hypertension because of its effects on suppressing renin release. Propranolol has other indications which must be kept in mind. It may be used for tachyarrhythmias in patients with angina pectoris to reduce heart rate and therefore decrease cardiac work, in patients with hypertrophic subaortic stenosis, or in patients with a pheochromocytoma who are also receiving α-blocking agents.

Propranolol is not a simple drug to use and there are certain absolute contraindications to its use. These include bronchial asthma, first degree AV block with sinus bradycardia, congestive heart failure unless the patient has an associated tachyarrhythmia, pulmonary hypertension with right ventricular failure, and allergic rhinitis. Complications of propranolol therapy are quite frequent and may be seen in as many as 10% of the treated population. Severe life-threatening reactions to propranolol have been described. These include hypotension, complete AV block, severe bradycardia with pulses of 40 or less, bronchospasm and acute respiratory distress, cardiac arrest, acute pulmonary edema, and congestive heart failure. Other complications include nausea, anorexia, and fatigue, confusion, vivid dreams, occasional depression, hypoglycemia, hyperosmolar coma, and impotence.

There are new β-blocking agents currently available and in general, their activities are very similar to propranolol. For instance, *sotalol* is unique in that it can be given once per day but its β-blocking activity is about one tenth that of propranolol. On the other hand, *practolol* is a cardioselective β-adrenergic blocking agent in that it is a predominantly β-1 receptor blocker. It has very little β-2 receptor blockade, thus it will significantly reduce the risk of bronchospasm. It must be remembered that any specific cardioselective β blocker, however, still has some bronchospastic characteristics. *Metoprolol* is very similar to practolol in that it is a β-1 receptor blocker agent. Other β-blocking agents such as *pindolol* have both β-1 and β-2 blocking activity but have particularly potent membrane-stabilizing characteristics. It must be remembered that these new β-blocking agents do not add significantly to the effects of the β blockade except that they may (1) be selective for β-1 receptors, (2) have more membrane-stabilizing activities, or (3) may be given once or twice per day rather than four times per day as is necessary with propranolol.

4. Peripheral α-Adrenergic Blockers

Two α-adrenergic blocking agents have been available for many years and these are *phentolamine* and *phenoxybenzamine*. They have received limited use in the treatment of hypertension because of significant side effects. Marked α-adrenergic inhibition is associated with weakness, fatigue, orthostatic hypotension, tachycardia, impotence, myosis, and nasal congestion. While phentolamine may be used as a diagnostic test for pheochromocytoma and is particularly helpful for the treatment of pheochromocytoma prior to surgery, its usefulness for other forms of hypertension is minimal. Thus, neither of these agents is recommended for the treatment of hypertension.

Prazosin is a quinazoline derivative which is an effective peripheral α-adrenergic blocking agent. Initially its mechanism of action was felt to occur through cyclic GMP generation and also possibly to vasodilatation peripherally. In fact, its most likely mechanism of action is as a postsynaptic α-adrenergic blocker. As such it produces vasodilatation without reflex tachycardia and no increase in renin release is seen.

Prazosin can be utilized as a single agent for the treatment of mild-to-moderate hypertension and may be effective on a twice daily dosage schedule. Care must be taken to initiate therapy at bedtime to obviate one of the more serious side effects, syncope. Prazosin can also be utilized with diuretic therapy for the control of moderate-to-severe hypertension. In severe hypertension, the use of a β blocker, a diuretic, and prazosin may be effective therapy. Because of its unique mechanism of action, prazosin will produce the peripheral vasodilatation seen with hydralazine without many of its side effects. Postural dizziness is seen frequently, although usually transiently with prazosin therapy. Palpitations and dyspnea may be seen on occasion. Rarely, headache, drowsiness, blurred vision, dry mouth, nausea, and vomiting are seen. More recent data would suggest that prazosin therapy may also be effective in congestive heart failure by reducing both preload and afterload since it is an arterial and venodilator. It would seem therefore that patients with hypertension and heart failure may be particularly good candidates for this form of therapy.

5. Peripheral Direct Vasodilators

Hydralazine is a direct vasodilator which produces its effect by interacting with sulfhydryl and carbonyl groups and also chelates certain metallic ions. Hydralazine is a phthalazine derivative whose activity requires a pyridazine ring. Hydralazine alone will reduce peripheral resistance by as much as 60%. While early studies suggested that there may be a decrease in sympathetic discharge, this contributes little to the net effect of reducing blood pressure. The major effect of hydralazine is the direct relaxation of smooth muscle. The areas affected are usually the vascular resistance vessels including the arteries and arterioles. There may be also a minimal reduction in resistance within the capacitance vessels. Recent evidence also suggests that the drug may be useful in the treatment of congestive heart failure by reducing afterload and in pulmonary hypertension by reducing pulmonary artery pressure. The major decrease in blood pressure seen with hydralazine is a reduction in the diastolic component. Because it is a direct vasodilator, reflex sympathetic activity may reduce its effectiveness by as much as 75%. There may be an increase in heart rate, an increase in force of ventricular contraction, an increase in plasma renin, and some sodium and water retention. All of these effects thus reduce the effectiveness of hydralazine when used alone and can be effectively counteracted by the use of β-blocking agents with or without diuretic therapy.

Hydralazine has many benefits and may be helpful in patients with congestive heart failure, renal impairment, or pulmonary hypertension. Furthermore, the drug does not reduce renal blood flow or glomerular filtration rate, so filtration fraction remains unchanged. The drug is contraindicated if there is known hypersensitivity to this agent, or in patients with coronary artery disease or mitral valvular rheumatic heart disease. Side effects of hydralazine therapy include headache, dizziness, nausea and vomiting, tachycardia and palpitations, occasional fatigue and lethargy, postural hypotension, anxiety, angina, and on rare occasions, the lupus syndrome.

In general hydralazine is indicated alone for treatment of mild hypertension and in combination with a diuretic or β blocker for moderate-to-severe hypertension.

Diazoxide is a potent vasodilator which is used exclusively in this country as an intravenous direct acting peripheral vasodilator agent in hypertensive crises. It is a benzothiadiazine derivative but does not have diuretic activity. Diazoxide is a potent antihypertensive agent and produces its effects by direct vasodilatation of peripheral arterioles. The primary mechanism of action appears to relate to an alteration in vascular calcium activity or content. Diazoxide is indicated in the use of hypertensive emergencies which were discussed earlier in this chapter. It is also indicated in cases with severe hypertension with impaired renal function and in certain forms of refractory hypertension in which oral agents have been ineffective. Diazoxide will significantly reduce mean arterial pressure but will also increase cardiac output due to an increase in sympathetic activity. Positive sodium balance may occur requiring the addition of a potent diuretic to enhance its effect. Thus it is recommended that both diazoxide and furosemide be given at the same time to produce maximal hypotensive effects. While diazoxide may be utilized for most types of hypertensive emergencies, certain contraindications for its use exist, including dissecting aortic aneurysm, hypertension with an acute myocardial infarction, or pulmonary edema, and hypertension with an intracerebral hemorrhage. It must also be remembered that diazoxide is not effective in patients with pheochromocytoma. The side effects of the use diazoxide are fluid retention, requiring the use of potent diuretic agents; hyperglycemia, which is usually transient; tachycardia, which may precipitate angina pectoris; hypotension; and very rarely, seizures and hypersensitivity reactions.

Minoxidil is a very potent antihypertensive agent which reduces blood pressure by direct arterial vasodilatation. It is a piperidinopyrimidine compound. While the exact mechanism of action is unknown, its effects are extremely potent and they last for as long as 12 hr, thus allowing for a twice daily dosage. Minoxidil is indicated for the treatment of refractory or severe hypertension and should not be used in mild-to-moderate hypertension or in severe hypertension that is responsive to other agents. Major side effects may occur with the use of this agent. Most notable is salt and water retention due primarily to the increase in renin release causing secondary hyperaldosteronism. Potent diuretics such as furosemide are required to control salt and water retention. Tachycardia is a frequent secondary effect of the sympathetic overactivity and may require the use of β blockade. Pericardial effusion and tamponade have been described in 3%–5% of the patients. The patients must be carefully followed for the presence of edema, occasional hypotension and the risk of pericardial effusion.

Sodium nitroprusside is the most potent antihypertensive agent available today. It is used exclusively as an intravenous product. Nitroprusside is a nitroso compound which produces its vasodilatory effect directly at the level of both the resistance and capacitance vessels. Of interest, little or no increase in heart rate is noted with the use of this compound. The drug is indicated for almost any form of hypertension and is essentially 100% effective. It is particularly helpful in all forms of hypertensive emergencies and since the degree of blood pressure reduction is dose dependent, titration is easily achieved with proper supervision. It is also effective in refractory congestive heart failure because of venodilatation, thus reducing preload, and because of arteriolar dilatation, thus reducing afterload. The major side effect of the use of this agent is hypotension. The patient must be carefully monitored and it is recommended that the drug be given with an automated pump and properly titrated. Thyocyanate, the by-product of nitroprusside metabolism, has occasionally been associated with toxicity but this is quite uncommon and is usually seen only in patients receiving the drug for more than five days or those with significant renal impairment. Other side effects include nausea, abdominal cramps, and some dizziness. Palpitations have been noted on occasion.

SUGGESTED READINGS

General Articles

Brunner, H. R., and Gavras, H.: Vascular damage in hypertension. *Hosp. Pract.* 38:97–108, 1975.

Davis, J. O.: The pathogenesis of chronic renovascular hypertension. *Circ. Res.* 40:439–443, 1977.

Dluhy, R. G., Barli, S. L., Leung, F. K., Solomon, H. S., Moore, T. J., Hollenberg, N. K., and Williams, G. H.: Abnormal adrenal responsiveness and angiotensin II dependency in high renin hypertension. *J. Clin. Invest.* 64:1270–1276, 1979.

Frohlich, E. D.: Essential hypertension, pathophysiological mechanisms and therapy. *Arch. Intern. Med.* 137:772–775, 1977.

Gavras, H., Brunner, H. R., Laragh, J. H., Sealey, J. E., Gavras, I., and Vukovich, R. A.: An angiotensin converting-enzyme inhibitor to identify and treat vasoconstrictor and volume factors in hypertensive patients. *N. Engl. J. Med.* 291:817–821, 1974.

Helgeland, A.: Treatment of mild hypertension: a five year controlled drug trial. The Oslo study. *Am. J. Med.* 69:725–732, 1980.

Lilley, J. J., Golden, J., and Stone, R. A.: Adrenergic regulation of blood pressure in chronic renal failure. *J. Clin. Invest.* 57:1190–1200, 1976.

McGrath, B. P., and Ledingham, J. G.: Renin, blood volume and response to saralasin in patients on chronic hemodialysis: evidence against volume and renin "dependent" hypertension. *Clin. Sci. Mol. Med.* 54:305–312, 1978.

Mills, I. H.: Kallikrein, kininogen and kinins in control of blood pressure. *Nephron* 23:61–71, 1979.

Moser, M., Chairman: Report of the Joint National Committee on Detection, Evaluation and Treatment of High Blood Pressure. A cooperative study. *JAMA* 237:255–262, 1977.

Sealey, J. E., Buhler, F. R., Laragh, J. H., and Vaughan, E. D.: The physiology of renin secretion in essential hypertension. *Am. J. Med.* 55:391–401, 1973.

Veterans Administration Cooperative Study Group on Antihypertensive Agents. *JAMA* 213:1143–1149, 1970.

Veterans Administration Cooperative Study Group on Antihypertensive Agents. *Circulation* 45:991–1001, 1972.

Wisgerhof, M., and Brown, R. D.: Increased adrenal sensitivity to angiotensin II in low-renin essential hypertension. *J. Clin. Invest.* 64:1456–1462, 1979.

Textbooks

Kaplan, N. M.: *Clinical Hypertension*, Second edition. Williams & Wilkins Co., Baltimore, 1978.

McMahon, F. G.: *Management of Essential Hypertension*, First edition. Futura Publishing Co., Mt. Kisco, New York, 1978.

Williams, R. H. (ed.): *Textbook of Endocrinology*, Sixth edition. Saunders, Philadelphia, 1981.

Review Articles

Birkenhager, W. H., and DeLeeuw, P. W.: Pathophysiological mechanisms in essential hypertension. *Pharmacol. Ther.* 8:297–319, 1980.

Brody, M. J., Haywood, J. R., and Touw, K. B.: Neural mechanisms in hypertension. *Annu. Rev. Physiol.* 42:441–453, 1980.

Brown, J. J., Fraser, R., Leckie, B., Lever, A. F., Morton, J. J., Podfield, P. L., Semple, P. F., and Robertson, J. S. Significance of renin and angiotensin in hypertension. *Cardiovasc. Clin.* 9:55–90, 1979.

Giese, J.: The renin–angiotensin system and the pathogenesis of vascular disease in malignant hypertension. A review. *Clin. Sci. Mol. Med.* 51:19–24, 1976.

Gonguly, A., and Weinberger, M. H.: Low renin hypertension: a current review of definitions and controversies. *Am. Heart J.* 98:642–652, 1979.

Hollenberg, N. K., and Williams, G. S.: Hypertension, the adrenal and the kidney: lessons from pharmacologic interruption of the renin–angiotensin system. *Adv. Intern. Med.* 25:327–361, 1980.

Kincaid-Smith, P.: Malignant hypertension; mechanisms and management. *Pharmacol. Ther.* 9:245–269, 1980.

Page, L. B., Yager, H. M., and Sidd, J. J.: Drugs in the management of hypertension. *Am. Heart J.* Part I-91:810–815, Part II-92:114–118, and Part III-92:252–259, 1976.

Report of the Hypertension Task Force of the National Heart, Lung and Blood Institute. Current research and recommendations from the Subgroup on Local Hemodynamics. *Hypertension* 3:342–369, 1980.

Simpson, F. O.: Principles of drug treatment for hypertension: indications for treatment and for selection of drugs. *Pharmacol. Ther.* 7:153–172, 1979.

Tobian, L.: Salt and hypertension. *Ann. N.Y. Acad. Sci.* 189:178–202, 1978.

IV

Pathophysiology of Proteinuric Renal Disease

This section contains two chapters. The first one, "Proteinuria and the Nephrotic Syndrome," describes the physiology of protein handling by the kidney and reviews the factors that prevent large amounts of protein from appearing in the urine. In addition, it describes the mechanisms responsible for pathologic proteinuria. Special emphasis is given to the development of heavy proteinuria that may result in decreases in plasma proteins and elevation of serum lipids (the nephrotic syndrome).

The second chapter of this section, "Pathology and Pathophysiology of Proteinuric Glomerular Disease," reviews the histologic classification of glomerular disease as well as the pathogenesis of such diseases. A series of clinicopathologic correlations are discussed that should familiarize the reader with most of the entities affecting the glomeruli and capable of causing proteinuria.

11

Proteinuria and the Nephrotic Syndrome

ALAN M. ROBSON

I. INTRODUCTION

Richard Bright drew attention to the association between renal disease and protein in the urine in 1827. Since that time proteinuria has become one of the major screening tests for pathology in the genitourinary tract. Recent work has greatly expanded our knowledge of the kidney's role in the metabolism of many proteins. It is now recognized that, in contrast to the larger plasma proteins, many smaller proteins in the plasma are readily filtered, that there are well-developed tubular mechanisms for reabsorption of proteins, that the kidney plays a major role in the elimination or catabolism of many proteins, and that proteins may be added to the urine as it traverses the renal tubules and lower urine tracts. Thus the amount and types of protein appearing in the urine represent the sum of the amounts filtered through the glomeruli and the amounts reabsorbed and added to the urine in the tubules and lower urinary tract.

Although the majority of pathologic proteinuria results from glomerular damage, the improved understanding of the renal handling of proteins has

ALAN M. ROBSON • Department of Pediatrics, Washington University School of Medicine, St. Louis, Missouri 63110.

helped to define other causes for increased loss of protein in the urine. In the future better characterization of urinary protein could represent an important noninvasive technique for accurate diagnosis of both systemic and renal diseases responsible for increased proteinuria. This chapter addresses each of these issues. It discusses the physiology of the normal renal handling of protein, the causes of abnormal proteinuria, and the consequences of proteinuria.

II. PHYSIOLOGY OF RENAL PROTEIN HANDLING

A. Glomerular Filtration of Proteins

1. Permeability of Glomeruli to Proteins

A volume of blood approximately equal to total blood volume perfuses the kidney every 5 min with 20%–25% of the fluid in this blood being filtered by the glomeruli. Despite this high rate of filtration, the glomerular filtrate is almost a true ultrafiltrate containing little protein, indicating that the glomeruli are remarkably impermeable to the larger plasma proteins. Micropuncture studies have demonstrated that *albumin* can be found in the glomerular filtrate of the mammalian kidney but only in low concentrations of 2 mg/dl or less, a value which represents approximately 0.05% the plasma albumin concentration of 4000–4500 mg/dl. Despite such low albumin concentrations in the glomerular filtrate, a normal human adult must filter more than 3.0 g of albumin into the glomerular filtrate each day if the values from experimental animals can be extrapolated to humans.

The kidney is even less permeable to *globulins*. These proteins cannot be detected in the majority of samples of glomerular filtrate that have been analyzed, contamination by plasma being thought to be responsible for the positive results found in the remaining samples.

In contrast, *smaller proteins* such as the peptide hormones, insulin, glucagon, growth hormone, or parathyroid hormone; enzymes such as ribonuclease or lysozyme; and fragments of immunoproteins such as β_2 microglobulin or light chains of immunoglobulins are able to penetrate the glomerular barrier more easily. Indeed, the glomerular sieving coefficient for proteins smaller than 23 Å in radius (25,000 daltons) is 0.5 or higher indicating that the concentration of these proteins in the glomerular filtrate is 50% or more of their plasma concentrations. The ability of these small proteins to enter the glomerular filtrate is dependant primarily on molecular size, shape, and rigidity. Thus small, deformable molecules penetrate the glomerular barrier more easily than do larger more rigid ones.

2. Nature of Glomerular Barrier to Proteins

The glomeruli function *as though* they are penetrated by pores with diameters of between 70 and 100 Å, the pores occupying approximately 5%

of the capillary surface. Such pores would prevent entry into the glomerular filtrate of globulins and other large proteins, would restrict, but not totally prevent, the transglomerular passage of albumin, and would allow small proteins to enter the filtrate quite freely.

The glomerular capillary wall is lined by a layer of endothelial cells the cytoplasm of which is penetrated completely by numerous openings or fenestrae which have an average diameter of about 400 Å (Figure 1). External to the endothelial cells is the glomerular basement membrane (GBM), which is embraced on its outer or urinary side by interdigitating foot processes from adjacent epithelial cells. In health these are separated from one another by slits 200–300 Å wide. Since only the GBM appears to separate completely the plasma in the glomerular capillary from the urine in Bowman's space, this structure would appear to be the principal barrier to the entry of proteins into the glomerular filtrate. Electron microscopy has failed however, to demonstrate pores in the GBM and it is proposed that the GBM is a hydrated gel with loose bonding between its protein and lipid components, this fluid structure having functional rather than anatomic pores to produce the filtration characteristics outlined above. Indeed glomerular filtrate is now thought to be formed by diffusion across the GBM as well as by bulk filtration through functional pores.

Studies with electron dense tracers suggest there may be a second mechanical barrier to filtration. This may be provided by the epithelial slit diaphragms which are located on the urinary side of the GBM where they bridge the spaces between adjacent podocytes of the epithelial cells (Figures 1 and 2). This membrane has a zipperlike structure containing rectangular pores 140 × 40 Å in size. These dimensions are similar to those of albumin, a cigar-shaped molecule with a length of 50 Å and a maximum diameter of 36 Å, suggesting that this membrane could be responsible for the glomerular

GLOMERULAR CAPILLARY

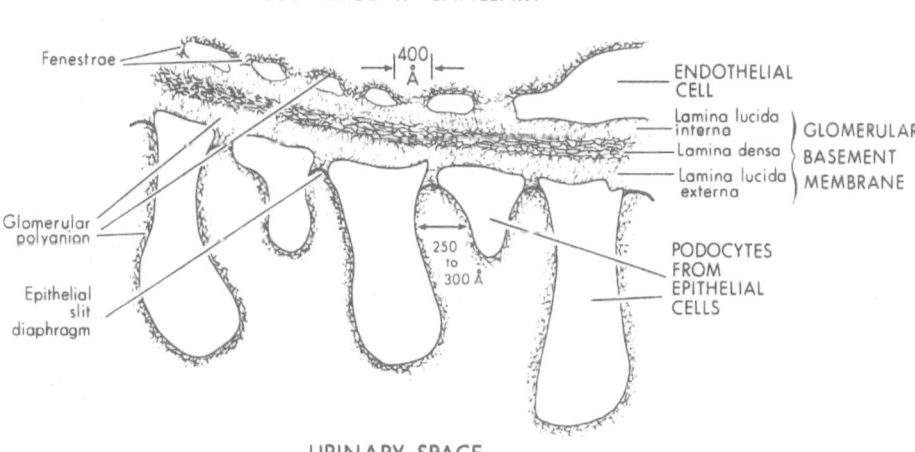

Figure 1. Diagrammatic representation of the structure of the glomerular capillary wall.

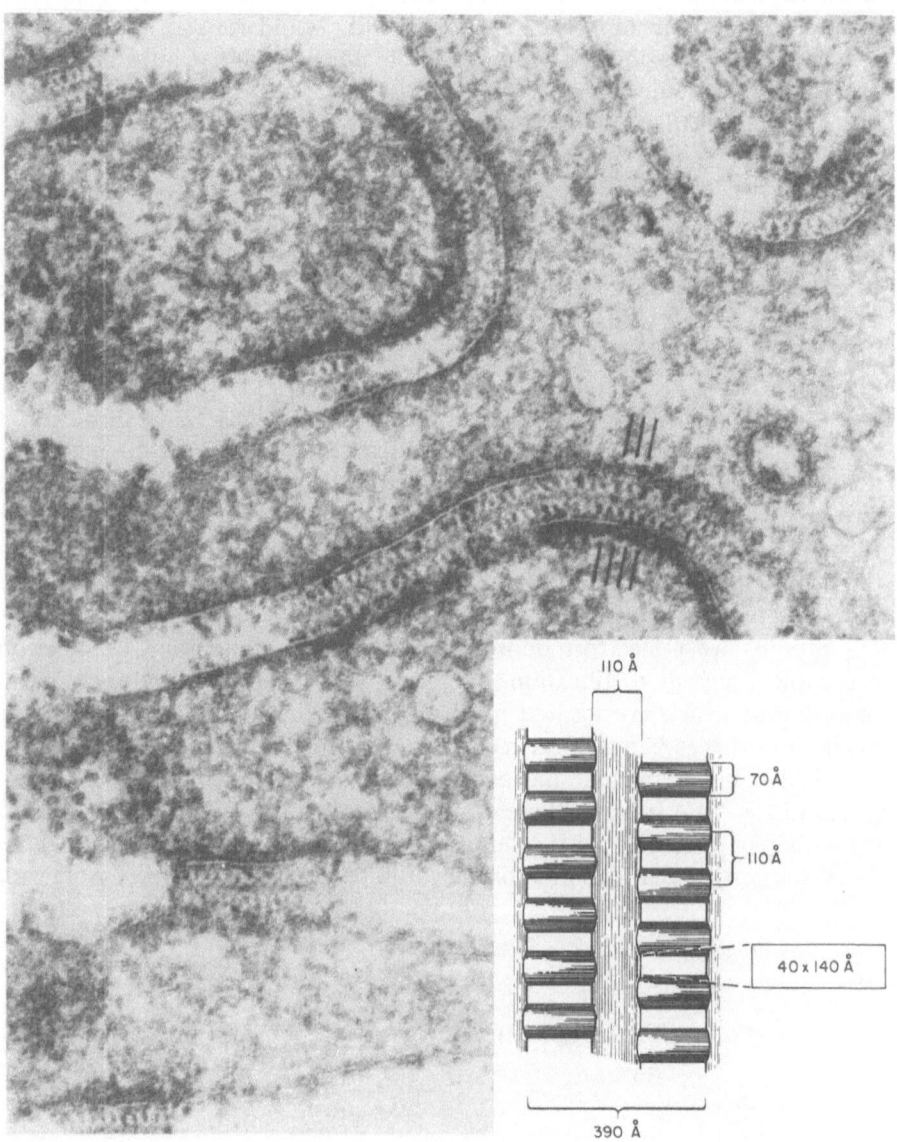

Figure 2. The epithelial split diaphragm from the rat glomerulus is shown bridging the gap between adjacent foot processes of epithelial foot processes (see marks). The insert illustrates the schematic drawing of the slit diaphragm and gives its dimensions. (Reprinted with permission from Rodewald, R., and Karnovsky, J. J.: *J. Cell. Biol.* 60:425–433, 1974.)

permeability characteristics to albumin. If, however, the slit diaphragms represent a major mechanical barrier to filtration one must explain what happens to molecules which penetrate the GBM but are unable to traverse the slit diaphragms. Without an efficient removal mechanism such molecules would accumulate between the two structures and would interfere with or eventually prevent filtration. Thus the functional role of epithelial slit diaphragms remains to be delineated.

Glomeruli appear to have electrical as well as mechanical barriers to filtration with molecular charge also affecting the ability of certain molecules to enter the filtrate. This was first proposed when patients with untreated minimal change nephrotic syndrome and marked albuminuria were found to have decreased, rather than increased, clearances of inert macromolecules

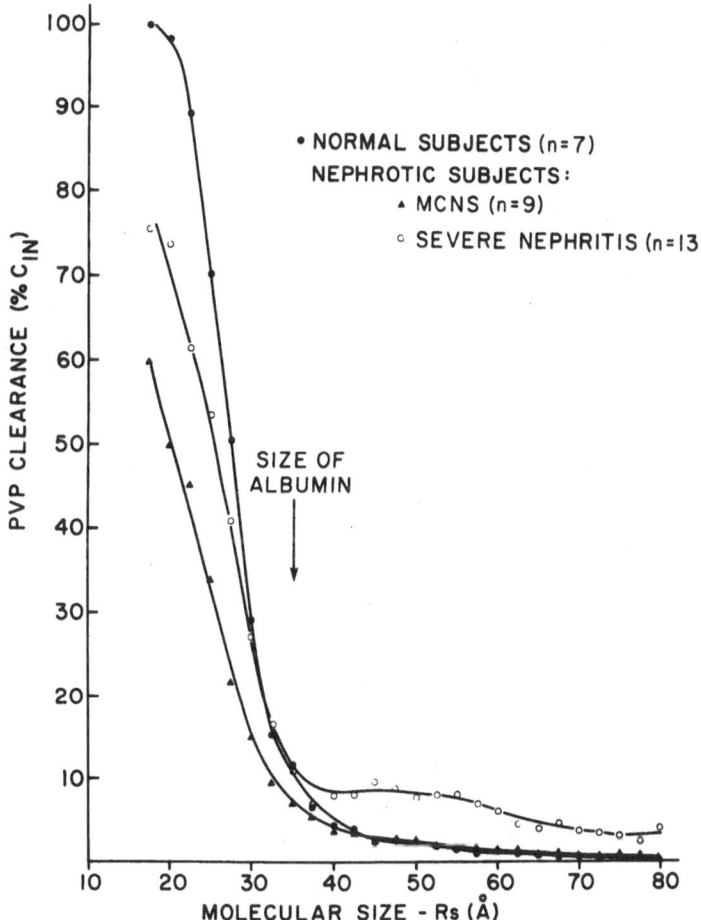

Figure 3. Patterns of permselectivity to polyvinyl pyrrolidone (PVP) observed in normal subjects and in those with nephrotic syndrome secondary to either chronic glomerulonephritis (CGN) or to minimal-change nephrotic syndrome (MCNS). In each group of subjects the clearances of fractions of PVP of known molecular size, expressed as a percentage of the clearance of inulin measured simultaneously, are plotted against molecular size. The relative size of albumin, which has a radius (Rs) of 35 Å, is shown. Even though patients with MCNS had marked albuminuria, the clearance of PVP molecules with a Rs of 35 Å was decreased. Indeed, both groups of nephrotic patients had relative decreases in the clearances of smaller molecules. Only the nephrotic patients with underlying glomerulonephritis had increased clearances of larger PVP molecules. (From A. M. Robson, unpublished observations.)

comparable in size to albumin molecules (Figure 3). Subsequently, the importance of charge in determining molecular clearance has been delineated by the elegant studies demonstrating that negatively charged dextrans have lower clearances, and positively charged dextrans higher clearances than uncharged dextrans of comparable size (Figure 4). These studies are particularly pertinent to the glomerular clearance of albumin which is negatively charged at pH 7.4. Histochemical studies have demonstrated also that the ability of tracers to penetrate the GBM depends in part on the charge of the tracer.

Glomerular polyanion (GPA), a negatively charged sialo-glycoprotein which is present in high concentrations on the surfaces of the foot processes of the epithelial cells and in lower concentrations on the surfaces of the endothelial cells (Figure 1), has been presumed to be responsible for glomerular charge selectivity. Evidence for its role in preventing proteinuria is, however, largely indirect. In both humans and animals, proteinuric glomerular diseases are characterized by reduced glomerular staining for GPA. In addition, in animals, the reduction of GPA in experimental glomerulonephritis is accompanied by loss of charge discrimination (Figure 4). Finally, infusing polycations into kidneys of normal animals results in neutralization of GPA, proteinuria, and epithelial cell foot process fusion (Figure 5), the histologic change characteristic of proteinuric states.

Until recently sialic acid was the only polyanion known to be present in the glomerulus. More recently anionic sites consisting of glycosaminoglycans (GAGs) rich in heparan sulfate have been demonstrated in both the laminae rara interna and lamina rara externa of the GBM. These sulfated GAGs are concentrated in particles thought to be proteoglycans (protein–polysaccharide complexes) and are distributed in a regular latticelike network. Removal of the heparan sulfate GAG by specific degrading enzymes has resulted in

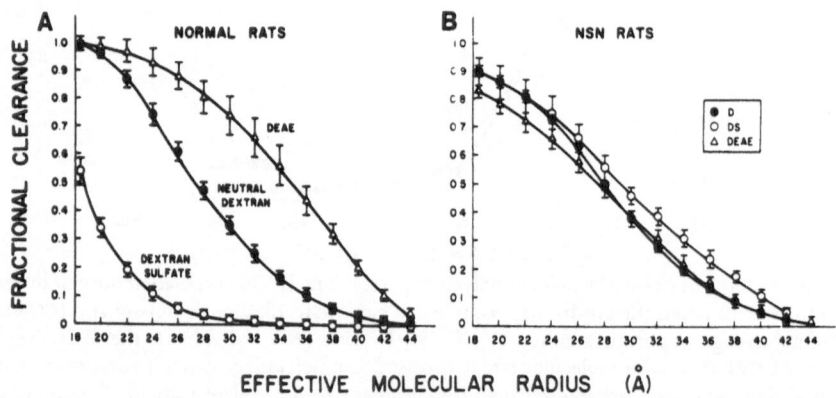

EFFECTIVE MOLECULAR RADIUS (Å)

Figure 4. (A) The influence of molecular charge on the renal clearance of molecules by the normal kidney. Dextran sulfate is negatively charged, DEAE dextrans are positively charged. (B) In animals with experimental nephritis (NSN) glomerular polyanion is lost as is the effect of charge on molecular clearance. (Reproduced with permission from Bohrer, M. P., *et al.: J. Clin. Invest.* 61:72–78, 1978.)

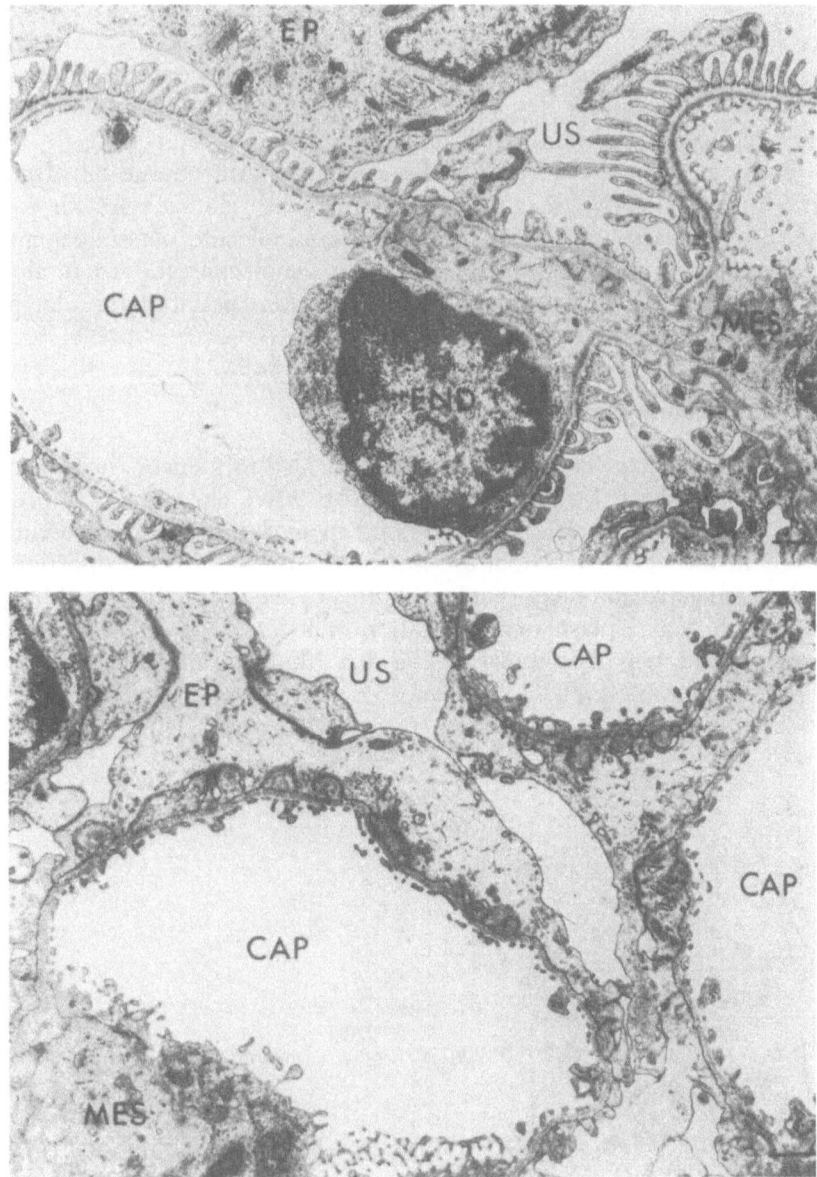

Figure 5. Effect of neutralization of glomerular polyanion by infusion of a polycation, protamine sulfate. (Top) normal rat glomerular capillary; (bottom) capillary after perfusion with protamine sulfate. The normally discrete foot processes of the epithelial cells have become blunted and appear fused. These changes can be reversed by the subsequent infusion of a polyanion, heparin. CAP, glomerular capillary; US, urinary space; EP, epithelial cells; MES, mesangium. (Reproduced with permission from Seiler, M. W., et al.: Science 189:390, 1975.)

increased permeability of the GBM. Whether this was due to removal of an electrostatic effect or a steric exclusion effect cannot yet be determined, but an influence on both seems likely. Based on studies with electron dense tracers, the main glomerular barrier to macromolecules occurs at the level of the lamina rara interna. A second barrier occurs between the lamina rara interna and the lamina densa. It was the latter which was eliminated or greatly reduced after removal of heparan sulfate.

Thus, molecular size, shape, deformability, and charge all affect the glomerular sieving coefficient for a protein. The relative roles for each of these factors depend on the size of the protein molecule, charge being much more important in modifying the clearance of molecules the size of albumin which have similar dimensions to those of the functional glomerular pores, than for smaller protein molecules.

3. Plasma Protein Concentration

The plasma concentration of a protein also influences the amount of that protein filtered by the glomeruli. Progressive elevation of a protein's plasma concentration results in increased urinary loss of that protein once threshhold has been exceeded, the loss increasing in direct proportion with the increasing plasma level (Figure 6). In normal man, the threshhold for albuminuria is at a plasma concentration of 6–7 g/dl, marked albuminuria occurring at higher plasma levels. The threshhold for smaller proteins is at much lower plasma levels.

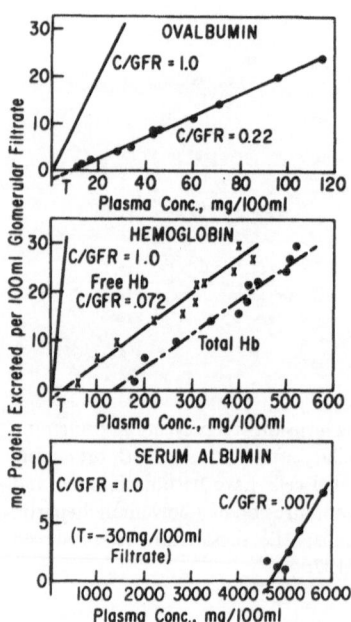

Figure 6. The effect of plasma concentration of a protein on its urinary excretion. The relationships shown suggest tubular reabsorption of some of the protein filtered with the ordinate intercept being an indication of the maximum rate of transport (T_m) for the protein. (Reproduced with permission from Renkin, E. M., and Gilmore, J. P.: *Renal Physiology*. American Society of Physiology, Washington, D.C., 1973, Chap. 9.)

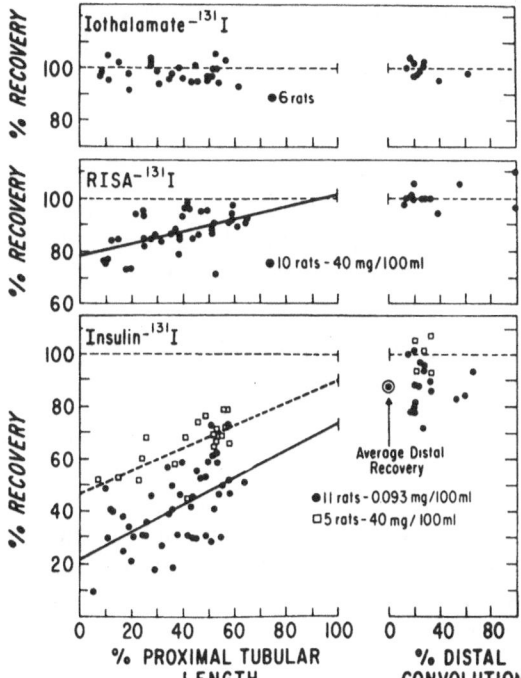

Figure 7. Recovery in the ureteral urine of radiolabeled iothalamate, albumin, and insulin after injection into the proximal or distal tubules of rat kidneys. The recovery of albumin injected into the proximal tubule is incomplete indicating its reabsorption. Recovery of insulin injected into either the proximal or distal tubule is less than 100%. (Reprinted with permission from Cortney, M. A., *et al.: J. Clin. Invest.* 49:1–4, 1970.)

B. Tubular Reabsorption of Proteins

1. Albumin

In normal man, the calculated filtered load of albumin greatly exceeds the rate of albuminuria. Thus, it is presumed that the renal tubules are able to reabsorb albumin. Histochemical and micropuncture studies support this thesis and indicate that albumin can be reabsorbed along the entire length of the accessible portion of the proximal tubule. Urinary recovery of ^{131}I-labeled serum albumin, injected into tubules of mammalian kidneys is incomplete, the percentage recovery being inversely related to the distance along the proximal tubule of the injection site (Figure 7). Under some circumstances, the distal tubule may be able to reabsorb albumin too, but at a much lower capacity than that of the proximal tubule. There probably is a maximum rate for tubular protein transport, this having been estimated to be as high as 30 mg/min for albumin.

2. Other Proteins

Most of the smaller proteins which are extensively filtered by the glomerulus undergo tubular reabsorption primarily in the proximal tubules. Proteins handled by these mechanisms include vasopressin, insulin (Figure 7), glucagon, ACTH, growth hormone, parathyroid hormone, lysozyme, and light-chain fragments or microglobulins. The tubular uptake mechanism, which is energy requiring, has a high capacity compared to the amount of protein filtered so that only minimal amounts of these proteins appear in normal urine.

Since most of the globulins in plasma are not filtered by the glomeruli, the ability of the tubules to transport these proteins remains uncertain. Small amounts of intact IgG and IgA have been found in normal human urine but most urinary proteins which react antigenically as globulins probably are fragments rather than intact plasma globulins.

3. Mechanisms for Tubular Reabsorption of Protein

Proteins and large polypeptides filtered through the glomeruli are bound to receptors on the luminal membrane of proximal tubular epithelial cells prior to absorption. The protein is then incorporated into apical vesicles in these cells by endocytosis (Figure 8). Vesicles fuse to form larger vacuoles in the cytoplasm where they combine with lysosomes to form phagolysosomes. Lysosomal enzymes released into the phagolysosomes hydrolyze the protein, this process beginning within 30 min of entry of most proteins into the apical vacuoles. The amino acids generated diffuse to the cells' contraluminal

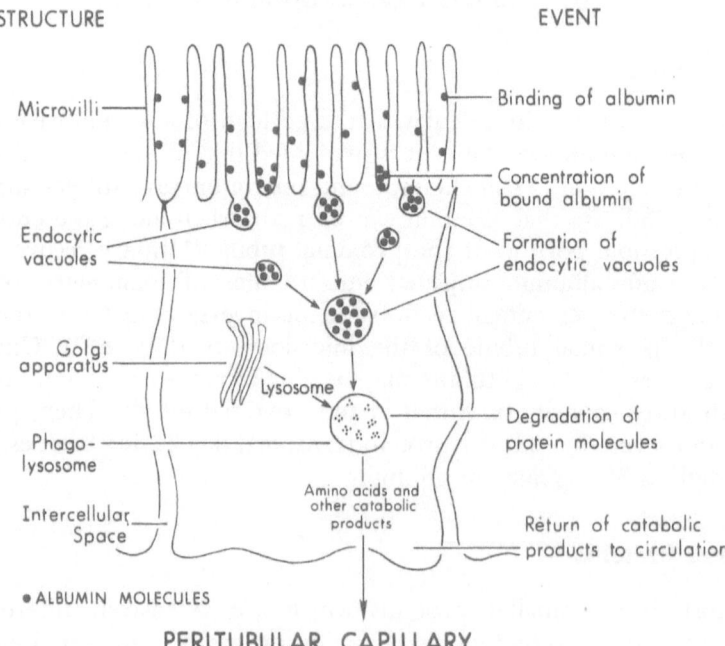

Figure 8. The proposed mechanism for protein reabsorption by cells of the proximal convoluted tubule.

membranes where they enter the interstitial space and are taken up into the renal circulation. Transport of intact protein from tubular fluid into the renal circulation by intracellular pathways has not been demonstrated. Nor in health is there any intercellular movement of intact protein from tubular lumen to peritubular blood.

4. Specificity of Protein Reabsorption

The infusion of albumin into man results not only in the increased urinary excretion of albumin but also in increased losses of α_1-, α_2-, and β-globulins. This suggests that the mechanism for tubular reabsorption of protein is nonselective with different proteins sharing the same transport sites. Presumably when the filtered load of one protein (in this case albumin) is greatly increased, reabsorptive sites are overwhelmed and urinary excretion of other proteins increases too. However, conflicting observations from subsequent studies have not excluded the possibility that different groups of proteins may be reabsorbed by separate transport systems. This could occur if there are specific receptors for individual proteins on the luminal membranes of the proximal tubular cells.

Indeed small, linear peptides do not appear to be taken up into apical vascuoles as are larger proteins. Rather they are degraded by hydrolytic enzymes present on the luminal surface of the brush border of proximal tubule cells. The amino acids liberated by this process are transported rapidly across the epithelial cells by active amino acid pumps on the apical cell membranes. The remaining partially hydrolyzed peptide fragments may be reabsorbed intact or undergo further degradation before being returned to the amino acid pool.

5. Peritubular Uptake of Proteins

Removal of some hormones from the circulation (see Chapter 3 on nonexcretory functions of the kidney) may occur by peritubular extraction and metabolism. If this mechanism does occur, it is of much less quantitative importance in overall metabolism of these proteins than is glomerular filtration with subsequent uptake by the luminal membranes of the proximal tubule cells.

6. Renal Role in Overall Turnover Rates of Small Proteins

Renal extraction may account for between 40% and 80% of the metabolic clearance rates of several small proteins and could be of great clinical importance. The rate-limiting step for renal removal of these proteins from the plasma is glomerular filtration rate, so that when nephron mass or glomerular filtration rate is reduced the plasma concentrations of these proteins can increase significantly.

C. Tubular Secretion of Proteins

1. Tissue Proteins

Approximately 40% of protein in normal urine does not react to antibodies prepared against plasma proteins. Although some of this protein may represent degraded plasma proteins which have lost their antigenic sites, much of it is tissue protein added to the urine in the tubules and lower urinary tract.

The major nonplasma protein is uromucoid (Tamm–Horsfall protein), which is excreted in amounts of 30–60 mg/day. This large glycoprotein has a molecular weight of 7 million and is the major constituent of urinary casts. Immunoelectron microscopy has shown that it is localized selectively among the surface membranes of the thick ascending limb of the loop of Henle. It has also been described in the distal tubule and the collecting duct although its location at these sites is disputed.

Trace amounts of numerous other proteins have been identified in the urine. Many are added to the urine in the lower urinary tract with several being derived from the accessory sex glands such as the prostate.

III. NORMAL PROTEINURIA

A. Quantitative Aspects

Normal human urine contains small amounts of protein. This should not exceed 60 mg/m^2 body surface area per day, except in the first month of life when normal proteinuria may be increased fourfold. Thus, urine protein excretion in the normal adult may be up to 100 mg/day. With a typical urine output of 1.5 liters/day, the concentration of this urinary protein would be less than 10 mg/dl. Such low concentrations of protein are not detectable by routine laboratory tests using the Esbach reagent, sulfosalicyclic acid, or dipsticks which have a sensitivity of 15 mg/dl at best.

Proteinuria may be increased markedly in the absence of renal disease, for example by fever, stress, the infusion of norepinephrine, the lordotic position, and congestive heart failure. Indeed, strenuous exercise may cause a dramatic increment in albuminuria by up to 5000%. Thus before ascribing proteinuria to pathologic processes in the kidney or urinary tract, it is important to learn the conditions under which the urine was collected and whether the patient has some other cause for increased proteinuria. If in doubt, the urine collection should be repeated when the patient is at rest and afebrile. Under these conditions urine protein excretion should not exceed 60 mg/m^2 per day.

B. Qualitative Aspects

Fifty to sixty percent of normal urine protein reacts to antibodies prepared against plasma proteins and presumably is of plasma origin. Of the more than 30 intact or partially degraded individual plasma proteins that have been identified in urine, albumin predominates approximating 40% of proteinuria in resting normal subjects and more than 80% following exercise. α_1- and α_2-globulins are next most abundant, approximating 9% and 2% of total urine protein, respectively. Numerous lower-molecular-weight proteins are present also including hormones, enzymes, immunoproteins, and peptides. Many are only presumed to be of plasma origin, their concentration in plasma being too low to be measured by current methodology. Their urinary concentrations are usually low too because of extensive tubular reabsorption of the filtered protein.

The remaining urinary protein is of tissue origin and consists of uromucoid, glycoproteins, globulins, enzymes, and organ specific antigens. Some originate from the cells lining the urinary tract, and from the accessory sex glands. Others are liberated from nonrenal tissues and organs, circulate in the blood, are filtered and excreted in the urine.

IV. PATHOLOGIC PROTEINURIA

A. Intermittent Proteinuria

Proteinuria is found in more than 1% of healthy subjects tested in routine screening studies, the incidence varying with both sex and age. An even greater percentage of normal, healthy subjects may spill protein in their urine intermittently. For example, in one large study, in which morning and evening urine samples were checked for proteinuria by dipstick on seven consecutive days, 19% of 15-year-old males had at least one positive test. None of these subjects had evidence of significant underlying disease in the urinary tract. Thus, proteinuria in a single urine sample does not necessarily indicate underlying renal disease and can result from fever, exposure to cold, exercise, or urinary contamination, for example, by vaginal secretions. In addition, drugs such as penicillins, sulfonamides, tolbutamide, Zephiran, Hibitane, or radiologic contrast media may give a positive dipstick test for protein.

More persistent proteinuria occurs less frequently. Usually less than 1% of any screened population will have protein in two or more samples of urine and if urines are collected with subjects at rest, the incidence of proteinuria in two or more urine samples falls to below 0.2% of subjects tested.

Asymptomatic intermittent proteinuria may be found in some cases of glomerulonephritis, with urine tract infection, or with genitourinary abnormalities such as obstruction. This abnormality, however, is rarely the sole manifestation of genitourinary tract disease and more often is accompanied by microscopic hematuria or other urinary abnormality when significant disease is present.

B. Postural Proteinuria

In orthostatic or postural proteinuria, urinary protein excretion is increased only when the patient assumes the upright position. Protein excretion in the recumbent position is normal. Total urinary protein excretion rarely exceeds 1 g/day. It is important to separate patients with true postural proteinuria from those with significant renal disease and an orthostatic component to their proteinuria. These latter patients have increased amounts of proteinuria in both the upright and recumbent positions with the upright values being higher than those in urines collected with the patients at rest.

The pathophysiology of postural proteinuria is not understood. Up to 10% of the patients may have renal biopsy abnormalities such as capillary wall thickening or glomerular hypercellularity and up to another 45% have more subtle abnormalities. These minor lesions, however, are not sufficient to explain the proteinuria. Indeed, similar mild histologic changes have been found in healthy populations with no proteinuria. Alternately it has been suggested that postural proteinuria could result from changes in renal hemodynamics which occur when the upright posture is assumed. To date, there is no experimental confirmation for this thesis. Selectivity of proteinuria (see Section IV.E.1) is altered in patients with orthostatic proteinuria when they are upright. The significance of this finding remains to be delineated. Even patients with persisting orthostatic proteinuria have an excellent prognosis. Despite the presence of histologic abnormalities on initial renal biopsy, progressive renal insufficiency has not been documented during ten or more years of followup.

C. Persistent Proteinuria

Renal diseases result most often in persistent proteinuria, a variety of pathophysiologic mechanisms being responsible (Table I). Glomerular diseases permit an increased leak of plasma proteins into the glomerular filtrate. Diseases which cause extensive damage to the proximal tubule result in decreased reabsorption of filtered protein. Proteinuria may also result from increased concentrations of the normal plasma proteins, abnormal proteins in the plasma, and increased addition of tissue protein to the urine. In some disease states, more than one mechanism may be responsible for proteinuria. Rather than analyze proteinuria according to the individual disease states causing this abnormality, the following discussion classifies it according to the primary mechanism responsible.

Table I. Proteinuria Classified According to Pathophysiologic Mechanisms
Responsible

I. Persistent proteinuria
    A. Increased glomerular permeability to plasma proteins
        1. Damage to basement membrane: glomerulonephritides
        2. Loss of glomerular polyanion: minimal-change nephrotic syndrome
        3. Other possible mechanisms: increased filtration fraction, loss of nephron mass with
           increased permeability in residual nephrons
    B. Decreased tubular reabsorption of filtered proteins
        Fanconi syndrome, hereditary tubular disorders, Balkan nephropathy, nephrotoxic
        drugs
    C. Overflow proteinuria
        1. Normal renal function. (a) Large plasma proteins; repeated albumin or blood
           transfusions. (b) Smaller plasma proteins: myeloma, macroglobulinemia
           (immunoglobulin fragments), leukemia (lysozyme), carcinoma of bronchus
           (orosumucoid)
        2. Decreased renal threshold: albumin infusions in nephrotic syndrome
    D. Secretory proteinuria
        1. Tamm–Horsfall proteinuria: neonatal period, pyelonephritis
        2. Kidney-specific antigens: analgesic nephropathy, heavy-metal poisoning, rapidly
           progressive glomerulonephritis
        3. Other proteins: diseases of prostate, other accessory sex glands
    E. Histuria
        1. Tissue antigens: urothelial carcinoma, melanoma, neuroblastoma
        2. Nonspecific antigens: diseases causing damage to basement membrane or collagen
II. Postural proteinuria
III. Intermittent proteinuria
    A. Random finding: no known pathologic cause
    B. Nonrenal abnormalities: fever, stress, e.g., exercise, exposure to cold
    C. Renal diseases (rarely an isolated abnormality): urine tract infection, genitourinary
        abnormalities, e.g., obstruction, chronic glomerulonephritis
    D. Contamination of urine: vaginal secretions
    E. False positive test: penicillins, sulfonamides, tolbutamide, Hibitane, radiologic contrast
        media

---

1. Glomerular Proteinuria

Glomerular diseases account for most, but not all, persistent proteinuria. Recent micropuncture studies have confirmed that there is increased glomerular permeability to plasma proteins in these diseases, the resulting increase in filtered load of protein overwhelming the tubular reabsorptive capacity and causing proteinuria (Figure 9). The principal underlying mechanism is damage to the GBM. In human glomerulonephritis glomerular histology is markedly deranged with abnormalities in the GBM being apparent on electron microscopy. This is accompanied by loss of normal glomerular permselectivity with larger macromolecules, that normally are excluded from the urine, having significantly increased clearances (Figure 3). Similar changes occur in animals with experimental forms of glomerulonephritis and are accompanied by alterations in the composition of the GBM and by loss of the normal ability of basement membrane fragments to segregate molecules

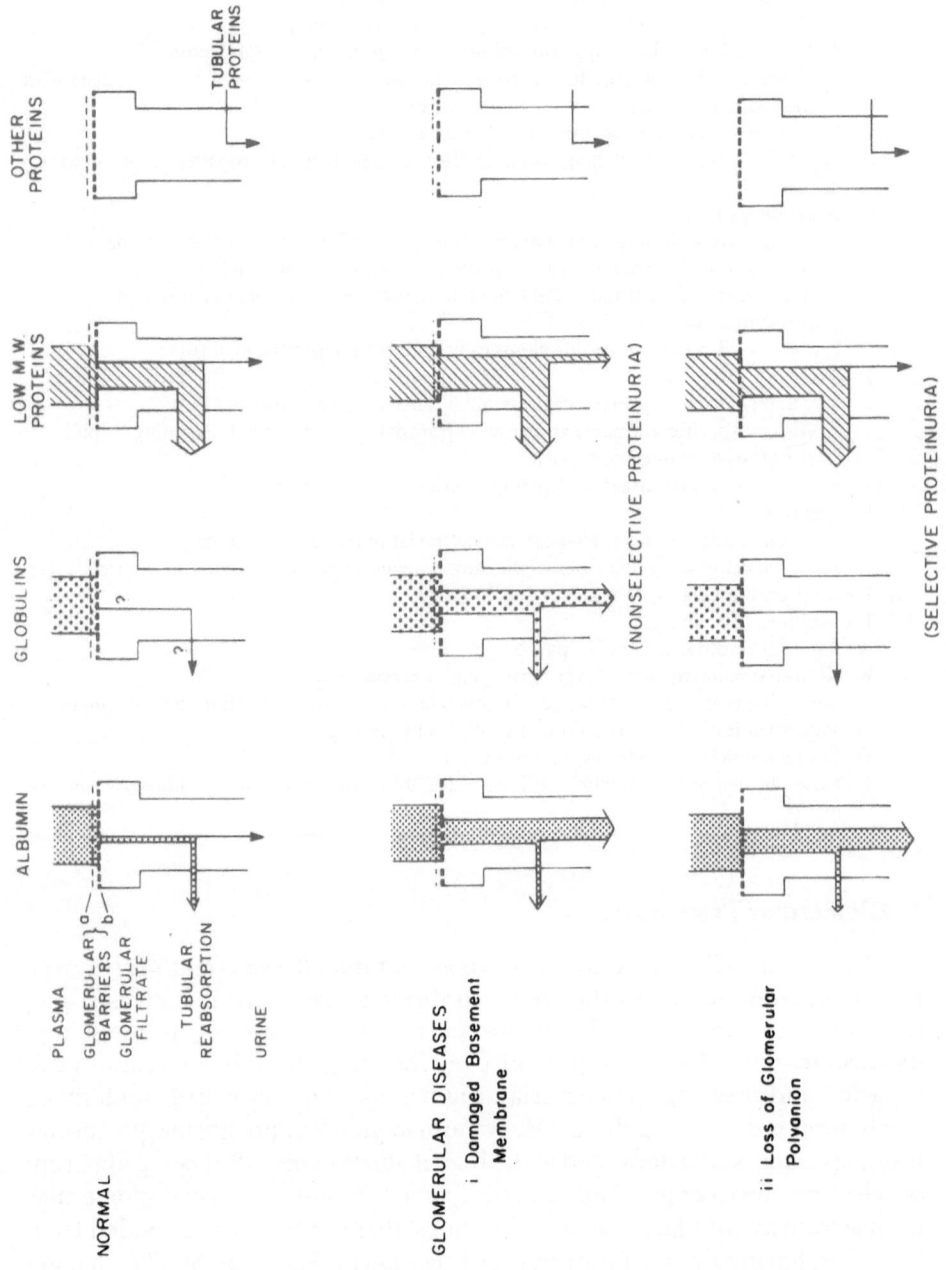

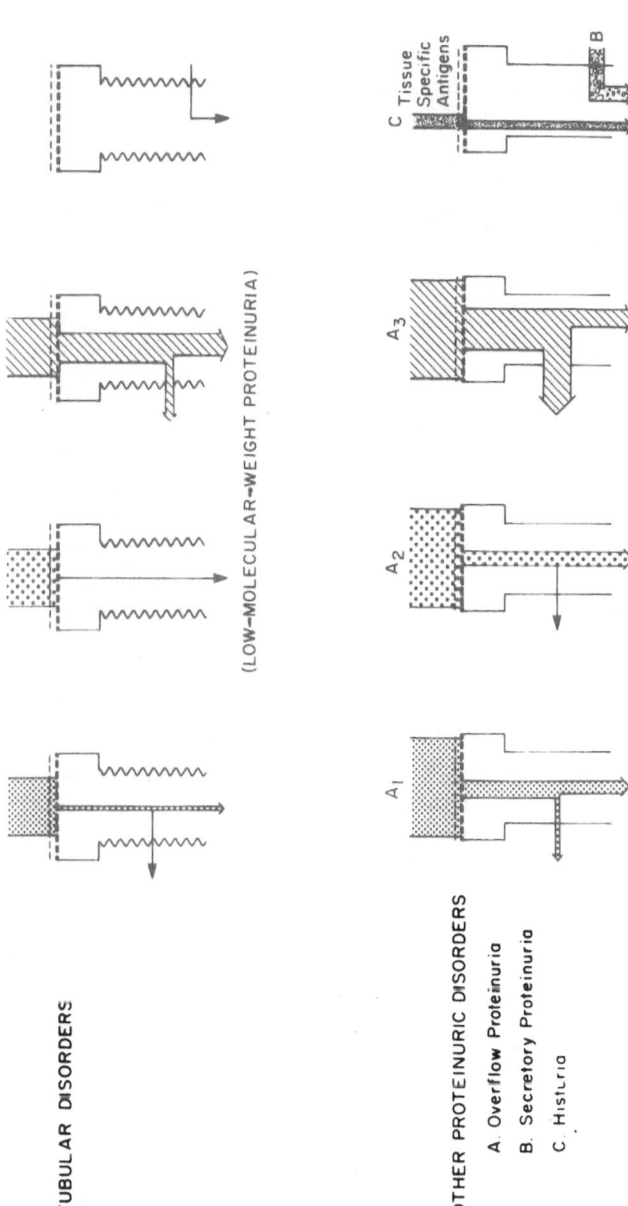

Figure 9. A diagrammatic representation of the handling of proteins by the normal kidney and the derangements in this normal physiology seen in each of the major causes of proteinuria. The widths of individual bars are not meant to indicate the relative blood concentrations of albumin, globulins, and low-molecular-weight proteins. They do, however, indicate variations in concentrations of each of these proteins in disease states, the approximate proportion of these proteins that are filtered, and the proportions of filtered protein that are reabsorbed by the tubules or secreted in the urine in each situation. Glomerular barriers: *a* refers to glomerular polyanion and *b* the glomerular basement membrane and epithelial slit diaphragm (see text for more details). Proteinuria may result from damage to the basement membrane or loss of glomerular polyanion. Tubular disorders result in low-molecular-weight proteinuria. Overflow proteinuria can occur when the concentration of either plasma albumin (A$_1$), plasma globulins (A$_2$), or low-molecular-weight proteins (A$_3$) are increased.

according to size. These observations suggest the damaged GBM permits increased loss of plasma proteins into the urine. Such damage could be induced by lytic enzymes released from polymorphonuclear leucocytes found in the glomeruli in acute glomerulonephritis, or it could be due to other causes such as abnormal metabolism of complement.

Evidence is accumulating that primary loss of the glomerular electrical barriers may be a primary cause of proteinuria too. Relapses of minimal change nephrotic syndrome are characterized by marked proteinuria even though the GBM appears to be normal. Fusion of epithelial cell foot processes and vacuolization of proximal tubule epithelial cells, which are the major histologic abnormalities seen during relapse, are now thought to be secondary to, rather than responsible for, the proteinuria. Loss of glomerular staining for polyanion is a consistent histologic feature during relapses also. This could be the primary renal event responsible for the proteinuria. Indeed, it is now known that infusions of polycations into kidneys of normal animals result in loss of staining for glomerular polyanion, fusion of epithelial foot processes and proteinuria, changes which are identical to those of human minimal change nephrotic syndrome. Loss of the glomerular charge barriers could contribute to the etiology of proteinuria in glomerulonephritis too. Alternately, since proteinuria induced by protein infusions results in loss of glomerular polyanion, the increased passage of plasma proteins across the damaged GBM in glomerulonephritis may cause secondary loss of staining for glomerular polyanion.

Reduction in renal mass is followed by increased proteinuria from the residual nephrons, the glomeruli in these nephrons having altered permselectivity characteristics with relatively increased permeability to larger-weight macromolecules (Figure 10). Presumably this change indicates an increase in effective pore size in these glomeruli. This could represent the pathophysiologic mechanism responsible for the proteinuria found with nonglomerular renal diseases that result in nephron loss and could contribute too to the proteinuria of glomerular diseases as nephron dropout occurs.

Since the glomerular filtrate is an ultrafiltrate of plasma, protein concentration increases progressively along the length of the glomerular capillary as fluid and crystalloid, but not colloid, solutes are filtered. If filtration fraction is high, the protein concentration at the distal end of the glomerular capillaries may be elevated sufficiently to exceed threshhold, a mechanism proposed as a cause of proteinuria in the absence of demonstrable renal disease.

2. Tubular Proteinuria

Diseases which cause extensive proximal tubular damage result in proteinuria by reducing tubular reabsorption of filtered protein. Small proteins, being filtered more readily than larger ones, require extensive tubular reabsorption to prevent their appearance in the urine, so that tubular disorders are characterized by proteinuria consisting primarily of the smaller proteins (Figure 9). Indeed, in these disorders clearances of many smaller proteins are similar to GFR, indicating little if any tubular reabsorption. This pattern of proteinuria is observed in diseases which result in a Fanconi syndrome, in the hereditary tubular disorders such as oculocerebrorenal syndrome and cystinosis, in Balkan nephropathy, after administration of nephrotoxic drugs such as phenacetin and the aminoglycoside antibiotics, after poisoning with heavy metals such as cadmium and mercury, and after renal homograft rejection.

3. Overflow Proteinuria

Intravenous infusions of protein will result in proteinuria in the absence of renal disease, once the plasma concentration of the protein increases above threshhold. Thus, the large plasma proteins may be excreted in the

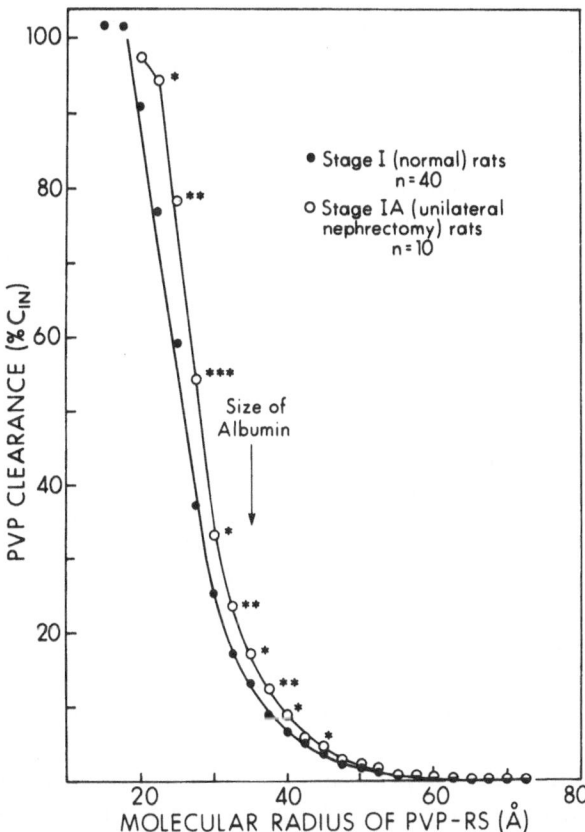

Figure 10. The effect of unilateral nephrectomy on glomerular permselectivity. The increase in permselectivity in residual nephrons following reduction in nephron mass is statistically significant (*$p < 0.05$, **$p < 0.005$, ***$p < 0.001$). Molecules the size of albumin show a greater than 30% increase in their relative clearances. Additional details are presented in Figure 3. (From A. M. Robson, unpublished observations.)

urine in increased amounts after repeated blood transfusions. Patients with the nephrotic syndrome may have a decreased threshhold for protein and be more susceptible to overflow proteinuria. Albumin infusions given to induce a diuresis in such patients are often followed by an increase in proteinuria equivalent in degree to the amount of albumin infused even though plasma albumin levels remain below normal.

Proteins with a low renal threshhold are more often responsible for overflow proteinuria than are albumin and globulins. In the monoclonal gammopathies multiple myeloma, macroglobulinemia, and heavy-chain disease, there is increased urine excretion of immunoglobulin fragments, expecially light and heavy chains. Increased production of these proteins elevates their blood levels and, along with the small size of the protein molecules, results in a high filtered load. This and possibly qualitative abnormalities of the proteins rapidly saturate tubular reabsorptive mechanisms. Proteinuria results and can be massive in amount. Albumin excretion increases along with that of the immunoglobulin fragments possibly because they compete for the same reabsorptive sites. Alternately, light chains, also referred to as Bence Jones protein, may be toxic to renal tubular cells, thus decreasing albumin reabsorption. Indeed, toxicity of light chains has been incriminated as the cause of the Fanconi syndrome, distal renal tubular acidosis, nephrogenic diabetes insipidus, or even acute or chronic renal failure observed some patients with multiple myelomatosis. Enhanced production of lysozyme in leukemia or orosomucoid in some patients with carcinoma of the bronchus increases the plasma levels and filtered loads of these proteins, causing proteinuria. Liberation of free hemoglobin into the plasma after intravascular hemolysis will be followed by its appearance in the urine once binding sites to haptoglobin, a plasma α_2-globulin, have been saturated.

4. Secretory Proteinuria

Proteinuria can be caused by the increased addition of protein to the urine by the renal tubular epithelial cells or in the lower genitourinary tract. For example, the increased urinary excretion of Tamm–Horsfall protein accounts in part for the relative proteinuria found in the neonatal period. There may be failure to visualize the kidneys by excretory urography during the first few days of extrauterine life, a self-limited problem which has been attributed to excessive formation of Tamm–Horsfall protein casts causing transient intratubular obstruction of urine flow. Kidney-specific antigens, possibly originating from degeneration of proximal tubular cells, have been found in the urine in a variety of diseases including the early stages of analgesic nephropathy, heavy-metal poisoning, and in both rapidly progressive and lupus glomerulonephritis. Urinary mucoprotein is increased with injury to the renal pelvis and lower urinary tract. Proteins originating from the kidney, ureter, urinary bladder, and urethra have also been found in increased amounts in patients with acute pyelonephritis and nephrolithiasis.

Diseases of the prostate and other accessory sex glands may be associated with proteinuria, much of which originates from these organs.

5. Histuria

Normal urine contains small amounts of proteins which are released from many nonrenal tissues and organs and are referred to as "tissue antigens." The increased urinary excretion of these proteins is referred to as histuria. They may be organ specific so that injury to individual organs such as the submaxillary glands, pancreas, liver, or testes can result in the increased urine excretion of a tissue-specific antigen from that organ. Alternately, these antigens may be of more widespread distribution originating, for example, from basement membrane or collagen.

Examples of this form of proteinuria are seen in patients with cancer. Proteinuria in these patients can result from minimal change nephrotic syndrome or from an immune complex glomerulonephritis secondary to an antitumor immune response. Alternatively, tissue proteins released from the malignancy itself or from normal tissue that is being destroyed by the neoplastic lesion may appear in the urine in appreciable quantities. Thus carcinoembryonic antigen has been found in the urine in significant amounts in patients with urothelial carcinoma as have specific antigens for melanoma, neuroblastoma, and bladder cancer in patients with these malignancies.

D. Consequences of Proteinuria

The effect of proteinuria on plasma protein concentrations is variable. It depends in large part on the ability of the body to synthesize new proteins to compensate for the urinary losses of plasma proteins. When proteinuria is relatively modest in amount, for example, less than 2 g/day in an adult patient, it may not result in any signs or symptoms and may be discovered as an incidental finding during a thorough routine examination. Conversely, if proteinuria is massive in amount and exceeds the patient's ability to synthesize new protein, it will result in hypoproteinemia. The prolonged loss of excessive amounts of protein in the urine typically results in the development of the nephrotic syndrome.

1. Nephrotic Syndrome

This clinical syndrome consists of proteinuria, hypoproteinemia (primarily hypoalbuminemia), edema, and hyperlipidemia. At one time thought to be a single entity, it is now recognized to be the result of a variety of disorders which have in common heavy proteinuria (Table II). Some are associated with progressive nephron loss, others are not. In addition to the clinical features common to all patients with nephrotic syndrome, many patients have additional clinical or laboratory abnormalities which are features

Table II. Diseases Associated with the Nephrotic Syndrome

I. Idiopathic glomerulopathies
   Minimal-change nephrotic syndrome, focal glomerular sclerosis, membranoproliferative glomerulonephritis, membranous glomerulonephritis
II. Collagen vascular disorders
   Systemic lupus erythematosus, periarteritis, dermatomyositis
III. Diabetes mellitus
IV. Infectious diseases
   Syphilis, malaria, subacute bacterial endocarditis, cytomegalic inclusion disease, toxoplasmosis
V. Malignancies
   Carcinoma, Hodgkin's disease, leukemias, multiple myelomatosis
VI. Cardiovascular disorders
   Thrombosis of renal vein or inferior vena cava, congestive heart failure, constrictive pericarditis
VII. Drugs: allergens
   Trimethadione, paramethadione, penicillamine, probenecid, heroin use; poison ivy, poison oak, bee stings, snake bites.
VIII. Nephrotoxins
   Mercurials (organic and inorganic), gold, bismuth
IX. Miscellaneous disorders
   Amyloidosis, congenital nephrotic syndrome, hereditary nephritis, pyelonephritis, sickle cell anemia, pregnancy, obesity, renal transplantation.

of the primary disease process that is causing the nephrotic syndrome. For example, those with glomerulonephritis may have hematuria, severe hypertension, and azotemia; others may have manifestations of a systemic disease such as systemic lupus erythematosus, which can result in glomerulonephritis and the nephrotic syndrome. Such abnormalities are not part of the nephrotic syndrome per se so that their absence does not exclude the diagnosis of this syndrome.

The pathophysiology of many of the features of the nephrotic syndrome are quite well understood. Common to most forms of the syndrome is an increase in glomerular permeability to proteins, the mechanism depending on the underlying disease process. Irrespective of etiology, it results in *albuminuria*, increased urinary losses of larger proteins occurring in addition in some diseases. When the rate of albumin loss exceeds the rate of synthesis,* *hypoalbuminemia* results. This reduces plasma oncotic pressure and permits net movement of fluid from the vascular to the interstitial fluid space. The resulting hypovolemia stimulates the increased secretion of renin, aldosterone, and antidiuretic hormone. Alterations in the levels of other hormones such as catecholamines and of the proposed natriuretic hormone may occur too. These changes are designed to promote retention of both sodium and

---

* Data on rates of albumin synthesis in nephrotic syndrome are conflicting. High, normal, or even reduced rates of synthesis have been obtained in different studies. Values can be interpreted in different ways, depending on how the data are expressed, e.g., whether absolute values are used or whether they are expressed per unit of albumin pool size, which is reduced in nephrotic syndrome. In addition, there are numerous causes for the nephrotic syndrome and values may vary in different disease states.

water so that *oliguria* and a very *low urine sodium* concentration results. Although such physiologic responses are appropriate for the low blood volume, the decreased plasma oncotic pressure prevents most of the retained sodium and water being maintained in the vascular space, most enters the interstitial fluid space where it contributes to increasing amounts of *edema* (see Section V.B.1 on edema).

Less clear is the etiology of *hyperlipidemia*. The magnitude of changes in the lipid levels correlates with the reduction in serum albumin and infusion of albumin reverses the hyperlipemia. Current wisdom suggests that hypoalbuminemia either stimulates synthesis of all proteins or that albumin shares a common synthetic pathway in the liver with other plasma proteins. As a consequence, there are increased production and plasma levels of the lipoproteins which are α_2- and β-globulins. Since lipids exist in the plasma as lipoproteins, secondary hyperlipidemia results. Recent observations have prompted a new hypothesis to explain how hypoalbuminemia may result in hypertriglyceridemia. These studies have demonstrated that in proteinuric patients the activity in the plasma of autologous lecithin:cholesterol acyl transferase (LCAT) is reduced in proportion to the decrease in plasma albumin levels. Values correlated well with those of high-density lipoprotein cholesterol too. LCAT catalyzes the esterification of cholesterol in human plasma and is a potential modulator of the plasma triglyceride pathway. Thus low autologous LCAT activity may lead to diminished clearance of plasma triglyceride in the nephrotic syndrome through the effect of cholesterol on lipoprotein lipase. Although LCAT has been found in the urine of animals with experimentally induced nephrotic syndrome, the diminished autologous LCAT activity in proteinuric patients is not necessarily due to loss in the urine. Rather it may result from substrate or acceptor limitation of the reaction consequent upon albumin depletion.

Even though the mechanisms responsible for the changes are not fully understood, the alterations in lipid levels in the nephrotic syndrome have been well described. Plasma levels of total fat, cholesterol, and phospholipids are consistently increased, with the levels of cholesterol and phospholipids being increased in proportion to the severity of the hypoalbuminemia. The elevation in cholesterol is greater than that of the phospholipids so that the cholesterol to phospholipid ratio is increased. Triglycerides increase when the hypoalbuminemia becomes severe. When values exceed 400 mg/dl, or more than four times normal, they produce the characteristic lactescence seen in the plasma of patients with a marked nephrotic syndrome. Free fatty acid levels are normal with an increased proportion bound to lipoproteins. Both type II and type IV lipoprotein profiles have been described depending on whether or not the nephrotic syndrome is associated with renal failure. High- and low-density lipoproteins are increased early in the course of the nephrotic syndrome but tend to return to normal or to below normal levels with increasing degrees of hypoalbuminemia. Very-low-density lipoprotein also rises early in the nephrotic syndrome, levels increasing with progressing severity of the disease. *Lipiduria*, demonstrable as doubly refractile fat bodies

Table III. Consequences of Urinary Protein Loss in the Nephrotic Syndrome[a]

Protein deficiency	Physiologic consequence	Clinical manifestation
Albumin	↓ Plama oncotic pressure ↓ Drug binding sites	Edema, hypovolemia, orthostatic hypotension, hyperlipidemia, ↑ toxicity of albumin-bound drugs
Antithrombin III	Impaired thrombin inactivation	Thromboembolic tendency
Complement factor B	Impaired complement-dependent opsonization of bacteria	Impaired resistance to infection
High-density lipoprotein	Impaired cholesterol transport	Accelerated atherogenesis
IgG	Hypogammaglobulinemia	Impaired resistance to bacterial infection
Metal-binding proteins (e.g., transferrin)	Urinary loss of Cu and Zn, impaired transport of Fe	Dysgeusia, hypochromic microcytic anemia (refractory to Fe), poor wound healing, ?impotence
Orosomucoid	Defective lipoptotein lipase, impaired conversion of VLDL to LDL	Hypertriglyceridemia
Procoagulant proteins	Factors IX, XI, XII	?Hemorrhagic tendency
Thyroxine-binding globulin	↑ Free thyroxine	↑ T_3 resin uptake, ↓ T_4 (chemical hypothyroidism)
Transcortin	↑ Free cortisol	↑ ?Susceptibility to exogenous Cushing's syndrome
Vitamin-D-binding protein	↓ 25-hydroxycholecalciferol, 1,25-dihydroxycholecalciferol, impaired GI calcium absorption, secondary ↑ parathormone secretion	Hypocalcemia, osteomalacia, 2° hyperparathyroidism, osteititis fibrosa cystica, muscle weakness, ?impotence

[a] Data taken from Glassock, R. J.: The nephrotic syndrome. *Hosp. Practice* 14(11):105–129, 1979.

or maltese crosses by polarized light microscopy, may be seen. This urinary lipid may be present in casts, as oval fat bodies which are degenerative epithelial cells or as free lipids in the urine.

Although albumin is the protein lost in greatest amounts in the urine of patients with nephrotic syndrome, the urinary loss of other proteins, albeit in smaller amounts, can result in significant clinical consequences. Examples include Factor B, the binding proteins for 25-OH vitamin D, thyroid-binding globulins, transferrin, and the smaller-molecular-weight coagulation factors. Their loss may contribute respectively to the increased susceptibility to infection, to hypocalcemia, to apparent hypothyroidism, to iron deficiency anemia, and to the hypercoagulable states which occur with increased frequency in patients with the nephrotic syndrome. A more detailed analysis is presented in Table III.

E. Clinical Evaluation of Proteinuria

1. Quantitative Measurements

Measurements of total urine protein are important in both the initial evaluation and follow-up of patients with renal disease. Factoring protein excretion by the simultaneous excretion of creatinine reduces errors from incomplete urine collections. Even more important is to express protein excretion per unit of GFR to avoid misinterpretation of the significance of changes in proteinuria. For example, in progressive glomerulonephritis, a falling GFR may result in a decreased filtered load of protein so that proteinuria can fall even though the underlying disease process is progressing. Factoring protein excretion by GFR avoids misinterpreting such changes. Rates of proteinuria do not always parallel changes in glomerular filtration rate. Typically, heavy proteinuria persists in patients with diabetes mellitus, amyloidosis, and renal vein thrombosis, even though GFR may be markedly reduced to very low levels.

2. Qualitative Measurements

Qualitative analysis of urine protein may become an even more important clinical tool than quantitative measurements of protein excretion in the future. From the proposed mechanism for proteinuria in minimal-change nephrotic syndrome, one would anticipate that the urine protein would consist primarily of albumin. Conversely, in nephrotic syndrome secondary to glomerulonephritis extensive disruption of the GBM would permit passage of larger proteins across the glomerular barrier and increased urinary losses of both albumin and globulins. Measuring the relative clearances of proteins of different molecular sizes should provide a noninvasive method to separate patients with these two causes for the nephrotic syndrome. This forms the basis for measurement of *protein selectivity* (Figure 11). In minimal-change nephrotic syndrome, proteinuria is *highly selective* with the clearances of globulins or other large proteins being small when compared to the clearance of albumin. In contrast, in patients with glomerulonephritis, proteinuria is *nonselective*, with the ratio of globulin-to-albumin clearance being higher.

Although measurements of selectivity can separate groups of patients with different causes for their nephrotic syndrome, the test has not found widespread clinical acceptance. Unfortunately results from groups of patients with different disease entities overlap (Figure 11) so that the test has limited value in an individual patient. This may not be because the concepts on which measurements of protein selectivity are based are invalid, rather it may result from technical difficulties. Accurate measurement of individual protein concentrations is not easy. Even immunoassay values may be misleading since they can measure immunoreacting protein fragments as well as intact protein. Moreover, factors other than molecular size are now known

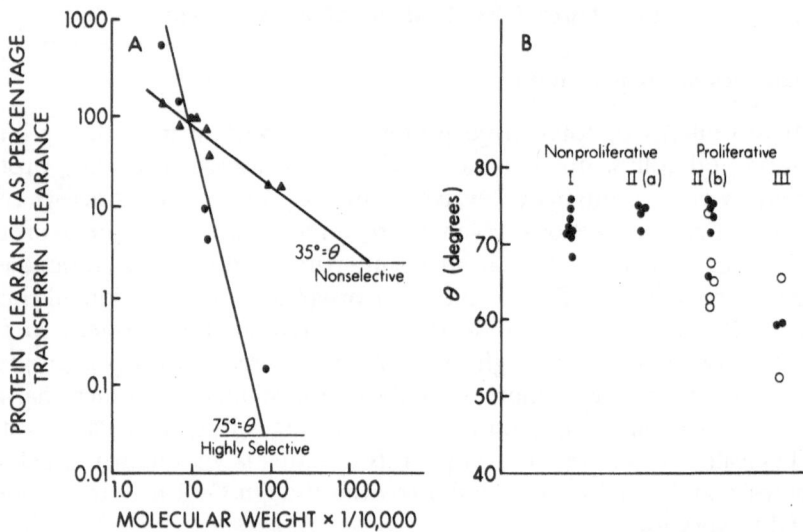

Figure 11. Protein selectivity. (A) Demonstrates one method for depicting selectivity in which the clearance of individual proteins is plotted against that protein's molecular weight. The angle of the regression line (θ) indicates the degree of selectivity; the higher the angle the more highly selective is the proteinuria. (B) Depicts results from a group of children with nephrotic syndrome. Although those children with proliferative renal diseases tend to have nonselective proteinuria (low values for θ), the overlap of the results from the different groups children is apparent. (Reprinted with permission from Cameron, J. S., and White, R. H. R.: *Lancet* 1:463–465, 1965.)

to affect entry of proteins into the glomerular filtrate. In addition, because of considerable tubular reabsorption of protein, the pattern of proteinuria does not necessarily reflect the pattern of protein crossing the glomerular barrier. These and possibly other problems may explain why the relationship between protein clearance and size applies only to selected urinary proteins.

In contrast to glomerular disease where the larger plasma proteins comprise most of the urinary protein, tubular disorders are characterized by the urinary excretion of low-molecular-weight proteins. This is referred to as *tubular proteinuria* with more than 20 small-molecular-weight proteins, including lysozyme, β_2-microglobulin, ribonuclease, and light chains, having been identified in increased amounts in the urine. Of these, lysozyme, an enzyme with a molecular weight of between 14,000 to 15,000, has been studied most extensively. Its excretion is increased by many diseases associated with tubular damage including heavy-metal poisoning, administration of nephrotoxic drugs, and renal homograft rejection. Unfortunately, not all patients with tubular disorders have lysozymuria and values may be increased in other disease limiting the diagnostic usefulness of lysozymuria. Thus, in sarcoidosis or some leukemias there are increased serum levels secondary to high production rates, and in genitourinary tract infections lysozymuria results from increased synthesis of the protein in the urinary tract.

The development of a commercially available antiserum to β_2-micro-globulin has facilitated its measurement and has prompted extensive study of this protein as a marker for tubular disorders. The origin and functions of β_2-microglobulin are uncertain. Its structure is relatively simple consisting of a single polypeptide chain, with a molecular weight of 11,800 and a molecular radius of only 16 Å. It is readily filtered through the glomerulus, with more than 99% of the filtered protein being reabsorbed and catabolized by the normal proximal tubule. As with most smaller proteins, tubular damage results in decreased reabsorption and increased losses in the urine of β_2-microglobulin. Unfortunately, it too has more than one mechanism for increased urinary excretion and it may prove necessary to measure blood concentrations and clearance rates of β_2-microglobulin before attempting to interpret the significance of increased urinary excretion rates of this protein.

All of these techniques warrant continued study. In addition, further delineation of the significance of histuria by identification of specific tissue antigens in the urine has the potential of resulting in qualitative analysis of proteinuria becoming an increasingly important diagnostic tool in the future permitting accurate diagnosis of nonrenal diseases by noninvasive methods.

V. TREATMENT

A. Treatment of Primary Disease

The obvious goal in the management of proteinuria is to treat the underlying disease process and eliminate further protein losses. In some entities, such as minimal-change nephrotic syndrome, effective treatment is available. More than 90% of children, and a somewhat smaller percentage of adult patients, with this entity respond to treatment with steroids. The drug usually employed is prednisone, given in a single daily dose of 2 mg/kg body weight. Typically, proteinuria is reversed within two or three weeks although some patients may take up to four weeks to respond. If patients do not respond by this time, they are considered to be steroid resistant. Fifty percent or more of patients who respond to steroids subsequently experience one or more relapses. Those patients who have frequent relapses, three or more a year, or those who develop severe side effects from steroids, may benefit from a three-month course of either cyclophosphamide or chlorambucil. Use of one of these drugs reduces the subsequent risk of relapse, with up to two thirds of children treated with such a regimen apparently entering into long-term or permanent remission.

Patients with focal glomerulosclerosis may present as though they had minimal-change disease, the correct diagnosis being established after the patients have been found to be resistant to treatment with steroids. In some, treatment with prednisone may reduce the degree of proteinuria, but not eliminate it. Cytotoxic drugs typically do not help these patients either. Preliminary observations have suggested that the use of anticoagulant drugs combined with antiplatelet agents may be beneficial in preventing or delaying the development of end-stage renal failure in patients with focal glomerulosclerosis.

Membranoproliferative glomerulonephritis is difficult to treat, too. Patients with a fulminant form of this disease associated with marked loss of renal function may benefit from steroids given intravenously in very high "pulse" doses. Less severe cases have been reported to benefit from long-term therapy with prednisone given every other day in low doses (0.3 − 0.5 mg/kg body weight) on alternate days.

Recent studies have shown that prednisone given every other day in a dose of approximately 2 mg/kg body weight for at least eight weeks and then tapered may improve the prognosis for patients with membranous glomerulonephritis. Although proteinuria frequently remitted or was decreased with treatment, many of the remissions were not sustained.

In patients with the more severe form of proliferative glomerulonephritis, it often is difficult, if not impossible, to lessen the degree of proteinuria by drug treatment. Some, with necrosis in the glomerular tuft and/or extensive crescent formation, may benefit from treatment with either anti-coagulants or steroids in "pulse" dosage.

In summary, proteinuria can be reversed in many patients with minimal-change disease. It is much more difficult to accomplish the task in patients with other glomerulopathies. One can still help these patients, however, by symptomatic treatment. This is designed to minimize the consequences of proteinuria especially when it is complicated by a nephrotic syndrome.

B. Symptomatic Treatment

1. Hypoproteinemia

Serum protein concentrations can be increased in patients with heavy proteinuria by providing a diet rich in protein. The dietary protein should be of high biologic value with the intake equal to at least 1.5 g of protein per kg body weight. In patients with heavy proteinuria and advanced renal failure, a high protein intake will increase the degree of azotemia and is not indicated. Such patients may become protein malnourished and have severe symptoms from marked contraction of intravascular volume. If their proteinuria is massive in amount, they may benefit from early nephrectomy as a treatment of last resort, especially if they are candidates for hemodialysis and transplantation. Renal arterial embolization has been shown to be effective for this purpose if the patient's condition precludes surgical nephrectomy.

Loss of proteins other than albumin may necessitate specific treatments. Examples include the use of anticoagulants to prevent thrombotic lesions, or administration of vitamin D metabolites to reduce the risk of osteomalacia. Doses of drugs which bind to albumin may have to be modified.

2. Edema

The treatment of edema has been detailed in Chapter 5. It is important to reemphasize here, however, that one should resist the temptation to use diuretics when treating mild degrees of edema in nephrotic patients. Such patients are especially susceptible to the side effects of diuretics.

Patients with anasarca, especially if there is massive ascites, may benefit from a diuresis induced by albumin infusion combined with diuretics. If such treatment is contemplated, it is advisable to start the patient on Aldactone in an oral dose of approximately 1 mg/kg body weight per day, given in three divided doses. This takes about three days to develop maximum effectiveness. To induce a diuresis, we commence with an intravenous dose of furosemide, 0.5 mg/kg body weight, followed by an intravenous infusion of salt-poor human albumin in a dose of either 0.5 or 1.0 g/kg body weight given over 1 to 1.5 hr. It is followed by a second intravenous infusion of fuorsemide in a dose of 0.5 mg/kg body weight. This regimen usually induces a diuresis, but may have to be repeated daily for two, three, or more days. We use the smaller dose of albumin if the patient is hypertensive, has compromised cardiac function, or impaired renal function. However, if the initial dose is tolerated well, the higher dose can be administered subsequently. The albumin has little long-term effect on serum albumin concentration. Proteinuria typically increases dramatically following the albumin infusion.

3. Hyperlipidemia

The long-term value of cholestyramine, clofibrate, or tryptophan to reduce lipid levels in nephrotic patients has not been proven. Nor has there been extensive experience with the new lipid-lowering agents. Indeed, their poor tolerance and toxic side effects when used longterm, limit their potential usefulness.

SUGGESTED READINGS

Proteinuria

Reviews

Boylan, J. W., and Van Liew, J. B. (eds.): Symposium on proteinuria and renal protein catabolism. *Kidney Int.* 16:247–429, 1979.

Brenner, B. M., Hotstetter, T. H., and Humes, H. D.: Molecular basis of proteinuria of glomerular origin. *N. Engl. J. Med.* 298:826–833, 1978.

Heineman, H.: Proteinuria. *Am. J. Med.* 56:71–82, 1974.

Manuel, Y., Revillard, J. P., and Betuel, H. (eds.): *Proteins in Normal and Pathological Urine.* University Park Press, Baltimore, 1970.

Pesce, A. J., and First, M. R.: *Proteinuria. An Integrated Review.* Marcel Dekker, New York, 1979.

Specific Topics

Farquhar, M.: The primary glomerular filtration barrier—basement membrane or epithelial slits? An editorial review. *Kidney Int.* 8:197–211, 1975.

Kanwar, Y. S., Linker, A., and Farquhar, M. G.: Increased permeability of the glomerular basement membrane to ferritin after removal of glycosaminoglycans (heparan sulfate) by enzyme digestion. *J. Cell Biol.* 86:688–693, 1980.

Nephrotic Syndrome

Reviews

Glassock, R. J.: The nephrotic syndrome. *Hosp. Practice* 14(11):105–129, 1979.

Heptinstall, R.: The nephrotic syndrome, in *Pathology of Kidney*, Second edition. Little, Brown and Co., Boston, 1974.

Hutt, M., and Glassock, R. J.: Proteinuria and the nephrotic syndrome, in Schrier, R. W. (ed.): *Renal and Electrolyte Disorders*, Second edition. Little, Brown and Co., Boston, 1979, Chap. 14.

Martinez-Maldonado, M., and Garcia, A.: A practical approach to the nephrotic syndrome. *Drug Therapy* 11(3):79–94, 1981.

Specific Topics

Bernard, D. B., and Alexander, E. A.: Edema formation in the nephrotic syndrome: pathophysiologic mechanisms. *Cardiovasc. Med.* 4:605–625, 1979.

Cohen, S. L., Cramp, D. G., Lewis, A. D., and Tickner, T. R.: The mechanism of hyperlipidemia in nephrotic syndrome—role of low albumin and the LCAT reaction. *Clin. Chim. Acta* 104:393–400, 1980.

Dorhout Mees, E. J., Roos, J. C., Boer, P., Yoe, O. H., and Simatupang, T. A.: Observations on edema formation in the nephrotic syndrome in adults with minimal lesions. *Am. J. Med.* 67:378–384, 1979.

Treatment

Coggins, C. H.: A controlled study of short-term prednisone treatment in adults with membranous nephropathy. *N. Engl. J. Med.* 301:1301–1306, 1979.

Cole, B. R., Brocklebank, J. T., Kienstra, R. A., Kissane, J. M., and Robson, A. M.: "Pulse" methylprednisolone therapy in the treatment of severe glomerulonephritis. *J. Pediat.* 88:307–314, 1976.

Robson, A. M., Cole, B. R., Kienstra, R. A., Kissane, J. M., Alkjaersig, N., and Fletcher, A. P.: Severe glomerulonephritis complicated by coagulopathy: treatment with anticoagulant and immunosuppresive drugs. *J. Pediat.* 90:881–892, 1977.

Simon, N. M., and Rosenberg, M. J.: Medical treatment of glomerular disease. *Med. Clin. N. Am.* 62:1157–1181, 1978.

12

Pathology and Pathophysiology of Proteinuric Glomerular Disease

BARBARA R. COLE and ANDRES J. VALDES

I. INTRODUCTION

Renal glomerular diseases began to be reasonably understood during the first part of this century when the major emphasis for classification shifted from pure clinical grounds to clinicopathological correlations. The popularization of renal biopsies, the refinements of laboratory methods for detection of possible etiological factors, the availability of electron microscopy, the development of experimental models, and the wealth of immunologic information accumulated during the last two or three decades all have contributed greatly to advance our knowledge; yet as of now there is not one generally accepted classification of glomerular diseases. The reason for this is multifactorial. The glomerulus has very limited ways of reacting to injury; therefore, different etiological insults might express indistinguishable structural and functional alterations. Furthermore, the humoral and cellular response may vary from patient to patient and similar etiological challenge may result in different morphological and clinical pictures. Most glomeru-

BARBARA R. COLE • Department of Pediatrics, Washington University School of Medicine, St. Louis, Missouri 63110.   ANDRES J. VALDES • Department of Pathology, Washington University School of Medicine and St. John's Mercy Medical Center, St. Louis, Missouri 63110.

lonephritides are of unknown etiology and usually present as primary renal disease. Similar glomerular alterations, however, may develop during the course of systemic diseases or may rarely precede them. Whether primary or associated with systemic disease the majority of glomerulonephritides are mediated by humoral immunologic mechanisms, as proven by the presence of glomerular deposits of immunoglobulin and complement demonstrable by immunofluorescence microscopy and rarely by the identification of specific antibody or antigen in the glomerular eluates. The etiopathogenesis of the remaining is not clear with the participation of cellular immunity, coagulation system, kinin system, and others at best just suspected. Finally, in practice. there is the not too infrequent problem of having to classify diseases discovered at the end stage, congenital diseases, and morphological alterations in transplanted kidneys.

It is therefore evident that no inclusive classification of glomerular diseases can be based on clinical, etiological, histological, ultrastructural, or immunologic grounds alone and that an adequate understanding can only be achieved from a multidisciplinary approach.

II. IMMUNOFLUORESCENCE TECHNIQUES

Fluorescence is the property of a substance of emitting a secondary light of a specific wavelength when excited by a primary light of a different wavelength. Immunofluorescence microscopy is based on the fact that antibodies can be labeled with a fluorochrome (e.g., fluorescein isothyocianate, tetramethyl rhodamine isothyocianate) and their presence in tissues can be demonstrated utilizing a microscope equipped with an adequate light source and different filters. Direct immunofluorescence microscopy allows the investigation of the presence of immunoglobulin, complement components, multiple plasma protein, or antigens in the kidney or other tissues. Frozen sections of the tissue are layered with a solution containing fluorescein-labeled antibodies specific for the protein or antigen investigated. The exciting light is suppressed by inserting a barrier filter in the optical path. The secondary light is visible if and where the antibodies are attached to the tissue. Indirect immunofluorescence microscopy allows the investigation of the presence of specific antibodies in the serum or tissue eluates by reacting the serum or the eluates with frozen sections of normal tissue known to contain antigen capable of binding the antibodies in question. After washing, the frozen section is layered with fluorescein-labeled antibodies to human immunoglobulin and examined as before.

Deposition of immunoglobulin and C3 in the glomerulus is usually granular and less frequently linear. Granular deposits in general identify diseases mediated by immune complexes. It is possible to discern whether

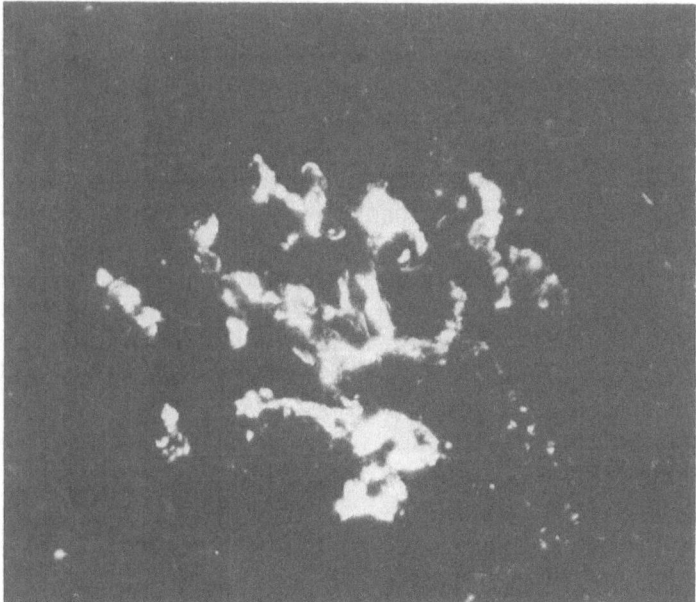

Figure 1. Mesangial pattern. Granular deposits of immunoglobulin in axial region. Berger's IgG-IgA nephropathy. Goat anti-human IgA (×516).

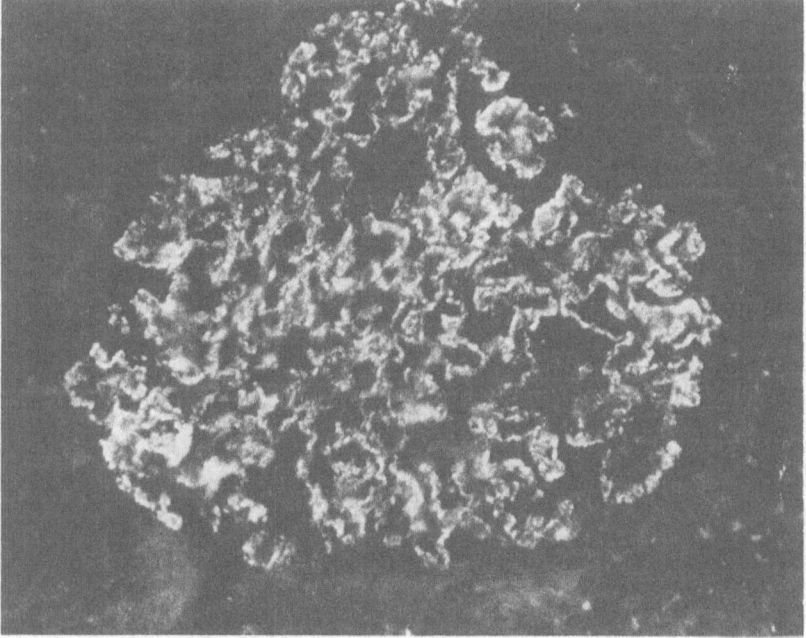

Figure 2. Peripheral pattern. Granular deposits of immunoglobulin outlining glomerular loops. Idiopathic membranous glomerulonephritis. Goat anti-human IgG (×516).

the deposits are in the mesangium or in the loop by their axial or peripheral distribution (Figures 1 and 2). The size and concentration of granular loop deposits vary in different diseases and the pattern is sometimes characteristic. By immunofluorescence microscopy, however, it is not possible to determine if the peripheral deposits are in the subepithelial or subendothelial zone. Linear deposits of immunoglobulin and C3 along the peripheral loop are usually associated with diseases mediated by antibodies to the glomerular basement membrane (Figure 3).

The mechanism of activation of the complement system responsible for the C3 deposits can be evaluated by immunofluorescence microscopy. The presence of C1q and C4 suggest activation through the classical pathway. Absence of early complement components and presence of properdin suggest activation through the "alternate" pathway.

Participation of the coagulation system can also be evaluated by immunofluorescence microscopy demonstrating the presence or absence of fibrinogen deposition in the glomerulus.

Similar techniques can be used to study the tubules, blood vessels, and interstitial tissue of the kidney.

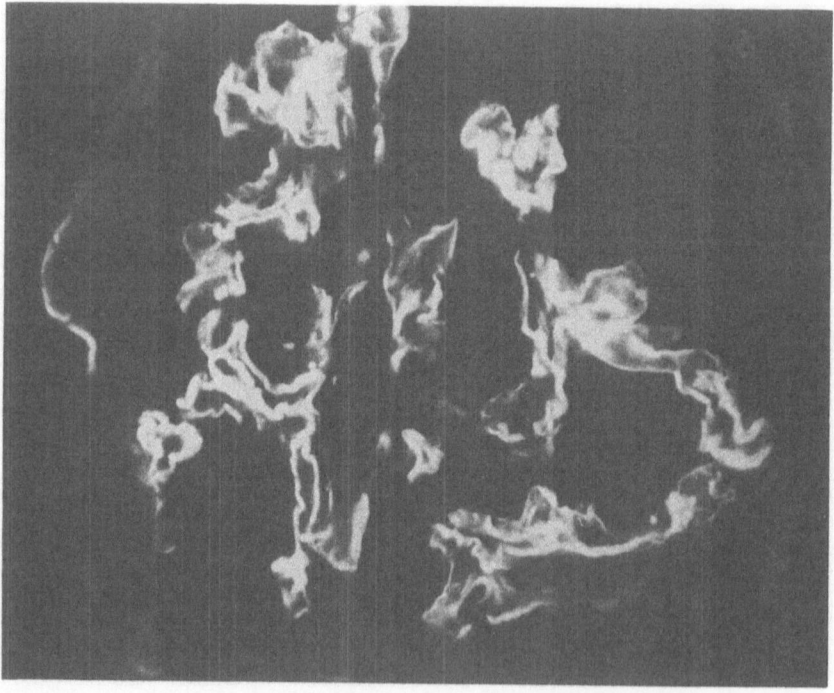

Figure 3. Linear pattern. Linear, ribbonlike deposits of IgG along glomerular basement membrane. Goodpasture's syndrome. Goat anti-human IgG (×516).

III. CHARACTERISTIC GLOMERULAR ALTERATIONS DEMONSTRABLE BY ELECTRON MICROSCOPY

The presence of subepithelial, intramembranous, subendothelial, or mesangial electron-dense deposits demonstrable by electron microscopy characterizes glomerular diseases mediated by immune complexes (Figures 4–6). The deposits, albeit rarely, might show pathognomonic features (e.g., fingerprint deposits in lupus nephritis). Large dense intramembranous deposits probably not related to immune complexes are typically found in type II membranoproliferative glomerulonephritis, so-called dense deposit disease. Diseases mediated by antibodies to glomerular basement membrane do not have diagnostic electron microscopic alterations. Discontinuities or "gaps" in the glomerular basement membrane are only rarely seen. Extensive splitting of the glomerular basement membrane is often encountered in patients with Alport's syndrome (Figure 7). Thinning of the basement membrane might be associated with benign familial hematuria. Thickening of the basement membrane is characteristic of diabetes nephropathy (Figure 8). Collagen fibrils may be found in the glomerular basement membrane of patients with the nail-patella syndrome. Myelinlike fibrils can be identified in the glomerular cells of patients with Fabrey's disease (Figure 9). Extensive fusion of foot processes of epithelial cells is characteristic but not diagnostic of Nil disease (Figure 10). The presence of fibrin or amyloid fibrils can be documented by electron microscopy. Viruslike inclusions, crystalloid structures, and many other less specific alterations can also be identified.

IV. PATHOGENESIS OF GLOMERULAR DISEASES

The participation of humoral immunity in the pathogenesis of glomerulonephritis has been amply documented by a vast number of experimental studies and clinical observations during the last 70 years. In the early experimental models, glomerular disease was evoked by injecting animals with heterologous serum or heteronephrotoxic antikidney serum. It was subsequently demonstrated that lesions of serum sickness could be induced by the injection of highly purified proteins such as bovine serum albumin (BSA) or γ-globulin (BGG). The use of a chemically homogeneous antigen instead of a mixture of antigens (e.g., serum) made possible the application of rigorous immunochemical techniques. This, together with the availability of electron microscopy and immunohistochemical methods (fluorescent and enzymatic) for detecting deposition of immunoglobulin, complement, and other plasma proteins within renal tissue, has provided the necessary information for delineating two basic immunologic mechanisms of glomerular injury (immune complex mediated and antiglomerular basement membrane mediated).

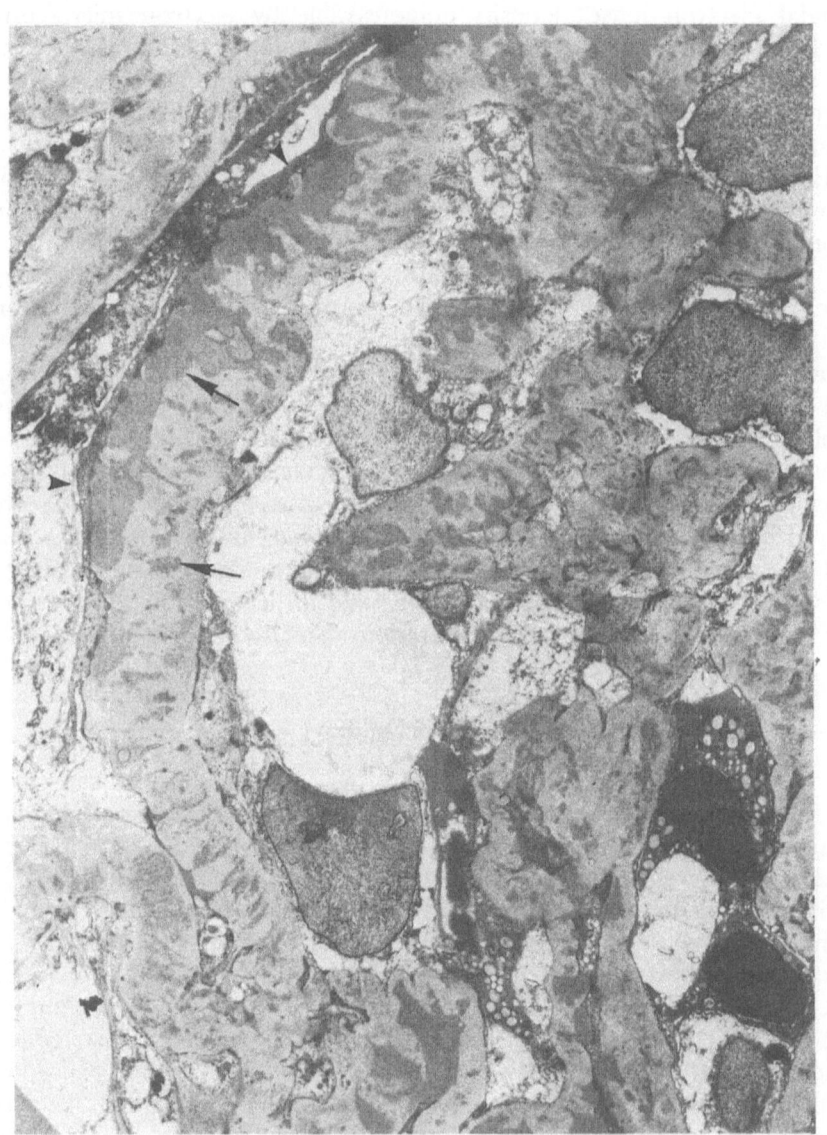

Figure 4. Subepithelial and intramembranous electron-dense deposits (↑). Note extensive fusion of foot processes (▲). Idiopathic membranous glomerulonephritis (×5600).

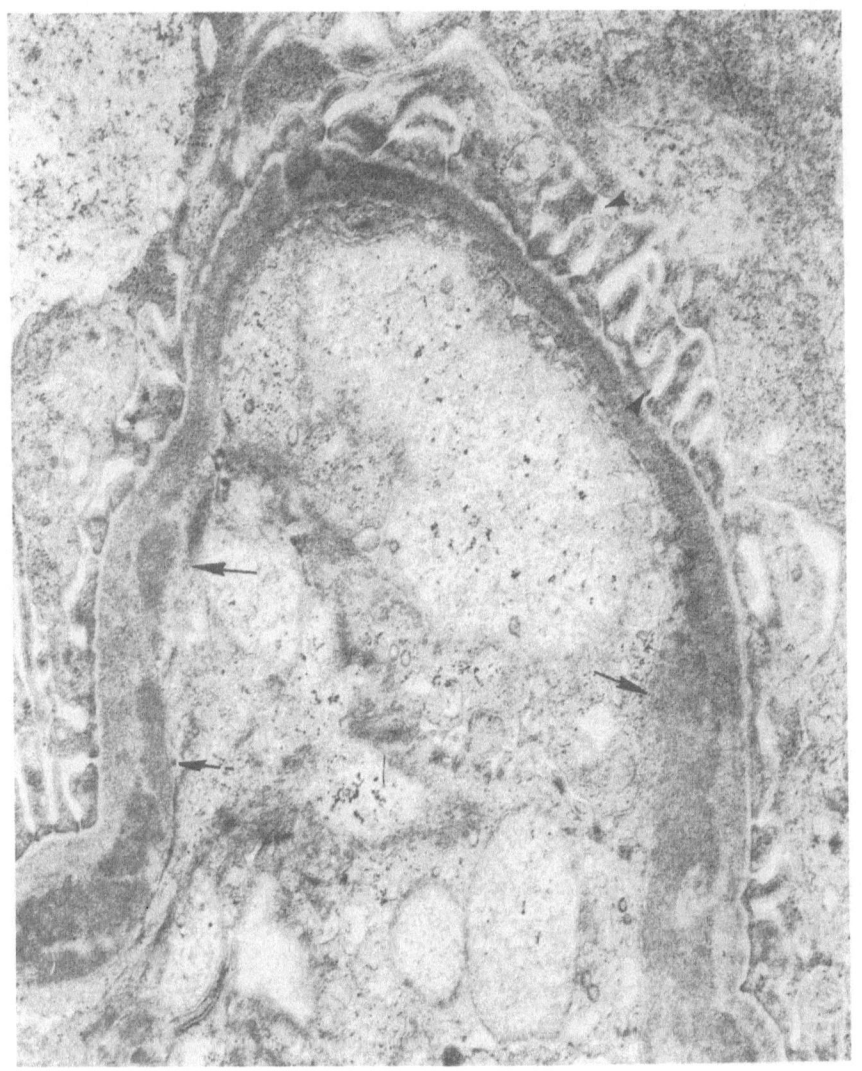

Figure 5. Subendothelial electron-dense deposits (↑). Note preservation of foot processes (▲). Type I membranoproliferative glomerulonephritis (×13,429).

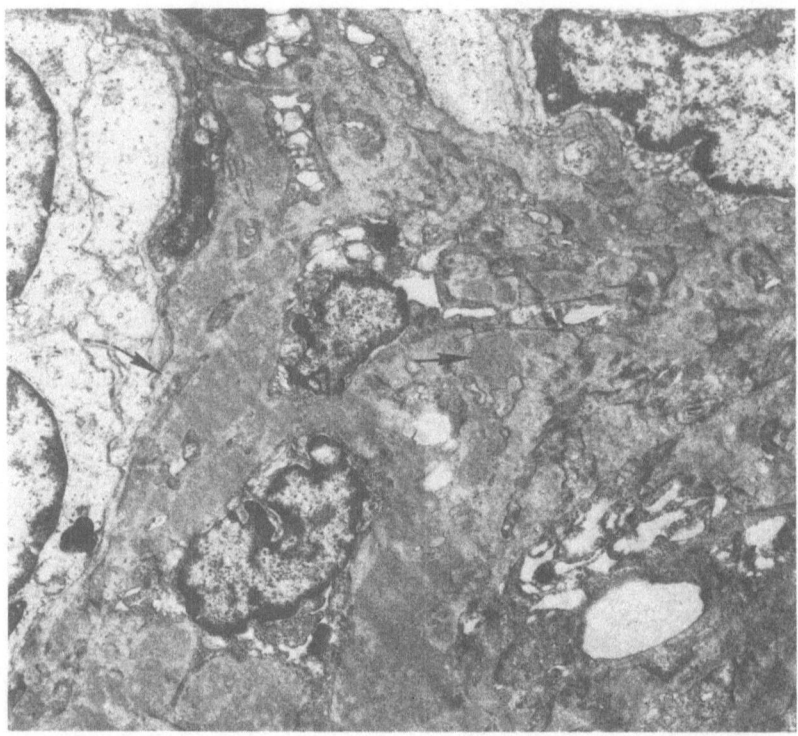

Figure 6. Mesangial electron-dense deposits (↑). Lupus mesangiopathic glomerulonephritis (×5833).

V. EXPERIMENTAL GLOMERULAR INJURY MEDIATED BY SOLUBLE IMMUNE COMPLEXES

A. Exogenous Antigen

If increasing amounts of antigen are added to a given amount of antibody in test tubes, the amount of resulting antigen–antibody precipitate increases progressively (zone of antibody excess) up to a maximum (equivalence) and then begins to decrease (zone of antigen excess). In the last test tube therefore most of the immune reactants remain in solution (soluble immune complexes).

When an antigen (BSA) is injected into a normal animal, it is eliminated in three well-defined phases, usually followed by the appearance of free antibody in the serum. The first phase of rapid loss results from equilibration of the antigen between the vascular and the extravascular fluids. The second phase represents the normal rate of catabolism of the antigen by the body. The third phase, the so-called "immune phase," is a result of a more rapid catabolism of the antigen following its combination with newly formed

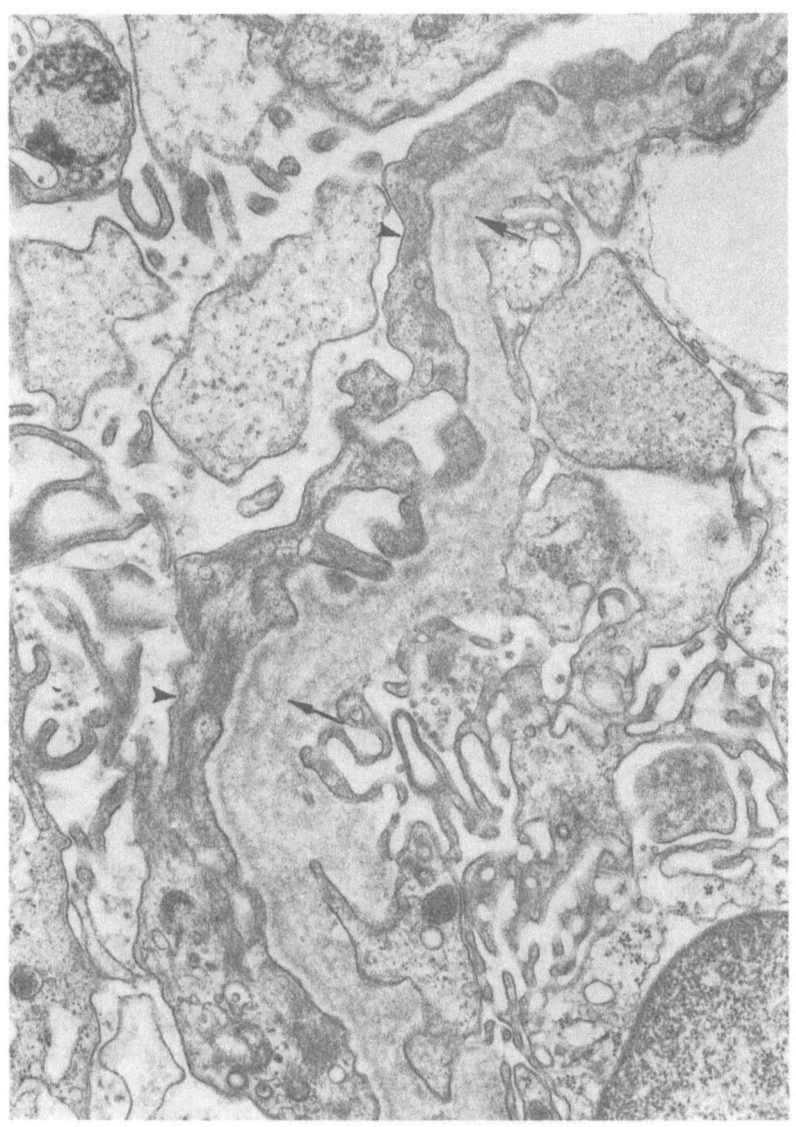

Figure 7. "Splitting" of the glomerular basement membrane into multiple layers (↑). Note segmental fusion of epithelial foot processes (▲). Hereditary nephritis (Alport's syndrome) (×17,000).

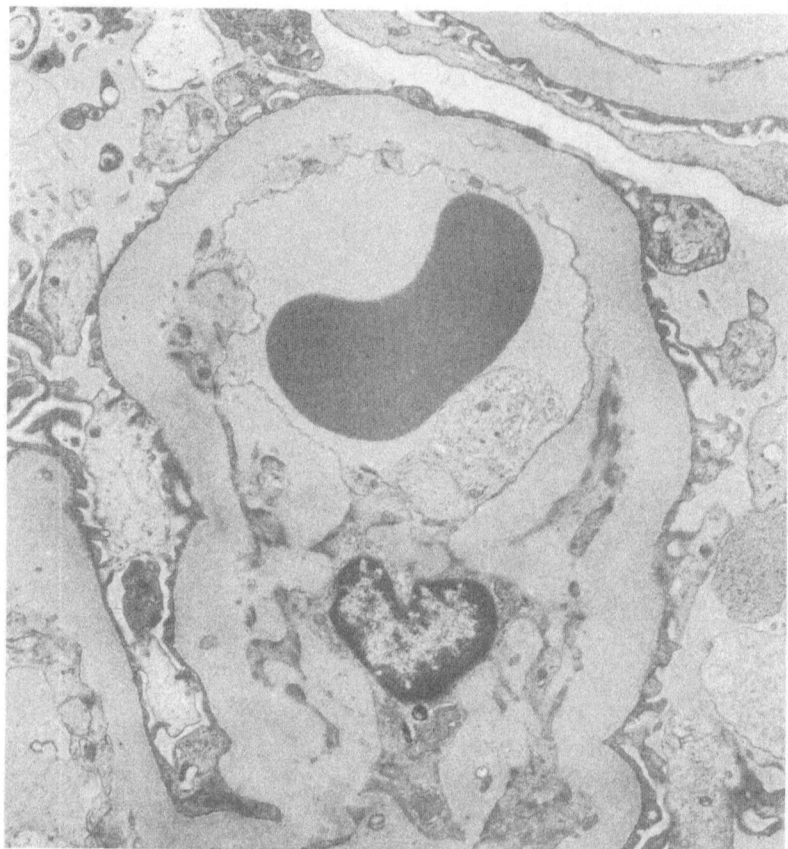

Figure 8. Diffuse thickening of glomerular basement membrane. Diabetic glomerulosclerosis ($\times$6800).

antibody. The tissue damage that may ensue was initially thought to result after the antigen became fixed to the tissue and the antibody reached the site transported in cells such as lymphocytes and monocytes. In 1953, F. Germuth studied the time of development of renal and other lesions in rabbits injected with one large dose of BSA in relation to the blood clearance of antigen and the time of appearance of circulating antibody. In this model of acute serum sickness, the tissue lesions were found to develop during the "immune phase" of antigen elimination and regressed after the antigen had been completely eliminated and free antibody had appeared in the circulation. In view of this temporal relationship he postulated that the tissue damage had been mediated by circulating soluble antigen–antibody complexes. Further proof of this was provided in subsequent studies which demonstrated that soluble antigen–antibody complexes form *in vitro* are indeed biologically active and may initiate a variety of tissue reactions in normal animals. Passive transfer experiments also proved that glomerular and other lesions could be evoked in normal animals by the passive transfer of antibody in the presence of previously injected antigen.

It is now widely held that the proliferative glomerulonephritis of acute serum sickness is mediated by soluble antigen–antibody complexes which penetrate the glomerular capillary walls and during their passage undergo progressive changes to larger, less soluble aggregates which are finally deposited in the subepithelial zone. Indeed, by immunofluorescence microscopy the glomerular lesions are characterized by granular deposits of immunoglobulin, antigen, and complement along the glomerular loops and numerous electron dense subepithelial deposits are demonstrated by electron microscopy. It has been reported that these deposits are in dynamic equilibrium with the circulation and can be resolubilized and made to disappear by the administration of large amounts of antigen. The latter is further proof of their immunologic specificity.

Considerable information on the pathogenesis of glomerulonephritis has also been obtained from a model of chronic serum sickness described by F.

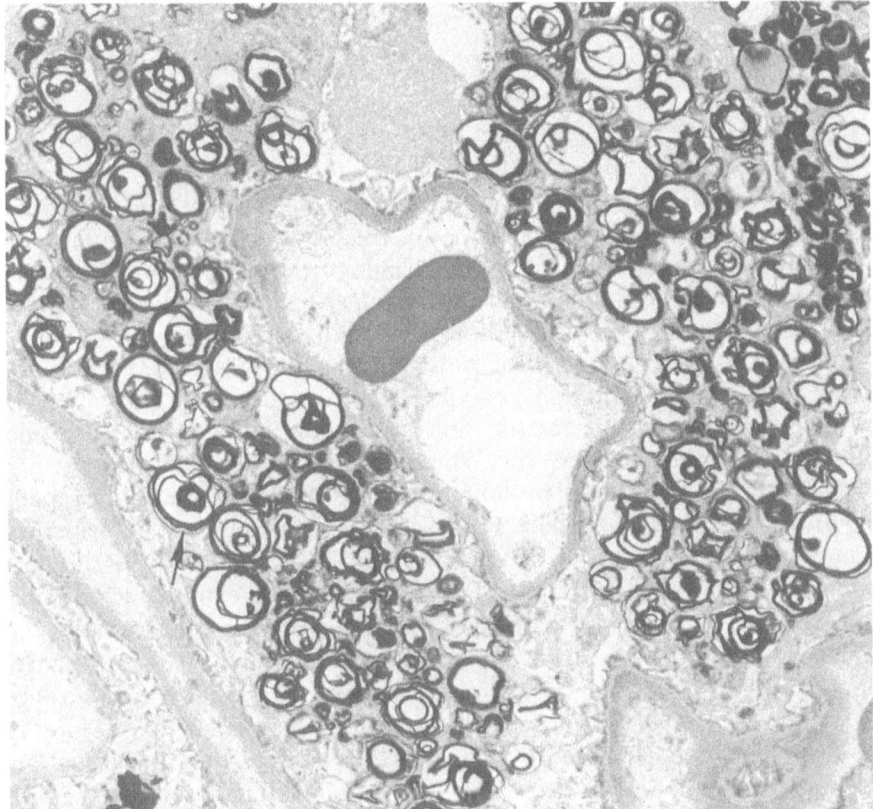

Figure 9. Enlarged epithelial cells containing numerous myelinlike figures (↑). Fabrey's disease (×2800).

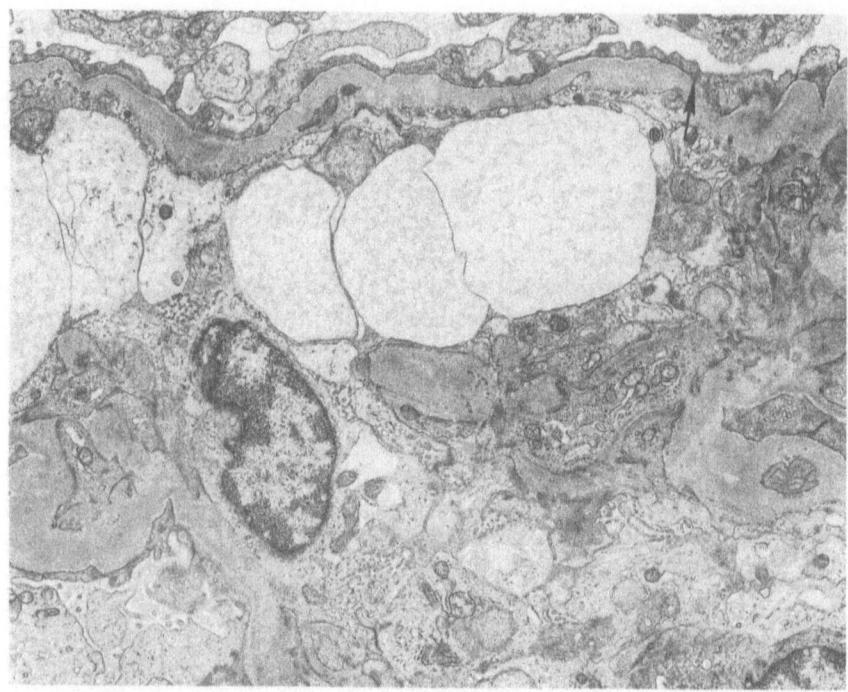

Figure 10. Extensive "fusion" of epithelial foot processes (↑). Nil disease (× 5250).

Dixon and extensively manipulated and studied by Dixon and associates, Germuth, and many others. In this model, the antigen (BSA) is administered in small daily dosages for prolonged periods of time. Some of the animals are incapable of mounting an antibody response and do not develop lesions. Other animals respond with either very high or very low amounts of antibodies. The high antibody responders produce very large, poorly soluble complexes formed in antibody excess which are rapidly removed by the reticuloendothelial system and do not cause renal lesions. The very poor antibody responder develop very small, highly soluble complexes which remain in the circulation for prolonged periods of time, but are not capable of inducing renal lesions. The remaining animals show an intermediate antibody response conducive to the formation of soluble antigen–antibody complexes. In the latter group, the glomerular lesions evoked include most of the entire spectrum of patterns of glomerular injury associated with human glomerulonephritis. Results of further experiments suggest that the primary determinant of the site of immune complex deposition and therefore of the pattern of tissue response is the size of the immune complex. The size of the complex is determined by many factors, such as the ratio of antigen to antibody, the size of the antigen, the antibody class, and the antibody avidity. Immune complexes with molecular weights of 500,000–700,000 are associated with proliferative glomerulonephritis and subepithelial deposits. Complexes larger than 1,000,000 daltons are associated with focal glomerulonephritis and subendothelialmesangial deposits. It has also been reported that the occurrence of membranous glomerulonephritis is favored by the prolonged presence in the circulation of small concentrations of soluble immune complexes, whereas crescentic glomerulonephritis results from the presence of high concentrations of such complexes. In recent passive transfer experiments, the avidity of the antibody is emerging as a very important determinant of the type of lesions evoked. Mice injected with soluble immune complexes of highly avid antibody to egg albumin in large antigen excess developed mesangial deposits and mesangiopathic glomerulonephritis, while mice injected with soluble complexes of poorly avid antibody to egg albumin in large antigen excess developed diffuse proliferative glomerulonephritis with subepithelial deposits. Penetration and deposition in the glomerular walls of immune complexes is also influenced by host factors such as the high hydrostatic pressure within glomerular capillaries and the release of vasoactive amines. It has been reported that reduction of renal hydrostatic pressure produced by constricting the main renal artery reduces or abolishes the development of glomerulonephritis. Vasoactive amines are known to increase the vascular permeability, and treatment with antagonists of histamine and serotonin have been shown to markedly inhibit the localization of immune complexes in glomeruli. Cortisone treatment has also been shown to abolish or modify serum sickness glomerulonephritis not by its antiinflammatory or immunosuppressive effects but by decreasing the permeability of the basement membrance to the immune complexes. Factors which determine serum levels and clearance kinetics of complexes including lattice formation, reticuloendothelial function, and structural changes in the antibody component of circulating complexes have also been shown to play an important role. Other glomerular properties such as the presence of glycoproteins, charged structures, and complement receptors may participate.

Spontaneous glomerulonephritis mediated by immune complexes have been found to develop in mice with long-standing lymphocytic choriomeningitis virus infection and immunoglobulin, complement, and LCM viral antigens have been demonstrated in the glomerular deposits. A similar mechanism appears to be operative in the glomerular lesions associatedwith Aleutian mink disease and in the glomerulonephritis associated with other viral infections in animals.

B. Autologous Antigen

Glomerulonephritis may be induced in rats by repeated intraperitoneal injections of rat kidney in Freund's adjuvant (Heymann nephritis). By immunofluorescence microscopy, granular deposits of immunoglobulin and complement are demonstrable along the glomerular loop, and electron microscopic examination reveals electron dense subepithelial deposits. The antigen taking part in complex formation resides in the brush border of the epithelial cells lining the renal tubules but small quantities of this antigen are present within the circulation in normal animals. Following immunization, antibodies are formed which combine with normally circulating autologous antigen to form the antigen–antibody complexes subsequently deposited in the glomerulus. In this model the subepithelial deposits have been reported to develop in marked antibody excess. This feature is difficult to reconcile with a circulating immune complex pathogenesis; therefore, the possible participation of a different mechanism has been suggested (see the following section). Even though the initial stimulus is not autologous the disease results from autologous immune complexes and could correctly be termed autoimmune or *autologous immune complex glomerulonephritis.*

Spontaneous autoimmune glomerulonephritis mediated by immune complexes is known to occur in NZB-NZW mice. These animals develop autosensitization to DNA and a lupus erythematosuslike syndrome.

VI. EXPERIMENTAL GLOMERULAR INJURY MEDIATED BY *IN SITU* IMMUNE COMPLEX FORMATION

It is becoming apparent that immune complex deposits may also be formed locally and without the participation of circulating, soluble antigen–antibody complexes. Rabbits injected with heat-aggregated human IgG developed nonimmunologic localization of the aggregates in the mesangium. Kidneys from those animals were transplanted into normal rabbits that were then given antihuman IgG. The mesangial aggregates (planted antigen) rapidly bound circulating antibody resulting in local immune complex formation, deposition of C_3, and histologic evidence of glomerulonephritis.

The plant lectin concanavalin A (Con A) has glycoprotein-binding properties and can be attached diffusely to the glomerular walls by renal perfusion. The subsequent administration of anti-Con A has evoked glomerulonephritis mediated by locally formed antigen–antibody complexes and C3.

The ability of free DNA to bind *in vitro* to collagen and collagenlike structures in the glomerular basement membrane has also allowed the production *in situ* of DNA–anti-DNA complexes.

Recent studies have provided evidence for an *in situ* mechanism of formation of subepithelial deposits. Frozen sections of normal rat kidneys bound antibody to rat tubular epithelial brush border antigen (Fx1A) in a granular pattern along glomerular loops. Isolated kidneys of normal rats perfused with 7 S anti-Fx1A developed scattered granular deposits of IgG along the capillary walls within 10 min. A full-blown membranous immunofluorescence pattern developed by 2 hr and electron microscopy revealed small electron-dense deposits in the subepithelial space and slit pores. Studies conducted in passive Heymann nephritis produced by administration of heterologous antibody to Fx1A demonstrated that glomerular changes identical to those seen in the autologous immune complex nephritis developed within hours. The results of these experiments suggest that rat glomeruli posses antigenic determinants capable of directly binding free anti-Fx1A antibody to produce subepithelial deposits in the absence of circulating immune complexes. It is therefore possible that a similar mechanism of *in situ* immune complex formation might be operative in autologous immune complex nephritis.

The previously summarized experiments and many others have conclusively demonstrated that the hallmark of immune complex glomerulonephritis is the granular deposition of immunoglobulin and complement in the glomerular loop or mesangium demonstrable by immunofluorescence microscopy and the presence of subepithelial, intramembranous, subendothelial, or mesangial deposits by electron microscopy. The mechanism by which immune complexes mediate the tissue damage is not completely clear. Significant participation of complement is implied by the demonstration that serum complement levels are consistently reduced during serum sickness at the time of development of lesions and that complement deposits are almost invariably present in immune complex glomerulonephritis. Sequential activation of the complement system is known to result in the formation of biologically active products capable of increasing vascular permeability and attracting neutrophils. Upon reacting with immune complexes neutrophils have been shown to release multiple enzymes capable of injuring the tissues. The proteinuria associated with passive Heymann nephritis is inhibited by decomplementing the animals with cobra venom but it is not prevented by depleting the animals of neutrophils. The glomerulonephritis of acute serum sickness, however, is not prevented by depletion of either complement or neutrophils; therefore, other mechanisms are also involved. Antigen–antibody complexes can trigger coagulation through activation of both Hageman factor and platelets. Hageman factor in turn can activate kinins. The participation of the coagulation and kinin systems, although likely, remains to be further elucidated.

VII. EXPERIMENTAL GLOMERULAR INJURY MEDIATED BY ANTIBODIES TO GLOMERULAR BASEMENT MEMBRANE

A. Nephrotoxic Nephritis (Masugi Nephritis)

Animals injected with heterologous antiserum against glomerular basement membrane develop immediate proteinuria followed a few days later by the onset of progressive deterioration of renal function. The initial proteinuric phase results from the immediate attachment of heterologous antibody to the glomerular basement membrane. At this time, immunofluorescence

microscopy demonstrates linear accumulation of heterologous immunoglobulin and host C3 along the glomerular loop. Light microscopy reveals mild
neutrophilic infiltration. The only change observed by electron microscopy
is a separation of the endothelial cells from the basement membrane, which
allows the polymorphonuclear leukocytes to come into direct contact with
the basement membrane. The second phase is due to the formation of host
antibodies to the heterologous immunoglobulin attached to the glomerulus.
By immunofluorescence microscopy linear glomerular loop deposits of
heterologous immunoglobulin and host IgG and C3 are seen. Light microscopic examination shows variable degrees of capillary thickening, cellular
proliferation, polymorphonuclear infiltration, fibrin deposition, crescent
formation, or focal necrosis. Numerous studies on different variations of this
basic model have demonstrated that complement and neutrophils play a
prime role in the mechanism of glomerular injury. The first phase of the
disease is mediated by complement-dependent migration of neutrophils. It
does not develop in decomplemented animals or following the administration
to rabbits of duck antibody against rabbit kidney (avian antisera do not fix
mamalian complement). These manipulations might modify the second phase
but do not prevent its appearance. The latter, however, can be completely
inhibited if the animals are made leukopenic by nitrogen mustard or other
means. Activation of the coagulation system might also mediate tissue injury
in this model since deposition of fibrinogen is regularly demonstrated and
the severity of the glomerulonephritis has been reduced by anticoagulation
therapy. Other studies, however, have shown that animals which received
heparin before and throughout the period of immunologic insult developed
lesions which were as severe or perhaps more severe than animals that did
not receive heparin.

B. Autoimmune Anti-Glomerular Basement Membrane Nephritis (Steblay Nephritis)

Sheep and other animals receiving injections of homologous or heterologous glomerular basement membrane in complete Freund's adjuvant
develop glomerulonephritis mediated by the production of autoantibodies
reactive with glomerular basement membrane. Immunofluorescence microscopy shows linear deposition of host IgG and C3 along glomerular loops.
Circulating anti-glomerular basement membrane antibodies have been demonstrated and passive transfer of the disease into normal sheep has been
accomplished by using plasma from nephrectomized nephritic sheep. The
development of autoimmune glomerulonephritis in sheep immunized with
human lung in complete Freund's adjuvant has also been reported.

The hallmark of glomerulonephritis mediated by anti-glomerular basement membrane antibodies is the linear deposition of IgG and C3 along the
glomerular loop frequently accompanied by demonstrable fibrin deposits.

VIII. PATHOGENESIS OF HUMAN GLOMERULONEPHRITIS

It is estimated that 60%–80% of all human glomerulonephritides are mediated by humoral immunologic mechanisms which involve the formation of immune complexes in over 90% of the cases and the production of antiglomerular basement membrane antibodies in less than 10%. The pathogenesis of the remaining is not known. Subendothelial deposits of fibrinogen without demonstrable immunoglobulin or C3 are regularly found in the glomerular and vascular lesions associated with acute tubular necrosis, preeclamptic toxemia, hemolytic uremic syndrome, scleroderma, and malignant hypertension. Nonimmunologic activation of the coagulation system, therefore, may play an important role. The complement system can also be activated by nonimmunologic means through the "alternate" or Properdin pathway and this mechanism might be operative in some instances. The possible participation of cell-mediated immunologic mechanisms and the kinin system has been suggested but not well documented.

IX. HUMAN GLOMERULAR INJURY MEDIATED BY IMMUNE COMPLEXES

Several lines of evidence indicate the participation of an immune complex mechanism in the pathogenesis of most human glomerulonephritis: (1) By immunofluorescence microscopy, granular deposits of immunoglobulin and

Table I. Antigens Associated with Glomerulonephritis (Identified or Presumed)

I. Exogenous
  A. Infectious agents
    1. Bacteria: β-streptococci, staphylococci, *Streptococcus pneumoniae*, *Treponema pallidum*, *Mycobacterium leprae*, *Enterococcus*
    2. Virus: hepatitis B, Epstein–Barr, Rubeola, Varicella
    3. Parasites: malaria, toxoplasma, Schistosoma, Filaria
  B. Drugs: gold, mercury, heroin, penicillamine, Mesantoin, Hydralazine, procainamide, probenecid, trimethadione, etc.
  C. Others: foreign serum, insect venom
II. Endogenous
  A. Autoantigens
    1. Various antigens (DNA) (systemic lupus erythematosus)
    2. Thyroglobulin (thyroiditis)
    3. Renal tubular brush border antigens (sickle cell disease)
    4. Glomerular basement membrane antigens (Goodpasture's)
    5. Immunoglobulin (Cryoglobulinemia)
  B. Tumor antigens
    Antigens in carcinoma of the lung, colon, cervix, and in Hodgkin's disease and non-Hodgkin's lymphoma

---

C3 are demonstrable in glomerular loops or mesangium. (2) Subepithelial, intramembranous, subendothelial, or mesangial deposits are seen by electron microscopy. (3) Decreased serum complement levels are regularly present in acute "poststreptococcal" glomerulonephritis, lupus nephritis, and some cases of membranoproliferative glomerulonephritis. (4) Circulating immune complexes have occasionally been demonstrated. (5) Specific antibody and antigens have been rarely identified in glomerular eluates. With very few exceptions, however (see Table I), the antigen or antigens participating in complex formation remain unknown. Most of the identified antigens are exogenous and unrelated to the kidney. The causative agent is sometimes implied by the temporal relationship between the initial clinical event and the subsequent development of glomerulonephritis (e.g., acute glomerulonephritis following a streptococcal infection). The participation of endogenous antigen has also been demonstrated (e.g., DNA in lupus nephritis, brush border of epithelial cells of renal tubules in sickle cell nephritis).

X. HUMAN GLOMERULAR INJURY MEDIATED BY ANTIBODIES TO GLOMERULAR BASEMENT MEMBRANE

The pathogenesis of glomerular injury in Goodpasture's syndrome and in certain cases of idiopathic rapidly progressive glomerulonephritis involves the production of autoantibody reactive with glomerular basement membrane. This is indicated by (1) presence of linear deposits of IgG and sometimes C3 along the glomerular loop, (2) demonstration that immunoglobulin eluted from the glomeruli frequently reacts with normal human glomerular basement membrane, (3) frequent demonstration of circulating antibodies reactive with glomerular basement membrane, and (4) production of glomerulonephritis in monkeys injected intravenously with immunoglobulin eluted from diseased glomeruli. The mechanism responsible for the production of the autoantibodies to glomerular basement membrane is not known. There is evidence to suggest that altered pulmonary alveolar basement membrane provides the initial stimulus that results in the formation of antibodies cross reactive with glomerular basement membrane. Indeed, pulmonary hemorrhages often precede the renal manifestations in Goodpasture's syndrome and IgG deposits have been reported in the alveolar walls. Goodpasture's syndrome has been related within inhalation of hydrocarbons and other irritants. It is also noteworthy that antibasement membrane glomerulonephritis was reported to have been induced in sheep by immunization with human lung in Freund's adjuvant. The mechanism of mediation of tissue damage is mostly inferred from experimental studies. The participation of the complement system, the polymorphonuclear leukocytes, and the coagulation system appear more than likely.

XI. PATHOGENESIS OF HUMAN GLOMERULAR DISEASES OTHER THAN GLOMERULONEPHRITIS

Very little is known about the mechanism of production of glomerular injury in other diseases such as diabetes mellitus and most hereditary nephritides. The glomerular lesions in amyloidosis are related to the accumulation of amyloid in the mesangium and other portions of the glomerulus. Glomerular damage in allograft rejection is complex and seems to involve humoral and cellular immunity, complement, neutrophils, and the coagulation system.

XII. PATHOGENESIS OF INTERSTITIAL NEPHRITIS

It is becoming increasingly apparent that tubular and interstitial damage may result from the interplay of immunologic mechanisms as suggested by experimental studies and certain clinical observations. Animals receiving injections of homologous renal tissue in adjuvant have been found to develop tubular cell and basement membrane damage, interstitial fibrosis, and mild inflammatory cell infiltration, sometimes accompanied by glucosuria and aminoaciduria. Granular deposits of immunoglobulin and complement were seen along the basement membrane of proximal convoluted tubules. Tubular and interstitial alterations with granular deposits of IgG and C3 have also been found in rabbits after injections of large amounts of BSA. The granular pattern of deposition of immunoglobulin and complement and the absence of antitubular basement membrane antibodies in the circulation or in renal eluates suggest that the damage was produced by immune complexes. The mechanisms leading to accumulation of immune complexes in this location and the mediators of the associated tissue damage are not clear. Deposits of immunoglobulin and complement along tubular basement membrane are frequently seen in lupus nephritis and are usually associated with evidence of tubular cell damage, interstitial fibrosis and inflammation. Comparable lesions may accompany other forms of glomerulonephritis and have also been seen in patients with unexplained tubular and interstitial disease.

Experimental production of antitubular basement membrane antibodies has been associated with tissue damage and linear glomerular loop deposits of immunoglobulin and complement in multiple models. In humans, antitubular basement membrane antibodies are often demonstrable in Goodpasture's syndrome and certain idiopathic rapidly progressive glomerulonephritides. It is difficult to assess their role in these diseases but it seems likely that they may contribute to the tubular and interstitial damage which is frequently present. Antitubular basement membrane antibodies have occasionally been found in association with other glomerulonephritides, in patients with renal allografts, and in methicillin-associated interstitial nephritis. Antitubular basement membrane antibodies were also found in one patient with interstitial nephritis unassociated with glomerulonephritis.

The presence of interstitial mononuclear cell infiltration in various renal diseases and the demonstration of migration inhibitory factor production or blastogenic response when lymphocytes from those patients were incubated with renal tissue suggest that cell-mediated immune mechanisms may also play a significant role in the pathogenesis of interestitial nephritis.

XIII. MORPHOLOGIC PATTERNS OF GLOMERULAR INJURY

Structural alterations may be seen in every glomerulus (generalized), or only in a few (focal). The alterations may involve the entire glomerulus (diffuse or global) or only a portion of it, often less than one half (local or segmental). Several basic morphologic patterns can be identified by light microscopy and can be further characterized by immunofluorescence microscopy and electron microscopy. Some of these are listed in Tables II–V. Others include the following:

1. Granular deposits of C3 in mesangium and sometimes in loop by immunofluorescence microscopy with large intramembranous dense deposits by electron microscopy, e.g., in membranoproliferative glomerulonephritis, Type II (dense-deposit disease).
2. Linear deposits of IgG and sometimes C3 along basement membrane, e.g., in Goodpasture's syndrome and idiopathic rapidly progressive glomerulonephritis.
3. Focal glomerular deposits of Ig (mostly IgM) and C3, e.g., in focal sclerosing glomerulopathy with segmental hyalinosis and focal glomerulosclerosis in heroin addicts.
4. No granular deposits by immunofluorescence or electron microscopy, e.g., in minimal-change disease and diabetic glomerulonephropathy.

Table II. Granular Deposits of Ig and C3 in Glomerular Loop

I. With subepithelial humps by electron microscopy
   Acute diffuse proliferative glomerulonephritis (poststreptococcal and others)
II. With subepithelial and intramembranous deposits by electron microscopy
   Membranous glomerulonephritis (e.g., idiopathic, lupus-associated)
III. With subendothelial deposits by electron microscopy
   A. Membranoproliferative glomerulonephritis (Type I)
   B. Membranoproliferative glomerulonephritis (associated with, e.g., lupus erythematosus, sickle cell disease, Waldenström's macroglobulinemia, mixed essential cryoglobulinemia).

Table III. Granular Deposits of Ig and C3 in Mesangium by Immunofluorescence and Electron Microscopy

Focal proliferative glomerulonephritis associated with:
1. Recurrent hematuria syndrome
2. Berger's nephropathy
3. Schoenlein–Henoch nephropathy
4. Lupus erythematosus nephropathy
5. Others (less constant): embolic nephropathy, microscopic variant of PAN, Wegener's granulomatosis, resolving stage of diffuse proliferative glomerulonephritis

A. Diffuse Proliferative

The glomeruli are hypercellular and bloodless owing to diffuse proliferation of enodthelial, mesangial, and, rarely, epithelial cells. Increased number of polymorphonuclear leucocytes and monocytes may also contribute to the hypercellularity. This pattern is characteristic of acute (poststreptococcal and others) proliferative glomerulonephritis.

B. Focal Proliferative

This pattern is characterized by focal proliferation of glomerular cells with or without necrosis and inflammatory cell infiltration. The lesions are most of the time segmental and the remaining portion of the glomerulus is not significantly altered. Lesions of this sort are found in patients suffering from the so-called recurrent hematuria syndrome, in Berger's IgG-IgA nephropathy, and in the nephropathy associated with Schoenlein Henoch purpura. The glomerular alterations in the latter two diseases are remarkably similar, often with IgA as the predominant immunoglobulin in the mesangial

Table IV. Extracapillary Fibrin Deposits (in Crescents)

I. With linear deposits of IgG along glomerular basement membrane
   A. Goodpasture's syndrome
   B. Idiopathic rapidly progressive glomerulonephritis
II. With granular deposits of Ig and C3 in loops by immunofluorescence and electron microscopy.
   A. Idiopathic rapidly progressive glomerulonephritis
   B. Poststreptococcal crescentic glomerulonephritis
   C. Crescentic glomerulonephritis associated with sarcoidosis
III. With granular deposits of Ig and C3 in mesangium
   A. Progressive forms of Schoenlein–Henoch nephritis
   B. Progressive forms of lupus erythematosus nephritis
   C. Others (less constant): crescentic glomerulonephritis associated with PAN, Wegener's granulomatosis, embolic nephropathy, etc.
IV. With no deposits of Ig or C3
   Idiopathic rapidly progressive glomerulonephritis

Table V. Subendothelial Fibrin
Deposits

I. With no deposits of Ig or C3
  A. Acute tubular necrosis
  B. Preeclamptic toxemia (most cases)
  C. Hemolytic uremic syndrome
  D. Scleroderma kidney
  E. Malignant hypertension
II. With variable deposits of Ig and C3
  A. Glomerulonephritis (in general)
  B. Allograft rejection
  C. Some cases of preeclamptic toxemia

deposits. Similar pattern of glomerular involvement is frequently encountered in the nephropathy associated with lupus erythematosus.

C. Mesangiopathic

This is characterized by generalized accentuation of the glomerular stalk regions secondary to proliferation of mesangial cells and/or increased mesangial matrix. This pattern might be present alone (i.e., idiopathic or in patients with mild forms of lupus nephritis); however, most of the time it is associated with one of the variants of focal proliferative glomerulonephritis. It is often the only clue to such a diagnosis since the focal proliferative lesions might not necessarily be present in the small needle biopsy sample.

In minimal-change glomerulopathy (e.g., Nil disease, lipoid nephrosis), the glomeruli usually appear histologically normal. In some instances, particularly after multiple relapses of the nephrotic syndrome, the glomeruli may show slight increase in mesangial cells and matrix.

Glomerular involvement in diabetes mellitus is often characterized by diffuse increase in mesangial matrix (diffuse glomerulosclerosis). Progressive accumulation of mesangial matrix in the center of the glomerular lobules might result in the formation of typical Kimmelstiel–Wilson nodules (nodular glomerulosclerosis).

Amyloid deposits might also produce enlargement of mesangial regions. Identification of amyloid is possible by demonstrating silvery green fluorescence under ultraviolet light in sections stained with thioflavin T or yellow-green birefringence under polarized light in sections stained with congo red.

Glomerular mesangial thickening might also be found in association with cirrhosis of the liver (so-called cirrhotic glomerulosclerosis).

D. Focal Sclerosis

Sclerosis is a segmental or global increase in mesangial matrix that leads to capillary obliteration. Focal sclerosing glomerular lesions are characteristic of idiopathic focal sclerosing glomerulonephropathy with segmental hyalinosis. Focal sclerotic lesions might also be encountered in heroin addicts with the nephrotic syndrome and in patients with malignant lymphoma and nephrotic syndrome.

Focal sclerotic lesions have diagnostic value only in the context of a given patient with nephrotic syndrome or proteinuria and no other morphologic alteration of the glomeruli. The lesion by itself is a nonspecific finding since similar lesions can be found in multiple conditions such as hypertension, pyelonephritis, Alport's syndrome, and various resolving or active glomerular diseases.

E. Membranous

This pattern consists of diffuse and uniform thickening of glomerular capillary walls without significant hypercellularity, inflammatory infiltration, or necrosis. On standard hematoxylin and eosin stains, the cause of this thickening cannot usually be resolved. With the aid of special stains such as periodic acid–shiff (PAS) or PAS–silver methenamine, the presence of thickening of the true basement membrane and/or epimembranous or intramembranous deposits might be demonstrable; however, most of the time, an accurate evaluation is not possible without immunofluorescence and electron microscopy. This pattern is characteristic of membranous glomerulonephritis (e.g., idiopathic or associated with lupus erythematosus, Australian antigen, gold).

Glomerular involvement in diabetes mellitus may show a membranous pattern by light microscopy. This can readily be differentiated from membranous glomerulonephritis by immunofluorescence and electron microscopy.

F. Membranoproliferative

This pattern is composed of mesangial cell proliferation and increased mesangial matrix associated with capillary wall thickening. Such lesions are characteristic of idiopathic membranoproliferative glomerulonephritis, Types I, II, and III. The thickening and "double contour" appearance of the capillary walls is due to the presence of deposits and extension of mesangial matrix between endothelial cells and basement membrane (mesangial interposition).

Advanced lupus erythematosus associated nephritis might show a membranoproliferative pattern with marked thickening of the capillary walls (wire loop).

A few cases of membranoproliferative glomerulonephritis associated with sickle cell anemia have been described.

Glomerulonephritis with membranoproliferative pattern may be rarely associated with Waldenstrom's macroglobulinemia and mixed essential cryoglobulinemia.

G. Crescentic

This is characterized by the presence of epithelial crescents in *many* glomeruli. Crescents are extracapillary masses of proliferating cells in the Bowman's space which partially or sometimes completely encircle and compress the tuft. The proliferating cells are derived mostly from the parietal epithelium of the Bowman's capsule with some participation of the visceral epithelium (cellular crescents). The etiopathogenic mechanism for the development of crescents has not been conclusively proven; however, the presence of fibrin in the Bowman's space is generally regarded as the main factor which incites the cellular proliferation.

Crescentic pattern is typical of antibasement membrane mediated glomerulonephritis with pulmonary involvement (Goodpasture's syndrome).

Large numbers of crescents are typically found in the so-called idiopathic rapidly progressive glomerulonephritis. The latter is probably not one but rather a group of diseases of different etiology but common clinical and light microscopic features. In some patients, the disease is mediated by antiglomerular basement membrane antibodies. In other patients, the disease is mediated by immune complexes. Very often, however, no immunoglobulin, complement, or electron-dense deposits are found and therefore the etiopathogenesis of the disease is not even suspected.

The microscopic variant of polyarteritis nodosa might present with extensive crescent formation. Fibrinoid necrosis and transmural inflammation of small intralobular arteries, arterioles, capillaries, and venules are characteristic but might not necessarily be present or easily identifiable in a small needle biopsy sample.

There are many reported examples of crescentic glomerulonephritis in patients with clinical history and serologic evidences of previous streptococcal infection.

The glomerulonephritis associated with sarcoidosis usually has a proliferative and occasionally a membranous pattern. Progressive proliferative glomerulonephritis with crescentic pattern has rarely been described.

Extensive crescent formation might be found in the progressive form of Schoenlein–Henoch nephritis. A crescentic pattern might also be seen in the glomerulonephritis associated with lupus erythematosus, in the so-called embolic glomerulonephritis, and in Wegener's granulomatosis.

H. Subendothelial Fibrin Deposition

This is characterized by the presence of subendothelial deposits of fibrin in glomerular capillaries and often in renal arteries and arterioles. The glomerular lesions might be reversible (i.e., acute tubular necrosis and preeclamptic toxemia) or persistent and progressive (i.e., thrombotic microantiopathies, scleroderma, and malignant hypertension). Intracapillary fibrin accompanied by immunoglobulin deposits is often found in glomerulonephritis and in allograft rejection.

I. End Stage

This pattern is characterized by markedly decreased number of nephrons. Most glomeruli are obsolete or show variable degree of sclerosis. The remaining glomeruli might be irregularly enlarged. Focal or diffuse hypercellularity, thickening of the capillary walls, periglomerular fibrosis, and scattered crescents might also be found. At this stage, the original disease cannot usually be identified.

J. Miscellaneous Alterations

In many congenital and hereditary diseases the glomeruli may show particular alterations which do not fit in any of the previous patterns. Their salient morphological features will be mentioned in the section dealing with clinicopathological correlations.

XIV. PATHOPHYSIOLOGY OF GLOMERULAR DISEASE

The glomerular abnormalities just described may result in (1) leakage of substances, such as blood and protein, so that patients may present with gross hematuria or be found on examination to have microscopic hematuria and/or proteinuria, and (2) reduction in filtration, so that fluid and normal serum constituents, such as sodium and potassium, cannot be excreted normally. In general, four kinds of clinical presentations may be observed, resulting from the above pathophysiological changes.

A. Asymptomatic Hematuria and/or Proteinuria

Not uncommonly, patients may be discovered to have microscopic hematuria and/or proteinuria on routine urinalysis without any accompanying symptoms. While the disease producing such findings may be nonprogressive, this is not always true. Diseases such as membranous glomerulonephritis may be indolent for many years before producing decreased renal function.

The pathogenesis of hematuria is not completely understood. Fragmented basement membranes may be seen in electron microscopic biopsy sections in some disease processes but this is not universally true. Whether red cells are able to traverse seemingly intact basement membranes in some processes is unknown. However the process occurs, hematuria is a fairly constant finding in glomerular diseases. A hallmark of glomerulonephritis is red blood cell casts in the urine, but these are usually found only with repeated observation in acute diseases or exacerbations of chronic ones.

In general, the number of cells in the urine does not correlate with the severity of disease. In acute poststreptococcal glomerulonephritis gross hematuria, appearing as dark brown or rust-colored urine, is frequently seen early in the course. Within a few days, the hematuria becomes microscopic. In chronic glomerulonephritis, the hematuria may be very mild even though there may be considerable glomerular damage. Finally, in some diseases, the nephritis of systemic lupus erythematosus being perhaps the most notable, few to no red blood cells may be found in the urine. This, plus the fact that hematuria occurs with many other urinary tract abnormalities, necessitates evaluation when hematuria is discovered.

Early in the course of inflammatory glomerular disease, many white blood cells may be seen in the urine. In fact, the number of white cells may exceed the number of red cells, particularly very early in acute poststreptococcal glomerulonephritis.

The quantity of protein may be somewhat more prognostic of severity of disease, although it too is frequently misleading. Generally, proteinuria in excess of 3 g/24 hr reflects severe disease, the exception being that of minimal-change nephrotic syndrome. As discussed in the chapter on proteinuria (Chapter 11), determination of the type of urinary protein excreted may be helpful. The presence of mostly albumin (highly selective proteinuria) conveys a better prognosis than the presence of proteins with varied molecular sizes.

B. The Symptom Complex of Acute Glomerulonephritis

Inflammation of glomeruli resulting in an abrupt decrease in glomerular filtration rate (GFR) produces fluid and salt retention and its many complications. A major reduction in GFR may occur by inflammatory swelling with capillary occlusion in some glomeruli. In addition, studies in experimental animals have determined that the reduction in single-nephron GFR is related to a decrease in the permeability coefficient of the glomerular capillary wall, and in most cases, a reduction in glomerular plasma flow, probably owing to vasoconstriction of the afferent arterioles. Why the permeability coefficient is reduced is still somewhat obscure, although the electron microscopic findings suggest that swelling of endothelial cells and their increased distance from the basement membrane may produce some of this change. The presence of polymorphonuclear leukocytes suggests that their chemical influences on the basement membranes may also play a part in the reduction of the permeability coefficient.

Since glomerular filtration rate is reduced, water and salts cannot be filtered normally, resulting in increased vascular volume. Since most patients are not sufficiently ill to discontinue eating and drinking, intake is relatively normal in the face of decreased excretion. The increase in vascular volume results in systemic hypertension, headaches, occasional encephalopathy, congestive heart failure, and edema. Since symptoms and signs may be full blown within a few days when GFR falls abruptly, these patients usually seek medical care early.

Urinalysis usually reveals hematuria, proteinuria, pyuria, and casts (granular, white cell and sometimes red cell).

C. The Symptom Complex of Chronic Glomerulonephritis

The many manifestations of chronic renal failure are discussed in Chapter 14. It is notable that if glomerular inflammation proceeds slowly so that reduction in GFR is gradual, the kidney adjusts with an increase in fractional excretion of salt and water. Thus, the symptoms seen in acute glomerulonephritides are usually not seen in the patient with chronic glomerulonephritis. There may be acute exacerbations of chronic diseases with an abrupt fall in GFR, producing similar symptoms.

The usual presentation of the patient with chronic glomerulonephritis occurs when GFR has reached a level of approximately 20% of normal, at which time, despite increased fractional excretion, the dietary intake of salt and fluid cannot be excreted, and hypertension or other signs of volume overload may appear. Anemia may be another presenting sign, and in children, growth failure is common.

Finally, as noted above, an occasional patient is found to have abnormal urinalysis on routine examination.

D. Nephrotic Syndrome

The constellation of edema, proteinuria, hypoalbuminemia, and hyper-cholesterolemia may be found in association with either the acute or chronic symptom complex. Its presence in a patient suspected of having acute postinfectious glomerulonephritis or the nephritis of Schoenlein–Henoch purpura suggests a more severe inflammatory process and may suggest to the physician that a renal biopsy is warranted to confirm his clinical diagnosis. The onset of the nephrotic syndrome in the patient with chronic glomerulonephritis may bring him to the doctor, and then again, histologic diagnosis is warranted.

XV. CLINICOPATHOLOGIC CORRELATIONS

A. Diffuse Proliferative Glomerulonephritis

Acute Postinfectious Glomerulonephritis (Poststreptococcal Most Common). Patients, most commonly children over the age of four, present 10–14 days postinfection with acute nephritic symptoms and occasionally, nephrotic syndrome. C3 is decreased, C4 normal. Electron microscopy of biopsy tissue

shows subepithelial deposits ("humps"). The clinical course shows spontaneous resolution in 90% of children with sequelae of decreased function,
hypertension, and proteinuria in 30%–50% of adults.

B. Focal Proliferative Glomerulonephritis

i. Schoenlein–Henoch Purpura with Nephritis. Patients, most commonly
children, present with purpuric lesions of legs, buttocks, and extensor
surfaces of arms, abdominal pain, melena or hematochezia, acute nephritic
symptoms, and occasionally nephrotic syndrome. Rash and/or hematuria
may occur late. C3 is normal to elevated; C4 normal. Renal biopsy findings
range from mild mesangiopathy to severe diffuse proliferation with mesangial
accentuation. The clinical course shows a better prognosis in the younger
patient with usual resolution of the acute nephritic picture. Those with
nephritic plus nephrotic components more frequently have permanent
sequelae or renal failure.

ii. Embolic Glomerulopathy. Patients who have subacute bacterial endocarditis or infected ventriculoatrial shunts present with hematuria, proteinuria, and mild azotemia. Staphylococci are frequent pathogens. C3 is reduced.
The biopsy picture varies from focal proliferation of endothelial and mesangial cells to diffuse proliferation with crescents and necrosis. The clinical
course is usually favorable, with resolution of the glomerular process when
the infection is cleared.

iii. IgA-IgG Nephropathy (Berger's Disease). This disease predominates in
adolescent and young adult males, manifesting with gross hematuria at times
of infections. Microscopic hematuria and proteinuria may persist; decreased
GFR is occasional. Complement levels are normal. The clinical course shows
spontaneous resolution in 3–14 days, reappearing with another intercurrent
infection. Occasional patients, especially older ones, develop chronic renal
failure.

iv. Recurrent Hematuria Syndrome (see benign familial hematuria also). Again
seen primarily in children and young adults, this condition is typified by
repeated attacks of hematuria, not uncommonly following upper respiratory
infections. Since it is often seen in several family members, it is important to
differentiate from familial nephritis (Alport's syndrome). Microscopic hematuria and/or proteinuria may persist between attacks, but the prognosis is
generally excellent. Light microscopy usually shows only mild mesangial
hypercellularity and stalk thickening, if anything. Electron microscopy in
some cases shows thinning of the basement membrane.

C. Membranoproliferative Glomerulonephritis—Types I, II, and III

This disease is most common in children and young adults, presenting
as (1) an acute nephritic complex with azotemia, (2) insidious onset of

azotemia, (3) incidental microscopic hematuria and proteinuria, or (4) nephrotic syndrome. C3 is greatly reduced; C4 is normal. Type I disease is typified by subendothelial deposits and mesangial interposition, Type II by electron-dense deposits within the basement membrane, and Type III by a combination of the two. The clinical course of all shows a variable decline in renal function with many developing chronic renal failure.

D. Crescentic Glomerulonephritis

i. Rapid Progressive Glomerulonephritis (also called subacute glomerulonephritis). The idiopathic disease usually presents in young to middle-aged adults with acute nephritic symptoms or insidiously with development of nephrotic syndrome. When presenting acutely, no pulmonary manifestations are present, but severe oliguria, thrombocytopenia, and microangiopathic hemolytic anemia are common. Complement levels are normal. Severe nephritic symptoms may dictate acute dialysis. In those patients whose biopsy specimens show crescents surrounding more than 70% of glomeruli, there is progressive deterioration to chronic renal failure within 18–24 months. High-dose steroids and/or anticoagulants appear to have alleviated the disease in some patients.

ii. Goodpasture's Syndrome. This syndrome is most common in young adult males, presenting with an acute nephritic complex and pulmonary hemorrhage. Circulating anti-GBM antibody is detectable and complement levels are generally normal. Clinically, the course is typified by a rapid downhill course which may be alleviated by nephrectomies, high-dose steroids, and/or plasmapheresis.

E. Membranous Glomerulonephritis

This disease often presents insidiously with proteinuria, nephrotic syndrome, or chronic renal failure. It is most common in adults, and may be associated with SLE and other systemic diseases, as well as renal vein thrombosis. C3 may be decreased. Patients suffer indolent renal deterioration, often as long as 20 years. The nephrotic component may be hard to control. Occasionally the disease remits spontaneously.

F. Minimal-Change Nephrotic Syndrome

This condition is most common in young children, often presenting after an upper respiratory infection. It is associated with highly selective proteinuria and complement levels are normal. The clinical course is typified by response to steroid therapy in the majority, with relapses in 60%–70%.

G. Focal Sclerosing Glomerulopathy

This condition usually presents with nephrotic syndrome, distinguishable clinically only by its frequent nonresponse to steroid therapy. Proteinuria is frequently nonselective. Patients who respond to steroids usually manifest relapses or steroid dependence. Those who do not respond to steroids frequently develop chronic renal failure in 2–5 years.

H. Glomerulopathy of Systemic Disease

i. Systemic Lupus Erythematosus. This disease, most common in adolescent young adult females, frequently presents with extrarenal manifestations including "butterfly" malar rash, arthralgias, fever, malaise, easy fatigability, weight loss, pneumonitis, myo- or pericarditis, leukopenia, anemia, thrombocytopenia, mood changes, seizure disorder, and chorea. The renal manifestations may be hematuria, proteinuria, nephrotic syndrome, and/or acute nephritic complex. Laboratory investigation shows antinuclear antibody, anti-DNA antibody, depressed C3 and C4, occasional circulating immune complexes, and "telescoped" urine sediment. The clinical course varies. The biopsy shows a mesangiopathic pattern. In general, the worse the glomerular lesion the worse the prognosis. Extrarenal manifestations may be controlled by nonsteroidal antiinflammatory agents but steroids are often necessary to control glomerulonephritis. Cytotoxic agents and plasmapheresis may be helpful.

ii. Diabetic Nephropathy. Glomerular involvement appears in many insulin-dependent diabetes mellitus patients after some 10 years of glucose intolerance. It is associated with generalized vascular disease, including retinopathy. The patient may present with edema, hypertension, nephrotic syndrome, or chronic renal failure. Once nephrotic syndrome has developed, the prognosis is poor, with a five-year survival rate of only about 30%. Transplantation has been attempted with varying success.

iii. Sickle Cell Nephropathy. Patients, both homozygotes and heterozygotes, may present with gross or microscopic hematuria secondary to papillary necrosis rather than glomerulopathy. Homozygotes with glomerulopathy may have hematuria, proteinuria, and/or nephrotic syndrome. The clinical course is commonly slowly progressive with eventual renal failure in those with membranoproliferative findings.

iv. Amyloidosis. This disease is rarely primary but far more commonly seen in patients with rheumatoid arthritis, tuberculosis, syphilis, ulcerative colitis, malignancies, and familial Mediterranean fever. Massive proteinuria, nephrotic syndrome, and renal failure are seen. The patient generally progresses slowly to renal failure. Once nephrotic syndrome or azotemia has developed, the prognosis is poor.

v. Hypertensive Kidney Disease, Including Malignant Hypertension. Patients may present asymptomatically with elevated blood pressure and proteinuria, mild symptoms, such as headache, or with florid symptoms of headache, blurred vision, encepahlopathy, and have azotemia (malignant). The clinical course depends on the degree of severity of the changes, those with malignant hypertension often developing chronic renal failure. Renal failure improves in some patients with control of hypertension. Biopsy findings include glomerular sclerosis, and fibrinoid necrosis is seen in malignant hypertension.

vi. Hemolytic-Uremic Syndrome. This syndrome is most common in children in whom gastrointestinal symptoms, including bloody diarrhea, are followed by hematuria, proteinuria, oliguria, pallor, CNS symptoms, hemolytic anemia, and thrombocytopenia. In adults the syndrome may be associated with pregnancy, oral contraceptive use, or postpartum. Renal failure is not uncommon. Fibrin thrombi are seen extensively in glomeruli, arterioles, and arteries. Supportive care in children usually results in recovery, but sequelae are seen in about 20%. Prognosis is less optimistic in adults.

vii. Preeclamptic Toxemia. This condition occurs during the last trimester of pregnancy, usually in primiparous women, and is clinically typified by hypertension, proteinuria, and edema. Microscopic hematuria, pyuria, and a mild decrease in GFR may be seen. The severity of the hypertension and proteinuria correlates with the severity of the glomerular lesion, which is a diffuse proliferative one involving endothelial and mesangial cells, with swelling of those cellular elements. Occasionally intimal proliferation is noted in arterioles, and basement membrane thickening may be observed. Fibrin deposits are frequently seen. Most patients do well following delivery, although hypertension may persist. The glomerular lesion resolves in most women.

viii. Scleroderma. Some 15%–50% of patients with scleroderma have been reported to have renal involvement. In some, the involvement is indolent, with proteinuria and mildly decreased renal function present, while others present with an acute nephritic syndrome and develop renal failure rapidly. In those patients whose disease is rapidly progressive, light microscopy of renal tissue shows small, compact glomeruli with widespread basement membrane thickening, so-called "wire loops." Interlobular arteries have extensive intimal thickening and afferent arterioles demonstrate fibrinoid necrosis. Those patients with indolent renal involvement show sclerotic intimal thickening of the interlobular arteries. These patients generally die from nonrenal causes, whereas those with acute nephritic presentations may develop renal failure rapidly, necessitating dialysis.

ix. Polyarteritis Nodosa (PAN), Wegener's Granulomatosus (WG), and Hypersensitivity Angiitis (HA). These diseases usually occur in adults. The typical presentation in PAN is with fever, hypertension, polyarthralgia, and neuritis. Renal involvement occurs in the majority with hematuria, proteinuria, and azotemia. In patients with WG, granulomas appear in the upper and lower respiratory tracts along with angiitis. Azotemia rapidly appears. In those with HA, microangiopathic hemoltic anemia is common. In PAN, inflammation of medium-sized arteries, fibrinoid necrosis of glomeruli, and hyperplasia of the juxtaglomerular apparatus are seen. In WG diffuse or segmental glomerular necrosis accompanies findings of granulomas in vessel walls. In HA small vessels, including glomerular capillaries, are infiltrated with inflammatory cells. Fibrinoid necrosis appears and hypercellularity of endothelial and epithelial cells is seen. Without treatment, the clinical course is a rapid, downhill one. Steroids and cytotoxic agents improve life expectancy markedly (especially in WG).

x. Diseases of Abnormal Protein Production (Essential or Mixed Cryoimmunoglobulinemia, Benign Monoclonal Gammopathy, Multiple Myeloma, Waldenström's Macroglobulinemia). Proteinuria and hematuria are frequent clinical manifestations in these diseases. In some, azotemia and the nephrotic syndrome may develop. The clinical course of the these diseases is variable.

I. Glomerulopathy of Congenital and Hereditary Disease

i. Congenital Glomerulonephritis. Infants present with hematuria, proteinuria, enlarged kidneys, hypertension, and/or azotemia. Serum IgM may be elevated if an intrauterine infection has been associated. Light microscopy shows diffuse proliferation and crescents, necrosis, and sclerosis. The clinical course is variable. The infant may recover or develop renal failure.

ii. Congenital Glomerulosclerosis. This condition is usually found incidentally in necropsy tissue and may be due to glomerular involution during development. It may be seen in congenital rubella. Biopsy material reveals scattered glomeruli totally obliterated by hyalin.

iii. Congenital Nephrotic Syndrome. This condition is inherited as an autosomal recessive, most commonly in those of Finnish ancestry. Patients present with gross edema in the first few weeks of life. Microscopic hematuria may be present. The areas of hyalinosis in some glomeruli extend with time. There is patchy hypercellularity, occasional areas of GBM thickening, and dilatation of proximal tubules. Most develop chronic renal failure and die within the first year of life, although some live to 3–4 years of age.

iv. Congenital Syphilis. Proliferative glomerulonephritis and nephrotic syndrome have also been reported in association with congenital syphilis. By immunofluorescent microscopy, granular loop deposits of Ig and C3 have been seen. By electron microscopy, subepithelial and intramembranous deposits have been reported.

v. Alport's Syndrome (Hereditary Nephritis). This syndrome usually presents in childhood with hematuria and proteinuria. High-frequency nerve deafness is present in some, as are ocular defects such as cataracts and spherophakia. Males are usually more severely affected. It is thought to be an autosomal dominant with variable expressivity. On biopsy, the glomeruli might appear normal. Focal, segmental hyalinosis with patchy GBM thickening may be present, or hypercellularity may occur. Tubular atrophy, interstitial fibrosis, inflammatory cell infiltration, and foam cells (lipid-laden macrophages) are not uncommon. C3 deposits have been reported. On electron microscopy, the GBM is frayed and split with small granular particles interposing.

Occasionally the mesangium may interpose the GBM also. Females with hematuria and proteinuria often, though not always, have a normal life expectancy. The course in males is variable with some having no renal dysfunction to a deterioration to renal failure within 5–10 years.

vi. Nail-Patella Syndrome. This condition is inherited as an autosomal dominant with skeletal abnormalities (hypoplastic patella, subluxed radial heads, iliac horns, dysplastic fingernails) bringing attention to the patient. Proteinuria is fairly common; nephrotic syndrome is rare. The biopsy findings may vary from patchy GBM thickening to glomerular obliteration. Tubular atrophy and arteriolar hyalinization may accompany. On EM, the GBM is thickened with electron-lucent areas containing fibrils of collagen. These fibrils may also be seen in subendothelial and mesangial regions. The clinical course of these patients is generally benign, with rare progression to chronic renal failure.

vii. Benign Familial Hematuria. This condition usually presents with recurrent gross hematuria in childhood. Microscopic hematuria and proteinuria occasionally persist. The family history may be positive or microscopic hematuria may be found in family members. Electron microscopy shows marked diffuse or segmental thinning of the lamina dense of the glomerular basement membrane. Focal areas of mild splitting of the basement membrane may be occasionally found. The clinical course is benign with the bouts of gross hematuria receding in time.

viii. Fabry's Disease (Angiokeratoma Corporis Diffusum Universale). This is a rare condition in which the skin demonstrates dark red papules, frequently clustered on the lower trunk and thighs, which are dilated capillaries. Associated with the skin disorder is nervous system, liver, and kidney involvement. The abnormality is an X-linked inborn error of metabolism in which there is deficiency of α-galactosidase activity, so that ceramide trihexoside accumulates in cells, especially of the organs noted above. The disease generally presents during puberty, leading to renal failure in the fourth and fifth decades. The disease can be diagnosed by assaying α-galactosidase in blood. Examination of the kidney by light microscopy shows foamy vacuolations of the cells of the glomerular tuft, particularly the epithelial cells. These changes are also seen in tubular cells and fine vacuolations are seen in the muscle cells of arterial media. As the disease progresses, glomeruli become sclerotic and tubular atrophy increases. The foamy vacuolated cells stain positively with lipid stains. Electron microscopy of those cells shows laminated bodies. In recent years, renal transplantation has been advocated for these patients since the renal transplant appears to provide sufficient α-galactosidase to alleviate the disease in some patients.

J. Glomerulopathy of Renal Transplantation

i. Hyperacute Rejection. This phenomenon occurs within minutes to hours following placement of the transplanted kidney. Function ceases. The histologic features are those of cortical necrosis, heralded by the presence of thrombi, PMNs, and platelet aggregates along capillary walls.

ii. Acute Rejection. This type of rejection may occur 1–2 weeks following transplantation, when it is mediated by cellular immunity, or much later in the course. It may respond to steroids or cytotoxic agents. A widespread invasion of mononuclear cells typifies the histologic picture.

iii. Chronic Rejection. This state may be seen in the first few weeks but usually occurs later with gradual functional deterioration. It does not usually respond to drugs. Narrowing of renal vessels with severe intimal thickening is seen. GBM thickening follows.

iv. Recurrence of Original Disease. In patients whose original disease was some variant of glomerulonephritis, the original disease may recur in the transplanted kidney. In some 60% of patients whose original disease was focal sclerosing glomerulopathy, the disease recurs weeks to years later. Dense deposit disease, Berger's, and membranous glomerulonephritis (one case) have also recurred in transplanted kidneys.

K. Interstitial Nephritis

This is a condition typified by the infiltration of mononuclear and, much less commonly, polymorphonuclear cells into the interstitium of the kidney. It usually is accompanied by tubular atrophy and occasionally by periglomerular fibrosis. The etiology of interstitial nephritis is varied. Probably the most commonly seen cause is exposure to drugs, with methicillin a frequent offender. Other drugs, such as phenindione and diphenylhydantoin, have also been implicated. Infectious agents may also cause the disease; infectious hepatitis has been cited as one cause. In Eastern Europe a peculiar type of chronic interstitial nephritis, known as Balkan nephropathy, is encountered. In most cases, interstitial nephritis is an acute illness which is self-limited. When drugs are the etiologic agents, their removal permits healing. Occasionally, steroids are used when the disease is so severe as to reduce GFR.

L. Treatment of Glomerular Disease

i. Supportive Therapy. This is the mainstay of all types of renal failure. Salt and fluid restriction is indicated when fluid overload is producing hypertension, edema, and congestive heart failure. Diuretics and digitalis may also be needed. Control of hypertension may be gained only when pharmacologic agents are added to salt and fluid restriction. Such agents as phosphate binders, calcium supplements, and vitamin D preparations help to maintain calcium–phosphorus balance in renal failure. Such resins as Kayexalate may aid in binding potassium in mild hyperkalemia. In severe or prolonged renal failure, dialysis may be the best supportive therapy. In addition to helping maintain fluid and electrolyte balance, the removal of uremic toxins may increase the feeling of well-being in the patient, as well as allow him to eat, alleviating massive catabolism (see Chapter 14).

ii. Steroids. In some glomerular diseases, steroids have been successful in alleviating disease. In minimal-change nephrotic syndrome, the administration of Prednisone permits diuresis and remission of proteinuria in the majority of patients. Patients with systemic diseases such as systemic lupus erythematosis benefit from steroids. The use of alternate-day steroids for membranoproliferative glomerulonephritis has been advocated. Usually, steroid medications are administered orally but the recent use of intravenous high-dose steroids is gaining popularity. It has been advocated particularly in the severe, diffuse proliferative glomerulonephritis of lupus, in rapidly progressive glomerulonephritis, and in some cases of focal sclerosing glomerulopathy. Its greatest use remains in the treatment of acute transplant rejection.

iii. Cytotoxic Agents. Agents such as azothiaprine and cyclophosphamide have been given to patients with a wide variety of glomerular diseases. In addition to their use as prophylactic agents in renal transplantation, their administration in systemic lupus, frequently relapsing minimal-change nephrotic syndrome and some cases of focal sclerosing glomerulopathy, appears helpful.

iv. Anticoagulants. The histologic findings of fibrin deposition as well as serologic evidence of increased intravascular coagulation in some patients with glomerular disease has prompted the use of both anticoagulants and antiplatelet agents. These drugs have been used primarily in crescentic glomerulonephritis, and some have claimed considerable success. In addition, they may be helpful in the hemolytic-uremic syndrome seen in adults, although there is little evidence of their efficacy in that syndrome in children.

v. Plasmapheresis. Circulating immune complexes have been demonstrated in the collagen vascular diseases as well as in some other glomerulonephritides. The removal of plasma, containing the immune complexes, and its replacement by albumin and saline, have been tried in a number of severe glomerulonephritides. There are numerous anecdotal accounts of success of the procedure, most notably in patients with systemic lupus.

vi. Combination Therapy. In those patients whose glomerulonephritis is so severe as to lead to certain renal failure, some physicians have advocated the use of multiple drugs. Thus, steroids, cytotoxic drugs, anticoagulants, and antiplatelet agents have been combined. Obviously, the risk of superimposed infection and the possibilities of hemorrhage must be weighed against the possible benefit of the drugs.

SUGGESTED READINGS

Pathogenesis of Glomerular Diseases

Hawn, C. V., and Janeway, C. A.: Histological and serological sequences in experimental hypersensitivity. *J. Exp. Med.* 85:571–590, 1947.

Experimental Glomerular Injury Mediated by Soluble Immune Complexes

Exogenous Antigen

Dixon, F. J., Buckantz, S. C., Dammin, G. J., and Talmadge, D. W.: Symposium on labelled antigens and antibodies; fate of ^{131}I labelled bovine gamma globulin in rabbits. *Fed. Proc.* 10:553–557, 1951.

Dixon, F. J., Feldman, J. D., and Vasquez, J. J.: Experimental glomerulonephritis. The pathogenesis of a laboratory model resembling the spectrum of human glomerulonephritis. *J. Exp. Med.* 113:899–920, 1961.

Dreesman, G. F., and Germuth, F. G.: Immune complex disease. IV. The nature of the circulating complexes associated with glomerulonephritis in the acute BSA-rabbit system. *Johns Hopkins Med. J.* 130:335–343, 1972.

Germuth, F. G.: Comparative histologic and immunologic study in rabbits of induced hypersensitivity of serum sickness type. *J. Exp. Med.* 97:257–282, 1953.

Germuth, F. G., and McKinnon, G. E.: Studies on the biological properties of antigen-antibody complexes. I. Anaphylactic shock induced by soluble antigen-antibody complexes in unsensitized normal guinea pigs. *Bull. Johns Hopkins Hosp.* 101:13–44, 1957.

Germuth, F. G., and Pollack, A. D.: The production of lesions of serum sickness in normal animals by the passive transfer of antibody in the presence of antigen. *Bull. Johns Hopkins Hosp.* 102:245–262, 1958.

Germuth, F. G., Keleman, W. A., and Pollack, A. D.: Immune complex disease. II. The role of circulatory dynamics and glomerular filtration in the development of experimental glomerulonephritis. *Johns Hopkins Med. J.* 120:252–261, 1967.

Germuth, F. G., Senterfit, L. B., and Pollack, A. C.: Immune complex disease. I. Experimental acute and chronic glomerulonephritis. *Johns Hopkins Med. J.* 120:225–251, 1967.

Germuth, F. G., Valdes, A. J., Senterfit, L. B., and Pollack, A. D.: A unique influence of cortisone on the transit of specific macromolecules across vascular walls in immune complex disease. *Johns Hopkins Med. J.* 122:137–153, 1968.

Germuth, F. G., Taylor, J. J., Siddique, S. Y., and Rodriguez, E.: Immune complex disease. VI. Some determinants of the varieties of glomerular lesions in the chronic bovine serum albumin-rabbit system. *Lab. Invest.* 37:162–169, 1977.

Germuth, F. G., Rodriguez, E., Lorelle, C. A., Trump, E. I., Milano, L., and Wise, O.: Passive immune complex glomerulonephritis in mice: models for various lesions found in human disease. II. Low avidity complexes and diffuse proliferative glomerulonephritis with subepithelial deposits. *Lab. Invest.* 41:366–371, 1979.

Haakenstad, A. O., Striker, G. E., and Mannik, M.: The glomerular deposition of soluble immune complexes prepared with reduced and alkylated antibodies and with intact antibodies in mice. *Lab. Invest.* 35:283–292, 1976.

Knicker, W. T., and Cochrane, C. G.: The localization of circulating complexes in experimental serum sickness. *J. Exp. Med.* 127:119–135, 1968.

Oldstone, M. B., and Dixon, F. J.: Pathogenesis of chronic disease associated with persistent lymphocytic choriomeningitis viral infection. I. Relationship of antibody production to disease in neonatally infected mice. *J. Exp. Med.* 129:483–505, 1969.

Salant, D. J., Belok, S., Stilmant, M. M., Darby, C., and Couser, W. G.: Determinants of glomerular localization of subepithelial immune deposits: effects of altered antigen to antibody ratio, steroids, vasoactive amine antagonists, and aminonucleoside of puromycin on passive Heymann nephritis in rats. *Lab. Invest.* 41:89–99, 1979.

Valdes, A. J., Senterfit, L. B., Pollack, A. D., and Germuth, F. G.: The effect of antigen excess on chronic immune complex glomerulonephritis. *Johns Hopkins Med. J.* 124:9–17, 1969.

Autologous Antigen

Couser, W. G., and Salant, D. J.: In situ immune complex formation and glomerular injury. *Kidney Int.* 17:1–13, 1980.

Glassock, R. J., Edgington, T. S., Watson, J. I., and Dixon, F. J.: Autologous immune complex nephritis induced with renal tubular antigen. II. The pathogenetic mechanism. *J. Exp. Med.* 127:573–588, 1968.

Hunter, J. L., Hackel, D. B., and Heymann, W.: Nephrotic syndrome in rats produced by sensitization to rat kidney proteins: immunologic studies. *J. Immun.* 85:319–327, 1960.

Lambert, P. H., and Dixon, F. J.: Pathogenesis of the glomerulonephritis of NZB/W mice. *J. Exp. Med.* 127:507–522, 1968.

Naruse, T., Fukasawa, T., Umegae, S., Oike, S., and Miyakawa, Y.: Experimental membranous glomerulonephritis in rats: correlation of ultrastructural changes with the serum level of autologous antibody against tubular antigen. *Lab. Invest.* 39:120–127, 1978.

Experimental Glomerular Injury Mediated by *In Situ* Immune Complex Formation

Couser, W. G., Steinmuller, D. R., Stilmant, M. M., Salant, D. J., and Lowenstein, L. M.: Experimental glomerulonephritis in the isolated perfused rat kidney. *J. Clin. Invest.* 62:1275–1287, 1978.

Feenstra, K., van den Lee, R., Greben, H. A., Arends, A., and Hoedemaeker, P. J.: Experimental glomerulonephritis in the rat induced by antibodies directed against tubular antigens. I. The natural history: a histologic and immunohistologic study at the light microscopic and the ultrastructural level. *Lab. Invest.* 32:235–242, 1975.

Golbus, S. M., and Wilson, C. B.: Experimental glomerulonephritis induced by in situ formation of immune complexes in glomerular capillary wall. *Kidney Int.* 16:148–157, 1979.

Henson, P. M.: Interaction of cells with immune complexes: adherence, release of constituents, and tissue injury. *J. Exp. Med.* 134:114, 1971.

Isui, S., Lambert, P. H., and Miescher, P. A.: In vitro demonstration of a particular affinity of glomerular basement membrane and collagen for DNA. A possible basis for a local formation of DNA-anti-DNA complexes in systemic lupus erythematosus. *J. Exp. Med.* 144:428–443, 1976.

Knicker, W. T., and Cochrane, C. G.: Pathogenic factors in vascular lesions of experimental serum sickness. *J. Exp. Med.* 122:83–98, 1965.

Mauer, S. M., Sutherland, D. E., Howard, R. J., Fish, A. J., Najarian, J. S., and Michael, A. F.: The glomerular mesangium. 3. Acute immune mesangial injury: a new model of glomerulonephritis. *J. Exp. Med.* 137:553–570, 1973.

Salant, D. J., Belok, S., Madaio, M. P., and Couser, W. G.: A new role for complement in experimental membranous nephropathy in rats. *J. Clin. Invest.* 66:1339–1350, 1980.

Thyne, M. B., and Germuth, F. G.: The relationships between serum complement activity and the development of allergic lesions in rabbits. *J. Exp. Med.* 114:633–646, 1961.

VanDamme, B. J. C., Fleuren, G. J., Bakker, W. W., Vernier, R. L., and Hoedemaeker, P. J.: Experimental glomerulonephritis in the rat induced by antibodies directed against tubular antigens. V. Fixed glomerular antigens in the pathogenesis of heterologous immune complex glomerulonephritis. *Lab. Invest.* 38:502–510, 1978.

Experimental Glomerular Injury Mediated by Antibodies to Glomerular Basement Membrane

Nephrotoxic Nephritis (Masugi Nephritis)

Bone, J. M., Valdes, A. J., Germuth, F. G., and Lubowitz, H.: Heparin therapy in anti-basement membrane nephritis. *Kidney Int.* 8:72–79, 1975.

Cochrane, C. G., Unanue, E. R., and Dixon, F. J.: A role of polymorphonuclear leukocytes and complement in nephrotoxic nephritis. *J. Exp. Med.* 122:99–116, 1965.

Germuth, F. G., Rodriguez, E., Shah, H. J., Lorelle, K., McGee, S., Milano, L., and Wise, O.: Antibasement membrane disease. II. Mechanism of glomerular injury in an accelerated model of Masugi nephritis. *Lab. Invest.* 39:421–429, 1978.

Hammer, D. K., and Dixon, F. J.: Experimental glomerulonephritis. II. Immunologic events in the pathogenesis of nephrotoxic serum nephritis in the rat. *J. Exp. Med.* 117:1019–1034, 1963.

Lange, K.: Delayed nephritis due to avian antiserum, in Metcoff, J. (ed.): *Proceedings of the Ninth Annual Conference on Nephrotic Syndrome.* National Kidney Foundation, New York, 1958, p. 13.

Unanue, E. R., and Dixon, F. J.: Experimental glomerulonephritis: immunological events and pathogenetic mechanisms. *Adv. Immunol.* 6:1–90, 1967.

Vasalli, P., and McCluskey, R. T.: The pathogenic role of the coagulation process in rabbit Masugi nephritis. *Am. J. Pathol.* 45:653–689, 1964.

Autoimmune Antiglomerular Basement Membrane Nephritis (Steblay Nephritis)

Lerner, R. A., and Dixon, F. J.: Transfer of ovine experimental allergic glomerulonephritis (EAG) with serum. *J. Exp. Med.* 124:431–442, 1966.

Steblay, R. W.: Glomerulonephritis induced in sheep by injections of heterologous glomerular basement membrane and Freund's complete adjuvant. *J. Exp. Med.* 116:253–272, 1962.

Steblay, R. W., and Rudofsky, U.: Autoimmune glomerulonephritis induced in sheep by injections of human lung and Freund's adjuvant. *Science* 160:204–205, 1968.

Pathogenesis of Human Glomerulonephritis

Germuth, F. G., and Rodriguez, E.: *Immunopathology of the Renal Glomerulus: Immune Complex Deposit and Antibasement Membrane Disease.* Little, Brown, Boston, 1973.

Gotze, O., and Muller-Eberhard, H. J.: The role of properdin in the alternate pathway of complement activation. *J. Exp. Med.* 139:44–57, 1974.

Kincaid-Smith, P.: Participation of intravascular coagulation in the pathogenesis of glomerular and vascular lesions. *Kidney Int.* 7:242–253, 1975.

Human Glomerular Injury Mediated by Immune Complexes

Koffler, D., Schur, P. H., and Kunkel, H. G.: Immunological studies concerning nephritis of systemic lupus erythematosus. *J. Exp. Med.* 126:607–624, 1967.

Strauss, J., Pardo, V., Koss, M. N., Griswold, W., and McIntosh, R. M.: Nephropathy associated with sickle cell anemia: an autologous immune complex nephritis. I. Studies on nature of glomerular-bound antibody and antigen identification in a patient with sickle cell disease and immune deposit glomerulonephritis. *Am. J. Med.* 58:382–387, 1975.

Human Glomerular Injury Mediated by Antibodies to Glomerular Basement Membrane

Beirne, G. J.: Glomerulonephritis induced by chronic exposure of rats to gasoline vapors: a model of Goodpasture's syndrome. *Abstracts of the Fifth Annual Meeting of the American Society of Nephrology,* Washington, D.C., 1971.

Koffler, D., Sandson, J., Carr, R., and Kunkel, H. G.: Immunologic studies concerning the pulmonary lesions in Goodpasture's syndrome. *Am. J. Pathol.* 54:293–306, 1969.

Lerner, R. A., Glassock, R. J., and Dixon, F. J.: The role of antiglomerular basement membrane antibody in the pathogenesis of human glomerulonephritis. *J. Exp. Med.* 126:989–1004, 1967.

Wilson, C. B., and Dixon, F. J.: Anti-glomerular basement membrane antibody-induced glomerulonephritis. *Kidney Int.* 3:74–89, 1973.

Pathogenesis of Interstitial Nephritis

Andres, G. A., and McCluskey, R. T.: Tubular and interstitial renal disease due to immunologic mechanisms. *Kidney Int.* 7:271–289, 1975.

Bergstein, J. M., and Litman, N.: Chronic interstitial nephritis with anti-tubular basement membrane antibodies, in *Abstracts of the Third International Symposium of Pediatric Nephrology.* Washington, D.C., 1974.

Border, W. A., Lehman, D. H., Egan, J. D., Sass, H. J., Glode, J. E., and Wilson, C. B.: Antitubular basement-membrane antibodies in methicillin-associated interstitial nephritis. *N. Engl. J. Med.* 291:381–384, 1974.

Brentjens, J. R., Sepulveda, M., Baliah, T., Bentzel, C., Erlanger, B. F., Elwood, C., Montes, M., Hsu, K. C., and Andres, G. A.: Interstitial immune complex nephritis in patients with systemic lupus erythematosus. *Kidney Int.* 7:342–350, 1975.

Klassen, J., McCluskey, R. T., and Milgrom, F.: Nonglomerular renal disease produced in rabbits by immunization with homologous kidney. *Am. J. Pathol.* 63:333–358, 1971.

Klassen, J., Kano, K., Milgrom, F., Menno, A. B., Anthone, S., Anthone, R., Sepulveda, M., Elwood, C. M., and Andres, C. A.: Tubular lesions produced by autoantibodies to tubular basement membrane in human renal allografts. *Int. Arch. Allergy Appl. Immunol.* 45:675–689, 1973.

Koffler, D., Sandson, J., Carr, R., and Kunkel, H. G.: Immunologic studies concerning the pulmonary lesions in Goodpasture's syndrome. *Am. J. Pathol.* 54:293–306, 1969.

Lehman, D. H., Lee, S., Wilson, C. B., and Dixon, F. J.: Induction of antitubular basement membrane antibodies in rats by renal transplantation. *Transplantation* 14:429–431, 1974.

Lehman, D. H., Wilson, C. B., and Dixon, F. J.: Interstitial nephritis in rats immunized with heterologous tubular basement membrane. *Kidney Int.* 5:187–195, 1974.

Levy, M., Gagnadoux, M. F., and Habib, R.: An immunologic Fanconi syndrome, in *Third International Symposium of Pediatric Nephrology*, Washington, D.C., 1974.

Mahieu, P., Dardenne, M., and Bach, J. F.: Detection of humoral and cell-mediated immunity of kidney basement membranes in human renal diseases. *Am. J. Med.* 53:185–192, 1972.

Morel-Maroger, L., Kourilsky, O., Mignon, F., and Richet, G.: Antitubular basement membrane antibodies in rapidly progressive poststreptococcal glomerulonephritis: report of a case. *Clin. Immunol. Immunopathol.* 2:185–194, 1974.

Rocklin, R. E., Lewis, R. J., and David, J. R.: In vitro evidence for cellular hypersensitivity to glomerular-basement-membrane antigens in human glomerulonephritis. *N. Engl. J. Med.* 283:497–501, 1970.

Steblay, R. W., and Rudofsky, U.: Renal tubular disease and autoantibodies against tubular basement membrane induced in guinea pigs. *J. Immunol.* 107:589–594, 1971.

Sugisaki, T., Klassen, J., Milgrom, F., Andres, G. A., and McCluskey, R. T.: Immunopathologic study of an autoimmune tubular and interstitial renal disease in brown Norway rats. *Lab. Invest.* 28:658–671, 1973.

Unanue, E. R., Dixon, F. J., and Feldman, J.D.: Experimental allergic glomerulonephritis induced in the rabbit with homologous renal antigens. *J. Exp. Med.* 125:163–176, 1967.

Morphologic Patterns of Glomerular Injury

Diffuse Proliferative

Germuth, F. G., and Rodriguez, E.: Class I immune complex deposit disease in humans: transmembranous (diffuse) glomerulonephritis, in *Immunopathology of the Renal Glomerulus: Immune Complex Deposit and Antibasement Membrane Disease*. Little, Brown, Boston, 1973, pp. 61–79.

Focal Proliferative

Jenis, E. H., and Lowenthal, D. T.: *Kidney Biopsy Interpretation*. F. A. Davis Co., Philadelphia, 1977, p. 145.

McCoy, R. C., Abramowsky, C. R., and Tisher, C. C.: IgA neonephropathy. *Am. J. Pathol.* 76:123–144, 1976.

Urizar, R. E., Michael, A., Sisson, S., and Vernier, R. L.: Anaphylactoid purpura. II. Immunofluorescent and electron microscopic studies of the glomerular lesions. *Lab. Invest.* 19:437–450, 1968.

Vernier, R. L., Resnick, J. S., and Mauer, S. M.: Recurrent hematuria and focal glomerulonephritis. *Kidney Int.* 7:224–231, 1975.

Mesangiopathic

Germuth, F. G., and Rodriguez, E.: *Immunopathology of the Renal Glomerulus: Immune Complex Deposit and Antibasement Membrane Disease*. Little, Brown, Boston, 1973, p. 133.

Focal Sclerosis

Hyman, L. R., and Burkholder, P. M.: Focal sclerosing glomerulonephropathy with segmental hyalinosis. A clinicopathologic analysis. *Lab. Invest.* 28:533–544, 1973.

Hyman, L. R., Burkholder, P. M., Joo, P. A., and Segar, W. E.: Malignant lymphoma and nephrotic syndromes: a clinicopathologic analysis with light, immunofluorescence, and electron microscopy of the renal lesions. *J. Pediatr.* 82:207–217, 1973.

Sreepada, T. K. R., Nicastri, A. D., and Friedman, E. A.: Natural history of heroin-associated nephropathy. *N. Engl. J. Med.* 290:19–23, 1974.

Velosa, J. A., Donadio, J. V., Jr., and Holley, K. E.: Focal sclerosing glomerulonephropathy: a clinicopathologic study. *Mayo Clin. Proc.* 50:121–133, 1975.

Membranous

Brzosko, W. J., Krawczynski, K., Nazarewicz, T., Morzycka, M., and Nowoslawski, A.: Glomerulonephritis associated with hepatitis-B surface antigen immune complexes in children. *Lancet* 2(7879):477–482, 1974.

Pollack, V. E., and Pirani, C. L.: Renal histologic findings in systemic lupus erythematosus. *Mayo Clinic Proc.* 44:630–644, 1969.

Rosen, S.: Membranous glomerulonephritis: current status. *Hum. Pathol.* 2:209–231, 1971.

Membranoproliferative

Germuth, F. G., and Rodriguez, E.: Class II immune complex deposit disease in humans: endomembranous (membranoproliferative or lobular) glomerulonephritis, in *Immunopath-*

V

Renal Failure

This section contains three chapters. The first one, Chapter 13, describes the pathophysiology of acute renal failure. This chapter discusses the differential diagnosis of acute renal failure, the clinical consequences of this entity, as well as the clinical course of acute intrinsic renal failure.

The next chapter, Chapter 14, describes the pathophysiology of chronic renal failure. It reviews the incidence and prevalence of chronic renal disease and the changes in renal function that occur as renal mass decreases. It also summarizes the consequences of chronic renal failure on the homeostasis of water and electrolytes. In a separate portion, the consequences of chronic renal disease on multiple organ systems are discussed. The endocrine and nutritional abnormalities that develop as a consequence of renal failure are analyzed and a discussion is presented regarding the possible pathogenesis of the uremic syndrome.

The last chapter of this section, Chapter 15, presents the pathophysiological principles in the treatment of patients with renal failure. The therapeutic modalities of dialysis and transplantation are discussed, as is the conservative management of chronic renal failure. The effects of these modalities of treatment on specific pathophysiologic alterations produced by renal failure are considered.

V

Renal Failure

13

Pathophysiology of Acute Renal Failure

KEVIN MARTIN

I. INTRODUCTION

Acute renal failure is a clinical syndrome of diverse etiology characterized by a marked and rapid reduction in glomerular filtration rate (GFR), which impairs the ability of the kidneys to maintain the composition of body fluids. GFR falls from the normal values of 100–140 ml/min to 1–10 ml/min. Classically, the decrement in renal function is associated with a marked reduction in GFR to less than 5 ml/min and a fall in urine output to less than 500 ml/24 hr (oliguria). It is being increasingly recognized, however, that acute renal failure may occur without such severe reductions in GFR (usually to levels of 5–10 ml/min) and under these conditions urine output may be greater than 500 ml/day giving rise to the term *nonoliguric acute renal failure*. The definition of oliguria (<500 ml/24 hr) arises from the fact that this approximates the minimum volume of urine required to excrete the 600 mOsm of solute generated from normal diet and metabolism under conditions of maximal urine osmolality which seldom exceeds 1200 mOsm/kg water in man. The term *anuria*, which literally means "no urine output," is often applied to urine volumes of less than 100 ml/24 hr.

KEVIN MARTIN • Department of Medicine, Washington University School of Medicine, St. Louis, Missouri 63110.

The sudden reduction in renal function results in a variety of clinical and biochemical consequences, the severity and magnitude of which depend on the duration and degree of the acute renal failure. The clinical significance of these abnormalities requires an understanding of the pathophysiological mechanisms involved in the generation and maintenance of the acute renal failure such that definitive diagnostic procedures and management can be instituted without delay.

II. CAUSES OF ACUTE RENAL FAILURE

It is convenient to consider the causes of acute renal failure in three major categories, i.e., prerenal, renal, and postrenal. The entities responsible for acute renal failure and their classification into major categories are summarized in Table I.

The common denominator to all the circumstances leading to prerenal acute renal failure is a decrease in renal perfusion. There is no abnormality of the renal parenchyma and the kidney responds to this decrease in perfusion by maximizing the reabsorption of salt and water, resulting in a

Table I. Principal Causes of Acute Renal Failure

I. Prerenal
  A. Decreased intravascular volume: hemorrhage, burns, vomiting, nasogastric suction, diarrhea, diuretics
  B. Increased intravascular capacity: sepsis, vasodilators, anaphylaxis
  C. Myocardial failure: myocardial infarction, pulmonary embolism, congestive heart failure
II. Renal
  A. Ischemia: all conditions in A above, postoperative shock
  B. Nephrotoxins: antibiotics, heavy metals, organic solvents, radiographic contrast materials
  C. Pigment release: traumatic or nontraumatic rhabdomyolysis, intravascular hemolysis
  D. Inflammatory: acute interstitial nephritis, acute glomerulonephritis, vasculitis
  E. Pregnancy-related conditions: septic abortion, eclampsia, postpartum hemorrhage, abruptio placenta, cortical necrosis, postpartum renal failure
  F. Hepatorenal syndrome
  G. Major renovascular disease: renal artery thrombosis and embolism, dissecting aortic aneurysm, renal vein thrombosis (bilateral)
  H. Miscellaneous: acute uric acid nephropathy, hypercalcemia
III. Postrenal
  A. Obstruction to ureters
    1. Intraluminal: papillary necrosis, calculi, clots
    2. Intramural: tumors
    3. Extraureteral: retroperitoneal fibrosis, lymph nodes, tumors
  B. Obstruction at bladder outlet
    Prostatic hypertrophy, carcinoma

Table II. Experimental Animal Models of Acute Renal Failure and Their Possible Counterparts in Human Disease

Experimental animal model	Acute renal failure in man
1. Renal artery clamping, intrarenal norepinephrine infusion	Ischemic acute renal failure
2. Uranyl nitrate administration, mercuric chloride administration	Nephrotoxic acute renal failure
3. Glycerol administration	Pigment release acute renal failure

decreased urine volume of low sodium content and high osmolality. Severe reductions in renal perfusion will result in a fall in GFR and the development of azotemia. This appropriate response of the kidney is important when considering the differential diagnosis of acute renal failure (see Section IV).

Postrenal causes of decreased urine output refer to obstruction to the flow of urine at any level of the urinary tract. In the presence of two kidneys obstruction to the ureters obviously must be bilateral to cause oliguria. It is important to realize that prolonged obstruction will lead to severe damage of the renal parenchyma.

The importance of these two categories (i.e., prerenal and postrenal) lies in the fact that with proper diagnosis and treatment the renal failure is readily reversible.

The remaining category of causes of acute renal failure involves intrinsic damage to the renal parenchyma. The terminology for the major causes of acute intrinsic renal failure due to ischemia, nephrotoxins, and pigment release has changed continually and such terms as acute tubular necrosis, lower nephron nephrosis, vasomotor nephropathy, and acute renal failure are commonplace in the literature. Many of these terms are unsatisfactory in view of the pathology and pathophysiology of this syndrome and it would appear preferable to refer to the syndrome by clinical circumstances, i.e., acute ischemic renal failure, acute nephrotoxic renal failure, or pigment release acute renal failure. The pathophysiological mechanisms operative in these causes of acute renal failure are complex and much of what is known has been learned from studies in experimental animals, particularly in relation to the development and maintenance of oliguria. The experimental models of acute renal failure which have been extensively studied and their possible counterparts in human disease are listed in Table II.

III. PATHOPHYSIOLOGY

Figure 1 illustrates the various sites within the kidney where abnormalities could potentially give rise to reduced GFR and oliguria. The evidence for

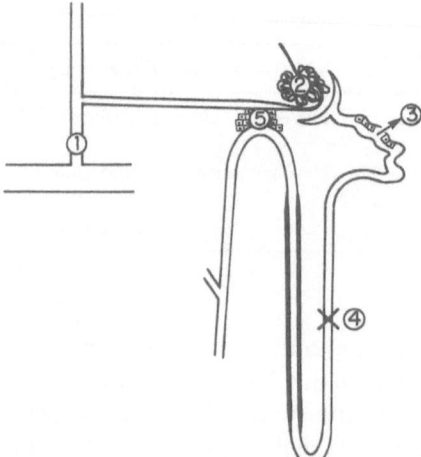

Figure 1. Potential sites within the kidney for the initiation or maintenance of reduced GFR. 1, Decreased renal blood flow; 2, decreased glomerular ultrafiltration coefficient (K_f); 3, leakage of filtrate; 4, tubular obstruction; 5, glomerulotubular feedback via macula densa.

participation of these sites in human and experimental disease will now be discussed in some detail.

A. Ischemic, Nephrotoxic, and Pigment Release Acute Renal Failure

1. Reduced Renal Blood Flow

Many investigators have measured renal blood flow in human acute renal failure by a variety of techniques. Although there are some potential problems with the interpretation of these measurements of renal blood flow, it would appear that renal blood flow is markedly reduced by 50%–75% in acute renal failure. Further knowledge of the role of the reduced blood flow in the development and maintenance of oliguria has been gained from experimental models. In the models utilizing renal artery clamping, norepinephrine infusion, and glycerol administration, renal blood flow is reduced in the early stages. In the nephrotoxic models renal blood flow may be normal or reduced. However, in all cases with reduced renal blood flow, volume expansion can restore renal blood flow without any appreciable effect on the reduced GFR. These studies indicate that while reduced renal blood flow may play an important role in the development of acute renal failure, it would appear that this mechanism is not essential for the maintenance of the renal failure.

Since acute renal failure commonly occurs in a setting of extracellular fluid volume contraction, there has been considerable interest in the role of the renin–angiotensin system in the pathogenesis of the reduced renal blood flow and oliguria. Although the effects of volume expansion in restoring renal blood flow and providing some protection against the development of acute renal failure are consistent with suppression of plasma renin activity, no cause–effect relationship has been shown. Furthermore, immunization of animals against renin or angiotensin II, thereby rendering endogenous renin or angiotensin II ineffective, or manipulation of the system with converting enzyme inhibitor SQ 20881 (which prevents the conversion of angiotensin I to angiotensin II) or with saralasin (a competitive inhibitor of angiotensin II) have not been shown to affect the course of the experimental acute renal failure. Although these studies provide strong evidence against the role of systemic renin–angiotensin, the possible role of intrarenal renin or angiotensin has not been excluded.

Similarly, there is considerable interest in the possible role of prostaglandins in modulating renal blood flow in acute renal failure, particularly the possibility of impaired production of the vasodilator prostaglandin E_2 (PGE_2). Thus, blockade of prostaglandin synthesis with indomethacin appears to increase the severity of acute renal failure in the glycerol model. Conversely, intrarenal infusion of PGE_2 offers some protection against the reduction of GFR in the norepinephrine model. No effect, however, is seen in the uranyl nitrate model. It must be remembered that the role of prostaglandins in the regulation of renal blood flow not only relates to the production of vasodilator prostaglandins but also to the production of vasoconstrictor prostaglandins, such as thromboxane A_2. Therefore, it is possible that the balance between vasoconstrictor and vasodilator prostaglandins is tipped toward the former in acute renal failure. Evidence has been presented for a role of the vasoconstrictor prostaglandin thromboxane A_2 in the pathogenesis of acute renal failure in the glycerol model.

2. Decreased Glomerular Ultrafiltration Coefficient

Recent investigations on the mechanisms of reduced GFR in acute renal failure have focused on the glomerular ultrafiltration coefficient (K_f) which is dependent on (1) the surface area of the glomerulus available for filtration and (2) the intrinsic permeability of the glomerular capillary wall, i.e., its hydraulic conductivity. The experimental conditions in which a reduction in K_f has been demonstrated are presented in Table III. It is not known at the present time if the reduction in K_f produced by the agents listed in Table III is due to a decrease in the glomerular surface area or to a change in the

Table III. Experimental Models of Acute Renal Failure in Which the Ultrafiltration Coefficient (K_f) is Decreased

1. Renal artery clamping	4. Mercuric chloride
2. Norepinephrine infusion	5. Gentamycin
3. Uranyl nitrate	6. Hypercalcemia

hydraulic conductivity, or whether both factors play a role. With regard to the possible role of the renin–angiotensin system discussed above, it is relevant to note that there are receptors for angiotensin II in the glomerulus and that an intrarenal production of this vasoconstrictor could decrease the glomerular surface area and, therefore, reduce the glomerular ultrafiltration coefficient.

3. Leakage of Filtrate

From early studies of renal histology in acute renal failure showing necrosis of tubular cells and disruption of basement membranes it has been postulated that tubular fluid could leak from the lumen into the interstitium. This leakage of filtrate could lead to an apparent decrease in GFR as a result of the loss of the marker for GFR (e.g., inulin, creatinine) from the tubular fluid to the interstitium. An additional possibility is that the leakage of filtrate into the interstitium would increase the hydrostatic pressure within the kidney and, thus, lead to a decrease in GFR. Evidence for leakage of tubular fluid has been provided in experimental acute renal failure. Thus, following microinjections of Lissamine Green (a colored dye) into the proximal tubule the dye can be seen exiting from the tubular lumen into the interstitium in the ischemic model of acute renal failure. Diffusion of horseradish peroxidase from the tubular lumen has been noted after microinjection into the proximal tubule or intravenous injection in a similar model. There is also evidence that tubular permeability is increased in the uranyl nitrate and mercury chloride models. Although leakage of tubular fluid does occur in acute renal failure and may play a role in reducing GFR, the actual contribution of this phenomenon to the decrease in GFR and oliguria is unclear.

4. Tubular Obstruction

Obstruction of the tubular lumen by necrotic debris or casts would result in an increase in tubular pressure reducing net filtration pressure and, therefore, causing a reduction in GFR and oliguria. While elevated intratubular pressures have been found in the renal artery clamp model early after release of the clamp, intratubular pressure returns to normal by 24 hr. It must be remembered that even "normal" intratubular pressures are compatible with tubular obstruction in the presence of a reduction in GFR which should cause a decrease in tubular pressure. Thus, although elevated intratubular pressures are not seen in other models of acute renal failure, rather than excluding tubular obstruction as a contributing event these data may indicate that additional factors are maintaining the reduced GFR. It is also possible that tubular obstruction may be secondary to decreased GFR in that cellular debris which would not normally cause obstruction may accumulate and impact in a state of low fluid flow through the tubules. In this regard, studies in the glycerol model have shown that tubular casts are easily dislodged by application of low pressure within the tubular lumen. A final consideration for the role of tubular obstruction may be that since prolonged ureteral obstruction results in a fall in renal blood flow, prolonged tubular obstruction may have hemodynamic consequences at the glomerular level leading to decreased glomerular blood flow.

5. Glomerulo-tubular Feedback

Over the last several years there has been increasing evidence for the role of the macula densa in the regulation of single-nephron GFR. Thus, it appears that the rate of sodium chloride reabsorption by the distal tubule in the region of the macula densa may modulate a local release of renin and angiotensin which in turn can regulate GFR by modifying afferent arteriolar tone. Recently it has been postulated that this mechanism may be operative in acute renal failure. According to this theory, damage of proximal tubular cells results in impaired NaCl reabsorption and increases its delivery to the distal tubule. This increased NaCl delivery is "sensed" by the macula densa, which then effects a marked reduction in GFR (via renin–angiotensin). Thus, the reduction in GFR may be an "appropriate compensation" by the kidney to prevent loss of fluids escaping proximal reabsorption due to impaired proximal tubular function. Although this theory is attractive in many ways, firm evidence that this mechanism is operative in acute renal failure is not available at the present time.

B. Integration of Experimental Data

A simplified scheme of the pathophysiology of acute renal failure is illustrated in Figure 2. The scheme is shown to consist of two phases, i.e., the initiation phase and the maintenance phase. The major factor(s) involved in the initiation of acute renal failure need not be the same as the factors which maintain the reduced GFR. For example, following clamping of the renal artery resulting in renal ischemia, which is the initiating event in the induction of acute renal failure, it has been shown that one to three hours after release of the clamp tubular pressures are elevated, indicating that an additional factor, tubular obstruction, was present. Moreover, renal blood flow can be restored in this model by volume expansion without an increase in GFR, thereby, providing further evidence that additional factors besides decreased renal blood flow are involved in the maintenance of the decreased GFR and acute renal failure.

In the majority of clinical circumstances, the initiating event is an ischemic insult to the kidneys and/or direct toxicity to the kidney by either endogenous or exogenous toxins. Each of the three main anatomical components of the kidney may be compromised, i.e., blood flow may be reduced,

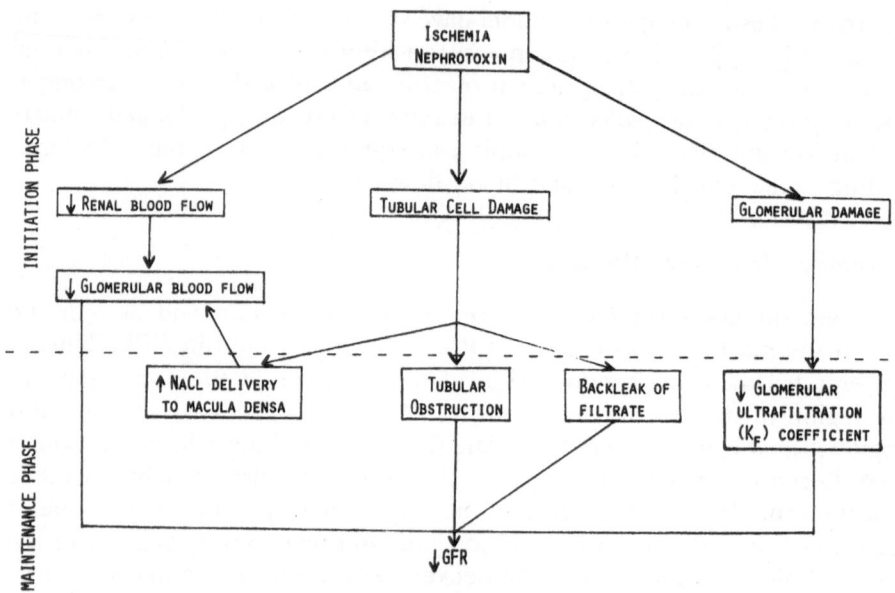

Figure 2. Pathogenesis of acute renal failure. For complete description, see text.

tubular function may be impaired, or the glomerulus may be damaged. It is likely then that the maintenance of the renal failure depends on additional factors which are the consequence of the initial insult. The factors may vary depending on the nature of the insult and the clinical circumstances, e.g., renal blood flow may not be reduced in acute renal failure of nephrotoxic origin or may be restored toward normal by volume expansion following an ischemic insult, yet the GFR remains markedly decreased, indicating the involvement of additional factors in this decrease. It must be remembered that our knowledge of the pathophysiology of acute renal failure has been gained to a large extent from experimental models which may not be totally analogous to human disease.

C. Inflammatory Acute Renal Failure

Acute renal failure may result from inflammatory processes involving the blood vessels of the kidney, the glomeruli or the renal interstitium alone or in combination. The inflammation is usually a consequence of an immunologic process due to a hypersensitivity reaction (e.g., penicillin administration), deposition of immune complexes (e.g., systemic lupus erythematosus), or the deposition of antibodies to renal structural constituents such as the glomerular or tubular basement membranes (e.g., Goodpasture's syndrome). While in most instances the inciting antigen is unknown, in some cases, however, it can be identified as a drug (e.g., sulfonamide) or a virus (e.g., hepatitis B antigen). The consequences of the inflammatory reaction are a reduction in renal blood flow, a decrease in the glomerular ultrafiltration coefficient (K_f), and a reduction in GFR. The differential diagnosis of these types of renal diseases from ischemic or nephrotoxic renal failure is extremely important in that the treatment and prognosis of these conditions (see Sections VII and VIII) differ markedly from the other types of intrinsic acute renal failure.

D. Acute Renal Failure Related to Pregnancy

Acute renal failure is a serious complication of pregnancy occurring once in approximately 5000 pregnancies. Septicemia resulting from septic abortion leading to acute renal failure is encountered less commonly nowadays. In late pregnancy, acute renal failure may follow eclampsia, abruptio placenta, or postpartum hemorrhage. In these instances, acute renal failure may be due to acute cortical necrosis in which arcuate arteries, interlobular arteries, afferent arterioles, and glomeruli of the kidney become thrombosed as a result of intravascular coagulation. Anuria rather than oliguria may be present in this condition and unless the cortical necrosis is patchy, renal function only rarely recovers.

In the postpartum period, acute renal failure may develop in association with evidence of intravascular coagulation. The etiology of this condition is unknown and may be similar to the adult hemolytic uremic syndrome. It is notable that a similar syndrome may occur in women taking oral contraceptives. The prognosis of these conditions is poor and recovery of renal function is rare. The term *renal cortical thrombotic microangiopathy* may better serve to describe these conditions.

E. Hepatorenal Syndrome

The hepatorenal syndrome refers to renal failure occurring in patients with severe liver disease in the absence of other known causes of renal failure. The cause of the renal failure is unclear but there is substantial evidence that the compromised renal function is functional in nature. Thus, these kidneys function normally when transplanted into patients without liver disease. In addition, these kidneys function normally *in situ* following hepatic transplantation. Accordingly, it appears that the hepatorenal syndrome is due to alterations in the renal circulation with afferent arteriolar vasoconstriction. The exact mechanism of this vasoconstriction is unknown. Possibilities include decreased "effective" blood volume, increased activity of the renin angiotensin system, increased vasoconstrictor prostaglandin production, or decreased catabolism and/or increased production of vasoactive substances by the liver.

Since the pathogenesis of the renal failure in the hepatorenal syndrome relates to an impairment in effective renal perfusion the urinary diagnostic indices of acute renal failure resemble those of prerenal azotemia (see Section IV).

F. Major Renovascular Disease

Acute renal failure may occur if the renal blood flow is reduced by renal arterial embolism or thrombosis or by involvement of the renal arteries by a dissecting aortic aneurysm. Precise diagnosis is imperative as the prognosis for recovery of renal function is poor unless renal blood flow can be restored by surgery.

G. Acute Uric Acid Nephropathy

Acute renal failure secondary to sudden and marked increases in the production of uric acid is a serious complication of the treatment of leukemia, multiple myeloma, and lymphomas. The destruction of large masses of malignant cells releases large amounts of nucleoprotein which is metabolized to uric acid. This substance is handled by the kidney by glomerular filtration, tubular reabsorption, and tubular secretion. The sudden marked increase in uric acid excretion following chemotherapy leads to precipitation of uric acid crystals within the terminal portions of the nephron. In this segment of the nephron the tubular fluid is concentrated leading to increased concentrations of uric acid and acidified leading to markedly decreased solubility of uric acid at pH values of tubular fluid below 5.7, thereby predisposing to precipitation of uric acid.

H. Hypercalcemic Nephropathy

Acute elevations in serum calcium of mild-to-moderate degree leads to polyuria, volume contraction, and azotemia unless salt and water deficits are replaced. More severe elevations of serum calcium may lead to acute renal failure and oliguria. The mechanisms of the acute renal failure include decreased renal blood flow, decreased glomerular ultrafiltration coefficient (K_f), and tubular obstruction by necrotic debris and calcium precipitation. With increased duration of the hypercalcemia, nephrocalcinosis develops. While the renal failure is reversible in the early stages by appropriate therapy, in advanced cases uremia may persist despite correction of the hypercalcemia.

I. Ureteral Obstruction

The consequences of ureteral obstruction depend on both the degree and duration of the obstruction. Partial obstruction results in slowly progressive decline in renal function often complicated by infection over many months to years. The syndrome of acute renal failure due to ureteral obstruction requires the obstruction to be severe and bilateral (if two kidneys are present). The mechanisms whereby obstruction decreases GFR is complex. A major component is that the rise in ureteral pressure is transmitted to the tubular fluid and to the glomerulus, therefore decreasing net hydrostatic filtration pressure at the level of the glomerulus. This mechanism would appear to be operative early after ureteral obstruction since renal blood flow increases initially. This initial increase in renal blood flow is due to increased synthesis of renal prostaglandin E_2 (a potent vasodilator). At later times after obstruction (>12 hr) when renal blood flow falls to subnormal levels glomerular blood flow could be decreased as a consequence of increased preglomerular vascular resistance due to effects of angiotensin II or the vasoconstrictor prostaglandin thromboxane A_2, and this mechanism may maintain the reduction in glomerular filtration rate. Therefore, in the later stages of obstruction the decrease in GFR is due mainly to a fall in intraglomerular hydrostatic pressure with a return of intratubular pressure toward normal.

IV. DIFFERENTIAL DIAGNOSIS OF ACUTE RENAL FAILURE

Since the prognosis and therapy of acute renal failure differ considerably depending on the etiology of the renal dysfunction, it is important to establish a firm diagnosis. A detailed discussion of the diagnosis of each specific cause of acute renal failure is beyond the scope of this chapter and only general principles are discussed. Emphasis is placed on the differentiation of prerenal failure and intrinsic renal failure. Diagnosis is made by careful medical history, physical examination, microscopic examination of the urinary sediment, and chemical analyses of urine and plasma. From the history, information regarding the occurrence of hypotension, ingestion of potential nephrotoxic agents, or the presence of immunological diseases may be obtained. Physical examination reveals not only the clinical consequences of acute renal failure but may also give information regarding possible etiology, e.g., state of hydration, blood pressure, presence of vasculitis in skin, and lymphodenopathy in leukemia and lymphoma. Microscopic examination of the urine sediment is of paramount importance. In prerenal azotemia moderate numbers of hyaline and finely granular casts may be seen. Coarse granular or cellular casts are uncommon. The presence of red blood cell casts is indicative of glomerular disease. The presence of a positive test for blood in the urine in the absence of red blood cells in the urine is suggestive of myoglobinuric or hemoglobinuric renal failure. The presence of a sediment containing cellular debris is suggestive of ischemic or nephrotoxic acute renal failure. Polymorphonuclear leucocytes or eosinophils in the urine sediment may indicate interstitial nephritis. Uric acid crystals may be seen in acute uric acid nephropathy. Chemical analysis of the urine provides information regarding the pathophysiology of acute renal dysfunction. In prerenal azotemia, with no intrinsic renal abnormality, the response of the kidney to decreased perfusion is to conserve salt and water. The marked reduction in single-nephron glomerular filtration rate seen with acute glomerular disease may result in similar findings early in the course (see below). In contrast, intrinsic tubular renal disease is associated with impaired ability to conserve salt and water. Conservation of salt is reflected by a low concentration of sodium and/or chloride in the urine. Water reabsorption by the kidney is assessed by the concentration of a nonreabsorable solute such as creatinine, usually expressed as the ratio of the concentration of creatinine in urine to that of plasma (U/P creatinine). A U/P creatinine ratio of 4 indicates that 25% of filtered water remains, U/P creatinine ratio of 100 indicates that 1% of the filtered water remains. Thus, in prerenal azotemia the U/P creatinine is high, whereas in the presence of intrinsic tubular renal disease the ability to conserve water is impaired so that the U/P creatinine ratio is low. The sensitivity of these tests of renal function can be improved by combining the information obtained from sodium concentrations and the U/P creatinine ratio to calculate the fractional excretion of sodium (FE_{Na}) (i.e., urine sodium excretion as a percent of the filtered load):

$$\% FE_{Na} = 100 \times \frac{\text{Na excreted}}{\text{Na filtered}} = \frac{U_{Na} \times V}{P_{Na} \times GFR} \times 100$$

$$= 100 \times \frac{U_{Na} \times V}{P_{Na} \times V(U_{cr}/P_{cr})} = \frac{U_{Na}}{P_{Na}} \Big/ \frac{U_{cr}}{P_{cr}} \times 100$$

The interpretation of these tests is summarized in Table IV.

While such calculations are extremely valuable, there are several potential pitfalls which must be remembered and are listed in Table V. There is no distinct pattern of urine chemistries in urinary tract obstruction. Acute obstruction may be associated with a prerenal picture, whereas in chronic obstruction a pattern resembling intrinsic renal failure may be obtained. Obstruction, therefore, must be excluded by other means such as intravenous pyelography, sonography, or computerized axial scanning. In some cases

Table IV. Urinary Chemistries in Acute Renal Failure

	Prerenal	Renal
U_{Na}[a]	<20	>20
$U_{Cr}P_{Cr}$[b]	>20	<20
FE_{Na}[c]	<1	>1

[a] U_{Na}, urinary sodium concentration.
[b] U_{Cr}/P_{Cr}, urine creatinine concentration divided by plasma creatinine concentration.
[c] FE_{Na}, fractional excretion of sodium (for calculation, see text).

Table V. Pitfalls in the Use of Urinary
Chemistries in ARF

1. Urinary tract obstruction
2. Acute glomerulonephritis
3. Prior administration of diuretics
4. Preexisting chronic renal disease
5. Residual urine–bladder irrigation fluid in bladder

with delayed dye excretion retrograde pyelography may be necessary. An important pitfall in the use of these urinary indices of acute renal failure may be present with acute glomerulonephritis and vasculitis. Early in the course of these diseases there is a marked reduction in single-nephron GFR while tubular function is intact. The kidney behaves in a similar fashion to that seen with decreased renal perfusion and the urine will have a low sodium concentration and high U/P creatinine ratio similar to that in prerenal azotemia. Later in the course, e.g., after 2–3 days, the pattern of the urinary indices will change to that of intrinsic renal failure as the adaptive changes of renal failure occur.

In evaluating urinary chemistries it is important to remember that prior administration of diuretics, particularly loop blockers, may result in a urine with a relatively low U/P creatinine ratio and high urine sodium even in the presence of prerenal azotemia. In the presence of preexisting chronic renal disease the damaged kidney cannot retain sodium avidly or concentrate the urine maximally even in the presence of prerenal factors so that urinary diagnostic indices are not useful in excluding a prerenal component which has led to further deterioration of function in chronic renal disease. Finally, the presence of fluid from prior bladder irrigation may not be representative of the current clinical situation.

With these pitfalls in mind, however, the use of urine Na concentrations and U/P creatinine ratios contributes valuable information regarding the pathophysiological mechanisms operative in states of acute renal dysfunction.

V. CLINICAL CONSEQUENCES OF ACUTE RENAL FAILURE

As a consequence of the decreased renal function there is an alteration in the composition of the volume of body fluids and electrolytes and in the excretion of the end products of metabolic functions. The potential clinical manifestations of acute renal failure are listed in Table VI. The most prominent of these is the inability to excrete salt and water such that expansion of the extracellular fluid volume occurs leading to peripheral edema, hypertension, congestive heart failure, and pulmonary edema unless the intake of salt and water is restricted. Ingestion of water in excess of salt will result in hyponatremia, which may become severe (110 mEq/liter) and

Table VI. Consequences of Acute Renal Failure

I. Cardiovascular	IV. Hematologic
A. Expansion of ECF	A. Anemia
B. Pulmonary edema	B. Platelet dysfunction
C. Hypertension	V. Gastrointestinal
D. Peripheral edema	A. Nausea
E. Cardiac arrhythmias	B. Vomiting
II. Metabolic	C. GI bleeding
A. Hyponatremia	VI. Infections
B. Hypocalcemia	A. Pulmonary
C. Hyperphosphatemia	B. Urinary tract
D. Hyperuricemia	C. Septicemia
E. Hypermagnesemia	
F. Hyperkalemia	
G. Azotemia	
H. Acidosis	
III. Neurologic	
A. Somnolence	
B. Asterixis	
C. Convulsions	
D. Coma	

may lead to convulsions unless managed appropriately. End products of metabolism such as urea and creatinine are retained and their measurement in blood serves as an index of residual renal function.

Creatinine, an end product of muscle metabolism, is handled by the kidney by glomerular filtration, is not reabsorbed, and may be secreted to some extent by the tubular cells in advanced renal failure. Thus, measurement of glomerular filtration rate by creatinine clearance will overestimate GFR when at values below 10 ml/min. In some cases of renal failure associated with muscle injury serum creatinine will rise rapidly as a consequence of a markedly increased production rate. Conversely, in situations with decreased muscle mass such as chronic debilitating illness, malnutrition, and cirrhosis, creatinine production is reduced, and therefore serum creatinine will rise slowly in spite of marked reductions in overall renal function.

Urea, an end product of protein metabolism, usually measured in blood as blood urea nitrogen (BUN) is handled by the kidney by glomerular filtration, but in contrast to creatinine is reabsorbed to an appreciable extent by the tubular cells. The reabsorption of urea is increased in conditions where renal blood flow is diminished. Thus, in prerenal azotemia BUN will rise out of proportion to the rise in serum creatinine. Similar findings are observed in severely catabolic states as a consequence of the breakdown of tissue proteins. By contrast, in acute renal failure due to rhabdomyolysis, there is a decrease in the BUN/Cr ratio due to a disproportionate increase in serum creatinine as a consequence of muscle destruction.

The kidney plays a central role in the regulation of potassium homeostasis. With severe renal failure and impaired ability to excrete potassium, elevations of plasma potassium are common and may become life threatening unless managed appropriately (see Chapter 7).

The failure of the damaged kidney to excrete nonvolatile acid results in the development of metabolic acidosis, which may become severe and require aggressive therapy. Hypocalcemia develops rapidly during acute renal failure as a consequence of retention of phosphorus leading to hyperphosphatemia, decreased intestinal calcium absorption secondary to decreased production of 1,25-dihydroxy vitamin D, and skeletal resistance to the actions of parathyroid hormone. The hypocalcemia is usually asymptomatic since the presence of acidosis increases the fraction of ionized calcium in serum. Rapid correction of acidosis with resultant fall in ionized calcium may precipitate tetany, painful muscle contractions, and, occasionally, laryngospasm.

Serum magnesium levels may rise, particularly if magnesium-containing antacids are being given. Hypermagnesemia may result in blockage of neuromuscular transmission due to presynaptic inhibition of acetylcholine release, depression of sinoatrial and atrioventricular nodes, lethargy, confusion, absent reflexes, CNS depression, and coma. It is important that these effects are not attributed to altered central nervous system function due to uremia per se so that appropriate treatment may be instituted.

Anemia develops rapidly within the first week of acute renal failure and is mainly due to impaired erythropoiesis presumably due to decreased erythropoietin production by the damaged kidneys. Hemodilution and hemolysis also contribute to the anemia as well as blood drawing for laboratory tests which are necessary in the management of a critically ill patient.

Gastrointestinal manifestations of uremia include nausea and vomiting, which may be extremely distressing to the patient with acute renal failure. Gastrointestinal hemorrhage may occur in acute renal failure and is a major cause of death in these patients.

There is an increased susceptibility to infection in acute renal failure, which, in addition to gastrointestinal hemorrhage, is a major cause of death. Infections of surgical wounds, urinary tract infections, and pulmonary injectons may all give rise to fatal septicemia.

VI. CLINICAL COURSE OF ACUTE INTRINSIC RENAL FAILURE

The clinical course of acute intrinsic renal failure of the ischemic or nephrotoxic variety can be described in four different phases:

1. The *initiation phase* extends from the time of the initial insult to the kidney to the development of oliguria. This phase may last from a few hours in the case of severe renal ischemia to several days to a week following nephrotoxins, e.g., carbon tetrachloride.

2. During the *oliguric phase* the GFR is markedly reduced and the clinical and biochemical manifestations of renal failure become

evident. This phase may last from a few days to several weeks. the mean duration is approximately two weeks.

3.   The *diuretic phase* is characterized by a gradually increasing urine volume. It is important to realize the BUN and creatinine may continue to rise for several days in spite of the increasing urine volume. This is explained by the fact that small changes in GFR insufficient to produce a decline in BUN or creatinine may, none-theless, produce large changes in urine volume. Thus, if GFR is 1 ml/min (severe renal failure) and urine output is 150 ml/day, then approximately 10% of the glomerular filtrate is being excreted per day. If GFR increases to 5 ml/min and the fraction of glomerular filtrate excreted remains the same 10%, then urine output will be 720 ml/day in spite of the fact that renal failure remains severe and serum creatinine will continue to rise toward the steady state level obligated by this GFR. Later in the diuretic phase, as GFR continues to increase, serum creatinine and BUN values decrease toward normal. There is often disparity between glomerular filtration rate and tubular function at this time such that the regulation of salt and water reabsorption and potassium excretion may remain abnormal for several days before returning toward normal. Accordingly, one must be aware that volume contraction and hypokalemia may occur unless appropriate measures are taken.

4.   The *recovery phase* refers to the period in which complete recovery of renal function occurs including the improvement of tubular function. Although renal function returns to normal in many patients over a period of weeks to months, mild-to-moderate decrease in GFR persists in some patients. Clinically insignificant abnormalities in renal acidification and in the concentrating and diluting mechanisms may also persist.

VII.   MANAGEMENT

The identification of prerenal and postrenal causes of ARF is of major importance since rapid correction of the compromised renal function may be achieved. With a knowledge of potential causes of acute renal failure, efforts can be made to prevent the occurrence of ARF. Preexisting renal insufficiency, the elderly patient, diabetes, multiple myeloma, major vascular surgery, and severe atherosclerosis are well recognized risk factors for ARF. Particular caution should be exercised with the use of radiographic contrast agents, preparation for surgery, the dosage of nephrotoxic antibiotics, and the prevention of volume contraction in these settings. The maintenance of a solute diuresis with mannitol or furosemide may offer some protection against the development of ARF as a consequence of surgery or radiographic procedures.

Once renal failure is established the general principles of management involve the assumption by the physician of the role of the kidneys in the maintenance of fluid and electrolyte balance, acid–base balance, endocrinologic and metabolic functions, and excretory function until renal function recovers or responds to specific treatment. Intake and output of salt and water should be monitored closely and confirmed by. daily weights and clinical examination. A weight loss of 0.25–0.5 kg/day is anticipated in the starving patient. Some enthusiasm exists for the administration of large doses of furosemide in established ARF. While urine output may increase somewhat and thus facilitate the maintenance of salt and water balance, there is controversy as to whether the clinical course and/or overall mortality is affected. Efforts should be made to supply sufficient nutrition to prevent endogenous protein catabolism and therefore minimize the rate of rise of BUN. Potassium intake should be restricted to minimize hyperkalemia. The administration of the cation exchange resin sodium polystyrene sulfonate may be of value in the control of hyperkalemia. The administration of magnesium-containing antacids should be restricted in order to prevent severe hypermagnesemia. Hypocalcemia due to phosphate retention, skeletal resistance to parathyroid hormone, and altered vitamin D metabolism generally does not require treatment unless tetany or other symptoms occur. The concomitant acidosis serves to increase the fraction of ionized calcium and should be treated slowly and cautiously to avoid volume overload and to avoid precipitating tetany. Anemia develops rapidly in ARF. In general, transfusions should not be given unless the hematocrit is less than 30%.

Infections, a major cause of death in ARF, should be treated promptly, with attention to the dosage of antibiotics in renal failure.

While ARF can be managed conservatively in some instances, there is an increasing role for the institution of dialysis therapy. Overall mortality may be improved by early dialysis, fluid and electrolyte balance may be easily achieved, hyperkalemia and acidosis controlled, and parenteral nutrition may be instituted since the large fluid loads are easily controlled. Specific indications for dialysis include volume overload, hyperkalemia, severe acidosis, neurologic abnormalities, severe hyponatremia, and hypercatabolism.

During the diuretic phase of ARF vigilance should not be relaxed since the regulatory capacity of the kidneys may be inadequate for several days and careful replacement of urinary losses of fluid and electrolytes is necessary.

VIII. PROGNOSIS

The prognosis for the patient with ARF depends upon the clinical circumstances, e.g., ischemic, traumatic, nephrotoxic, or obstetric causes and upon the severity of the ARF, e.g., oliguric or nonoliguric. Ischemic and traumatic ARF, most often occurring postsurgery, is associated with a mortality of 50%–70%, whereas the other categories are associated with a mortality of 10%–35%. Nonoliguric ARF is felt to be a less severe form of ARF and appears to have a better prognosis than the oliguric form (a mortality rate of 20%–30% vs. 50%–60% for nonoliguric ARF and oliguric ARF, respectively).

IX. SUMMARY

The central role of the kidney in the maintenance of the body's internal environment is readily appreciated when renal function is suddenly severely impaired. Since acute renal failure is associated with a high mortality rate (approximately 40%), it is essential to discover the cause of the acute renal dysfunction, to determine the reversibility of the insult, and to endeavor to prevent complications of acute renal failure. An understanding of the pathophysiology of oliguria in the various clinical settings is essential for the interpretation of laboratory tests which may indicate the cause and potential reversibility of the acute renal failure. A knowledge of the clinical consequences of acute renal failure is essential for prevention and treatment of complications. Much of our knowledge of the pathophysiology of acute renal failure has been gained from experimental animal models which may not be totally analogous to acute renal failure in humans. However, the similarities are such that these models provide an essential tool for the further study of the pathophysiology of acute renal failure. It is hoped that future investigations will lead to maneuvers which can prevent or ameliorate clinical acute renal failure.

SUGGESTED READINGS

Abel, R. M., Beck, C. H., Abbot, W. M., Ryan, J. A., Barnett, O. G., and Fischer, J. E.: Improved survival from acute renal failure after treatment with intravenous essential e-amino acids and glucose. *N. Engl. J. Med.* 288:695–699, 1973.

Anderson, R. J., Linas, S. L., Berns, A. S., Henrich, W. L., Miller, T. R., Gabow, P. A., and Schrier, R. W.: Non-oliguric acute renal failure. *N. Engl. J. Med.* 296:1134–1138, 1977.

Bennett, W. M., Muther, R. S., Parker, R. A., Ferg, P., Morrison, G., Golper, T. A., and Singer, I.: Drug therapy in renal failure: dosing guidelines for adults. I. *Ann. Intern. Med.* 93:62–89, 1980.

Bennett, W. M., Muther, R. S., Parker, R. A., Ferg, P., Morrison, G., Golper, T. A., and Singer, I.: Drug therapy in renal failure: dosing guidelines for adults. II. *Ann. Intern. Med.* 93:286–325, 1980.

Brenner, B. M., and Stein, J. H. (eds.): *Contemporary Issues in Nephrology: Acute Renal Failure*, Vol. 6. Churchill Livingstone, New York, 1980.

Byrd, L., and Sherman, R. L.: Radio-contrast induced acute renal failure. *Medicine* 58:270–279, 1979.

Kleinknect, D., Jungers, P., Chanard, J., Barbanel, C., and Ganeval, D.: Uremic and non-uremic complications of acute renal failure: evaluation of early and frequent dialysis on prognosis. *Kidney Int.* 1:190–196, 1972.

Kleinknect, D., Kornfer, A., Morel-Maroger, L., and Mery, J.: Furosemide in acute renal failure: a controlled trial. *Nephron* 17:51–58, 1976.

Levinsky, N. G.: Pathophysiology of acute renal failure. *N. Engl. J. Med.* 296:1453–1458, 1977.

Miller, T. R., Anderson, R. J., Linas, S. L., Henrich, W. L., Berns, A. S., Gabow, P. A., and Schrier, R. W.: Urinary diagnostic indices in acute renal failure. A prospective study. *Ann. Intern. Med.* 89:47–50, 1978.

Stein, J. H., Lipschitz, M. D., and Barnes, L. D.: Current concepts on the pathophysiology of acute renal failure. *Am. J. Physiol.* 243(3):F171–F181, 1978.

Thurau, K., and Boylan, J. W.: Acute renal success: the unexpected logic of oliguria in acute renal failure. *Am. J. Med.* 61:308–315, 1976.

14

Pathophysiology of Chronic Renal Failure

PHILLIP HOFFSTEN and SAULO KLAHR

I. INTRODUCTION

Chronic renal impairment usually refers to any permanent depression of glomerular filtration rate (GFR). The term, however, can also be used to describe abnormal tubular function which can occur on a permanent basis even in the face of a normal glomerular filtration rate. We will use the term *renal impairment* to signify a decrease in GFR. Impairment becomes "failure" when plasma composition becomes substantially abnormal and symptoms usually appear at a GFR of approximately 25% of normal (30 ml/min). Chronic renal failure can be divided descriptively into early (GFR around 30-10 ml/min), late (GFR 10-5 ml/min), and terminal (GFR less than 5 ml/min) phases. The symptoms and signs of uremia, as discussed in this chapter, become prominent in late chronic renal failure and life threatening in the terminal phase.

Regardless of the cause of the renal disease, decreased kidney function may occur through three major mechanisms: (1) a decrease in the number

PHILLIP HOFFSTEN • Department of Medicine, Washington University School of Medicine, St. Louis, Missouri 63110. *Present address:* Medical Associates Clinic, Pierre, South Dakota 57501.   SAULO KLAHR • Department of Medicine, Washington University School of Medicine, St. Louis, Missouri 63110.

of functioning nephrons (normal man has approximately 1 million nephrons in each one of his two kidneys); (2) a marked fall in filtration rate of each individual nephron without a decrease in their number; or (3) a combination of 1 and 2. The consequences of either one of these events will be a decrease in GFR. For example, at a physiologic GFR of 120 ml/min and with a normal complement of nephrons (2,000,000), the filtration rate per nephron is 60 nl. If the total number of nephrons is decreased to 500,000, the total GFR (assuming no adaptation in the remaining nephrons) will fall to 30 ml/min. The same GFR value may obtain when the total number of nephrons remains unaltered (2 million) but the single-nephron GFR is decreased to 15 nl/min, or when the total number of nephrons is 1 million and the single-nephron GFR is 30 nl/min.

The mechanisms of kidney injury are complex and diverse. They embrace abnormal immunological processes, disturbances in coagulation, infection, biochemical and metabolic perturbations, vascular disorders, congenital abnormalities, obstruction to urine flow, neoplasia, and trauma. Each of these mechanisms may interact with diseases (e.g., diabetes, hypertension) and intoxications in which renal failure is not infrequently a presenting feature.

As mentioned above, progressive chronic renal failure has a large number of etiologies, some of which produce evident urinary tract or systemic symptoms. Yet, in the vast majority of cases the early to moderately advanced stage of diffuse loss of renal function is a silent process, the patient being unaware that a serious disease process is ongoing. This silent stage of chronic renal disease may be recognized on a routine physical or laboratory examination, although the significance of such clues as high blood pressure, retinal changes, anemia, slight elevation of the blood urea nitrogen (BUN) or serum creatinine, minor abnormalities of the urinary sediment and slight proteinuria is, at times, overlooked. The first symptoms of chronic renal failure usually come late in the course of renal diseases and are also vague and nonspecific, the whole constellation of symptoms (and findings) being referred to as *uremia*.

A. Incidence and Prevalence of Renal Disease

No satisfactory data on the incidence of end stage renal disease in North America are available. Data based on mortality figures suggest an incidence of 150–200 per million population. With the exception of the Tecumseh Study, there are no direct estimates of the incidence of renal disease in the United States. The Tecumseh Study is based on small numbers, the number of blacks with renal disease in this population is not given, and the calculated figures would give an incidence for end stage renal disease of 190–250 per million population. It seems, therefore, that figures for incidence of end stage renal disease in the United States are somewhere between 150 and 200 per million. These figures, of course, may vary in certain regions depending on the proportion of blacks in the population. The incidence of renal disease in blacks is higher than in whites (presumably because of the higher incidence of hypertension, and its consequences, in blacks). The distribution of primary diseases leading to end stage renal disease and the percentage contributed by each one of these different disorders to end stage renal disease is as follows: glomerulonephritis, 38%; primary hypertensive disease, 12%; polycystic kidney disease, 8%; interstitial disorders, 15%; diabetic nephropathy, 7%; known miscellaneous, 5%; collagen and vascular disorders, about 3%; all other hereditary disorders, 2%; and diseases of unknown cause, about 10%. Again, these figures are difficult to substantiate, since there is great variability in those reports available.

B. Nature of the Kidney Adaptations in Chronic Renal Disease

Normal man is born with approximately 2 million nephrons. He probably can survive, albeit with difficulty, with less than 40,000 nephrons (2% of normal renal function). This reserve *capacity* is fortunate, indeed, for there are a large number of different disease entities with a predilection for nephron destruction. These processes vary in their pathogenetic and histologic detail and in their rate of progression, but they all evoke common alterations in renal functional and a common constellation of chemical and physiologic abnormalities. The challenge to survival posed by the loss of nephrons is met by a variety of adaptive mechanisms, most of which are not fully understood. Adaptations occur both at an intrarenal level, within the surviving nephrons, and at a whole body level. The success of the adaptation mechanisms is attested to most vividly by the fact that life persists after over 90% of the original nephron population has been destroyed. From a more quantitative point of view, the excretion rates of some of the principal solutes of body fluids (including sodium, chloride, and potassium) may be regulated with sufficient precision to permit the maintenance of external balance down to very low levels of renal function without either retention in body fluids or an increase in chemical concentration in the extracellular fluid. However, as the nephron population diminishes the GFR falls, solutes that are excreted primarily by glomerular filtration, such as urea and creatinine, will be retained in the blood. Indeed, the degree of retention of these two solutes provides a rough index of the percentage reduction in GFR. As GFR decreases below approximately 25% of normal, other solutes which are either filtered and reabsorbed or secreted may also be retained in body fluids. These include phosphate, sulfate, and urate. Finally, a host of other solutes accumulate in the blood when the renal disease is far advanced. The list includes organic acids, phenolic compounds, indols, guanidines, a variety of metabolic intermediates, and certain peptides. Certain of these retained solutes may have toxic potential; hence, they conceivably could contribute to the symptoms and signs of advanced chronic renal disease.

C. Limitations in Renal Function in Chronic Kidney Disease

In addition, as renal function decreases the ability of the individual to tolerate changes in dietary intake of sodium, potassium, and water is markedly restricted. Although the range of excretion per nephron may increase for specific solutes under renal regulation, the fewer the number of nephrons, the smaller is the total range of excretion achievable by the composite nephron population. Thus, the upper limit of excretion for many solutes and for water is less than that achieved by normal subjects, and for sodium (and perhaps other solutes) and water there is a restriction on the minimum amount that may be excreted. The overall effect is that the individual with chronic renal disease is subjected to decreased *flexibility* in his dietary intake as kidney failure progresses.

The *loss of synthetic functions* of the kidneys may also contribute to the abnormalities of uremia. For example, a decrease in erythropoietin, a substance which promotes the maturation of red blood cells in the bone marrow, plays a role in the anemia of uremia.

Alterations in the levels of blood-pressure-controlling factors (renin, angiotensin II) coupled with expansion of the extracellular fluid due to salt retention contribute to the high incidence of hypertension observed in individuals with chronic renal failure.

II. CONSEQUENCES OF CHRONIC RENAL FAILURE

In this portion the effects of chronic renal failure on the volume and composition of body fluids will be described. When possible, the mechanisms underlying these changes will be outlined.

A. Water Excretion

A major restriction in renal function in chronic renal disease relates to water excretion. With advancing disease, there is a progressive impairment in the urinary concentrating ability. Whereas in health, the urine may be excreted at an osmolality about four times greater than that of plasma, with progressive renal disease the maximum osmolality approaches that of plasma. If total solute to be excreted in uremia remains at about 600 mOsm/day and the urine osmolality is fixed at slightly over 300 mOsm/kg of water, about 1 liter of water will have to be excreted with every 300 mOsm of solute and obligatory water excretion will approximate 1½–2 liters/day. This restricts the capacity of patients with chronic renal disease to lower water excretion to the levels seen in normal individuals. There is also a restriction on the upper limit of water excretion which can be achieved with a decrease in the nephron population. Although diluting ability, that is, the capacity to lower urine osmolality to 60 mOsm/liter or less, is well preserved in chronic renal disease and free-water generation per 100 ml of GFR is normal or even slightly greater than normal in uremia, the total amount of free water that can be excreted decreases as the nephron population and GFR diminish. For example, if a water diuresis is induced in a normal person and a uremic patient and both excrete 10 ml of free water per 100 ml GFR, urine volume will increase in both, but the increments will be quite different in amounts. In the normal person (GFR = 120 ml/min) 24-hr urine volume will increase from 2 liters of isosmotic urine to 19.3 liters of dilute urine per day. In the uremic patient (GFR = 4 ml/min) the increase will be from 2 to 2.6 liters/day.

The obligatory increased excretion of water in the patient with chronic renal disease may lead to polyuria and result in the development of nocturia, which may be a manifestation of late renal insufficiency. Occasionally, particularly when extra fluids, containing almost exclusively dextrose and water, are administered in an effort "to flush the kidneys," hyponatremia may result owing to the inability of the patient with chronic renal failure to increase appropriately the excretion of water.

B. Sodium Excretion

As renal disease progresses, fractional sodium extretion increases in a manner which is adequate to maintain external balance (see Figure 1). This

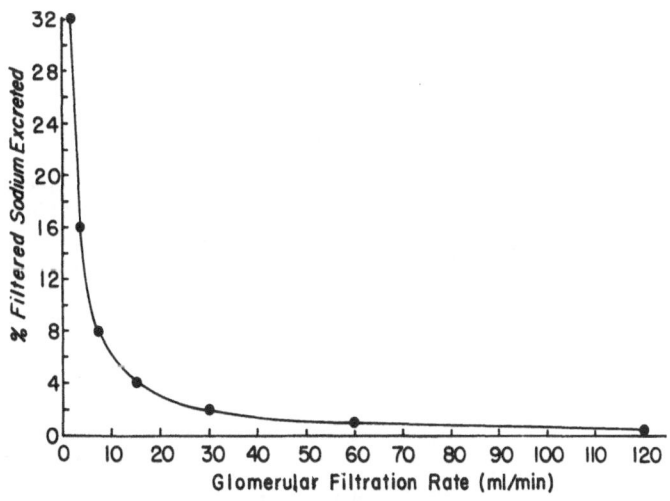

Figure 1. The patterns of sodium excretion, expressed as the percentage of filtered sodium excreted, are shown at different levels of glomerular filtration rate (from 120 to 2 ml/min) in subjects with normal renal function or chronic renal disease ingesting 7.0 g of sodium chloride daily. (Reproduced with permission from Bricker, N.S., Klahr, S., Lubowitz, H., and Slatopolsky, E.: *Pediatr. Clin. North Am.* 18:595, 1971.)

occurs until very late in the course of renal disease so that extracellular fluid volume is preserved. With changes in sodium intake, the fractional excretion of sodium will have to change substantially in the patient with chronic renal failure to maintain sodium balance. For example, in a normal individual doubling the sodium intake from $3\frac{1}{2}$ g/24 hr to 7 g will necessitate only a change in fractional excretion of sodium from 0.25% to 0.5%. The same increment in salt intake may require a change in fractional sodium excretion from 8% to 16% in a patient with a GFR of 4 ml/min (see Figure 2). Hence, the patient with chronic renal disease can vary sodium excretion over a rather restricted range and this range narrows as GFR declines. With chronic renal disease an upper and a lower limit of sodium excretion develops. The lower limit, or "floor," would result in the inability of patients with chronic renal disease to conserve sodium maximally. A patient with renal disease fed a low salt diet is often unable to reduce his sodium output so as to match intake over the usual time scale. He goes into negative sodium balance and excretes a corresponding volume of water. His ECF volume, plasma volume, and GFR all fall. This persistent natriuresis in the face of decreased salt intake has been attributed to the osmotic diuresis in the surviving nephrons which limits the ability of the patient to conserve sodium in response to normal hormonal controls. However, it has recently been shown that if sodium intake is reduced very gradually over weeks or months rather than days, most patients with chronic renal failure can reduce renal sodium excretion below 10 mEq/day without substantial reduction in GFR. About 1% or 2% of patients with early chronic renal failure have a urinary sodium leak which causes sodium depletion even on a normal salt intake. They are mainly individuals who have medullary cystic disease and analgesic nephropathy, but a few have obstructive uropathy, chronic interstitial nephritis, or polycystic kidney disease. They are typically normotensive or hypotensive at

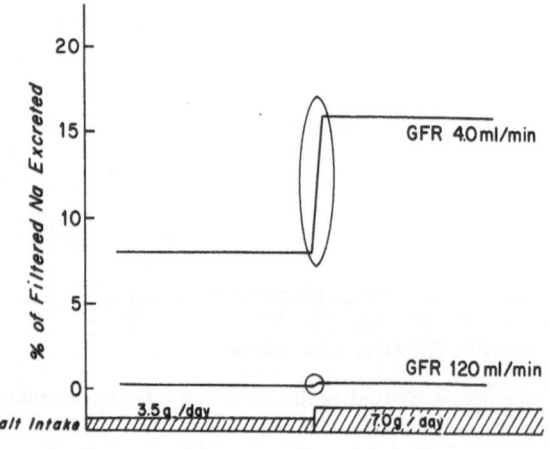

Figure 2. The patterns of sodium excretion, expressed as the percentage of filtered sodium excreted, are shown at a normal GFR (120 ml/min) and at a reduced GFR (4 ml/min). Notice that the baseline fractional excretion of sodium, necessary to maintain sodium balance, when ingesting either a 3.5-g or a 7.0-g salt diet, differs at the two levels of GFR. Notice also the marked change in fractional sodium excretion (from 8% to 16%), required to maintain sodium balance, in the case of a patient with a GFR of 4 ml/min, when dietary sodium intake is increased from 3.5 to 7.0 g/day. (Reproduced with permission from Bricker, N. S., Klahr, S., Lubowitz, H., and Slatopolsky, E.: *Pediatr. Clin. North Am.* 18:595, 1971.)

rest or have postural hypotension when sodium depleted. Sodium retention is a more common problem than sodium depletion in chronic renal failure. It may occur early in the course of chronic progressive renal disease when the nephrotic syndrome is present. Also in far advanced chronic renal disease, if some degree of salt restriction is not introduced, salt retention may occur resulting in increased positive sodium balance, expansion of the extracellular fluid volume and plasma volume, and sometimes an increase in GFR. However, congestive heart failure, increases in blood pressure, etc. may result as a consequence of volume overload.

C. Potassium Excretion

As discussed in Chapter 7, 90%–95% of ingested potassium is excreted via renal mechanisms with the remainder being excreted in the stool. In chronic renal failure a greater fraction of ingested potassium is excreted in the stool with 20%–50% of the ingested amount appearing in the stool when the GFR falls below 5 ml/min. In chronic renal failure increased potassium excretion per nephron also occurs and potassium excretion approaches and may even surpass filtered load of potassium. In chronic renal failure, therefore, these adjustments in renal mechanisms which increase potassium excretion plus the increased stool excretion of potassium are enough to maintain a normal plasma and potassium balance until the glomerular filtration rate reaches less than 10 ml/min, even on a normal intake of potassium (100 mEq/day). In contrast to sodium, potassium excretion depends upon tubular secretion to maintain balance. In health, aldosterone as well as other factors are the major mediators of potassium secretion in the distal tubule (see Chapter 7). In chronic renal failure, aldosterone and increased flow through the distal tubule may be important factors increasing potassium excretion per nephron. Enzymatic adaptations of Na–K-ATPase in the distal nephron may also underlie the increased capacity of the remnant nephrons to increase potassium excretion. Plasma potassium may rise in chronic renal disease as acidosis becomes progressive owing to redistribution of potassium between intracellular and extracellular compartments. Intracellular potassium will leave the cells and will be replaced by hydrogen and sodium. In addition, hormonal deficiencies such as lack of aldosterone or low aldosterone levels in hyporeninemic patients may result in hyperkalemia earlier in the course of renal insufficiency. Patients with diabetes, because of lack of insulin, may also develop hyperkalemia earlier in the course of chronic renal disease (see Chapter 7).

The maintenance of normal renal potassium excretion with a decreased number of functioning nephrons is dependent upon a large increase in the distal tubular capacity to secrete potassium. At very low rates of GFR, the secretory rate of potassium may be near maximal to maintain the steady state. Thus, very little functional reserve remains to respond to sudden changes in potassium intake. Situations such as oliguria, sudden increases in potassium intake, sudden metabolic acidosis, or catabolic states may result in life-threatening hyperkalemia in patients with far-advanced renal insufficiency.

Despite the tendency for hyperkalemia in far-advanced chronic renal failure, total body potassium may in fact be decreased. This apparent paradox is related to the fact that the vast majority of potassium in the body is located intracellularly. Decreased intake, increased catabolism, and decreased exchange of sodium for potassium in advanced uremia may lead to increased levels of intracellular sodium, decreased intracellular potassium, and hence some degree of potassium depletion despite an elevation in extracellular fluid potassium. Occasionally, hypokalemia may occur in patients with chronic renal failure. This usually signifies extreme total body potassium deficits, and alkalosis may be a coexistent abnormality.

D. Acid–Base Balance

The contribution of the kidneys to the preservation of acid–base balance in normal man requires the reabsorption of the daily filtered load of approximately 4000 mEq of bicarbonate and the excretion of 50–100 mEq of hydrogen ions in the form of ammonium and titratable acid (H^+ bound to phosphate and other buffer ions). As with many other nephron functions, there are remarkable compensatory responses in acid–base regulation by the residual functioning kidney mass as overall renal function declines. Except for a small group of patients with hyperchloremic acidosis, most subjects with renal disease do not show significant acidemia attributable to renal disease per se until GFR falls below roughly 20% of normal. Plasma bicarbonate concentration may be depressed at high levels of GFR but blood pH level remains normal or is only barely depressed due to ventilatory compensation. Even when GFR falls below 20 ml/min the extent of acidosis is highly variable. Causes of this variability include the nature of the intrinsic renal disease, diet, intake of acidic ion salts, extracellular volume status, potassium balance, and efficiency of respiratory compensation.

Hydrogen ion excretion is impaired in two ways in chronic renal failure. There is diminished capacity to excrete ammonia and a tendency to leak bicarbonate when the plasma bicarbonate level is restored to normal by infusion of bicarbonate. When bicarbonate infusion is stopped, renal excretion of bicarbonate continues until plasma bicarbonate falls back to its previous level. This resetting of the plasma level at which a bicarbonate leak occurs is also encountered in primary hyperparathyroidism. In chronic renal failure this resetting in bicarbonate reabsorption may be partly due to secondary hyperparathyroidism. As renal failure progresses, urine becomes more acid, eventually reaching a pH of about 5, close to the minimum achieved by normal subjects after acid loading. However, this does not imply normal urinary acidification since the patient with chronic renal disease achieves this urine pH at a much lower plasma bicarbonate level than the normal subject. Although ammonia excretion per residual nephron increases, total urinary ammonia excretion is lower than normal for the urinary pH. Titratable acid, on the other hand, is normal or only slightly reduced because the main buffers (phosphate and creatinine) are excreted in nearly normal amounts in the urine until very late in the course of renal disease (see Figure 3). Respiratory compensation for the acidosis occurs in a predictable manner. If there is no lung disease, the uremic subjects have a fall in P_{CO_2} of about 1.2 mm Hg for every 1.0-mEq fall in plasma bicarbonate. This does not completely correct blood pH, which falls in a roughly linear relationship to

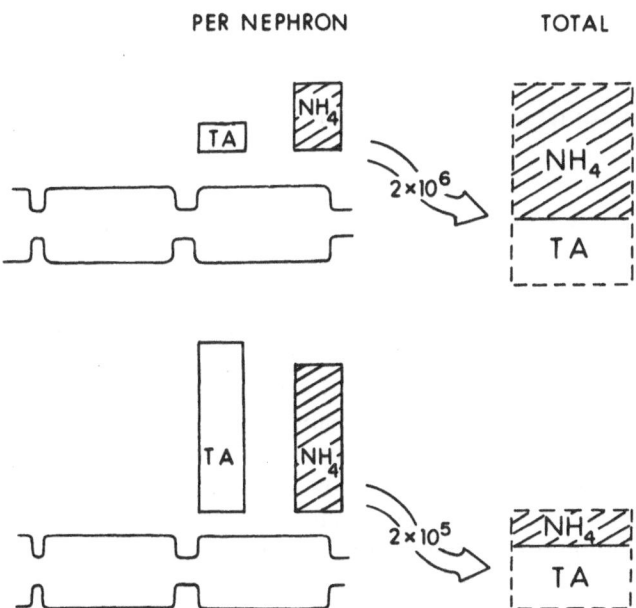

Figure 3. Excretion of titratable acid (TA) and ammonium (NH₄) by a representative nephron when the total complement of nephrons is normal (2×10^6) and when the total nephron population is decreased to 10% of normal (2×10^5). Notice that there is an increase in the excretion of titratable acid and ammonium per nephron as renal mass decreases. However, the increment in ammonium excretion per nephron is limited and the total excretion of ammonium in chronic renal disease is lower than in health. On the other hand, the excretion of titratable acid remains within normal levels until very late in the course of renal disease. Notice also that about two thirds of total acid excretion is accounted for by ammonium in health. However, the percent contribution of titratable acid to total acid excretion increases as renal disease progresses. The decrease in total ammonium excretion in chronic renal disease leads to positive hydrogen ion balance and the development of metabolic acidosis. (Reproduced with permission from Bricker, N. S., and Fine, L. G., in Maxwell M. H., and Kleeman, C. R. (eds.): *Clinical Disorders of Fluid and Electrolyte Metabolism,* Third edition. McGraw-Hill, New York, 1980, pp. 799–825.)

the plasma bicarbonate, reaching the lower limit of normal, 7.35, when the plasma bicarbonate is about 15 mEq/liter. In terminal renal failure plasma bicarbonate falls below 10 mEq/liter and there is deep sigh respiration which produces a low Pa_{CO_2} but blood pH is well below the normal range. A progressive fall in plasma bicarbonate below 15 mEq/liter does not occur in far-advanced renal insufficiency until GFR values are quite low, presumably because buffers such as carbonate of bone are then being utilized in buffering the hydrogen retention (positive H^+ balance) that occurs in patients with renal insufficiency. Two types of acidosis have been observed in chronic renal disease. One is characterized by hyperchloremic acidosis (normal gap acidosis) and occurs relatively early in the course of renal insufficiency in entities characterized mainly by tubulointerstitial involvement. Under most conditions, in the garden variety of patients with renal disease, there is an increase in the anion gap during the development of metabolic acidosis which is due to the accumulation of phosphate, sulfate, and other anions usually not measured during routine laboratory determinations (see Chapter 8). The development of acidosis, which will become severe as renal disease advances, may contribute to some of the abnormalities of uremia.

E. Magnesium

Most patients in chronic renal failure have normal or moderately elevated serum magnesium levels which seldom cause symptoms. Serum magnesium rises further in response to acidosis, tissue trauma, and the administration of vitamin D and its analogs. Only in patients receiving occasional enemas or antacids containing magnesium are there marked increases in serum magnesium levels which can lead to drowsiness, muscle weakness, and skin irritation. In patients with higher levels of magnesium dramatic symptoms may occur leading to muscle paralysis and respiratory failure (see also Chapter 9).

F. Phosphate and Calcium

Phosphate excretion changes little as GFR falls since there is a progressive decrease in tubular reabsorption of phosphate which is mediated mainly by an increase in the excretion of parathyroid hormone (Figure 4). However, when GFR falls below 30 ml/min, even a marked decrease in the reabsorption of phosphate is not enough to overcome the marked decrease in the filtered load and phosphate accumulation occurs. Hyperphosphatemia, therefore, is seen commonly on an unrestricted diet in patients with GFRs of 25 ml/min or less. It is also at this level of GFR that changes in serum calcium occur.

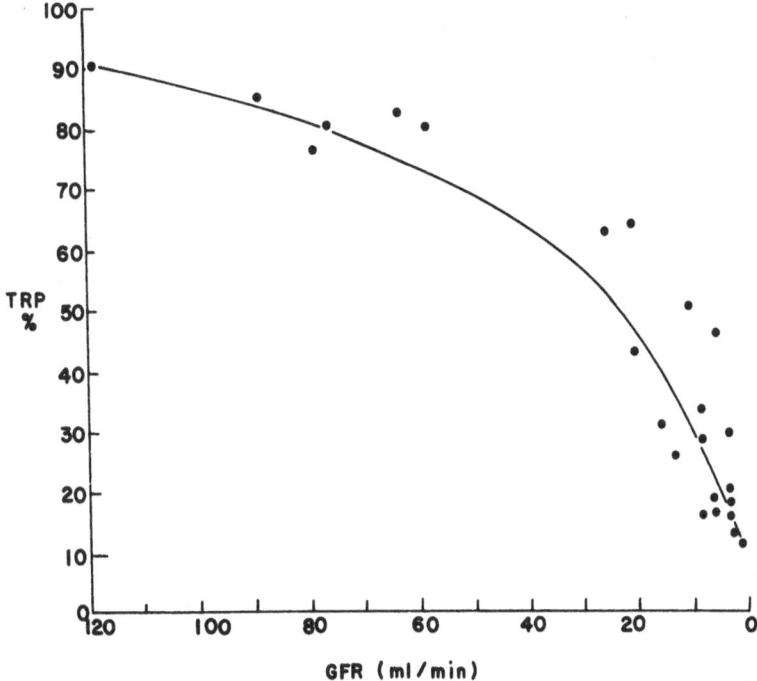

Figure 4. Tubular reabsorption of phosphate (TRP) is shown at different levels of glomerular filtration rate (GFR). Notice that TRP values are 90% at a GFR of 120 ml/min, indicating a fractional excretion of phosphate of 10%, and decrease to very low values as GFR decreases. The decrease in TRP values (or increase in the fractional excretion of phosphate) is mainly mediated by increased levels of circulating parathyroid hormone. (Reproduced with permission from Slatopolsky, E., Robson, A. M., Elkan, I., and Bricker, N. S.: *J. Clin. Invest.* 47:1864, 1968.)

These changes in calcium concentration presumably are related to several factors. The increase in serum phosphate produces a reciprocal decrease in serum-ionized calcium. There is also evidence that the levels of 1,25-dihydroxy D_3 fall at GFRs below 30 ml/min and the decreased production of $1,25(OH)_2D_3$ may result in decreased absorption of calcium from the gastrointestinal tract, a phenomenon that has been documented in patients with this level of GFR. The ability of parathyroid hormone to remove calcium from bone may be impaired and this "skeletal resistance" to the action of the hormone may also contribute to the development of hypocalcemia. It should be remembered that acidosis tends to increase the fraction of total calcium which is in the ionized form and thus prevents some of the clinical consequences of hypercalcemia (see Chapter 9). Rapid correction of acidosis leading to an elevation of plasma bicarbonate and pH may decrease suddenly the levels of ionized calcium and precipitate acute manifestations of hypocalcemia, including tetany and convulsions in patients with chronic renal disease.

III. SYSTEMIC INVOLVEMENT IN CHRONIC RENAL DISEASE

A. Hematological Disorders

1. Anemia

Perhaps the most consistent finding in chronic renal failure is anemia (see Table I). As the GFR falls below 40 ml/min the hematocrit decreases in proportion to the degree of renal insufficiency until a hematocrit of approximately 20% is reached with end stage renal failure. The primary event underlying the anemia is the absence of erythropoietin. As discussed in Chapter 3, erythropoietin is normally produced by the renal juxtaglomerular apparatus. As renal mass decreases, erythropoietin secretory capacity falls leading to decreased red cell production by the marrow. As end stage renal failure is reached, a mechanism other than renal erythropoietin apparently stimulates the marrow and a hematocrit of approximately 15%–20% is maintained, even in the anephric state.

Additional factors underlying the anemia of chronic renal failure include an increased rate of hemolysis, causing a decreased red cell life span. This is an extrinsic red cell defect and can be corrected by providing a nonuremic environment for the individual's red cells. In addition, uremia depresses the ability of the bone marrow to respond to erythropoietin, and thus even with a hypoxic stimulus and erythropoietin production, the marrow response is not normal. Finally, gastrointestinal blood loss is a common problem in individuals with chronic renal failure. The continued loss of blood from the gastrointestinal tract leads to iron deficiency, which is an additional factor predisposing to anemia in chronic renal failure. Neither vitamin B_{12} nor folic acid appear to be involved in the anemia of chronic renal failure unless an inordinately high rate of hemolysis results in relative folate deficiency.

2. Coagulation Abnormalities

Individuals with chronic renal failure have a qualitative defect in platelet function. This is manifest as a prolonged bleeding time although the partial thromboplastin time, prothrombin time, and clotting time are all within normal limits. The serum concentrations of the various proteins of the coagulation cascade are usually within normal limits unless the patient has the nephrotic syndrome in addition to chronic renal failure.

The factors in uremic serum which induce the qualitative platelet defect have been investigated. Guanidinosuccinic acid and hydroxyphenolacetic acid inhibit platelet function when present in concentrations normally found in uremic serum. Both of these compounds are dialyzable and their removal from uremic plasma corrects the qualitative platelet defect.

Table I. Features of the Uremic Syndrome

I. Neuropsychiatric features
  A. Psychiatric symptoms
    1. Impaired concentration
    2. Decreased ability for abstract thinking
    3. Agitation, restlessness, insomnia
    4. Depression–anxiety
    5. Psychosis (rare)
  B. Neurologic symptoms
    1. Fatigue
    2. Muscular irritability
    3. Headache
    4. Seizures
    5. Coma
  C. Peripheral nerve disturbances
    1. Peripheral nerves–ascending polyneuropathy
    2. Autonomic nerves
      a. Postural hypotension
      b. Neurogenic bladder
      c. Impotence
II. Cardiovascular features
  A. Volume overload, congestive heart failure
  B. Hypertension
  C. Pericarditis
  D. Accelerated atherosclerotic disease?
III. Gastrointestinal features
  A. Nausea, vomiting, anorexia
  B. Diarrhea
  C. Hiccoughs
  D. Abdominal pain
  E. Pancreatitis
  F. Melena
  G. Uremic colitis
  H. Oral and pharyngeal ulcers
IV. Failure of renal excretion
  A. Sodium retention
  B. Water retention
  C. Hyperkalemia
  D. Metabolic acidosis
  E. Hyperphosphatemia, hypocalcemia, hypermagnesemia
  F. Retention of nitrogenous waste products (see Table II)
V. Pulmonary features
  A. Pleuritis
  B. "Uremic pneumonitis"
VI. Dermatologic features
  A. Pruritis
  B. Uremic frost
  C. Darkening of pigmentation
VII. Hematologic
  A. Anemia
  B. Coagulation abnormalities
VIII. Skeletal
  A. Bone pain
  B. Spontaneous fractures
  C. Necrosis of femoral heads

B. Cardiopulmonary Complications

The cardiovascular system may be affected through the intervention of diastolic hypertension. The combination of hypertension, anemia, fluid overload, and acidosis all contribute to the increased propensity for congestive heart failure. Pericarditis, an inflammation of the serosal membranes covering the heart, occurs in approximately half of undialyzed patients with chronic renal disease who develop terminal uremia. Pericarditis is a complication of very-late-stage chronic renal failure. Prior to the availability of dialytical or transplantation therapy, pericarditis was a common event in the several days prior to death from uremia. The pathogenesis is not understood. However, correction of the uremic environment by dialytic therapy is usually effective in reversing the clinical manifestations of pericarditis. In certain individuals, the process may not be reversed by correction of uremia and pericardiectomy may be required to prevent cardiac tamponade.

Uremic pneumonitis has been suggested as a diagnosis for an entity which is seen in certain patients with late stage chronic failure and characteristic radiographic appearance of perihilar vascular congestion with clear peripheral lung fields. Several authors have suggested that this characteristic appearance occurs in uremic patients in the absence of circulatory overload. The concept of uremic pneumonitis has not gained wide acceptance and instead probably relates to circulatory overload in these individuals.

In comparison to the general population, uremic patients have a higher death rate due to cardiovascular disease and die at a younger age. Increased risk factors in the chronic uremic group include hypertension, hyperparathyroidism with vascular calcification, carbohydrate intolerance, hypertriglyceridemia, and hyperuricemia. Hyperkalemia, sufficient to cause cardiac disturbances, may occur in end stage chronic renal failure.

C. Hypertension

Over 50% of patients with end stage renal failure have hypertension. The mechanisms by which end stage renal disease causes an elevation of blood pressure are probably multiple. The kidney may release increased quantities of substances such as renin leading to the production of pressor substances (angiotensin) which cause peripheral vasoconstriction leading to hypertension. On the other hand, the diseased kidney may fail to produce substances that are vasodepressors and as such may play a role in lowering blood pressure. Prostaglandins and a neutral lipid produced in the kidney have been postulated to play such a role. In addition, the diseased kidney may have a relative inability to excrete salt as renal disease advances. Consequently, extracellular fluid volume may be expanded and this may lead to the development of a volume-dependent type of hypertension. In the treatment of hypertension in patients with renal failure, which has not reached end stage, there are two important considerations. The first is that hypertension should be adequately controlled because if left unchecked it will produce additional renal damage on the basis of progressive nephrosclerosis. The second consideration relates to the possibility of producing excessive sodium depletion during the treatment of hypertension in patients with renal disease. This may accelerate the decrement in glomerular filtration rate and augment the manifestations of the uremic syndrome. Under these conditions, prerenal acute renal failure may be superimposed on the picture of chronic renal failure.

D. Neurological–Muscular Abnormalities

The central nervous system and peripheral nerves are affected with diverse consequences. Nerve conduction time characteristically is prolonged, peripheral neuropathy may develop in advanced uremia, sleep patterns are disturbed, and asterixis, convulsions, and psychosis all may occur. The early changes of uremic encephalopathy are subtle. They consist of insomnia, inability to concentrate, lack of alertness, and slowing of cerebration. Ultimately, there may be loss of memory, confusion, hallucinations, and delirium or obtundation. Convulsions may occur in about 1/30 untreated patients nearing terminal uremia. The electroencephalographic changes seen in uremia ("slow wave pattern") may be related to increased brain calcium, which in turn may be caused by high levels of circulating parathyroid hormone. The changes in the electroencephalogram usually improve with adequate dialysis.

Muscle weakness and muscle irritability are characteristic of the late stages of chronic renal failure. The former is apparently related to a deficiency of 1,25-dihydroxy D_3 (see Chapter 3). It has been found that supplementation of this vitamin to patients with chronic renal failure improves muscle strength remarkably. Muscle irritability is apparently related to derangements in the composition of the extracellular and intracellular fluids. Transmembrane potential across muscle membranes is decreased in uremia. This is presumably related to decreased extrusion of sodium which results in increased sodium and decreased potassium concentrations in the intracellular fluid of muscles. Dialytic therapy and/or correction of the uremic environment by transplantation reverses the changes in transmembrane potential and muscle irritability.

E. Gastrointestinal Disturbances

Gastrointestinal symptoms attributable to chronic renal failure generally are not manifest until the GFR falls below 10 ml/min. In this range, early symptoms include anorexia, nausea, and vomiting. The latter two symptoms are most prominent in the early morning when vomiting may be a daily event. Early morning vomiting may be expected to alleviate further nausea during the day when appetite improves allowing adequate oral intake. Other symptoms and signs of gastrointestinal disturbances are presented in Table I.

It has long been felt that peptic ulcer disease is common in patients with chronic renal failure. Several studies have shown that gastric acid secretion is depressed in 40% of patients with chronic renal failure, while the other 60% have normal gastric acid secretion. Plasma gastrin values increase progressively with renal failure. This may represent small polypeptides with gastrinlike antigen structure accumulating in plasma because of the inability of the diseased kidney to metabolize low-molecular-weight proteins (see Chapter 3). Alternatively, it is possible that the increase in plasma gastrin levels represents a true increase in hormonal activity.

Gastrointestinal bleeding is very common in chronic renal failure, as previously mentioned. The bleeding may occur at any site from the stomach through the rectum. The most commonly noticed lesions are shallow small ulcers that bleed slowly. Occasionally, one of the ulcers will erode a small artery and lead to massive bleeding, but this is unusual. The pathogenesis of these ulcers is not understood. At least part of the problem seems to be due to the platelet defect associated with chronic uremia.

Pancreatitis and atrophic gastritis may occur in the late stages of severe chronic renal failure but this is unusual. Gastrointestinal-related hormones such as cholecystokinin, gastric inhibitory polypeptide, and glucagon all are elevated in the serum of patients with chronic renal failure. These elevations may be due to failure of the diseased kidney to metabolize these hormones or their fragments. Elevations in the plasma levels of hormones measured by radioimmunoassay may represent the accumulation of biologically inactive hormone or its fragments, or it may represent actual elevation of the metabolically active hormone.

F. Immunologic and Infectious Complications

Infection is a common cause of death in both acute renal failure and the terminal stages of chronic renal failure. In patients not receiving dialysis or transplantation, pulmonary infections are responsible for 50% of the deaths of end stage chronic renal patients. Most such infections are due to gram-positive organisms. An additional significant fraction of patients with late stage renal failure die of sepsis secondary to coliform bacilli. There does not appear to be an increased incidence of clinically significant infections or their consequences in chronic renal failure until the GFR falls to 5–10 ml/min.

A variety of factors have been implicated in the impaired ability of patients with terminal renal failure to cope with infections. The granulocytic leukocyte counts are usually normal in late stage renal failure although these patients do have an absolute lymphopenia. Total serum γ-globulin concentrations and complement concentrations are generally normal unless the patient has one of the forms of glomerulonephritis or nephrotic syndrome which are associated with low complement or low γ-globulin levels. Antibody responses to certain antigens (tetanus, diphtheria) are normal, whereas the response to certain other antigens (typhoid O, typhoid H, influenza) are clearly diminished. Delayed hypersensitivity reactions are subnormal in uremic patients. The few studies done regarding reticuloendothelial function in uremia have demonstrated slow clearance of particulate matter from the blood.

In vitro tests of lymphocytes from uremic patients have demonstrated that the mixed lymphocyte culture, stimulation by phytohemaglutanin, and stimulation by polk weed mitogen are all within normal limits. In contrast, normal lymphocytes are significantly inhibited by the presence of uremic plasma in regard to the response for the mixed-lymphocyte culture, phyto-hemaglutanin, and the phagocytic capacity of cultured monocytes.

As a general rule, diminished cellular immunity has been associated with a predisposition to viral and fungal diseases. This has not been observed in patients with chronic renal failure. In contrast, patients with defects in humoral immunity and phagocytic capacity are expected to have severe impairment in the ability to cope with bacterial infections. Uremics as a group have been demonstrated to have impaired antibody responses, opsonic activity, and *in vitro* phagocytic capacity. Thus, the susceptibility of patients with end stage uremia to bacterial infection may be explained by information presently available.

G. Renal Osteodystrophy

1. Hyperphosphatemia, Hypocalcemia, and Secondary Hyperparathyroidism

As renal mass decreases, phosphate excretion decreases resulting in an elevation of serum phosphate levels which, in turn, decrease ionized serum calcium. The latter stimulates the parathyroid glands to secrete more parathyroid hormone, which acts on the renal tubular cells to decrease phosphate reabsorption. When GFR falls below 25% of normal, evidence of this secondary hyperparathyroidism may become evident. The elevated levels of parathyroid hormone, a consequence of both increased secretion and decreased degradation, lead to increased bone resorption, and reduced bone density may be found on X-ray examination (see Chapter 9). Also, when renal functional mass is decreased to less than 25%, there is decreased conversion of the 25-hydroxy vitamin D to a more active form, 1,25-dihydroxy vitamin D. This results in decreased intestinal absorption of calcium and potentially in osteomalacia. Metabolic acidosis, the result of decreased renal excretion of hydrogen, also contributes to bone disease (Figure 5).

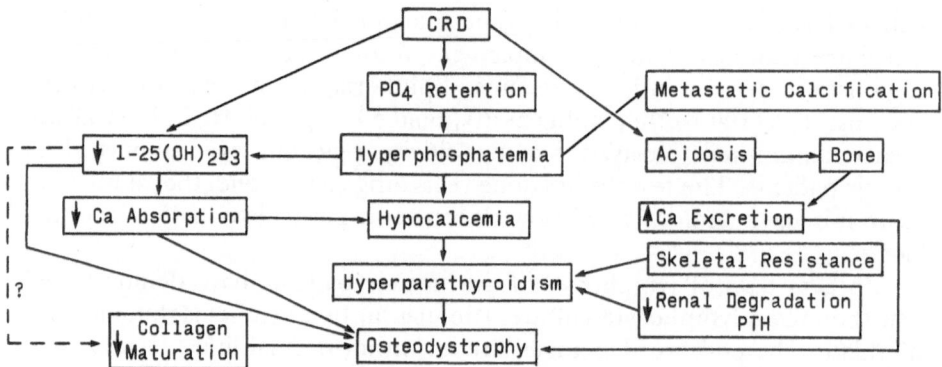

Figure 5. Pathogenesis of osteodystrophy in patients with chronic renal disease (CRD). The retention of phosphate leads to hyperphosphatemia and a decrease in serum calcium levels (hypocalcemia). The hyperphosphatemia may also decrease the levels of circulating $1,25(OH)_2$ vitamin D_3 by an effect on the renal 1-α-hydroxylase enzyme. The fall in the levels of $1,25(OH)_2$ vitamin D_3 results in decreased gastrointestinal calcium absorption which contributes to the hypocalcemia. The fall in serum calcium leads to increased secretion of parathyroid hormone (hyperparathyroidism). The levels of the hormone also increase as the consequence of decreased degradation by the kidney, as renal mass decreases, and skeletal resistance. The acidosis of CRD promotes the removal of calcium carbonate from bone and contributes to the osteodystrophy. Parathyroid hormone results in bone changes (osteitis fibrosa cystica). A negative calcium balance may result in osteomalacia. (Reproduced with permission from Slatopolsky, E.: *Kidney Int.* 7:S253, 1975.)

2. Osteodystrophy and Abnormal Calcification

Renal osteodystrophy includes osteitis fibrosa, osteomalacia, osteosclerosis, and osteoporosis. Secondary hyperparathyroidism results in the development of osteitis fibrosa cystica, which may present radiographically as subperiosteal bone resorption. Such lesions are most frequently seen in the middle phalanges of the hand, distal end of the clavicles, and proximal ends of the tibia. Histology of the bone reveals osteoclastic resorption with fibrosis. Elevated serum levels of alkaline phosphatase are commonly seen.

Osteomalacia is a disorder of bone in which the mineralization process of the organic bone matrix is impaired. The major symptoms of osteomalacia are diffuse bone and muscle pains, which cause disability and increasing needs for analgesic medication. Osteomalacia may be due to low serum levels of calcium and phosphorus or to a defect in mineralization related in some way to abnormalities in the organic matrix of bone. Osteomalacia accounts for a portion of the bone disease seen in uremic individuals and is responsible for a higher morbidity in patients undergoing hemodialysis.

Osteosclerosis, an increase in the density of bone, is a less common form of renal osteodystrophy. The etiology of this bone disorder is poorly defined.

Osteoporosis is also a disabling form of bone disease in the patient with uremia. The exact mechanisms responsible for the development of osteoporosis in chronic renal failure have not been elucidated adequately.

These bone changes can have devastating effects upon patients. In children there may be retardation of growth. In the adult, bone pain, fractures, collapse of vertebrae, necrosis of femoral heads, and skeletal deformities may occur. Along with osteitis fibrosa, there are metastatic calcifications, medial calcification of arteries with ischemic necrosis, calcification of soft tissues and skin with intractable pruritus, periarthritis from calcium hydroxyapatite precipitation, and conjunctival calcification.

H. Nutritional and Metabolic Alterations

1. Disorders of Nitrogen Metabolism

The metabolism of nitrogenous substances is of importance in chronic renal failure for several reasons. The empirical observation that many uremic symptoms are markedly reduced when dietary protein intake is limited implies that uremic toxins are either nitrogenous-containing solutes or derivatives of such solutes. Second, the occurrence of protein malnutrition in advanced uremia and persistence of this disorder in some patients on long-term dialysis has stimulated the study of nitrogen, amino acid, and protein metabolism in chronic renal failure. Protein malnutrition of severe degree is less common today than a decade ago when dialysis facilities were in short supply. A combination of inadequate caloric intake due to anorexia and prescription of a rigid reduction of protein intake over many months yielded patients with marked wasting. Patients were often 15%–30% below their customary weight during the early phase of dialysis after edema fluid had been removed. The nutritional status of patients with end stage renal disease and those on dialysis has no doubt been greatly improved in recent years because of early initiation of dialysis and better application of nutritional knowledge. There are a number of observations that indicate that a lesser but still significant degree of protein malnutrition may still be prevalent. Extravascular pools of albumin may be reduced, though serum albumin concentration is normal. Serum concentration of transferrin, possibly a more sensitive indicator of protein malnutrition, has been found to be low in many patients with moderate to advanced renal failure and was also subnormal in a group of patients on chronic dialysis despite ingestion of 1 g of protein per kg/day. Although inadequate protein or caloric intake or both may well be the major cause of malnutrition in chronic renal failure, the possibility that one or more steps in the complex process of protein synthesis is disturbed by renal failure per se has not received sufficient study. This possibility is supported by the finding of reduced alkali soluble protein in muscle from patients with only moderate renal failure.

2. Energy Turnover

A gradual onset of anorexia in chronic renal failure leads to inadequate intake of calories. In adults, this change leads to loss of caloric stores, consumption of body proteins, and diversion of dietary proteins for use as fuel. In children, a caloric deficit, in addition, contributes to impaired growth. Although few measurements have been made, it is a general clinical observation that both mental and physical activity progressively decline in advancing uremia and remain impaired in some patients on dialysis. There has been some success in improving caloric intake, especially by patients on long-term hemodialysis. There is, unfortunately, little information on energy turnover at the cellular level in chronic renal failure. Adenosine triphosphate levels are elevated in erythrocytes, whereas phosphorylating activity and ATPase activity may be reduced suggesting decreased energy turnover.

3. Disorders of Carbohydrate Metabolism

Carbohydrate tolerance is impaired in uremia. This is evident after oral or intravenous glucose loads. Several factors may be involved. Skeletal muscle shows resistance to the action of insulin on glucose uptake. Increased growth hormone levels in uremia may also contribute to the resistance of peripheral tissues to insulin. There is elevation of basal insulin levels presumably as a consequence of a decreased rate of renal degradation of insulin. The levels of glucagon are also increased and remain elevated as compared to controls even after a glucose load. Of interest is the fact that diabetic patients who develop progressive renal disease require diminishing doses of insulin as the disease progresses. Reduced caloric intake and weight loss plus a reduced degradation of insulin probably play a role in this decreased insulin requirement of diabetics with progressive renal disease.

4. Disorders of Lipid Metabolism

Uremic patients have hypertriglyceredemia and hyperlipoproteinemia. There is decreased rate of removal of triglycerides from the plasma as well as decreased activity of lipoprotein lipase and increased hepatic synthesis of very-low-density lipoproteins. There are also decreased plasma levels of high-density α-migrating lipoprotein and low-density cholesterol-rich lipoprotein. Plasma cholesterol levels are usually normal in uremia. It has been postulated, but not proven, that in renal failure these abnormalities of carbohydrate and lipid metabolism contribute to increased risk of accelerated atherogenesis that may be so troublesome in patients on chronic dialysis.

5. Vitamins

There is only limited information concerning vitamin nutrition in end stage renal disease. Evaluation of published reports is complicated by the frequent omission of information on precise dietary intake of protein, on use of vitamin supplements, the time of sampling in relation to dialysis treatment, and on intake of drugs that potentially may affect vitamin metabolism. Reduced concentrations in serum and/or in erythrocytes and leukocytes have been reported for a number of water-soluble vitamins. Hematologic evidence of folate deficiency has been found at several centers but not others. These differences probably reflect variations in dietary intake and use of vitamin supplements. In one report patients who were not receiving vitamin supplements had low plasma and leukocyte concentrations of vitamin C, and a few patients had signs suggestive of mild scurvy. The plasma concentrations of other water-soluble vitamins were normal in most reports. Since the kidney is one route of elimination of water-soluble vitamins and their metabolites, decreased elimination by the kidney may be a protective mechanism, especially for patients on hemodialysis in whom removal of water-soluble vitamins may occur during the procedure.

6. Trace Elements

The possible existence of deficiency of essential trace elements and of toxic accumulation of essential or nonessential trace elements has been suggested in end stage renal disease. The kidney is the major route of elimination for elements such as fluoride, bromide, and cobalt. Highly protein-bound elements, such as copper and zinc, are lost in excessive amounts with heavy proteinuria. Present available information on trace element metabolism comes from only a few geographical areas and is fragmentary. Most of the work on trace elements has been done in patients on dialysis and the information is even more limited in patients with end stage renal disease before the initiation of dialytic therapy.

I. Endocrine Alterations

Uremia alters virtually all hormones in the body either in the amount present or in their effect. Not only are hormones arising within the kidney affected by renal failure but so are also those being produced elsewhere. There are decreased levels of erythropoietin with consequent anemia. There is increased renal renin activity with increased plasma levels of angiotensin and resultant hypertension. There is decreased renal production of 1,25-dihydroxy D_3 leading to decreased intestinal calcium absorption. There is hypertrophy of the parathyroid glands and elevation of serum PTH levels. There is decreased degradation of this hormone by the kidney leading to its elevation. There is resistance to the action of antidiuretic hormone in the kidney and inability to concentrate the urine and to conserve water to the same extent as in normal individuals. Although uremic patients clinically do not have thyroid abnormalities, several tests of thyroid function are abnormal and a substantial number of chronic renal failure patients have goiters that are possibly the result of increased thyroid-stimulating hormone (TSH) levels. Uremic patients have elevated plasma calcitonin levels as determined by radioimmunoassay, probably as a result of decreased rate of metabolic clearance by the kidney. Elevated levels of gastrin, glucagon, growth hormone, and basal insulin are also present in end stage renal failure patients. The role of these abnormalities on the carbohydrate intolerance of uremia has not been adequately clarified (see page 482). It has been suggested that hypersecretion of aldosterone in advanced chronic renal failure by increasing distal tubular secretion of potassium is necessary to prevent lethal hyperkalemia.

Gonadal dysfunction is characteristic of late stage chronic renal failure. Menstrual irregularities are very frequent and menstruation may cease completely in late stage renal failure. With glomerular filtration rates below 20 ml/min, both conception and the ability to complete a pregnancy are severely impaired. Impotence and a diminished sperm count are expected in a major fraction of men with chronic renal failure.

These abnormalities in both men and women are secondary to gonadal resistance to the effects of follicle-stimulating hormone and luteinizing hormone. Men have diminished concentrations of testosterone in their plasma, and both progesterone and estrogen are diminished in women with chronic renal failure. In men, administration of testosterone has been shown to suppress plasma luteinizing hormone, although with a slightly delayed response. Thus, the individual with chronic renal failure has gonadal resistance to the effects of pituitary trophic hormones as the major lesion causing sexual inadequacy.

IV. THE UREMIC SYNDROME: DESCRIPTION OF PATHOGENESIS

Uremia is a term used to describe the symptomatic phase of chronic renal failure. As noted in a previous section, most symptoms attributable to decreased renal function begin after the GFR falls below 20 ml/min and become more disabling at GFR values below 10 ml/min. A tabulation of the various symptoms of uremia are presented in Table I; many of these are described in a previous section. Obviously, there is multisystem involvement in uremia. Most frequently, patients complain initially of gastrointestinal disorders including anorexia, nausea, and vomiting. However, it should be stressed that the hallmark of uremia is central nervous system dysfunction. Nondietary therapeutic intervention in uremia is most frequently instituted on a permanent basis to treat altered gastrointestinal and/or central nervous system function. When symptoms involving other organ systems occur in the absence of central nervous system symptoms, a search for complicating factors not related to uremia should be instituted.

The pathogenesis of the uremic syndrome has been the subject of intense study. It has been variously attributed to retention of nitrogenous waste products, excessive accumulation of several peptide hormones as a consequence of the loss of renal function or as a compensatory mechanism ("trade-off hypothesis"), and to deficiencies of essential compounds not produced in uremia.

A. Uremic Toxins

Over the past 150 years, numerous studies have attempted to identify substances that accumulate in end stage renal failure and ultimately reach levels that are toxic to vital functions. The increasing availability of dialysis during the past ten years has accelerated such efforts. The yield to date has been disappointingly limited. A number of approaches have been used to uncover such toxins. As better analytical methods became available for measuring specific organic compounds or classes of compounds, the concentration of such materials has been determined in body fluids and tissues. A vast number of compounds have been found to accumulate in renal failure (see Table II). Whole uremic serum, ultrafiltrates of serum, dialysate, or suspected toxins have been used in an attempt to produce in various test systems or in humans or animals symptoms, clinical findings, or functional disturbances resembling those seen in chronic renal failure. Most of the studies have yielded only disappointing results. In terms of specific chemical–clinical correlations, critical appraisal leaves us with few established "toxins" other than water, potassium, sodium, hydrogen ion, calcium, and mangesium.

B. Accumulation of Peptide Hormones

More recently, accumulation of peptide hormones or their metabolic by-products has been suggested as contributing to the uremic syndrome. Parathyroid hormone excess in uremia is associated with electroencephalographic abnormalities and abnormal elevation of central nervous system

Table II. Nitrogenous Waste Products Which Accumulate in Uremia

I. Urea
II. Guanidinium compounds
   A. Guanidine
   B. Methylguanidine
   C. Dimethylguanine
   D. Guanidinosuccinic acid
   E. Guanidinoacetic acid
   F. Creatine
   G. Creatinine
III. Aromatic compounds
   A. Phenolic and hydroxyphenolic acids
   B. Aromatic amines
   C. Indols
IV. Aliphatic amines
 V. Conjugated amino acids
VI. Low-molecular-weight polypeptides (mostly hormones and their metabolic products)

calcium content; parathyroidectomy prior to the induction of experimental uremia prevents these abnormalities. Many other peptide hormones are increased in uremia (see Chapter 3) but their single or collective role in the uremic syndrome remains speculative.

C. Deficiency of Essential Compounds

Examples of a deficiency attributed to uremia include decreased levels of erythropoietin and of 1,25-dihydroxycholecalciferol. Neither of these two hormones produces classic uremic symptoms and thus the individual or collective role of deficiencies in the pathogenesis of uremia is not established.

It is very likely that the pathogenesis of the uremic syndrome is multifactorial in nature. Accumulation of products normally excreted by the kidney, deficiency of essential compounds not produced in uremia, and excessive accumulation of several peptide hormones as a consequence of the loss of renal mass may all contribute to the symptoms and signs of uremia. Other factors such as malnutrition due to poor intake and alterations in intermediary metabolism may also play a role in the genesis of the uremic syndrome.

V. RATE OF PROGRESSION OF CHRONIC RENAL FAILURE AND CONSIDERATION OF REVERSIBLE FACTORS WHICH MAY ACCELERATE THE PROGRESSION OF CHRONIC RENAL FAILURE

Certain disease entities may result in a given decrease in GFR which then remains constant at this new level for an indefinite period of time. Examples of this include injuries whereby renal mass is permanently reduced, acute intoxications which result in severe renal failure with incomplete recovery of function subsequently, or the state that follows the relief of chronic obstruction. In the latter example, men with chronic bladder neck obstruction from prostatic hypertrophy may develop relatively severe renal failure, which may then stabilize at GFR levels of 10–20 ml/min for indefinite periods of time when the bladder neck obstruction is corrected.

Far more commonly, intrinsic renal disease, such as glomerulonephritis, diabetic glomerulosclerosis, or polycystic kidney disease, leads to a progressive loss of renal function. Most of the causes of progressive renal failure are summarized in Table III. The rate of loss of renal failure may vary among individuals with renal disease. Variations in the rate of progression occurs in individuals with similar illness and even occurs among family members with the same hereditary illness. However, for any one individual with a given disease causing progressive renal failure, the rate of decrease in renal function is constant and predictable in the absence of therapeutic intervention or underlying complicating factors. The linear rate of progression of chronic renal failure has been shown to be proportional to the logarithm of the serum creatinine in some individuals and to the reciprocal of the serum creatinine in others. The value of this information is that it may allow the detection of a complicating factor causing acceleration of the rate of progression of the renal failure or, alternatively, the response to a therapeutic intervention which potentially may modify the rate of progression of renal failure. These considerations apply to most cases of intrinsic renal disease which are progressive.

Chronic renal failure is characterized by relatively slow progression during which there may be long periods of clinical and functional stability. Episodes of more rapid renal functional deterioration, sometimes reversible and sometimes irreversible, may be superimposed. Proper management of chronic renal failure before the end stage is reached emphasizes the recognition and treatment of factors that can cause deterioration in renal function. The potentially reversible causes of deterioration in renal function are inadequate renal blood flow (often due to salt and water depletion), urinary tract obstruction, urinary tract infection, nephrotoxic drugs, hypercalcemia, and hyperuricemia. The prognosis is worse when more than one of these factors are present simultaneously, as frequently occurs, for example, in the immediate postoperative period.

The commonly encountered factors which accelerate the rate of progression of chronic renal failure are listed in Table IV. They include obstruction of the urinary tract such as might occur from ureteral calculi or

Table III. Differential Diagnosis of Chronic Progressive Renal Failure

I. Prerenal causes—renal artery obstruction
II. Intrinsic renal disease causes
  A. Proteinuric glomerular disease
    1. Idiopathic glomerulonephritis (several pathological types)
    2. Systemic lupus erythematosus
  B. Interstitial renal disease
    1. Infectious pyelonephritis
    2. Gout
    3. Nephrotoxins (e.g., analgesic nephropathy, cadmium poisoning, hypercalcemia)
    4. Idiopathic
  C. Hypertensive nephrosclerosis
  D. Hereditary renal diseases (e.g., polycystic kidney, Fabry's disease)
  E. Diabetes mellitus
  F. Amyloidosis
  G. Radiation nephritis
  H. Malignancy-related
    1. Multiple myeloma
    2. Carcinomas
    3. Lymphomas
    4. Leukemias
III. Postrenal causes—obstruction

Table IV. Causes of Acute Deterioration in Renal Function in Patients
with Chronic Renal Disease

  I. Obstruction
 II. Hypertension
III. Urinary tract infection
 IV. Nephrotoxins
     A. Endogenous (hypercalcemia, hyperuricemia, light-chain nephropathy)
     B. Exogenous (usually antibiotics)
  V. Volume abnormalities
     A. Dehydration and hypovolemia
     B. Extracellular fluid volume overexpansion with congestive heart failure

---

bladder neck obstruction. The occurrence of renal parenchymal infection leads to a very rapid decrease in renal function, especially in the setting of chronic renal failure. Hypertension, which is a very common accompaniment of chronic renal failure, especially when diastolic blood pressures exceed 120 mm Hg, also leads to an accelerated decrease in renal function. Since chronic renal failure is caused by a variety of different diseases, the patients are frequently on several different medications; nephrotoxic effects of drugs are quite common and accentuated if the patient already has decreased renal function. Either volume overload with congestive heart failure or extracellular fluid volume depletion can adversely affect renal function, although usually only for the time during which the volume abnormality exists. Whenever a patient with stable or slowly progressive chronic renal failure is noted to have a sudden acceleration in the rate of progression of his disease, as assessed by serial determinations of serum creatinine, the patient should be carefully evaluated and the above-listed factors considered. Correction of the complicating factor accelerating the rate of progression of the renal disease will frequently lead to return of renal function to the value present prior to the onset of the superimposed insult.

VI. CAUSES OF ACUTE DETERIORATION IN RENAL FUNCTION

A. Inadequate Renal Blood Flow

By far the commonest cause of diminished renal perfusion is extracellular volume depletion. Common causes for sodium and volume depletion in patients with chronic renal failure include gastrointestinal losses due to vomiting or diarrhea and renal losses due to diuretics or inadequate conservation in the face of dietary restriction.

The ability to conserve urinary sodium varies from patient to patient and also in the same patient. The term "salt-losing nephritis" is used when the impairment in sodium conservation is extreme. Certain disorders such as medullary cystic disease and phenacetin nephropathy are characterized a tendency to excrete large quantities of sodium. In general, sodium restriction should *not* be imposed in patients with chronic renal failure unless there is clear evidence of salt retention (such as in the nephrotic syndrome and congestive heart failure). In patients with very low glomerular filtration rates (less than 10 ml/min) congestive heart failure is a frequent complication and often results in diminished renal perfusion.

B. Urinary Tract Obstruction

In patients with established renal insufficiency superimposed urinary tract obstruction is easily overlooked because the further reduction in renal function and urine output that often results is readily ascribed to the underlying disease. Bladder-neck obstruction, the commonest cause, may result from benign prostatic hyperplasia, inflammation of the bladder neck, drugs that affect the autonomic nervous system, and neuropathy consequent to diabetes mellitus or uremia. Ureteral obstruction is most often due to renal stones but can also result from a sloughed papilla in patients with papillary necrosis.

C. Infection

Urinary tract infection rarely causes detectable renal functional impairment in patients with otherwise normal kidneys but may do so when there already is renal damage. Treatment of such infections may result in improvement in renal function or may prevent further decline.

D. Hypercalcemia

In chronic renal failure hypercalcemia often results from excessive treatment of renal osteodystrophy with vitamin D and calcium supplements. Other causes include sarcoidosis, multiple myeloma, and malignancy.

E. Hyperuricemia

Acute hyperuricemia most often results from the treatment of malignancies with cytolytic drugs.

SUGGESTED READINGS

Avioli, L. V., and Teitelbaum, S. L.: Renal osteodystrophy, in Earley, L. E., and Gottschalk, C. W. (eds.): Strauss and Welt's *Diseases of the Kidney*. Little, Brown and Co., Boston, 1979, pp. 307–370.

Bolton, C. F., Johnson, W. J., and Dyck, P. J.: Neurologic manifestations of renal failure, in Earley, L. E., and Gottschalk, C. W. (eds.): Strauss and Welt's *Diseases of the Kidney*. Little, Brown and Co., Boston, 1979, pp. 371–392.

Bricker, N. S.: On the pathogenesis of the uremic state. An exposition of the "trade-off hypothesis." *N. Engl. J. Med.* 286:1093–1099, 1972.

Bricker, N. S. and Fine, L. G.: The pathophysiology of chronic renal failure, in Maxwell, M. H., and Kleeman, C. R. (eds.): *Clinical Disorders of Fluid and Electrolyte Metabolism*, Third edition. McGraw-Hill, New York, 1980, pp. 799–825.

Bricker, N. S., Klahr, S., Lubowitz, H., and Slatopolsky, E.: The pathophysiology of renal insufficiency: on the functional transformation in the residual nephrons with advancing disease. Symposium on Pediatric Nephrology. *Pediatr. Clin. North Am.* 18:595, 1971.

Bultitude, F. W., and Newham, S. J.: Identification of some abnormal metabolites in plasma from uremic subjects. *Clin. Chem.* 21:1329, 1975.

Coburn, J. W., and Slatopolsky, E.: Vitamin D, parathyroid hormone and renal osteodystrophy, in Brenner, B. M., and Rector, F. C., Jr. (eds.): *The Kidney*, Second edition. W. B. Saunders, Philadelphia, 1981, pp. 2213–2305.

Cotton, J., Woodard, T. A., Carter, N., and Knochel, J. P.: Resting skeletal muscle membrane potential as an index of uremic toxicity. *J. Clin. Invest.* 63:501, 1979.

Erslev, A. J., and Shapiro, S. S.: Hematologic aspects of renal failure, in Earley, L. E., and Gottschalk, C. W. (eds.): Strauss and Welt's *Diseases of the Kidney*. Little, Brown and Co., Boston, 1979, pp. 279–306.

Feldman, H. A., and Singer, I.: Endocrinology and metabolism in uremia and dialysis: a clinical review. *Medicine (Baltimore)* 54:345, 1975.

Friedman, E. A., and Giordano, C. (eds.): Uremia: formulation and expectations. *Kidney Int.* (Suppl.) 8:1–202, 1978.

Holdsworth, S., Atkins, R. C., and de Kretser, D. M.: The pituitary–testicular axis in men with chronic renal failure. *N. Engl. J. Med.* 296:1245, 1977.

Holliday, M. A.: Calorie intake and growth in uremia. *Kidney Int.* (Suppl. 2) 7:S-73, 1975.

Knochel, J. P., and Seldin, D. W.: The pathophysiology of uremia, in Brenner, B. M., and Rector, F. C., Jr. (eds.): *The Kidney*, Second edition. W. B. Saunders, Philadelphia, 1981, pp. 2137–2183.

Lim, V. S., Auletta, F., and Kathpalia, S.: Gonadal dysfunction in chronic renal failure: an endocrinologic review. *Dial. Transplant.* 7:896, 1978.

Lim, V. S., Fang, V. S., Katz, A. E., and Refetoff, S.: Thyroid dysfunction in chronic renal failure: a study of the pituitary–thyroid axis and peripheral turnover kinetics of thyroxine and triiodothyronine. *J. Clin. Invest.* 60:522, 1977.

Lindner, A., Charra, B., Sherrard, D., and Scribner, B. H.: Accelerated atherosclerosis in prolonged maintenance hemodialysis. *N. Engl. J. Med.* 290:697, 1974.

McCosh, E. J., Solangi, K., Rivers, J. M., and Goodman, A.: Hypertriglyceredemia in patients with chronic renal insufficiency. *Am. J. Clin. Nutr.* 28:1036, 1975.

Rapoport, J., Aviram, M., Chaimovitz, C., and Brooks J. G.: Defective high-density lipoprotein composition in patients on chronic hemodialysis. *N. Engl. J. Med.* 299:1326, 1978.

Slatopolsky, E.: Recommendation for the treatment of renal osteodystrophy in dialysis patients. *Kidney Int.* 7:S253, 1975.

Slatopolsky, E., Robson, A. M., Elkan, I., and Bricker, N. S.: Control of phosphate excretion in uremic man. *J. Clin. Invest.* 47:1864, 1968.

15

Pathophysiological Principles in the Treatment of Patients with Renal Failure

JAMES A. DELMEZ

I. INTRODUCTION

It is estimated that, by 1984, 55,000–60,000 patients will be maintained on dialysis in the United States and a minimum of 5200 will be transplanted. The total yearly cost of medical care for these patients will exceed $3 billion. Because of the protean manifestations of renal failure, physicians not primarily trained in renal diseases are often involved in the care and management of the patient with impaired renal function. A basic knowledge of the treatment rationale is therefore critical.

This chapter will review the effects of three types of therapy, (1) conservative management, (2) dialysis, and (3) transplantation, on the known pathophysiological aberrations of severe renal failure. It is recommended that Chapter 14 be read prior to this discussion. Unfortunately, much of the pathophysiology of severe renal failure is poorly understood and therapy remains empirical. Those areas where knowledge is limited will not be

JAMES A. DELMEZ • Department of Medicine, Washington University School of Medicine, St. Louis, Missouri 63110.

emphasized. In order to adequately discuss the effects of conservative therapy, dialysis, and transplantation on the pathophysiology of uremia, a brief description of these procedures is necessary.

II. PRINCIPLES OF CONSERVATIVE THERAPY, DIALYSIS, AND TRANSPLANTATION

Patients with chronic renal failure share one common feature, a decreased glomerular filtration rate (GFR). How each patient responds to the physiological demands of a reduced GFR depends on the patient's age and general medical condition, as well as on the specific etiology, rate of progression, duration, and the severity of the renal disease. Despite this variability, the physician caring for these patients is faced with a number of problems common to most patients with a severely reduced GFR. Many of these problems can be treated successfully on the basis of known pathophysiological principles.

The aims of conservative therapy in a patient with chronic renal failure are to (1) treat any reversible forms of renal failure, (2) prevent or treat extrarenal complications of renal failure, and (3) formulate a plan for treatment (dialysis, transplantation) when conservative therapy can no longer control the clinical or biochemical manifestations of uremia. This requires not only the careful management of a skilled nephrologist or internist but also significant effort by dietitians, social workers, and nurses.

Dialysis is usually defined as the process of separating crystalloids (such as sodium or potassium) from colloids (such as albumin) utilizing the differences in their rates of diffusion through a semipermeable membrane. Crystalloids pass through the membrane readily whereas colloids do not. Although extensively modified, the process of removing particles from a solution, based on their permeability characteristics, is the fundamental mechanism for the treatment of patients with end stage renal disease (ESRD).

Dialysis of uremic patients is predicated on the assumption that toxic substances accumulate in the body during the course of progressive renal failure. Currently, over 36 compounds have been found to be elevated in the blood of uremic patients. Some of these substances have known harmful effects. Excess sodium and water retention, for example, may lead to edema and hypertension. High levels of serum potassium may cause cardiac arrhythmias. These substances readily diffuse from the patient's blood through the semipermeable membrane to the artificially prepared solution on the other side. Other easily dialyzable substances (urea, creatinine) that routinely can be shown to be elevated in severe renal failure probably do not cause uremic symptoms. It is also likely that several higher-molecular-weight substances which accumulate in uremic subjects but are impermeable through a specific semipermeable membrane are toxic. Unfortunately, despite intensive research effort, there is a poor understanding of which substances are "toxic" and which are of no pathological significance. Thus, during a dialysis treatment, substances are removed in an unselective manner; presumably, both toxic and nontoxic substances are removed. Some of the nontoxic substances which are removed may be essential for function and hence the diet must be supplemented with such substances so as to prevent a depletion state. For example, folic acid, a relatively low-molecular-weight water-soluble vitamin, is dialyzable. Without adequate oral supplementation, folic acid depletion and subsequent megaloblastic anemia may occur.

There are two major forms of dialysis currently available in the treatment of patients with terminal renal failure, hemodialysis and peritoneal dialysis.

A. Description of Hemodialysis and Determinants of Mass Transport

Hemodialysis involves the passage of a patient's blood continuously through an artificial dialyzer at the rate of 200–300 ml/min. In the dialyzer, the blood of the patient is separated by a semipermeable membrane from an artificial solution (dialysate) whose ionic composition resembles plasma. A portion of the substances in the blood diffuse across the semipermeable membrane and are removed by the circulating dialysate. The partially "cleansed" blood returns to the patient's circulation and the dialysate is discarded (see Figure 1). During a typical four-hour hemodialysis, 48–72 liters of blood will flow through the dialyzer. Thus, hemodialysis is a rapid and efficient (for low-molecular-weight solutes, see below) method to remove potential uremic toxins.

The rate of removal of a specific substance across a semipermeable membrane is influenced by several factors (Table I). Obviously, the permeability characteristics of the membrane are important. A membrane with a large pore surface area will allow removal of substances at a greater rate than a membrane with a relatively small pore surface area. For a given pore surface area, membranes with large pores will clear larger particles more efficiently than membranes with small pores.

The second major factor is the concentration gradient of a given solute between the blood side of the semipermeable membrane and the bath or dialysate side. Assuming there is no transmembrane hydrostatic pressure (discussed below) solutes will cross the semipermerable membrane in either direction proportional to their concentration gradients. The typical dialysate composition and an example of some of the solute concentrations in a uremic patient's serum are shown in Figure 2. The dialysate is continuously replenished to maintain a bidirectional concentration gradient. Nonetheless, as the patient's serum concentration of a dialyzed solute falls during the course of dialysis, so will the concentration gradient. Net transport will therefore diminish with time.

The third major factor which determines the net removal rate of a given solute is the physical property of that solute. In general, at any given

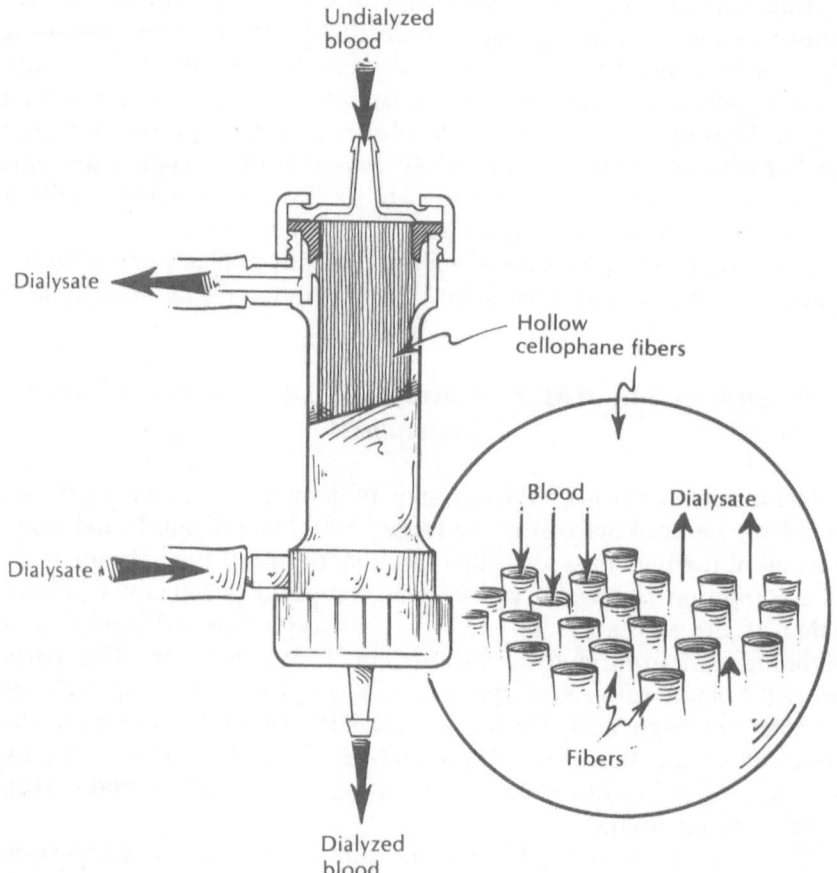

Figure 1. The patient's blood enters the dialyzer and flows within small cylinders whose walls comprise the semipermeable membrane. Solutes diffuse across the membrane into the dialysate which is discarded. The partially "cleansed" blood then returns to the patient's circulation. (Reprinted with permission from Knox, F. G. (ed.): *Textbook of Renal Pathophysiology.* Harper and Row, Hagerstown, Maryland, 1978.)

Table I. Factors Which Influence the Rate of Movement of a Solute across a Semipermeable Membrane during Hemodialysis

1. Permeability characteristics of the membrane
2. Concentration of the solute in the two compartments separated by the semipermeable membrane (concentration gradient)
3. Physical properties of the solute (e.g., molecular weight, shape)
4. Hydrostatic pressure differences across the semipermeable membrane
5. Blood flow rate throught the dialyzer
6. Dialysate flow rates

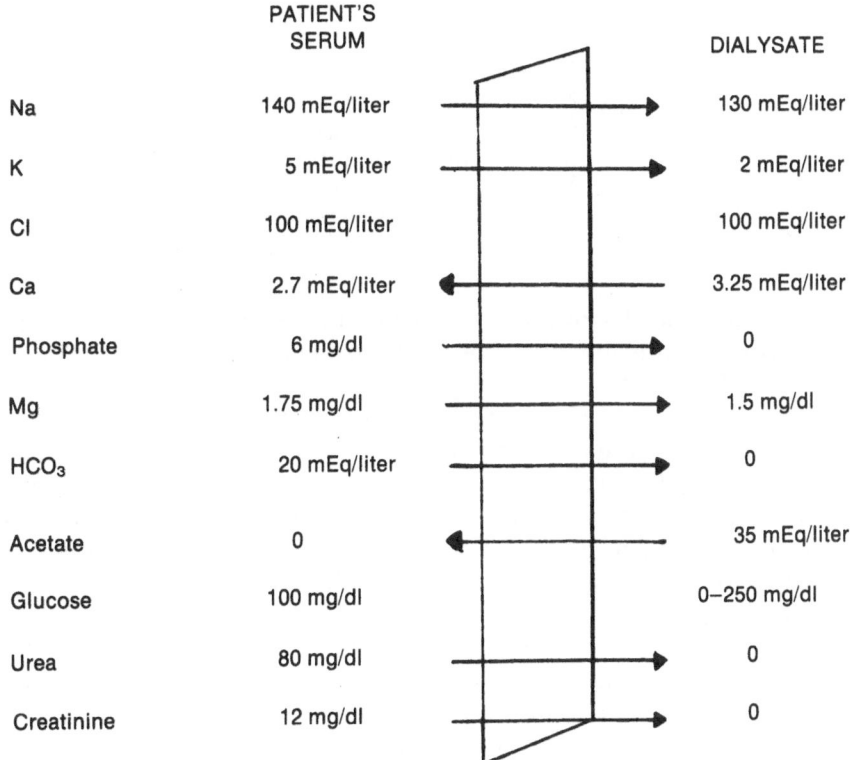

Figure 2. Diagram of the bidirectional diffusion of solutes across a dialyzer membrane based on the concentration gradients.

concentration, the lower the molecular weight of a solute, the greater the removal rate. This relationship is depicted in Table II. Most standard hemodialysis membranes remove efficiently low-molecular-weight molecules but the removal rates decrease dramatically with substances with a molecular weight of between 500 and 5000. This characteristic is important because it has been proposed that some substances with this range of molecular weights ("middle molecules") may be toxic.

Table II. Clearances of Different Solutes in Relation to Their Molecular Weights (U_2 Coil)

	Molecular weight	Clearance (ml/min)
Potassium	39	80–110
Urea	60	90–150
Creatinine	113	80–140
Uric acid	168	40–60
Vitamin B_{12}	1355	10–30

Blood   Membrane   Dialysate

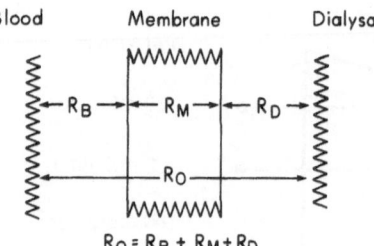

Figure 3. Representation of resistances to solute transport in hemodialysis. (Adapted from Sargent, J. A., and Gotch, F. A.: Principles and biophysics of dialysis, in Drukker, W., Parsons, F. M., and Maher, J. F. (eds.): *Replacement of Renal Function by Dialysis.* Martinus Nijhoff Medical Division, The Netherlands, 1978.)

The fourth major factor affecting membrane transport is the transmembrane hydrostatic pressure difference. The patient's blood is mechanically pumped past the membrane, creating hydrostatic pressure. If this pressure exceeds the hydrostatic pressure of the dialysis solution (assuming no osmotic pressure gradients), there will be a net flux of water from the patient's serum into the dialysate (ultrafiltration). The movement of water into the dialysate produced by ultrafiltration in turn increases the rate of removal of dissolved solutes from the patient's serum. This process is termed "solvent drag." By manipulating the transmembrane pressures, the physician can control the rate of ultrafiltration and degree of solvent drag.

The rate of the flow of blood or dialysate through the dialyzer is also crucial in determining the rate of mass transfer of solutes during a hemodialysis treatment. The reason is that the resistance (R_O) to transfer of a solute from the patient's blood to the dialysate is comprised not only of the

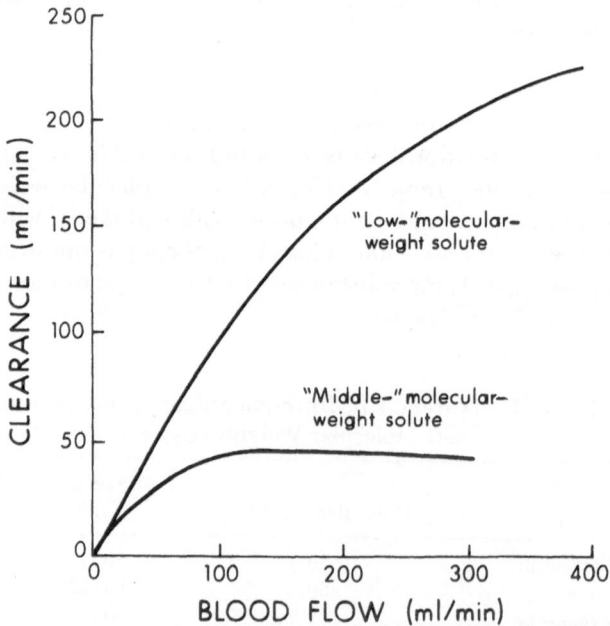

Figure 4. Schematic representation of the effects of blood flow on clearances of "low-" and "middle-"molecular-weight solutes in hemodialysis.

membrane resistance (R_M) but also the resistances derived from the blood (R_B) and dialysate (R_D) unstirred layers which line the membrane (Figure 3). With increasing rates of blood or dialysate flow, these layers (analogous to eddys in a river) are exposed to greater turbulence and become narrower. This results in a decrease in R_B or R_D and therefore in R_O (Figure 3). Eventually, increasing the flow rate does not result in further increasing solute clearances. This is because R_M (which is unaffected by flow) approaches R_O. The mass transfer of larger solutes is impaired to a greater degree by R_M and their clearances are therefore less affected by flow rates (Figure 4).

B. Description of Peritoneal Dialysis and Mass Transport Characteristics

The physiological principles of peritoneal dialysis are similar to those of hemodialysis. Instead of an artificial membrane, however, the lining of the peritoneum serves as the semipermeable barrier to solute transport. The dialysate is instilled within the peritoneal cavity and allowed to equilibrate with the solutes circulating through the peritoneal vessels. The composition of a typical dialysate solution is shown in Table III.

Since the osmolality of the dialysate exceeds that of the plasma of the uremic patient, water will leave the peritoneal circulation and enter the peritoneal cavity. Thus, with peritoneal dialysis, ultrafiltration is achieved because of the hyperosmolality of the dialysate fluid, whereas with hemodialysis ultrafiltration is the result of transmembrane hydrostatic differences. In both situations solvent drag occurs with ultrafiltration.

Peritoneal dialysis also differs from hemodialysis in the permeability characteristics of the membrane. The clearance rates of low-molecular-weight solutes across the peritoneal membrane are less than with hemodialysis. In contrast, the removal of middle-molecular-weight molecules is significantly greater with peritoneal dialysis. The peritoneal membrane behaves as if the total pore surface area is less than most membranes in artificial dialyzers but each individual pore is considerably larger. This transport characteristic has important clinical implications. If middle molecules are toxic, peritoneal

Table III. Typical Composition of Dialysate for Peritoneal Dialysis

Na	132 mEq/liter
Ca	3.5 mEq/liter
Mg	1.5 mEq/liter
Cl	102 mEq
K	0–3 mEq/liter
Lactate	35 mEq/liter
Glucose	1500 mEq/dl
Osmolality	357 mOsm/liter

dialysis may be more effective in removing these substances. On the other hand, high-molecular-weight nontoxic substances such as albumin (molecular weight 69,000) are lost in large amounts in peritoneal dialysis. If the patient does not compensate for this loss with increased protein synthesis, requiring a high protein intake, a protein depletion state may ensue.

Currently, there are two major forms of peritoneal dialysis treatment: intermittant peritoneal dialysis and continuous ambulatory peritoneal dialysis (CAPD). With the former, 2 liters of dialysate are instilled into the peritoneum by an automated peritoneal dialysis machine over 5–10 min. The fluid then "dwells" for 40 min and is subsequently allowed to drain from the peritoneal cavity over 10–15 min. This cycle is repeated on an hourly basis for a total duration of 8–10 hr per treatment. Usually four such treatments are performed per week.

CAPD is a recent form of peritoneal dialysis wherein the patient instills 2 liters of dialysate fluid into the peritoneal cavity. As opposed to intermittent peritoneal dialysis, the fluid remains in the peritoneum for 4–8 hr. Usually four such cycles are performed every day. Therefore, essentially 24 hr a day, seven days a week, there is slow but continuous removal of solutes from the patient's plasma into the dialysate. Between each bag exchange, the patient is ambulatory and able to carry out usual activities. The rationale for CAPD is based on kinetic analysis of solute transfer (Figure 5). Urea (molecular weight 60) diffuses from the patient's plasma rather rapidly into the dialysate and approaches an equilibrium between the two pools within about 3 hr. Larger solutes, such as inulin (molecular weight 5200), however, diffuse more slowly into the dialysate and ongoing removal from the plasma occurs even after 8–12 hr.

With CAPD the removal rates of small solutes is less than with either

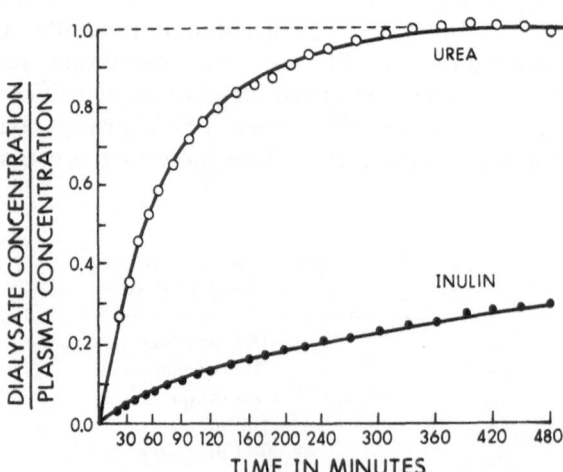

Figure 5. The effects of the duration of peritoneal dialysis dwell time on the equilibration of solutes of different molecular weights. (Adapted from Popovich, R. P., *et al.*: Continuous ambulatory peritoneal dialysis. *Ann. Int. Med.* 88:449, 1978.)

Table IV. Clearance Rates of Solutes with Continuous Ambulatory Peritoneal Dialysis, Intermittent Peritoneal Dialysis, and Two Normal Kidneys

	Milliliters per minute			Liters per week		
	CAPD	Hemodialysis	Two kidneys	CAPD	Hemodialysis	Two kidneys
Urea (60)[a]	8.3	150	60	84	135	604
B₁₂ (1355)[a]	5–6	33	100	50	30	1,008
Inulin (5200)[a]	3	5.5	100	30	5	1,008

[a] Numbers in parentheses are molecular weights.

hemodialysis or intermittent peritoneal dialysis. However, because it is performed continuously instead of intermittently, the net weekly removal rates are roughly comparable. Because removal of middle-molecular-weight solutes occur throughout the instillation, their net weekly removal rates actually exceed those of either hemodialysis or intermittent peritoneal dialysis (Table IV).

C. Description of Renal Transplantation

In renal transplantation the donor kidney is placed in the iliac fossa. Its renal artery is anastomosed to either the hypogastric or iliac artery and its distal ureter is anastomosed to the patient's bladder (Figure 6).

An adequately functioning renal transplant changes dramatically the internal milieu of the uremic patient. Renal excretory and nonexcretory function normalize to a large extent. By contrast, dialysis can only partially correct the former and has no direct effects on the latter defect. The early and late effects of an adequately functioning transplant on the pathophysiological abnormalities of uremia will be discussed. Most patients receiving a renal transplant require chronic immunosuppressive therapy to prevent rejection. The effects of these drugs, usually steroids and cytotoxic agents

Figure 6. In the technique of cadaveric renal transplantation, the donor renal artery is usually anastomosed, end to end, with the hypogastric artery, the renal vein is anastomosed end to side; with the hypogastric artery, the renal vein is anastomosed, end to side, with the external iliac vein, and the ureter is anastomosed to the bladder. (Reprinted with permission from Chatterjee, S. N. (ed.): *Manual of Renal Transplantation.* Springer-Verlag, New York, 1979.)

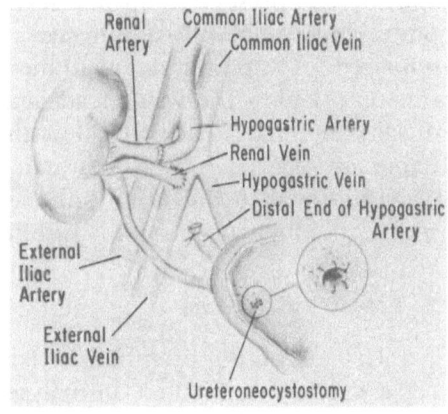

such as azathioprine or cytoxan, are complex and controversial. A discussion of the effects of these drugs is beyond the scope of this chapter.

III. EFFECTS OF TREATMENT ON SPECIFIC PATHOPHYSIOLOGICAL ALTERATIONS IN RENAL FAILURE
A. Treatment of Pathophysiological Alterations of Sodium and Water in Renal Failure

1. Conservative Management

As the GFR progressively declines, the percent of filtered sodium that each remaining nephron must excrete to maintain sodium balance on a constant salt diet increases. Thus, until the final stages of chronic renal failure, the patient is often in sodium balance. However, as the GFR decreases, the range of dietary sodium loads that the kidneys can excrete narrows. In addition, certain forms of renal diseases may be associated with a greater capacity to excrete a sodium load (e.g., medullary cystic diseases, interstitial nephritis). On the other hand, other renal diseases in which large amounts of protein are lost in the urine (nephrotic syndrome) are often associated with sodium retention. Thus, in estimating the optimal sodium content in the diet, one must avoid diets too low in sodium content, in which case the patient may become volume depleted, which may lead to a further decrease in GFR, or diets too high in sodium content, whereby the patient may develop severe edema, congestive heart failure, and hypertension. Quantitative measurement of a 24-hr urinary sodium excretion, when used in conjunction with the clinical situation, is often of value in determining the appropriate sodium intake for a given patient.

Patients with a low GFR also have a decreased range of water excretion rates. Fortunately, however, the secretion of ADH which controls serum osmolality and thirst mechanisms are intact in these patients. Even with severe renal failure, most patients will maintain an appropriate water intake and thereby preserve a normal serum sodium concentration. Occasionally a physician is tempted to administer a water load to the patient with a severely impaired GFR in an attempt to increase renal perfusion and improve renal function. Unless the water load is accompanied by an appropriate amount of salt, the renal capacity to dilute the urine is easily exceeded and profound hyponatremia may ensue. If water intake must be controlled, daily intakes of fluid equal to the urine volume plus 500 ml/day will usually maintain serum sodium concentrations within the normal range.

2. Effects of Dialysis

Urinary output often falls to trivial amounts when patients with chronic renal failure are initiated on dialysis. This is due in part to the lowering of serum urea levels, which decreases the osmotic diuresis produced by urea.

In addition, mild volume expansion often seen in uremic patients is partially corrected by ultrafiltration, leading to a lessened natriuretic stimulus (see Chapter 14). Progression of the patient's renal disease also occurs while an dialysis. Since at this stage of renal failure, the kidneys cannot concentrate or dilute urine, the urine output falls almost in proportion to the further fall in GFR. Therefore, as urine output falls or ceases, the salt and water the patient consumes must be balanced by salt and water removal during dialysis. This can be achieved during hemodialysis by increasing the hydrostatic pressure gradient across the artificial kidney membrane, by increasing the "leakiness" of the membrane, or by increasing the total duration of dialysis. Frequently, however, it is very difficult to remove more than 3 or 4 kg of fluid during any one hemodialysis period. The patients frequently develop cramps, nausea, and hypotension. The causes for this are multifactorial. During hemodialysis, there is a rapid fall in the extracellular urea concentration and serum osmolality. Therefore, not only is intravascular plasma volume decreased by ultrafiltration but there is a transient osmotic gradient favoring the shift of water from the extracellular to the intracellular compartment. Hypotension may be also potentiated by the effects of acetate entering the patient's systemic circulation from the dialysate. Acetate, at the serum concentrations achieved during hemodialysis, may cause peripheral vasodilation. If the patient cannot increase his cardiac output in response to the vasodilation, hypotension will ensue. With the institution of a moderate salt (4 g) and water (800–1000 ml) intake, the patient will not require high ultrafiltration rates and hemodialysis is usually better tolerated.

With compliance to dietary restrictions, adequate chronic hemodialysis and ultrafiltration, the extracellular fluid volume and total exchangeable sodium of the uremic patient falls. This usually occurs in the first few months of dialysis and remains stable thereafter (Figure 7).

Peritoneal dialysis removes salt and water through osmotic rather than through hydrostatic differences across the semipermeable membrane. Water enters the peritoneal cavity in proportion to the difference in osmolality between the dialysate and plasma. Sodium, despite being a highly permeable solute, does not transverse the membrane as freely as water. This may lead to hypernatremia. Most dialysis solutions now have a sodium concentration of approximately 132 mEq/liter. Assuming a normal serum sodium level (140 mEq/liter) in the patient, sodium will move from plasma into the dialysate across the peritoneal membrane not only because of solvent drag, but also because of a concentration gradient. Hypernatremia can thus be prevented. The removal of solutes is usually slower during peritoneal dialysis and the patient rarely has cardiovascular instability during treatment. Since the dialyses last longer, the total amount of fluid removed per week is comparable to hemodialysis.

3. Renal Transplantation

When the patient with end stage renal disease receives a well-functioning transplanted kidney, there is a profound natriuresis and diuresis. This is due

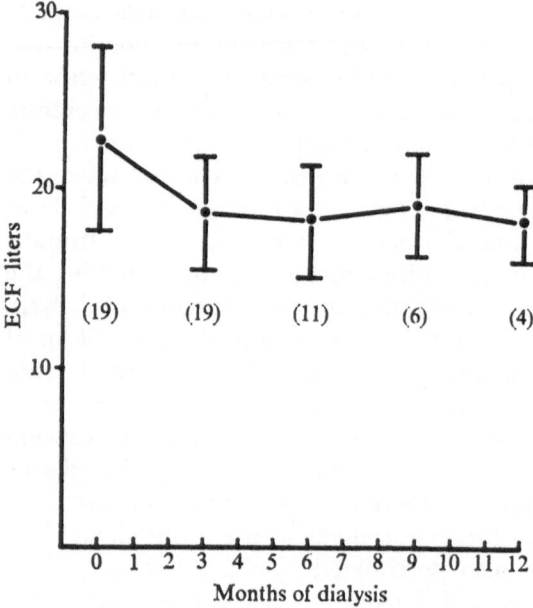

Figure 7. Reduction in the extracellular fluid compartment by chronic hemodialysis. (Reprinted with permission from Coles, G. A.: Body composition in chronic renal failure. *Q. J. Med.*, New Series, XLI, No. 161:25–47, 1972.)

to urea which is excreted (osomotic diuresis) and to an expanded extracellular space. The natriuresis, however, is under physiological control. Once the urea levels fall and the extracellular space contracts, the fractional excretion of sodium returns to normal (see Figure 8).

Satisfactory renal transplants maintain a GFR of 60–100 ml/min. Therefore, the intrinsic renal capacity to excrete a salt and water load is usually normal. However, because of its mineralocorticoid effects, large doses of prednisone which are administered to prevent rejection may lead to fluid retention. This is usually easily managed with diuretics.

B. Effects of Treatment on the Pathophysiology of Potassium in Renal Failure

1. Conservative Management

Most patients with chronic renal failure maintain near-normal serum potassium concentrations at GFR values of 10 ml/min or greater. This is primarily accomplished by increasing potassium secretion per nephron. Mild degrees of hyperkalemia (serum potassium less than 6.0 mEq/liter) may occur when the patient becomes symptomatic (GFR less than 10–15 ml/min). With the institution of a low-protein (40-g-high biological value) and potassium diet (less than 40 mEq/day), the uremic symptoms and hyperkalemia are often corrected. If the patient is acidotic, the institution of alkali therapy lowers the serum potassium levels by shifting potassium from the extracellular into the intracellular space.

Occasionally, the use of cation-exchange resins are required. Kayexalate taken orally removes approximately 1 mEq potassium per gram of resin administered. Since kayexalate is constipating, it should be given with a poorly absorbed carrier such as sorbitol. The recommended dose is 20–50 g kayexalate dissolved in 100–200 ml of 20% sorbitol solution. Since kayexalate exchanges 1.3–1.7 mEq of sodium for each millequivalent of potassium removed, it must be administered with caution in patients susceptible to cardiovascular overload.

Despite near-normal levels of serum potassium in patients with chronic renal failure, total body potassium stores and intramuscular potassium concentrations are often low. This may be due to impaired membrane transport mechanisms, acidosis, or malnutrition.

2. Dialysis Therapy

If the stable hemodialysis patient is able to restrict his potassium intake to 50–60 mEq/day, the serum potassium levels can be well controlled with hemodialysis (clearance often exceeds 100 ml/min). The amount of potassium removed during hemodialysis depends partially on the gradient of the patient's serum versus the dialysate potassium concentration. Dialysate with

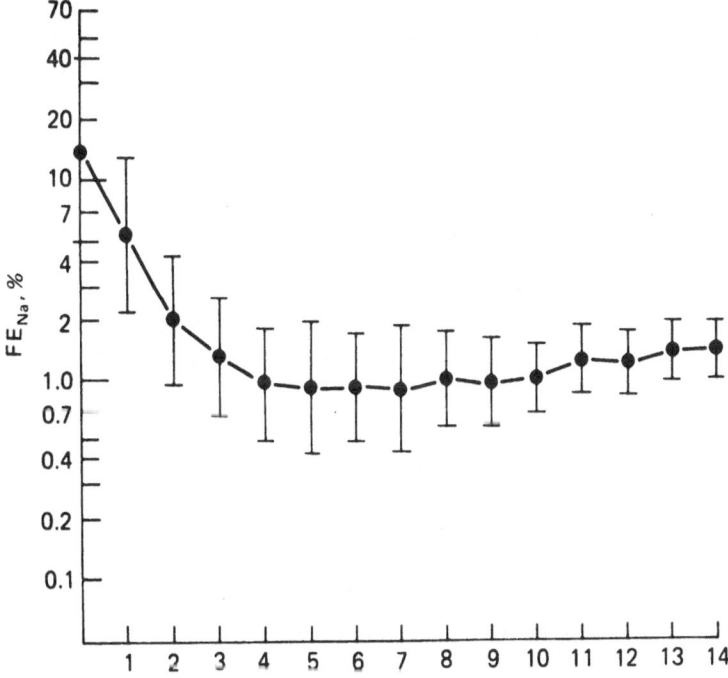

Figure 8. The effects of renal transplantation on the fractional excretion of sodium. %FE$_{NA}$ (mean ± 1 S.D.) after renal transplantation is plotted versus days posttransplant. (Reprinted with permission from Hong, C.D., *et al.*: Fractional excretion of sodium after renal transplantation. *Kidney Int.* 16:167–178, 1979.)

a very low potassium concentration may further reduce total body potassium and acutely lower serum potassium levels to such an extent that cardiac arrhythmias (especially if the patient is on digoxin) and muscle weakness may ensue. If the patient is dialyzed against a bath with the same concentration of potassium as the blood, there will be no net removal of potassium (assuming no ultrafiltration). With continued ingestion of potassium, severe hyperkalemia will occur. If the patient is adequately dialyzed for 7 weeks with a dialysate potassium concentration of 2.0 mEq/liter, the potassium concentration in the skeletal muscle increases to normal (Table V).

Peritoneal dialysis does not remove potassium from the body as rapidly as hemodialysis. For example, if 2 liters of potassium free dialysate fluid are instilled for 2 hr in the peritoneal cavity of a patient with a serum potassium concentration of 6 mEq/liter, a maximum of 12 mEq would be removed. If, as occurs with CAPD, 2 liters of dialysate are exchanged four times a day, approximately 48 mEq of potassium would be removed per day. This regimen usually maintains normal serum potassium levels. The effect of peritoneal dialysis on intracellular muscle potassium stores is not currently known. However, in those patients with adequate protein intake, total body potassium may increase slightly.

3. Renal Transplantation

Because of the osmotic diuresis in the early transplant period, there is decreased reabsorption of potassium by the proximal convoluted tubules. In addition, distal tubular secretion of potassium is flow dependent and thus would increase during an osmotic diuresis. Many patients with renal failure have high aldosterone levels. The sudden presence of a functioning kidney leads to an aldosterone-mediated increased potassium secretion by the cortical collecting ducts. This may lead to hypokalemia in the early posttransplant period. In addition, the mineralocorticoid effects of large doses of steroids may potentiate potassium secretion. However, all these effects leading to a kaliuresis are transient. The patient with a normally functioning renal transplant on low steroids usually maintains normal long-term potassium balance.

Table V. Effect of Hemodialysis on the Skeletal Muscle Concentration of Potassium in Renal Failure[a]

	Intracellular potassium concentration
Normal subjects	155 ± 4.3
Before dialysis	147 ± 3.1 ⎱ $p < 0.01$
After dialysis	155 ± 4.9 ⎰

[a] From Cotton, J. R., et al.: Resting skeletal muscle membrane potential as an index of uremic toxicity. J. Clin. Invest. 63:501–506, 1979.

C. Effects of Treatment on Acid–Base Pathophysiology in Renal Failure

1. Conservative Management

Patients with chronic renal failure do not ordinarily develop acidosis until the GFR falls below approximately 20% of normal. The degree of acidosis among individual patients varies considerably but serum bicarbonate levels less than 10–12 mEq/liter are unusual in the well-compensated nonoliguric patient. To avoid complications of acidosis, sodium bicarbonate is given in amounts (usually 1–3 g/day) great enough to maintain serum bicarbonate concentrations greater than 15 mEq/liter. Caution must be exercised in administering excessive amounts of $NaHCO_3$. Since sodium is primarily distributed in the ECF space, volume overload may occur. An expanded ECF compartment also leads to a decreased proximal tubular threshold for HCO_3 reabsorption and bicarbonaturia. Since endogenous acid production is, in part, related to dietary protein metabolism, protein restriction improves the systemic acidosis.

2. Dialysis Therapy

Most dialysate solutions contain between 35 and 40 mEq/liter of acetate. During dialysis about 150 mEq of acetate diffuses per hour into the systemic circulation and approximately 80% is metabolized to CO_2 and H_2O via the citric acid cycle:

$$H^+ + CH_3COO^- + 2O_2 \rightarrow 2H_2O + 2CO_2$$

The consumption of a hydrogen ion during the oxidative metabolism of acetate is equivalent to generating bicarbonate ion. Concurrent with acetate diffusing from the dialysate to the systemic circulation, bicarbonate also diffuses from the systemic circulation to the dialysate. The loss of bicarbonate from the plasma is more than compensated for by acetate utilization and "synthesis" of bicarbonate so that serum bicarbonate rises throughout dialysis. Most hemodialysis patients maintain serum bicarbonate concentrations between 18 and 22 mEq/liter.

All commercially available peritoneal dialysis solutions contain nonvolatile alkali equivalents (usually lactate) at concentrations of 35–45 mEq/liter. Like acetate, diffusion into the systemic circulation and metabolic conversion of lactate are required in order to generate an alkalinizing effect.

3. Acute Effects of Renal Transplantation

The acute effects of a well-functioning renal transplant on acid–base balance are somewhat variable. In a volume-expanded patient, proximal tubular reabsorption of HCO_3 decreases (see Chapter 8). High levels of parathyroid hormone are common in hemodialysis patients. This may also decrease proximal bicarbonate reabsorption. If the patient is hyperphosphatemic (see Chapter 9), however, the new kidney will be able to quickly generate large amounts of titrable acid. High levels of aldosterone will also enhance distal tubular hydrogen ion secretion. In the first month post-transplantation, the serum bicarbonate often normalizes, but in some patients the metabolic acidosis may not be corrected owing to persistent renal tubular acidosis in the transplanted kidney.

D. Effects of Treatment on the Anemia of Renal Failure

1. Conservative Management

The anemia of chronic renal failure is primarily due to decreased erythropoiesis. Early studies have shown that erythropoietin levels are low in severe renal failure, presumably because of decreased production by the diseased kidneys. More recently, however, slightly elevated serum erythropoietin levels have been detected in severe renal failure. Nevertheless, it is clear that the diseased kidneys are unable to produce erythropoietin at rates appropriate to the degree of anemia. *In vitro* studies also suggest that "inhibitors" which accumulate in uremia suppress the response of the bone marrow to erythropoietin. In addition, a mild hemolysis occurs when the blood urea nitrogen (BUN) exceeds 100 mg/dl. This may result in circulating red blood cells whose half life is roughly one-half normal.

The conservative management of the anemia of renal failure is similar to that of dialysis therapy (see Section III.D.2). Vitamin and iron therapy should be instituted if there is evidence of depletion. Overzealous blood drawing for diagnostic tests should be avoided.

2. Dialysis Therapy

The institution of regular hemodialysis usually improves erythropoiesis during the first 6–12 months of dialysis. Most patients entering hemodialysis have hematocrits between 15%–25%. With proper medical management most patients will subsequently increase their hematocrits to between 20% and 35% (Figure 9). The mechanism is unknown. Red cell survival and erythropoietin levels, however, do not appear to improve with standard dialysis regimens. Recent *in vitro* evidence suggests that a middle-molecular-weight (1000) fraction found in uremic patients' serum directly inhibits erythropoiesis. After 16 weeks on hemodialysis, the patients' serum demonstrates less inhibitory activity. Because of its molecular weight, it is likely that this fraction is partially removed with dialysis. Presumably because nephrectomized patients produce less renal erythropoietin than those with *in situ* kidneys, they are often more severely anemic and may require frequent blood transfusions.

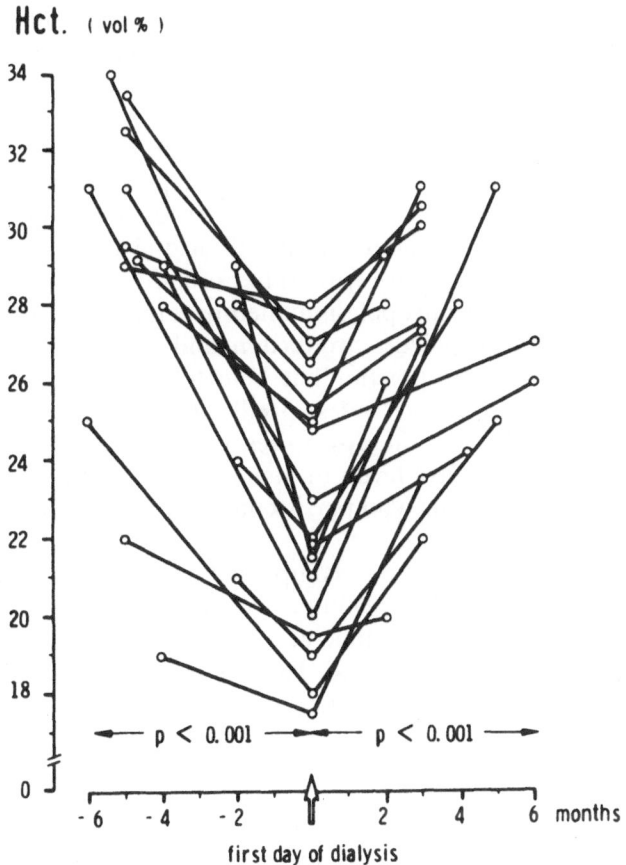

Figure 9. The effects of hemodialysis on the anemia of renal failure. The hematocrit is plotted versus time. (Reprinted with permission from Radtke, H. W., *et al.*: Serum erythropoietin concentration in chronic renal failure: relationship to degree of anemia and excretory renal function. *Blood* 54:877, 1979.)

Iron deficiency is present in approximately 25% of nontransfused chronic hemodialysis patients. Intestinal absorption of iron is usually normal, but may not fully compensate for accelerated exogenous losses of iron. Loss of blood which remains in the dialyzer after every treatment ranges from 4 to 50 ml. On a yearly basis this amounts to a loss of approximately 780 mg of iron. In addition, periodic blood tests and technical complications of dialysis leading to blood loss may acount for an additional loss of 1–1.5 g of iron per year. Because of systemic anticoagulation due to heparin infusion during hemodialysis, gastrointestinal or uterine bleeding occurs with a higher incidence in chronic hemodialysis patients than in normal subjects. Therefore, the diet of most patients on hemodialysis is supplemented with oral (usually 325 mg of ferrous sulfate given three times daily) or intravenous iron. Care must be taken to avoid iron overload and its consequences, parenchyma deposition of iron. Ferritin levels may be drawn periodically to assess total iron stores. Recent data suggest that ferritin levels may not reflect bone marrow iron content in those patients receiving intravenous iron. In patients in whom this information is crucial, a bone marrow aspirate with appropriate iron stains is indicated.

Folic acid is a small water-soluble vitamin which is dialyzable. Although a diet containing greater than 60 g of protein per day usually supplies enough folic acid to maintain body stores, it is customary to supplement the diet of chronic hemodialysis patients with folic acid (1 mg/day).

Most dialysis units use a variety of either oral or parenteral androgenic preparations to improve erythropoiesis in their patients (Table VI). Androgen therapy increases erythropoietin production and may also increase bone marrow sensitivity to erythropoietin. The hematologic response, which may take up to six months to detect, is less predictable and weaker in anephric patients. Because androgen therapy raises triglyceride and lowers high-density lipoprotein cholesterol levels in hemodialysis patients, its use should be reserved for those patients who persistently maintain a hematocrit of less than 25%.

Since peritoneal dialysis is not accompanied by blood loss during dialysis, iron deficiency is probably less common with peritoneal dialysis than with hemodialysis. Like hemodialysis, folic acid is lost during peritoneal dialysis and oral supplementation is required. Patients begun on peritoneal dialysis undergo a slow increase in the hematocrit to comparable levels as those on hemodialysis.

3. Renal Transplantation

The normally functioning renal transplant releases adequate amounts of erythropoietin and should completely remove "uremic substances" which

Table VI. Mean (± S.E.) Values for Red Cell Mass, Hematocrit, and Blood Transfusion Requirements before and after the Administration of Placebo and Androgen in 21 Patients on Maintenance Hemodialysis[a]

Treatment	Red cell mass (ml)	Hematocrit (%)	Blood transfusions (units/patient per month)
Placebo			
Before	1093 ± 44	26.0 ± 1.1	0.35 ± 0.13
After	964 ± 46	22.8 ± 1.2	
p value[b]	<0.01	<0.005	
Androgen			
Before	946 ± 56	23.1 ± 1.2	0.16 ± 0.07
After	1173 ± 70	27.0 ± 1.5	
p value[b]	<0.001	<0.005	0.05

[a] From Hendler et al.: Controlled study of androgen therapy in anemia of patients on maintenance hemodialysis. N. Engl. J. Med. 291:1046–1053, 1974.
[b] Paired t test.

inhibit bone marrow response to erythropoietin. The hematocrit is usually normal in these patients 6–12 weeks following transplantation. On rare occasions, polycythemia with a hematocrit greater than 55% occurs. This may be due to excess erythropoietin production by an ischemic area or renal artery stenosis of the transplanted kidney.

E. Effects of Treatment on the Hypertension of Renal Failure

1. Conservative Management

Approximately 80% of patients with terminal renal failure have hypertension. In most cases, the major pathogenetic factor is an expanded ECF volume due to retention of salt and water. In some patients, however, absolute or relative hyperreninemia and/or neurogenic factors may be responsible for the hypertension. Irrespective of the cause, it is imperative to control the patient's blood pressure because hypertension accelerates cardiovascular complications which are the most common cause of death in the renal failure population. In addition, uncontrolled hypertension can cause vascular damage and accelerate the progression of the renal failure.

Since hypertension in renal failure is usually due to salt and water accumulation, salt restriction and diuretic therapy are the initial measures to be employed. Loop diuretics, particularly furosemide, are preferable to thiazide diuretics. Furosemide does not decrease renal blood flow and, by virtue of impairing salt reabsorption in the ascending limb of the loop of Henle instead of the distal convoluted tubule, produces a greater natriuresis. Large doses may be required as the GFR falls. Care must be taken to prevent volume depletion and its consequences: lower GFR and renal blood flow. If the blood pressure is unresponsive to these measures, additional antihypertensive therapy should be added. This includes drugs which may decrease cardiac output. The choice of which drugs are to be utilized must be individualized for each patient. Each has the potential for serious side effects which may complicate the overall medical care (see Chapter 10).

2. Dialysis Therapy

Since dialysis removes salt and water, the hypertension of most chronic dialysis patients is well controlled with salt restriction and adequate fluid removal by ultrafiltration. The remaining 30%–50% of patients on dialysis require additional antihypertensive drug therapy. It should be emphasized that many of the side effects of these drugs may potentiate certain medical problems which occur frequently in the hemodialysis patient (see Table VII). Rarely, despite an optimal antihypertensive regimen, patients may remain hypertensive. These patients frequently have high rates of renin release by

Table VII. Side Effects of Common Antihypertensive Drugs Which May Worsen Symptoms Commonly Present in Chronic Hemodialysis Patients

Hydralazine
  1. Increased cardiac output leading to
     angina
  2. Headaches
  3. Nausea, anorexia, vomiting
Clonidine
  1. Dry mouth leading to increased fluid
     intake
  2. Increased somnolence
α-Methyldopa
  1. Postural hypotension, which may be
     severe following a hemodialysis
     treatment
  2. Impotence (present in 30% of male
     hemodialysis patients)
  3. Increased sommnolence
	Propranolol
	  May cause heart failure in those with
	    limited cardiac reserve
	Prazosin
	  Postural hypotension
	Guanetheline
	  1. Postural hypotension
	  2. Impotence
	Reserpine
	  1. Depression
	  2. Sedation
	Minoxidil
	  Increased cardiac output leading to
	    angina

their kidneys. This causes increased secretion of angiotensin II, a powerful vasoconstrictor (see Chapter 3). Bilateral nephrectomy is rarely necessary to eliminate these vasoconstrictor effects and facilitate blood pressure control if an aggressive medical regimen is maintained.

Preliminary reports suggest that blood pressure may be normalized in as many as 80% of patients undergoing CAPD. This may be due entirely to the effective removal of salt and water by this technique. One cannot however, exclude the possibility that vasoconstrictor substances such as angiotensin II may be removed by peritoneal dialysis.

3. Renal Transplantation

Hypertension is quite common in the renal transplant population. An incidence of 56% has been reported in those patients followed as long as six years. One third of the patients initially hypertensive become normotensive, whereas one third of the patients initially normotensive become hypertensive. The etiology of the hypertension is unclear. In most patients, the hypertension is due to salt and water excess. This may be due either to the transplanted kidney's inability to regulate salt and water balance or to the mineralocorticoid effects of steroids. Furosemide and salt restriction often suffice in the successful treatment of these patients. Hypertension may also be caused by renal artery stenosis of either the patient's diseased kidneys or the transplanted kidneys or by chronic rejection. The ischemic kidney releases inappropriately large amounts of renin, leading to vasoconstriction. Since renin secretion is increased by β-adrenergic stimulation, β-adrenergic blocking drugs such as propranolol are often efficacious.

F. Effects of Treatment on the Renal Osteodystrophy of Renal Failure

1. Conservative Management

The objectives of the conservative management of osteodystrophy in patients with impaired renal function are to (1) suppress secondary hyperparathyroidism and (2) mineralize osteoid normally. This primarily requires (1) prevention of hyperphosphatemia by dietary restriction of phosphate and the use of aluminum hydroxide or aluminum carbonate gels and (2) dietary supplementation of calcium and/or vitamin D.

Even in the early stages of renal failure, parathyroid hormone (PTH) rises (see Chapter 14). This causes phosphaturia and therefore maintenance of a normal serum phosphate. However, elevated levels of PTH also lead to bone resorption and histological changes of osteitis fibrosa cystica. If gastrointestinal absorption of phosphorus is decreased by dietary means or by the use of gels, the need for increasing phosphorus excretion by each remaining nephron may be eliminated; hyperparathyroidism will be prevented and the bone changes can be delayed or avoided.

The average daily intake of phosphorus is 1200 mg, and about 700 mg are absorbed from the gastrointestinal tract. The absolute amount absorbed can be significantly reduced by decreasing the dietary intake of phosphorus to 600–800 mg/day. The gastrointestinal absorption of phosphorus can also be reduced by aluminium hydroxide gels. These gels bind phosphorus in the gastrointestinal tract and prevent absorption. By dietary phosphorus restriction and the use of aluminum hydroxide binders, daily fecal phosphorus excretion can actually exceed the daily dietary intake of phosphorus.

As the patient progresses to severe renal failure, the ability of the diseased kidneys to hydroxylate 25-hydroxy vitamin D_3 (25-hydroxy-cholecalciferol) to 1,25-dihydroxy vitamin D_3 becomes impaired. 1,25-dihydroxy vitamin D_3 is the most potent metabolite of vitamin D in stimulating calcium absorption by the intestine. A decreased intestinal fractional absorption of calcium is well documented in patients with severe renal failure. This may lead to hypocalcemia and potentiate secondary hyperparathyroidism.

The total daily intestinal absorption of calcium may be increased by either supplementing dietary calcium intake or by the initiation of vitamin D therapy. The daily intake of elemental calcium is approximately 800–1000 mg. If one supplements this with 500 mg to 1500 mg of elemental calcium per day in the severely uremic patient, the absolute amount of calcium absorbed will increase significantly despite a low fractional absorption. Administration of 1,25-hydroxy-cholecalciferol is an attractive alternative to oral calcium supplementation. A recently synthesized vitamin D_3 analog, 1α,25-dihydroxy vitamin D, is orally absorbable and has a biologic activity comparable on a weight basis to 1,25-dihydroxy vitamin D. With any regimen designed to improve calcium balance, care must be taken to avoid hypercalcemia and its consequences (see Chapter 9). The effects of treatment on the bone disease of secondary hyperparathyroidism (osteitis fibrosa cystica) are summarized in Table VIII.

The second major disorder of bone histology in patients with chronic renal failure is osteomalacia. This is characterized by low rates of bone mineralization and excess osteoid. Unfortunately, the pathophysiological events leading to this disorder are less clearly understood than osteitis fibrosa cystica (see Chapter 14). It is likely that vitamin D therapy is most advantageous to uremic patients with osteomalacia as the predominant form of bone disease. It is postulated that vitamin D directly increases the mineralization front. It is interesting, in this regard, that 25-hydroxy vitamin D_3 may be more potent than $1\alpha,25$-dihydroxy vitamin D_3.

Overly aggressive dietary phosphorus reduction and aluminum hydroxide gel administration may lead to hypophosphatemia. Prolonged phosphate depletion may impair bone mineralization and lead to osteomalacia. In addition, hypophosphatemia causes a decline of 2,3-diphosphoglycerate (2,3-DPG) and ATP levels in erythrocytes. Hemoglobin and 2,3-DPG interact chemically so as to promote the release of oxygen. Low levels of 2,3-DPG may decrease the release of oxygen to peripheral tissues. Thus hypophosphatemia may limit oxygen release at the cellular level and thereby create anoxia.

Table VIII. Effects of Conservative Treatment on the Pathophysiological Alterations of Osteitic Fibrosa Cystica in Severe Renal Failure

Altered serum levels of hormones and minerals in severe renal failure	Causes of altered serum levels	Effect of altered serum levels on mineral hemostasis	Treatment	Effect of treatment
1. ↑ Phosphate	↓ Renal excretion	↓ Ca	Phosphorus restriction Aluminum hydroxide gels	↓ P
2. ↓ Calcium	↑ Phosphate levels ↓ GI absorption	↑ PTH secretion	Treat ↑ P, calcium supplements	↑ Ca
3. ↓ 1,25-Dihydroxy vitamin D_3	↓ Renal synthesis	↓ Ca	Vitamin D and/or calcium supplements	↑ Ca
4. ↑ PTH	↑ Secretion ↓ Catabolism	Osteitis fibrosis cystica Phosphaturia	All of the above	Improve osteitis fibrosa cystica

Chronic acidosis may also cause bone disease (see Chapter 14). Oral sodium bicarbonate therapy increases the serum pH and thus reduces the "leaching" of calcium carbonate from the bone to buffer the hydrogen ion excess.

2. Dialysis Therapy

The pathophysiological events leading to renal osteodystrophy in patients with end stage renal failure also occur in patients on dialysis and therapy is quite similar. Additional factors, however, also play a role. The gradient between the concentration of calcium in the dialysate versus the concentration of unbound calcium in the serum determines whether the patient will have a net gain or loss of calcium during the period of dialysis treatment. It is estimated that the permeability of calcium across the artificial membrane is approximately 60%–70% that of urea. Therefore, the total quantity of calcium transferred into a patient from the dialysate can reach 400–600 mg during 5 hr of hemodialysis when dialysate calcium levels exceed the plasma free calcium by 1.5–2.0 mg/dl. If the dialysate contains calcium at a lower concentration than the patient's unbound serum calcium level, there will be a net loss of calcium during dialysis.

The dialysate fluid contains no phosphate and therefore phosphate levels decrease during dialysis. The magnitude of phosphate removal, however, is insufficient to preclude the use of phosphate restriction and aluminum hydroxide binders as the cornerstones in the control of hyperphosphatemia.

The infusion of heparin into the patient during chronic hemodialysis may have a role in the development of bone disease (osteomalacia?). It is of interest that peritoneal dialysis, which requires no heparin, may not be associated with a progressive osteomalacia. Peritoneal dialysis, however, may also remove high-molecular-weight substances in uremic serum which inhibit the calcification of bone.

Fluoride is a common additive to tap water. If dialysate is not adequately ridded of this ion, fluoride will accumulate in the bone. Dialysis patients treated in this fashion appear to be prone to the development of osteomalacia.

If the patient develops severe bone changes secondary to uncontrolled secondary hyperparathyroidism, a partial parathyroidectomy is indicated. In the immediate postoperative period, there is usually a profound fall in the serum PTH and calcium levels. The hypocalcemia results from the decreased PTH stimulation of bone resorption and from the shift of calcium into bone in the process of remineralization. Under constant hypocalcemic stimulation the remnant parathyroid gland becomes more hyperplastic and parathyroid secretion increases. With calcium and vitamin D supplements the serum calcium level often returns to near normal levels within several months. Over the ensuing several months there is healing of the changes of osteitis fibrosa cystica. On the other hand, osteomalacia worsens following parathyroidectomy.

3. Renal Transplantation

Dramatic changes in bone metabolism occur with a successful renal transplant. High levels of PTH will produce an immediate phosphaturia which may result in hypophosphatemia. Severe hypophosphatemia may induce a reciprocal increase in serum calcium levels. In addition, the capacity to hydroxylate 25-hydroxy vitamin D_3 to 1,25-dihydroxy vitamin D_3 is quickly available. This process is further stimulated by high levels of PTH and low levels of serum phosphate. Thus intestinal absorption of calcium increases and serum calcium levels rise. This, in turn suppresses parathyroid hormone release. Since PTH and its polypeptide fragments are partially metabolized by the kidney, parathyroid hormone levels also fall due to a decreased half life. The effects of renal transplantation on mineral metabolism in renal failure are summarized in Table IX. In addition, the potential untoward effects of acidosis and heparin administration on the osteomalacic component of the osteodystrophy disappear.

Thus with a successful renal transplantation, the pathophysiological aberrations tend to return toward normal. In most instances, renal osteo-dystrophic lesions heal over a period of several months. However, in some patients, particularly those with severe hyperparathyroidism, hypersecretion cannot be adequately suppressed despite years of normal renal function and high levels of serum calcium. Because of sustained hyperparathyroidism, phosphaturia and hypophosphatemia may persist. It is likely that the sustained hyperparathyroidism results from severe hyperplasia which can only be partially suppressed with hypercalcemia. Subtotal parathyroidectomy is occasionally necessary in these patients.

A selective phosphate "leak" in the transplanted kidney may also be present in some patients. Hypophosphatemia increases 1,25-dihydroxy vitamin D_3 production leading to hyperabsorption of calcium and hypercalcemia. In these patients the PTH levels are low. The treatment is oral

Table IX. Effects of Transplantation on Mineral Metabolism in Severe Renal Failure[a]

---

1. $\uparrow$ PTH catabolism by kidney $\rightarrow$ $\downarrow$ serum PTH levels
2. Phosphaturia $\rightarrow$ $\downarrow$ serum P $\rightarrow$ $\uparrow$ serum Ca $\rightarrow$ $\downarrow$ PTH secretion
3. $\uparrow$ 1,25-Dihydroxy vitamin D_3 synthesis $\rightarrow$ $\uparrow$ Ca GI absorption $\rightarrow$ $\uparrow$ serum Ca $\rightarrow$ $\downarrow$ PTH secretion

---

[a] $\uparrow$, Increase; $\downarrow$, decrease; GI, gastrointestinal; P, phosphorus; Ca, calcium; PTH, parathyroid hormone.

phosphorus supplementation. One or two capsules of Neutra-phos® (250–500 mg phosphorus) or 5 ml of Phospho-soda® (1 ml contains 129 mg phosphorus) two or three times a day may be used.

G. Effects of Treatment on the Lipoprotein Abnormalities of Renal Failure

1. Conservative Management

Patients with severe chronic renal failure develop a variety of lipoprotein abnormalities including high concentrations of the triglyceride-rich, very-low-density lipoprotein (VLDL) and low levels of high-density lipoprotein (HDL) cholesterol. The major cause for elevated triglyceride levels in uremia is an impaired rate of removal from the circulation by lipoprotein lipase. A number of therapeutic practices employed in the treatment of patients with renal failure may additionally alter lipid metabolism. Androgens, used to increase hematopoiesis, and propranolol, a β-sympathetic blocker used for hypertensive or anginal control, both elevate triglyceride levels through unknown mechanisms.

2. Dialysis Therapy

The lipid abnormalities do not improve with the institution of hemodialysis. Sera from hemodialysis patients inhibit lipoprotein lipase activity *in vitro*. The inhibitor of lipoprotein lipase may be a protein with a molecular weight in the "middle-molecule" range. One might anticipate therefore that peritoneal dialysis may improve the lipid abnormalities of uremia. Most studies have shown, however, that triglyceride levels in peritoneal dialysis patients are either higher than or the same as hemodialysis patients. This may be due to hyperinsulinism in response to the large amounts of glucose systemically absorbed from the dialysate, which may in turn cause increased hepatic triglyceride synthetic rates. Exercise training has been shown to improve the lipid abnormalities in selected chronic hemodialysis patients.

3. Renal Transplantation

Lipoprotein lipase activity is corrected with a successful renal transplant. However, high triglyceride levels may persist. The mechanism is controversial. Some studies show that increased triglyceride production rates, perhaps secondary to steroid-therapy-induced hyperinsulinism, are responsible for the abnormality. Others, however, have reported a defect in VLDL-triglyceride degradation despite normalization of lipoprotein lipase activity.

H. Effects of Dialysis on the Carbohydrate Abnormalities of Renal Failure

Chronic uremia is associated with carbohydrate intolerance. Although some patients have elevated fasting glucose concentrations, most patients have normal levels. Following a carbohydrate load, elevated peak glucose levels are observed in approximately 50% of patients with severe renal failure. Based on the findings of elevated fasting and peak immunoreactive insulin levels and an impaired glucose response to an exogenous insulin load, it has been suggested that this abnormality is due, at least in part, to insulin resistance. It is not clear which organ is primarily responsible for this defect. An impaired forearm glucose uptake in response to an insulin infusion suggests peripheral insulin resistance. Recently, increased rates of gluconeogenesis from alanine have been demonstrated in patients with chronic renal failure.

Many of the pathophysiological alterations of carbohydrate metabolism in patients with severe renal failure improve but do not entirely correct with chronic hemodialysis. Following a glucose load, the glucose and insulin responses return toward normal (Figure 10). The pathophysiological mechanisms responsible for this change are complex. Recent studies demonstrate

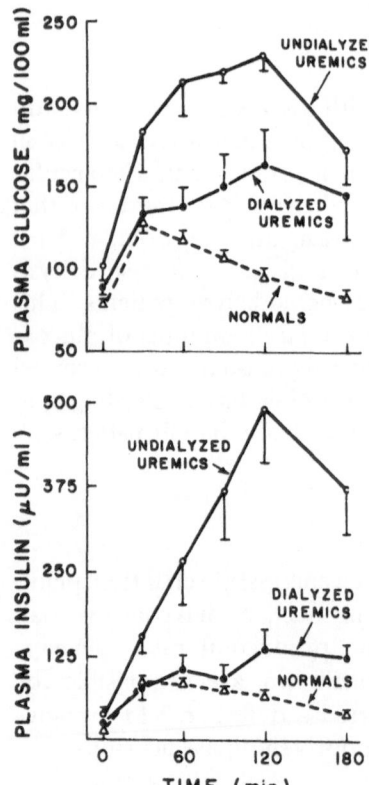

Figure 10. The effect of chronic hemodialysis on plasma glucose and insulin levels following an oral glucose tolerance test. (Reprinted with permission from Sherwin, R. S., *et al.*: Influence of uremia and hemodialysis on the turnover and metabolic effect of glucagon. *J. Clin. Invest.* 57:722, 1976.)

that the peripheral tissue sensitivity to insulin is improved with dialysis. Paradoxically, serum from both dialyzed and undialyzed uremic patients suppresses the insulin stimulated uptake of glucose by the *in vitro* rat hemidiaphragm to the same extent. This suggests that the removal of a dialyzable substance during chronic hemodialysis therapy may not account for the improvement in peripheral tissue sensitivity to insulin. Hemodialysis also decreases the rates of glucose production and gluconeogenesis from alanine but does not return them to normal.

Patients in severe renal failure are often on a markedly restricted diet and are inactive. These factors may also promote carbohydrate intolerance. It is possible that hemodialysis improves carbohydrate metabolism in part because of its indirect effects allowing improved nutrition and greater levels of activity.

I. Effects of Dialysis on the Alterations of Protein Metabolism in Renal Failure

Protein metabolism is significantly disturbed in patients with severe renal failure. It is likely that some alterations are due to the uremic process itself and some are due to malnutrition. Low-protein diets, decreased protein intake resulting from nausea or depression, and accelerated rates of protein catabolism secondary to intercurrent illness often result in a protein-deficient state. The hemodialysis procedure itself may potentiate this deficit. Approximately 5–8 g of free amino acids and 3–4 g of bound amino acids are removed during one standard dialysis procedure. If no glucose is present in the dialysate, 20–50 g of glucose may be lost during the course of hemodialysis. This loss may potentiate gluconeogenesis from protein catabolism. These losses can be countered with the institution of an adequate protein and caloric diet. An intake of 0.9 g of protein per kilogram of ideal body weight and 35 cal/kg daily will result in a positive nitrogen balance. Peritoneal dialysis results in losses of albumin. With four 2-liter exchanges per day performed during CAPD, for example, 5–10 g of protein may be lost in the dialysate. These losses may increase to 20 g/day if the patient develops peritonitis. Therefore a diet providing a 1.25 g of protein/kg per day is often necessary to promote a positive nitrogen balance while patients are undergoing peritoneal dialysis. A high caloric diet is usually unnecessary since most peritoneal dialysis solutions contain from 1.5 to 4.25 g of glucose per dl. While undergoing the peritoneal dialysis regimen described above, between 125 and 200 g of glucose are absorbed per day.

J. Summary

The clinical manifestations of severe renal failure result from the inability of the diseased kidneys to adequately perform critical excretory and nonexcretory functions. Many of these alterations can be controlled with the institution of conservative, dialytic, or renal transplantation treatment. By proper conservative management, certain excretory demands placed on the kidneys are lessened. Dietary salt, water, potassium, and phosphorus control, for example, may avoid the net accumulation of these substances in uremic subjects. Dialysis is basically an attempt to replace the excretory function of the kidney in those patients with advanced renal failure. However, the effects of dialysis differ from the task accomplished by normally functioning kidneys in a number of ways. First, on a weekly basis, it is far less efficient. The average weekly creatinine clearance via hemodiaysis is less than 10% of that of normal kidneys. Second, dialysis removes substances from the patient's serum based primarily on their molecular weight. This unselective process thus removes both potentially harmful as well as beneficial substances. Third, dialysis involves the net addition of substances to the patient's circulation. Some substances, such as acetate, are beneficial in that they help maintain acid–base balance. Other substances, which are critical to the performance of hemodialysis, such as heparin, may be detrimental. Furthermore, non-excretory renal functions, such as $1,25$ vitamin D_3 or erythropoietin production, are not replaced by dialytic procedures. Nevertheless, with adequate knowledge of the pathophysiological alterations in renal failure, these defects may be at least partially treated. Impaired gastrointestinal calcium absorption, for example, may be easily treated with calcium or vitamin D supplements. Unfortunately, some beneficial effects of hemodialysis are poorly understood. Why does carbohydrate intolerance improve on hemodialysis whereas lipoprotein abnormalities do not? Or more importantly, why do some patients feel well on dialysis and others do not?

Transplantation offers the attractive alternative of replacing both excretory and nonexcretory renal function to the patient. However, pathophysiologic alterations such as hypertriglyceridemia also occur in these patients. Presumably these alterations are due, in part, to the medicines given to prevent rejection of the renal allograft and the presence of one functioning kidney instead of two.

SUGGESTED READINGS

Textbooks

Brenner, B. M., and Rector, F. C., Jr. (eds.): *The Kidney*, Vol. 2. W. B. Saunders Co., Philadelphia, 1981.

Drukker, W., Parsons, F. M., and Maher, J. F. (eds.).: *Replacement of Renal Function by Dialysis.* Little, Brown and Co., Boston, 1979.

Early, L. E., and Gottschalk, C. W. (eds.): *Strauss and Welt's Diseases of the Kidney*, Vol. 3. Little, Brown and Co., Boston, 1979.

Friedman, E. A. (ed.): *Strategy in Renal Failure.* John Wiley and Sons, New York, 1977.

Morris, P. J. (ed.): *Kidney Transplantation, Principles and Practice.* Academic Press, London, 1979.

Articles

Bell, J. D., Kincaid, W. R., Morgan, R. G., Bunce, H., III, Alperin, J. B., Sarles, H. E., and Remmers, A. R. Jr.: Serum ferritin assay and bone marrow iron stores in patients on maintenance hemodialysis. *Kidney Int.* 17:237–241, 1980.

Blumenkrantz, M. J., Gahl, G. M., Kopple, J. D., Kamdar, A. V., Jones, M. R., Kessel, M., and Coburn, J. W.: Protein losses during peritoneal dialysis. *Kidney Int.* 19:593–602, 1981.

Cohn, S. H., Cinque, T. J., Dombrowski, C. S., and Letteri, J. M.: Determination of body composition by neutron activation analysis in patients with renal failure. *J. Lab. Clin. Med.* 79:978–994, 1972.

Coles, G. A.: Body composition in chronic renal failure. *Q. J. Med.* 41:25–47, 1972.

Cotton, J., Woodard, T. A., Carter, N., and Knochel, J. P.: Resting skeletal muscle membrane potential as an index of uremic toxicity. *J. Clin. Invest.* 63:501–506, 1979.

DeFronzo, R. A.: Pathogenesis of glucose intolerance in uremia. *Metabolism* 27:1866–1880, 1978.

DeFronzo, R. A., Alvestrand, A., Smith, D., Hendler, R., Hendler, E., and Wahren, J.: Insulin resistance in uremia. *J. Clin. Invest.* 67:563–568, 1981.

Fisher, J. W., Ohno, Y., Barona, J., Martinez, M., and Rege, A. B.: The role of serum inhibitors of erythroid colony-forming cells in the mechanism of the anemia of renal insufficiency, in Murphy, M. J., Jr. (ed.): *In Vitro Aspects of Erythropoiesis*, Springer-Verlag, New York, 1978.

Goldberg, A. P., Applebaum-Bowden, D. M., Bierman, E. L., Hazzard, W. R., Haas, L. B., Sherrard, D. J., Brunzall, J. D., Huttunen, J. K., Ehnholm, C., and Nikkila, E. A.: Increase in lipoprotein lipase during clofibrate treatment of hypertriglyceridemia in patients on hemodialysis. *N. Engl. J. Med.* 301:1073–1076, 1979.

Goldberg, A. P., Hagberg, J. M., Delmez, J. A., Haynes, M. E., and Harter, H. R.: Metabolic effects of exercise training in hemodialysis patients. *Kidney Int.* 18:754–761, 1980.

Grodstein, G. P., Blumenkrantz, M. J., Kopple, J. D., Moran, J. K., and Coburn, J. W.: Glucose absorption during continuous ambulatory peritoneal dialysis. *Kidney Int.* 19:564–567, 1981.

Guttmann, R. D.: Renal transplantation. *N. Engl. J. Med.* 301:975–982, 1038–1048, 1979.

Hodsman, A. B., Sherrard, D. J., Wong, E. G. C., Brickman, A. S., Lee, D. B. N., Alfrey, A. C., Singer, F. R., Norman, A. W., and Coburn, J. W.: Vitamin D resistant osteomalacia in hemodialysis patients lacking secondary hyperparathyroidism. *Ann. Intern. Med.* 94:629–637, 1981.

Hong, C. D., Kapoor, B. S., First, M. R., Pollak, V. E., and Alexander, J. W.: Fractional excretion of sodium after renal transplantation. *Kidney Int.* 16:167–178, 1979.

Hruska, K. A., Teitelbaum, S. L., Kopelman, R., Richardson, C. A., Miller, P., Debman, J., Martin, K., and Slatopolsky, E.: The predictability of the histological features of uremic bone by non-invasive techniques. *Metab. Bone Dis. Rel. Res.* 1:39–44, 1978.

Kim, K. E., Onesti, G., Schwartz, A. B., Chinitz, J. L., and Swartz, C.: Hemodynamics of hypertension in chronic end stage renal disease. *Circulation* 46:456–464, 1972.

Landsman, M. K.: The patient with chronic renal failure: a marginal man. *Ann. Intern. Med.* 82:268–270, 1975.

Linas, S. L., Miller, P. D., McDonald, K. M., Stables, D. P., Katz, F., Weil, R., and Schrier, R. W.: Role of the renin–angiotensin system in post-transplant hypertension in patients with multiple kidneys. *N. Engl. J. Med.* 298:1440–1445, 1978.

Lipchitz, M. D., Kischenbaum, M. A., Rosenblatt, S. G., and Gibney, R.: Effect of saralasin in hypertensive patients on chronic hemodialysis. *Ann. Intern. Med.* 88:23–27, 1978.

Neff, M. S., Goldberg, J., Slifkin, R. F., Eiser, A. R., Calamia, V., Kaplan, M., Baez, A., Gupta, S., and Mattoo, N.: A comparison of androgens for anemia in patients on hemodialysis. *N. Engl. J. Med.* 304:871–875, 1981.

Nolph, K. D.: Continuous ambulatory peritoneal dialysis. *Am. J. Nephrol.* 1:1–10, 1981.

Radtke, H. W., Frei, U., Erbes, P. M., Schoeppe, W., and Koch, K. M.: Improving anemia by hemodialysis: effect on serum erythropoietin. *Kidney Int.* 17:382–387, 1980.

Rosenbaum, B. J., Coburn, J. W., Shinaberger, J. H., and Massry, S. G.: Acid–base status during the interdialytic period in patients maintained with chronic hemodialysis. *Ann. Intern. Med.* 71:1105–1111, 1969.

Rosenbaum, R. W., Hruska, K. A., Korkor, A., Anderson, C., and Slatopolsky, E.: Decreased phosphate reabsorption after renal transplantation: evidence for a mechanism independent of calcium and parathyroid hormone. *Kidney Int.* 19:568–578, 1981.

Rubenfeld, S., and Garber, A. J.: Impact of hemodialysis on the abnormal glucose and alanine kinetics of chronic azotemia. *Metabolism* 28:934–942, 1979.

Saudie, E., Gibson, J. C., Crawford, G. A., Simons, L. A., and Mahony, J. F.: Impaired plasma triglyceride clearance as a feature of both uremic and post-transplant triglyceridemia. *Kidney Int.* 18:774–782, 1980.

Slatopolsky, E., Martin, K., and Hruska, K.: Parathyroid hormone metabolism and its potential as a uremic toxin. *Am. J. Physiol.* 239:F1–F12, 1980.

Van Ypersele de Strihou, C.: Potassium homeostasis in renal failure. *Kidney Int.* 11:491–504, 1977.

Wilson, D. R., and Siddiqui, A. A.: Renal tubular acidosis after kidney transplantation. Natural history and significance. *Ann. Intern. Med.* 79:352–360, 1973.

Wright, L. F., and Myers, W. D.: Medical management of home hemodialysis patients. *Ann. Intern. Med.* 89:367–372, 1978.

VI

Pathophysiology of Nephrolithiasis

This section contains a single chapter concerned with the pathophysiology of nephrolithiasis. It describes the incidence and composition of stones frequently seen in clinical practice. It describes the physicochemistry of stone formation, and the different entities responsible for the development of stone formation (hypercalciuria, hyperoxaluria, hyperuricosuria, cystinuria) are described in detail.

IV

Pathophysiology of Schizophrenia

16

Pathophysiology of Nephrolithiasis

JEFFREY FREITAG and KEITH HRUSKA

I. INTRODUCTION

Urolithiasis is a significant cause of morbidity with an incidence in the American population of about 1%, accounting for approximately one of every 1000 hospital admissions. For the United States there are "stone belts" (e.g., the Southeast) where the prevalence of urolithiasis is considerably higher. Because of this high incidence, urolithiasis is a major cause of patient suffering both economically (medical costs and time lost from work) and physically. Urolithiasis is a frequent cause of renal colic. The scars and urinary tract obstruction caused by urolithiasis may lead to chronic urinary tract infection and pyelonephritis.

Despite the frequency and morbidity associated with urolithiasis, most of the advances in the diagnosis and treatment of the underlying causes have been made in recent times. Even today, stones are often not analyzed upon removal or passage, diagnostic searches for etiology are frequently not performed, and the only treatment prescribed is a low-calcium diet and high fluid intake. This chapter is designed to outline the physical chemistry and pathogenesis of urolithiasis and to produce an awareness of the medical

JEFFREY FREITAG • Department of Medicine, Washington University School of Medicine, St. Louis, Missouri 63110. *Present address*: Saginaw General Hospital, Saginaw, Michigan 48602.   KEITH HRUSKA • Department of Medicine, Washington University School of Medicine and The Jewish Hospital of St. Louis, St, Louis, Missouri 63110.

advances in this area. Understanding these principles is necessary for the proper diagnosis and subsequent therapy of the specific disorders associated with urolithiasis.

II. DESCRIPTION OF TERMS

A. Crystals (Crystalluria)

Although crystalluria is often associated with urolithiasis, it can also be a common finding in normal urine. Its significance is that, in patients with documented or suspected urolithiasis, the identification of a particular crystal may aid in the diagnosis of an underlying disease process associated with stone formation. The discreet structure and characteristic form of crystals may not be readily apparent by routine light microscopy, and a more detailed microscopic examination using polarized light techniques may be required for crystal identification.

The site of crystal formation within the urinary tract is not known, but it is suggested that this occurs within the collecting system of the nephron. It is also unclear what size crystals or stones must be before they are retained in the collecting system and thus assume clinical importance.

Since the majority of stones from patients with lithiasis are composed of calcium phosphate, calcium oxalate, cystine, uric acid, or magnesium ammonium phosphate, these are also the urine crystals which the physician should be able to identify using light microscopy. Some of the characteristic forms of these crystals are shown in Figure 1. It should be noted that formation of many of the crystals is pH dependent, and determining the urinary pH at the time of examination will help in the differentiation of the various types of crystals.

B. Stones

1. Composition

Kidney stones are a heterogenous group with regard to composition and structure. All urinary tract stones have two basic components: crystal (crystallike composition) and matrix.

Stones vary in crystallike composition with age, geographical area, frequency of urinary tract infection, economic status, and date of study; therefore, any one set of statistics is only of general informational value. Figure 2 presents the composition of stones as compiled from several series reported in the literature. From these data several general statements can be made. The vast majority of all stones contain calcium (>70% and probably

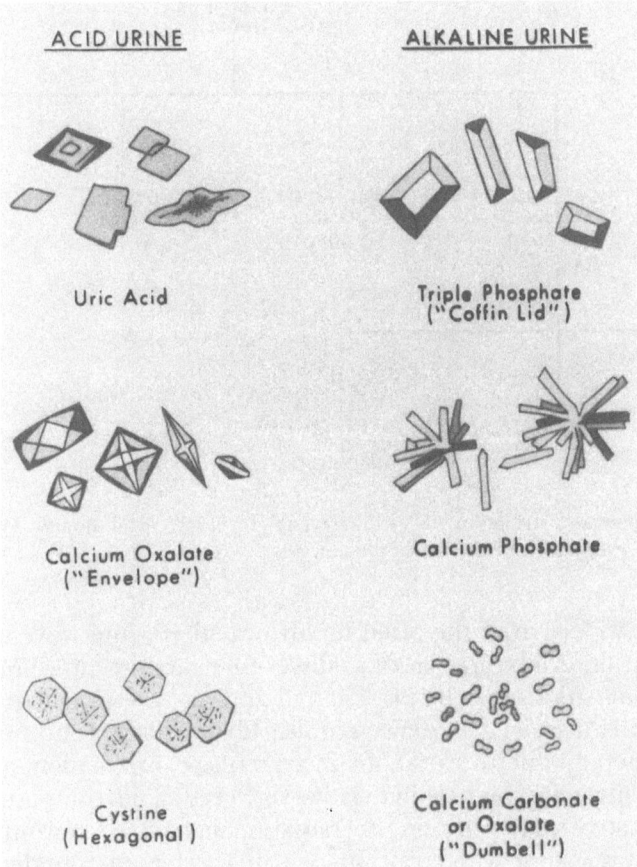

Figure 1. Drawings of crystals commonly seen in urine of patients with renal nephrolithiasis. These crystals may also be seen in normal urine except for cystine crystals, which are never a normal finding and diagnostic of cystinuria.

approaching 90%); approximately two thirds of these stones contain oxalate (as calcium oxalate), and many stones are of mixed composition. The incidence of triple-phosphate (magnesium ammonium calcium phosphate) stones, for practical purposes, reflects the role of urinary tract infection with urea-splitting organisms in the production of urolithiasis (see page 545).

The biochemical composition of stone matrix is predominantly mucoprotein with smaller amounts of nonamino sugars, glucosamine, and bound H_2O. The matrix protein contains no hydroxyproline and less than 2% proline, thus distinguishing it from collagen and elastin. The major protein in stones appears to be an acidic, low-molecular-weight protein (30,000–40,000) termed *matrix substance A*.

The relationship between the crystalloid and matrix composition of

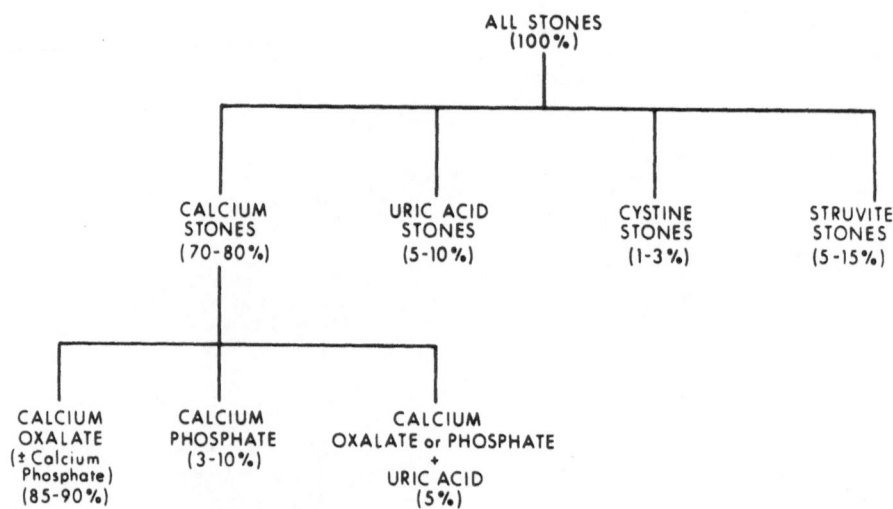

Figure 2. Frequency distribution of various crystal forms in renal stones. The data were compiled from several series reported in the literature.

stones varies widely from the often highly organized, interwoven pattern to a disordered intermixture lacking discernible architecture. Macroscopic concentric laminations may be present and appear to represent growth rings with the matrix arranged in dense parallel fibers. These concentric laminations are generally due to variations in crystal size, orientation, and density rather to changes in composition. However, crystalloid composition within the stone matrix may vary in its radial sequence. An example of this phenomenon is a stone with a calcium oxalate (center) surrounded by a shell of magnesium ammonium phosphate, reflecting the superimposition of urine infection on the underlying stone-forming process.

2. Stone Analysis

The first step in stone analysis is the determination of crystal composition since this is often the most important clue to the etiology of the urolithiasis. Stone analysis methodology should meet several rigid criteria: (1) accurate (with ability to identify substances as compounds); (2) sensitive (ability to identify small amounts of material from many areas of the stone); (3) semiquantitative; (4) discriminating (able to identify mixtures); (5) rapid, simple, and convenient; and (6) inexpensive. The methods available for stone analysis include chemical analytic methods, X-ray defraction, infrared spectroscopy, and optical crystallography combining the use of dissecting and polarizing microscopes. Only the latter method meets the above criteria and is the optimal method of stone analysis. It can present a topographic analysis of stone architecture and provide a time sequence of stone formation, especially for stones of mixed crystal composition. Of all the listed techniques, simple chemical qualitative analysis of stones provides the least information and should be discarded.

3. Areas of Formation

As for crystals, the exact location of initial stone formation within the urinary tract is not known. Several series indicate the collecting system (collecting tubules, calyceal system) as a likely site.

4. Metabolic–Surgical Activity

Stone formation varies among patients, even among those with the same disorder. Therefore, there must be criteria to determine the metabolic activity of stone formation if therapy is to be used and assessed appropriately. Urolithiasis is metabolically active when (1) there is X-ray evidence of new stone formation within the past year, (2) there is X-ray evidence of stone growth within the past year, or (3) there is passage of documented gravel within the past year. With previous X-ray evidence of urolithiasis, the absence of any of the criteria described above indicates metabolically inactive urolithiasis. In the absence of any of the above criteria and previous roentgenograms, the metabolic activity is considered indeterminant and the patient is followed with periodic X-ray studies until the true metabolic activity can be determined.

Passage of a renal stone or the development of renal colic does not indicate metabolically active renal stone disease. When patients with renal stones experience renal colic, urinary tract obstruction, or urinary infections secondary to urolithiasis, this is generally considered to be a urological problem and defined as surgical activity of the stone disease.

5. Stone Recurrence

The data suggest that recurrent stone formation is common with about one half of the patients having a recurrence within five years, and two thirds within nine years. However, recent data suggest that recurrent urolithiasis decreases with time and that remissions are common beyond the age of 50 years, especially in the absence of roentgenologic evidence of intrarenal calcification.

III. PHYSICAL CHEMISTRY OF STONE FORMATION

Development of a renal stone is a culmination of two related but separate processes. Initially, a solid phase nucleus develops in the solution (urine), and serves as the nidus for subsequent growth of the nidus by aggregation

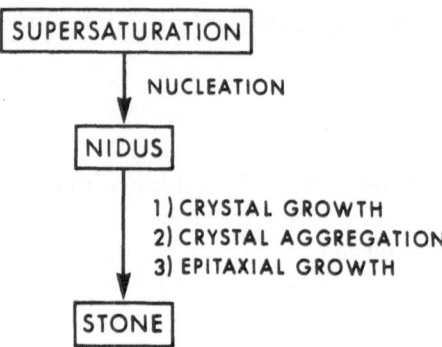

Figure 3. Schematic representation of the development of a renal stone beginning with formation of a nidus in a super-saturated solution through crystal precipitation (nucleation) and growth of the nidus.

of new crystals on the nidus. The end result of these two processes is the formation of a renal stone. As shown in Figure 3, the development of a nidus in a supersaturated urine is referred to as nucleation. Nucleation represents precipitation of crystals from the supersaturated solution which serve as the nidus for the stone development. Growth of the nidus is dependent upon crystal growth within the nidus, aggregation of new crystals on the nidus, and even the development of crystals of a different species in the nidus by the process of epitaxial growth. Nucleation may be homogenous or heterogenous. Homogenous nucleation indicates that the ion species precipitating from the supersaturated solution is the same species for which the solution was supersaturated. Heterogenous nucleation indicates that the precipitating species is different from the ionic species for which the solution was supersaturated. An example of heterogenous nucleation would be precipitation of calcium oxalate crystals from a solution supersaturated with sodium urate. The processes of crystal nucleation and nidus development depends on many factors. The major factors to be considered here are (1) supersaturation of the tubular fluid beyond its limits of stability, (2) inhibitors of supersaturation, and (3) promoters of crystal precipitation and growth.

A. Supersaturation of Urine

Supersaturation of the urine with various ionic species eventually leads to precipitation as urinary crystalloids and subsequent crystal growth, culminating in the formation of a stone. Urine and other solutions, saturated with an ion pair, are completely equilibrated with the solid (crystalline) form of the ion pair. The activity product (the product of the chemical activities of the two ionic species) of the solution at this point is equal to the solubility product (K_{sp}) (Figure 4). An increase in the activity product of a given ionic species above the K_{sp} (supersaturation) will eventually result in spontaneous precipitation (homogenous nucleation). At this level of supersaturation the activity product equals the formation product (K_{fp}) (Figure 4). For a given ionic pair (e.g., calcium and oxalate), the solution is undersaturated below the K_{sp}; unstable with spontaneous precipitation above the K_{fp}, and metastable between the K_{sp} and K_{fp}. Crystals of a given ionic pair added to an undersaturated solution of the same ionic species will dissolve; if added to a metastable supersaturated solution, they will grow. In other words, a metastable solution can support crystal growth (including epitaxial growth) and aggregation, but spontaneous nucleation does not occur. Various crystals of different ionic species with a structure similar to the ionic pair for which a solution is metastably supersaturated can induce heterogenous nucleation and result in crystal growth. Crystal growth via this latter mechanism is referred to as epitaxial growth (Figure 3).

The activity product of an ion pair in solution may be less or greater than its solubility product (K_{sp} in Figure 4), and may be expressed as a ratio (AP/K_{sp}). This is referred to as the activity product ratio (APR) and values less than 1 indicate undersaturation and values greater than 1 indicate supersaturation of the solution.

In addition to the degree of saturation, other factors which affect the solubility of an ionic species in a complex solution (urine) include its ionic strength, its complexation, the solution pH, and the flow rate of the solution. The ionic strength of any chemical is inversely related to its solubility in solution. Thus, oxalate salts as an ionic species with low solubility exhibit a high ionic strength. Many ionic species exist in solution in a complexed form. For instance, calcium ions are complexed with citrate ions in a molar ratio of 4 : 1, and in this complexed form do not contribute to the state of saturation of a solution for calcium. Urine pH affects the solubility of several constituents involved in stone formation as shown in Figure 5. The pH has important effects on the solubility of uric acid, calcium phosphate, and triple-phosphate salts. At acid urinary pHs, uric exists in solution largely as the undissociated acid. Undissociated uric acid is quite insoluble and readily precipitates from solution. This is the basis for urinary alkalinization in the treatment of uric acid stones. The deleterious effects of an alkaline urine in the solubility of calcium phosphate salts (calcium monohydrogen phosphate, brushite) are shown. Brushite is an unstable crystalline form and is rapidly hydrogenated to calcium dihydrophosphate (apatite), which is stable as a precipitate and is

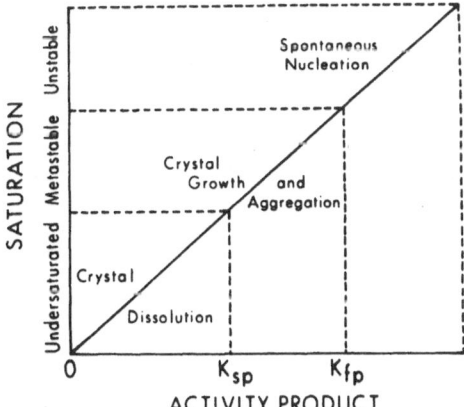

Figure 4. The relationship between the activity product of an ionic species and the saturation of a solution of the ion pair.

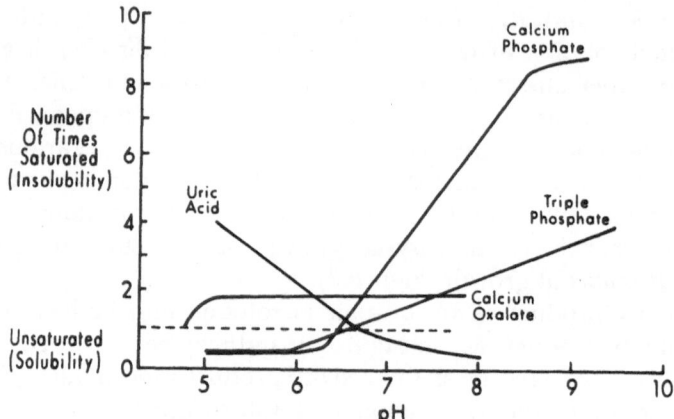

Figure 5. The effect of urine pH on crystalloid solubility.

a common stone constituent. Apatite is also the crystalline form seen on intravenous pyelograms when nephrocalcinosis is discovered. Triple-phosphate crystals are phosphate crystals associated with a mixture of ammonium ion (NH_4^+), magnesium, and calcium. Precipitation of triple-phosphate crystals results when bacteria present in the urinary space hydrolyze urea to ammonia salts in an acid urine. The ammonium ion is formed in high concentrations and results in precipitation of the triple-phosphate crystal. Thus, triple phosphate crystals are representative of urinary tract infections and are never seen clinically in other instances.

Stasis also favors crystallization probably because of its contribution of time to the process of stone formation. For example, the formation product ratio (K_{fp}/K_{sp}) for brushite *in vitro* decreases with increasing time of incubation (Figure 6). Stones which occur repeatedly from only one kidney suggest the possibility of urinary stasis in a hydronephrotic, partially obstructed urinary tract.

The urine of many non-stone-forming people is often supersaturated and, as noted above, crystalluria may even be a normal finding. When stone-forming patients as a group are compared to normal, non-stone-forming

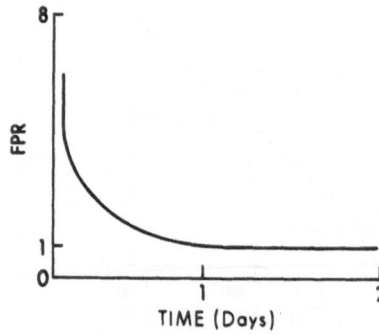

Figure 6. The effect of stasis on the formation product ratio (FPR) for brushite.

people, they have higher activity product ratios (APR) and lower formation products. The increased APRs may be due to their tendency to excrete more calcium. The lower formation products may be due to the presence of various impurities (heterogenous nuclei with the resultant tendency for epitaxial growth) or perhaps the absence of some inhibitors of stone formation (see below). However, the ability to determine APR and formation products is not widespread. The ability of these determinations to discriminate an individual stone subject from the normal population is not of great accuracy. Thus, the use of these measurements remains, for the present, as concepts in the understanding of the physicochemistry of stone formation.

A major role of crystal nucleation from supersaturated solutions is involved in the formation of cystine, magnesium ammonium phosphate, xanthine, brushite, and uric acid stones. Application of this pathogenesis to calcium oxalate stones has been more difficult because the excretion rates for both substances are often within the normal range in stone patients. Thus, in these patients the activity product ratio for calcium oxalate does not exceed the formation product, and invocation of nucleation from a super-saturated solution cannot be made. However, there is some evidence that short transient periods of supersaturation with calcium oxalate exceeding its formation product control crystal formation and aggregation. Furthermore, it may be that small changes in urinary oxalate due to its high ionic strength are more important than we can currently assess.

B. Inhibitors of Supersaturation in Urine

Since the capacity of urine to hold crystalloids in solution is greater in the presence of certain substances (inhibitors), inhibitor absence has been proposed to explain stone formation, particularly in patients with normal excretion of urinary crystalloids. Although normal urine may contain crystals, the crystals in urine from stone-forming patients tend to be larger and occur more frequently; and, as suggested earlier, this may be due to a deficiency of an inhibitory substance of growth and aggregation. The known inhibitor substances include citrate, magnesium, pyrophosphate, mucopolysacharides, diphosphonates, small peptides, urea, and pH (via its ability to decrease precipitation of various crystalloids by increasing their solubility).

Although some urine inhibitors (especially pyrophosphate) can retard spontaneous calcium phosphate precipitation *in vitro*, it appears that the major mechanism by which inhibitors decrease stone formation is by binding to the crystal surface and thereby slowing crystal growth and decreasing crystal aggregation. Pyrophosphates, magnesium, citrate, and other low-molecular-weight substances (less than 1000) are important inhibitors of calcium phosphate stone formation, whereas pyrophosphates and high-molecular-weight substances (10,000–20,000) are important inhibitors of calcium oxalate stone formation.

There are data to suggest that stone formers have less inhibitory substance in their urine. Consistent absence of any single inhibitor substance, however, has not been consistently demonstrated in a group of stone formers with a few exceptions. These exceptions are altered urinary pH in uric acid and magnesium ammonium phosphates stone formers and low urinary citrate in patients with renal tubular acidosis.

C. Promoters of Crystallization and Crystal Growth

Recent discoveries in the area of stone research concern the role that certain substances play in promoting nucleation of other ionic species and aggregation of urinary crystalloids. One such promoter substance is sodium urate. This salt of uric acid is present in the urine when the urinary pH exceeds 5.7 (pK_a uric acid = 5.7). The lattice structure of sodium urate crystals has similar dimensions to those of calcium oxalate, and several studies have shown that the addition of sodium urate to a metastable solution of calcium oxalate results in calcium oxalate nucleation and crystal aggregation. This observation may explain the clinical finding of a high incidence of hyperuricosuria among calcium oxalate stone formers and the decrease in the formation activity (metabolic activity) of calcium stones in these patients during treatment with allopurinol. Other substances may play a similar role as sodium urate in the promotion of heterogeneous nucleation, but have been largely discarded as being significant in stone pathogenesis. These include the matrix substance A of Boyce and possibly brushite ($CaHPO_4 \cdot 2H_2O$).

Other significant promoters of stone formation include urinary tract infection with urease-producing organisms and altered urinary pH. The former process results in increased urinary concentrations of ammonium ion, an alkaline urine, and the formation of calcium magnesium ammonium phosphate (triple-phosphate) stones. Patients with inflammatory bowel disease have a persistently acid urine, and they are prone to the formation of uric acid stones, owing to decreased solubility of uric acid in an acid milieu. In this latter example, the acid pH promotes stone formation.

IV. TYPES OF UROLITHIASIS

The etiologic classification of urolithiasis into types according to stone constituents is shown as follows: (1) calcium, (2) oxalate, (3) uric acid, (4) triple phosphate, and (5) cystine. The pathogenesis of clinical urolithiasis discussed below is based on these major stone constituents.

A. Calcium Urolithiasis

Greater than 70% of all stones contain calcium (Figure 2). Of the factors responsible for stone formation and growth, no single factor appears to be universally involved in calcium urolithiasis. Rather, it appears that some patients have problems with heterogenous nucleation and epitaxial growth of calcium oxalate induced by sodium urate, while other patients may suffer from lack of urinary inhibitors of saturation. However, in calcium urolithiasis, the most general problem appears to be supersaturation of the urine for calcium salts related to abnormally elevated excretion rates of calcium itself. Sixty percent of the patients with calcium containing stones will be hypercalciuric on a 1-g/day calcium diet (urinary calcium greater than 300 mg/day for males and 250 mg/day for females or greater than 4 mg/kg per day for both). Despite large variations in calcium intake (400–2000 mg/day), the urinary calcium excretion in normal people fluctuates very little (less than threefold) and does not reach hypercalciuric levels (Figure 7). On the other hand, hypercalciuric patients are characterized by an elevated fractional absorption of dietary calcium and their urinary calcium excretion increases markedly with increases in dietary calcium. Thus, while on low calcium intakes (400 mg/day or less), this latter group of patients may be normocalciuric and overlap with the normal population (Figure 7). Their separation from normal subjects can be achieved by increasing the dietary calcium to 1 g/day. Therefore, in the evaluation of calcium stone disorders the dietary history is essential to determine the significance of a measurement of calcium excretion.

Also the understanding of calcium excretion requires knowledge of the mechanism of calcium reabsorption. The renal handling of calcium by the kidney is very similar to that of sodium. Thus, of the 9–10 g of calcium filtered each day, fractional excretion is 1–2%. The bulk of calcium (60%) is reabsorbed in the proximal tubule similar to sodium, and possibly through the same mechanisms and pathways. This reabsorption is isotonic so that the tubular fluid to plasma concentration ratio (TF/P calcium) is one at the end of the accessible portion of the proximal tubule. Calcium reabsorption also occurs in the loop of Henle (20–25%), again in parallel with sodium reabsorption. Thus, calcium is greatly concentrated in the medullary portion of the kidney as is sodium by the countercurrent multiplier system. It is this medullary concentration that leads to the typical distribution of calcium

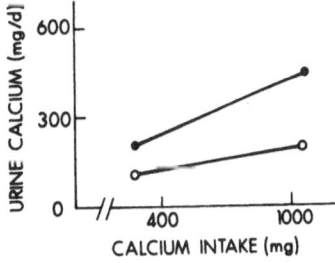

Figure 7. Influence of dietary calcium on urinary calcium excretion: normal (○) vs. hypercalciuric (●) patients.

deposition in the kidney in disease states associated with nephrocalcinosis. In the distal tubule, 5–10% of the filtered calcium load is reabsorbed, and here fine modulation of calcium reabsorption occurs. Here, also, calcium reabsorption can be dissociated from sodium reabsorption. Two means of producing this dissociation are the actions of parathyroid hormone and the use of thiazide diuretics (see Chapter 9).

Parathyroid hormone (PTH) increases calcium reabsorption in the nephron distal to the proximal tubule, while its effect on sodium reabsorption is minor. PTH causes a decreased reabsorption of both calcium and sodium in the proximal tubule, but most of the increased delivery of sodium to the distal tubule is reabsorbed so that the natriuresis is quite small. PTH stimulates distal tubular (and possibly thick ascending level of Henle's loop) calcium reabsorption and this leads to a fall in calcium excretion. However, PTH-induced bone resorption eventually leads to hypercalcemia, resulting in an increased amount of filtered calcium which subsequently overwhelms the PTH-stimulated increased distal reabsorption leading to increased calcium excretion. Thus, although PTH increases distal tubular calcium reabsorption, it may increase calcium excretion because of the increased filtered load of calcium.

The effect of thiazide diuretics is chiefly on the diluting segment of the early distal tubule. They decrease distal tubular reabsorption of sodium while slightly increasing calcium absorption, thereby resulting in an initial natriuresis and a decrease in calcium excretion. Chronically, mild volume contraction tends to minimize the natriuresis and enhance further the decreased calcium excretion by increasing proximal tubular reabsorption. The exact mechanism(s) by which thiazide diuretics reduce urinary calcium excretion is not entirely clear, but this effect is almost always sustained.

1. Hypercalciuric States

There are three general mechanisms of hypercalciuria: (1) accelerated bone turnover resulting in excess release of calcium containing salts into the circulation (resorptive hypercalciuria), (2) intestinal hyperabsorption of dietary calcium (absorptive hypercalciuria), and (3) defective renal reabsorption of calcium or phosphorus (reabsorptive hypercalciuria). Classification of the differential diagnosis of hypercalciuria based on these mechanisms is presented in Table I.

a. Nonidiopathic Hypercalciurias

Many of these disorders are also associated with hypercalcemia. As can be seen from the classification, disease states associated with increased bone turnover (resorptive) comprise frequent causes of hypercalciuria. Metastatic cancer and multiple myeloma must especially be remembered as causes of hypercalciuria, although urolithiasis is an unusual complication of these diseases. Vitamin D intoxication has dual effects on calcium excretion since

Table I. Differential Diagnosis of Hypercalciuria

I. Hypercalciuria associated with known disease states
  A. Resorptive
    1. Metastatic cancers
    2. Multiple myeloma
    3. Vitamin D intoxication
    4. Cushing's disease
    5. Sarcoidosis
    6. Hyperthyroidism
    7. Distal renal tubular acidosis
    8. Hyperparathyroidism
  B. Absorptive
    1. Milk alkali syndrome
    2. Vitamin D intoxication
    3. Sarcoidosis
II. Idiopathic hypercalciuria
  A. Resorptive
  B. Absorptive
  C. Reabsorptive
    1. Defective calcium absorption
    2. Defective phosphorus reabsorption

it modulates both active intestinal calcium absorption and bone mineral metabolism. Part of the effect of vitamin D on bone is the stimulation of the resorptive process. The mechanism through which adrenal cortical steroids stimulate bone reabsorption is not known, but hypercalciuria is seen in patients with Cushing's disease. Yet steroids, by their antagonism of the effects of vitamin D at the level of the gut, are useful in treating sarcoidosis where an apparent sensitivity to vitamin D results in hypercalciuria.

Hyperthyroidism is associated with accelerated bone turnover, osteoporosis, and elevated urinary calcium but progression to urolithiasis is uncommon.

Distal renal tubular acidosis (RTA) is associated with hypercalciuria and often results in nephrocalcinosis and nephrolithiasis (calcium phosphate). The renal calcium deposition is typically medullary. The basis for the hypercalciuria is presumably systemic acid retention which reduces tubular calcium reabsorption. There is also elevated calcium mobilization rates from bone, elevated PTH levels, and abnormal intestinal calcium absorption resulting in a negative calcium balance. Furthermore, patients with distal RTA excrete decreased amounts of citrate (a calcium chelator and inhibitor of calcium phosphate stone formation). Treatment of this disorder is correction of the systemic acidosis with bicarbonate which results in restoration of normocalciuria as well as normal urinary citrate excretion.

Hyperparathyroidism accounts for 5–10% of all stones in a hospital setting. Renal manifestations of nephrocalcinosis and calculi are the most common clinical symptoms of primary hyperparathyroidism, occurring in more than 40% of the cases in some series, while bone symptoms, radiologic abnormalities, and elevated alkaline phosphatase are only present in approximately 20% of the cases. The stones in this disorder are primarily calcium oxalate, although there is an increased frequency of calcium phosphate and mixed stones as well. The elevated APR and reduced formation product ratios for calcium phosphate and calcium oxalate probably account for the increased frequency of urolithiasis in this disorder; but other factors, such as the absence of inhibitors or the presence of promoters, cannot be excluded since many patients with this disorder do not form stones despite being hypercalciuric.

The milk alkali syndrome is a rare entity seen in patients who ingest large volumes of milk and antacids (especially calcium-containing antacids) for treatment of peptic disease. These patients are usually hypercalciuric and often hypercalcemic, and may present with calcium-containing stones.

b. Idiopathic Hypercalciurias

When all other causes of hypercalciuria have been excluded, there remains a large group of patients (40% of calcium stone formers) with normal serum calcium, phosphorus, and alkaline phosphatase levels who comprise the single most frequent diagnosis made in a stone-forming population—idiopathic hypercalciuria. Stones from these patients consist primarily of calcium oxalate although calcium phosphate and uric acid (generally mixed with calcium and oxalate) may also be present. Patients with idiopathic hypercalciuria all manifest mildly accelerated rates of bone turnover, intestinal calcium hyperabsorption and hypercalciuria (when on an average calcium intake of 1 g calcium/day). It is not entirely clear which of these defects is primary since the mechanism leading to one defect causes secondary adjustments in the others.

c. Resorptive Idiopathic Hypercalciuria

Resorptive idiopathic hypercalciuria has as its primary defect the increased secretion of PTH. The increase in PTH secretion may be insufficient to increase total plasma calcium, but plasma-ionized calcium may be abnormal. The pathogenesis of hypercalciuria is the combined effect of increased bone resorption and production of 1,25-dihydroxy vitamin D_3, resulting in increased intestinal calcium absorption (Figure 8). Treatment is subtotal parathyroidectomy. The hypercalciuria, however, may not correct postoperatively, and it has recently been suggested that some of these patients also have a long-standing, primary renal calcium leak (see page 537) that resulted in stimulation of PTH secretion which gradually became autonomous.

d. Absorptive Hypercalciuria

Absorptive hypercalciuria probably has as its primary defect the overproduction of 1,25-dihydroxy vitamin D_3 or an enhanced sensitivity to

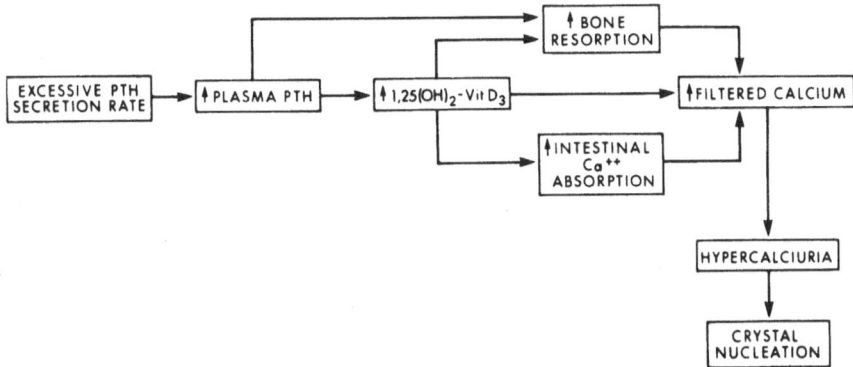

Figure 8. Proposed pathogenesis of resorptive hypercalciuria due to increased secretion of parathyroid hormone.

normal amounts of this vitamin D metabolite. This causes increased intestinal calcium absorption and increased bone turnover, both of which result in increased serum calcium (although not hypercalcemia), consequent suppression of PTH secretion, and associated hypercalciuria (Figure 9). Treatment should be aimed at decreasing calcium hyperabsorption through dietary modification of calcium intake and, as recently suggested, by the use of chronic thiazide diuretic therapy.

e. Defective Renal Calcium Absorption

Defective renal calcium absorption is a primary metabolic disorder which results in hypercalciuria with secondary increases in serum PTH and 1,25-dihydroxy vitamin D_3 levels (Figure 10). Here, thiazide therapy is the treatment of choice since it corrects the hypercalciuria with a subsequent return of PTH secretion and 1,25-dihydroxy vitamin D_3 levels to normal. This is in contrast to the effects of thiazide on patients with idiopathic hypercalciuria of the resorptive variety, in whom it produces frank and sustained hypercalcemia.

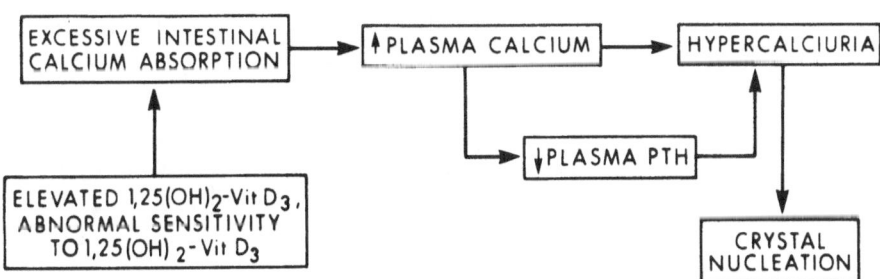

Figure 9. Proposed pathogenesis of absorptive hypercalciuria.

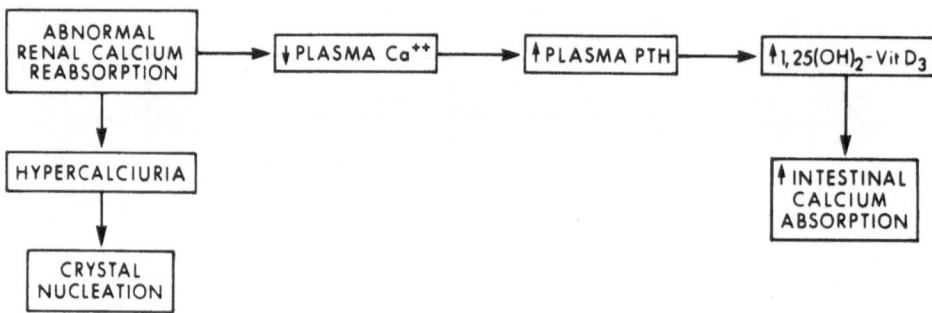

Figure 10. Proposed pathogenesis of renal hypercalciuria due to abnormal renal calcium reabsorption.

f. Defective Renal Phosphorus Absorption

Defective renal phosphorus absorption leads to low serum phosphorus concentrations and the subsequent stimulation of 1,25-dihydroxy vitamin D_3 production. This metabolite increases intestinal calcium absorption and bone turnover, both effects combining to result in hypercalciuria (Figure 11). Suppression of PTH secretion decreases distal tubular calcium reabsorption. Treatment with phosphorus reverses the phosphate depletion thus correcting the basic defect.

2. Normocalciuric Calcium Urolithiasis

Forty to fifty percent of calcium stone formers will not manifest detectable hypercalciuria on an average calcium intake, yet will form calcium oxalate or mixed calcium oxalate–calcium phosphate stones. Although the exact basis for the urolithiasis in these patients remains an enigma, at least four mechanisms have been proposed to account for this (Figure 12). Each of these mechanisms has some experimental data to support it and two (excess oxalate and hyperuricosuria) have clinical support as well.

The first possible mechanism suggests that these patients are deficient in inhibitory substance(s). As noted earlier, however, documentation of a

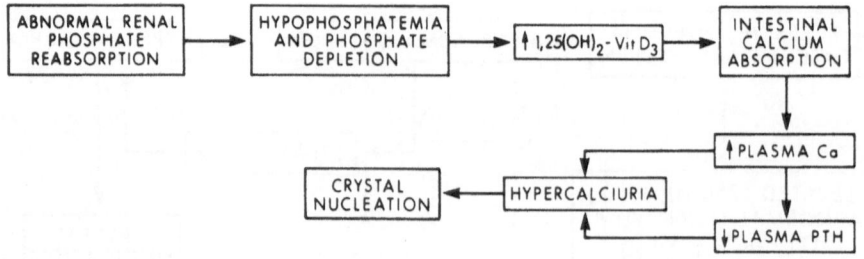

Figure 11. Proposed pathogenesis of renal hypercalciuria due to abnormal renal phosphate reabsorption.

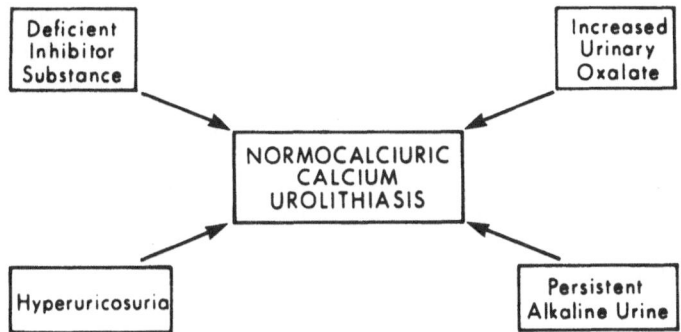

Figure 12. Pathogenesis of normocalciuric calcium urolithiasis.

consistent deficiency has not been possible. A second mechanism is the hyperuricosuria (commonly on a dietary basis) that some of these patients display. It may induce calcium oxalate stone formation by inducing epitaxial growth of calcium oxalate on a sodium urate nidus. It may also promote heterogenous nucleation although this has not been demonstrated clinically. That hyperuricosuria could be important in calcium urolithiasis is suggested by clinical data which show an apparent decrease in metabolic activity of urolithiasis in these patients when treated with allopurinol alone.

A third mechanism postulated to explain the calcium urolithiasis in these normocalciuric patients is increased excretion of urinary oxalate. Even increases of oxalate within the normal range may be important, since oxalate has a high ionic strength and is very insoluble as the calcium salt. This mechanism is supported by the clinical data which show that urine from these patients does have a higher than normal activity product of calcium oxalate and is often oversaturated with respect to calcium oxalate. Thiazide therapy has been reported to decrease oversaturation of calcium oxalate and to reduce the incidence of urolithiasis in these patients.

Finally, a persistently alkaline urine may favor the formation of calcium phosphate stones in some of these normocalciuric patients. This may occur because (1) periodically, urine may be normally oversaturated with respect to calcium phosphate, and (2) calcium phosphate solubility is decreased in an alkaline urine.

B. Oxalate Urolithiasis

1. Role of Oxalate in Calcium Oxalate Urolithiasis

About two thirds of all stones contain oxalate, as pure calcium oxalate or often mixed with other stone constituents. Most calcium oxalate stones occur in patients with no detectable disorder of oxalate metabolism or excretion but rather disordered calcium metabolism (hypercalciuric patients) or as part of the spectrum of patients with normocalciuric urolithiasis. Since oxalate is a metabolic end product, any oxalate absorbed from the gut (normally about 1%–2% of intestinal oxalate is absorbed) or produced endogenously requires excretion. Oxalate is completely filtered at the glomerulus and undergoes subsequent tubular reabsorption and secretion. The normal urinary excretion of oxalate is between 10 and 50 mg/24 hr. Because of its marked insolubility as the calcium salt and because of the high ionic strength of oxalate, conditions which result in hyperoxaluria cause calcium oxalate urolithiasis.

2. Hyperoxaluric States

The conditions (Table II) which result in hyperoxaluria do so either by increasing intestinal absorption of oxalate or by increasing endogenous oxalate production. A simplified scheme of endogenous oxalate metabolism is shown in Figure 13. There are two precursors to oxalate production, ascorbic acid and glyoxalate. The importance of ascorbic acid as an oxalate precursor is solely in those patients who ingest large amounts of vitamin C and have renal stone disease. Generally, oxalate is produced from glyoxalate, which is in turn produced from glycolate. Pyridoxine deficiency impairs the conversion of the oxalate precursor, glyoxalate to glycine, thus increasing oxalate production. Ethylene glycol markedly increases the levels of glycolate which have an end result of increasing oxalate production. The primary hyperoxalurias are autosomal recessive inborn errors of metabolism and are rare.

Type I primary hyperoxaluria is due to the absence of a thiamine-pyrophosphate-dependent carboligase enzyme resulting in increased urinary excretion of glycolate and glyoxalate as well as oxalate. Type II primary

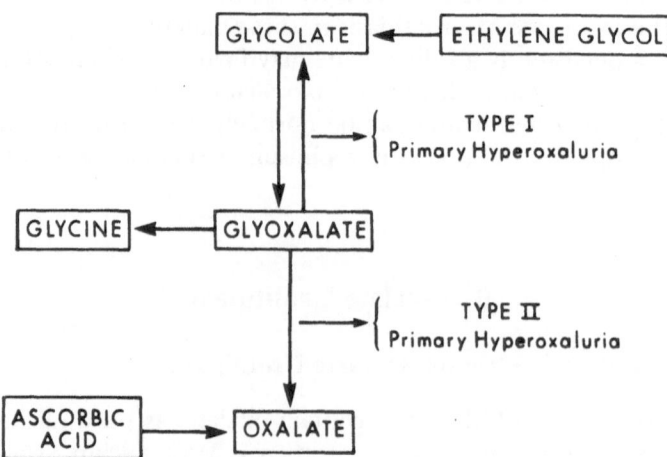

Figure 13. A simplified diagrammatic representation of endogenous oxalate production and the effects of known stimulants of oxalate production.

Table II. Known Causes of Hyperoxaluria

I. Increased oxalate absorption
   A. Elevated dietary intake
   B. Inflammatory bowel disease (Crohn's
      disease, ulcerative colitis)
   C. Intestinal bypass
II. Increased endogenous production
   A. Ascorbic acid (vitamin C)
   B. Pyridoxine (vitamin B_6 deficiency)
   C. Ethylene glycol
   D. Primary hyperoxaluria

---

hyperoxaluria has an enzymatic defect in the gluconeogenic pathway of serine metabolism and results in the excess urinary excretion of oxalate with normal urinary glycolate and glyoxalate levels. The enzyme defect results in increased production of L-glyceric acid, which has been linked to increased production of oxalate.

Enteric abnormalities (ileal resection of greather than 50 cm, inflammatory bowel disease, chronic pancreatic and biliary tract disease, blind loops, bacterial overgrowth, jejunoileal bypass procedures) are presently the most common causes of hyperoxaluria. The abnormality in these disorders is the hyperabsorption (probably colonic) of dietary oxalate, which appears directly related to the degree of fat malabsorption in these patients. The free fatty acids in the bowel lumen bind calcium, thus leaving more oxalate available for absorption. Also, abnormally high delivery of bile salts to the large intestine in these patients appears to stimulate oxalate absorption. The oxalate hyperabsorption associated with intestinal bypass may be reversed by the dietary use of medium-chain triglycerides, reduction of dietary oxalate, the administration of oral calcium supplements, or the use of cholestyramine. Finally, there is some evidence that hepatic oxalate production from glycolate is increased in these patients (Figure 13).

Calcium is an important chelator of oxalate in the gut and is probably responsible for the normally low intestinal absorption of dietary oxalate. Maneuvers which lower intestinal luminal calcium (e.g., marked dietary calcium restriction or use of cellulose phosphate in the treatment of hypercalciuric calcium urolithiasis) may have a paradoxical effect on stone activity because of the consequent increase in oxalate absorption.

C. Uric Acid Urolithiasis

1. Uric Acid Metabolism

Uric acid is the metabolic end product of purine metabolism and its production is determined by dietary purine intake, endogenous purine production, and the efficiency of purine conversion of uric acid. Figure 14 illustrates the major pathways of purine metabolism and uric acid production. Dietary purines, following several enzymatic degradation steps within the gut, enter the purine metabolic cycle as free purine bases adenine and guanine. Endogenous production of the parent purine product (inosine 5'-phosphate, IMP) results from two main pathways: (1) addition of glutamine to phosphoribosylpyrophosphate (PRPP) enzymatically by PRPP amidotransferase and (2) enzymatic conversion of the purine nucleotides adenosine 5'-phosphate (AMP) and guanisine 5'-phosphate (GMP). There is feedback inhibition of the PRPP amidotransferase enzyme by the purine nucleotides (GMP and AMP). Free purine bases of either dietary or endogenous origin can be reutilized to form their respective nucleotides. IMP, once formed, can be interconverted back to AMP of GMP or can proceed to hypoxanthine. Xanthine oxidase (XO) then catalyzes the formation of xanthine and subsequently uric acid. Hypoxanthine-guanine phosphoribosyl transferase

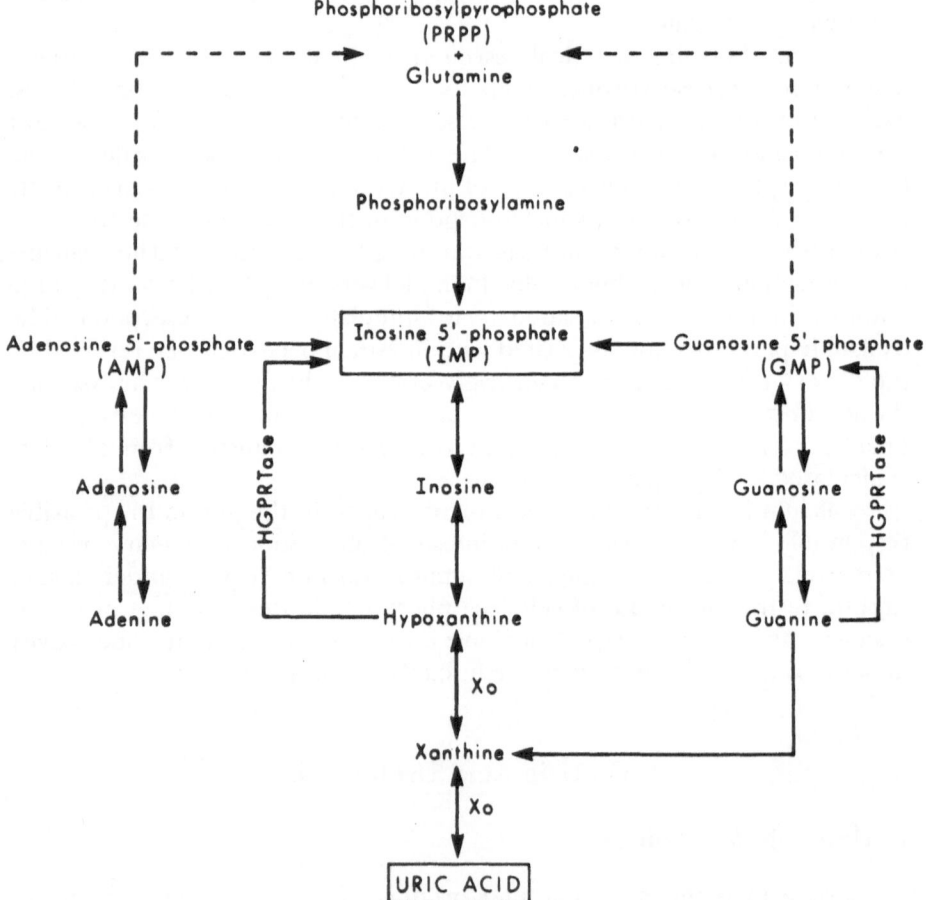

Figure 14. Pathways of uric biosynthesis—interconversion as indicated by the solid lines, inhibitory controls by the dashed lines.

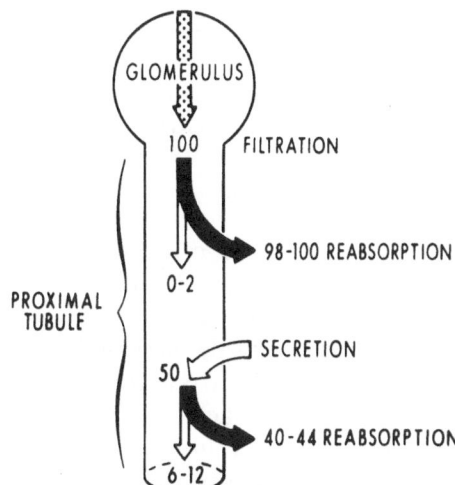

Figure 15. Diagrammatic representation of normal renal handling of uric acid. The numbers represent the percentage of the filtered load undergoing transport.

(GHPRTase) catalyzes the conversion of hypoxanthine and guanine to IMP and GMP, respectively. Inherited deficiency of this enzyme results in a self-mutilating childhood disease that is referred to as the Lesch–Nyhan syndrome.

The renal handling of uric acid (Figure 15) is complex and involves glomerular filtration and tubular reabsorption and secretion. Of the normal daily uric acid synthesis (750–1000 mg/day), about one third is secreted into the gut and destroyed by bacteria. Following essentially complete filtration at the glomerulus, the remaining two thirds of the daily uric acid load undergoes carrier-mediated bidirectional transport within the tubule, normally resulting in the excretion of 6%–12% of the filtered load (Figure 15).

2. Pathogenesis of Uric Acid Stones

There are three main determinants of uric acid crystallization and subsequent stone formation: (1) urinary pH, (2) daily uric acid excretion, and (3) urine volume. Uric acid has two dissociable protons, but only the first, with pK_a of 5.57, is of physiologic importance. Uric acid in the undissociated form is relatively insoluble (60–120 mg/liter), but, in the dissociated urate form, the solubility increases markedly (1580 mg/liter at pH 7.0). This was illustrated earlier in Figure 5. Because urate is so soluble, urate stones rarely occur. This effect of pH on uric acid dissociation, and hence uric acid–urate solubility, is dramatic and is an important factor in uric acid stone formation. Hyperuricosuria or decreased urine volume (increased uric acid concentration) may also result in supersaturation of the urine at a given pH (especially acid pH) but a small increase in urinary pH could easily negate both these effects (e.g., pH change from 5 to 6 could decrease the concentration of undissociated uric acid sixfold). These three determinants, hyperuricosuria, concentrated urine, absence of alkaline tide (see page 546), combine their effects during the night (sleeping hours), making susceptible patients especially prone to uric acid urolithiasis during this time period.

Uric acid stone formers can be separated into two general groups: (1) those with hyperuricosuria and (2) those with a persistently acid urine.

a. Hyperuricosuric States

Hyperuricosuria can result from increased endogenous purine metabolism (enzyme defects such as HGPRTase deficiency, lymphoproliferative, or myeloproliferative disorders), from increased purine ingestion, from renal tubular defects causing increased uric acid excretion (hyperuricosuria without hyperuricemia), or from the use of uricosuric medications. The overall incidence of uric acid urolithiasis in patients with gout is about 22%. Approximately 25% of gouty patients are overproducers of uric acid, while the remaining patients are normal producers but underexcretors of uric acid. The pathogenesis of uric acid stone formation in these latter patients probably relates to their tendency to have low urinary pHs. The mechanisms by which some patients with gout overproduce uric acid are not clearly defined, but increased availability or decreased utilization of PRPP has been suggested as a potential etiology.

b. Persistently Acid Urine

A postprandial alkaline tide (urine pH greater than 6.0) results from the excretion of excess bicarbonate generated as gastric acid (HCl) secreted with meals. This homeostatically appropriate alkalinization of the urine persists for several hours postprandially, keeping the urine above pH 6 throughout much of the day. However, as noted above, at night the urine pH decreases. Many gouty and nongouty uric acid stone formers have a defect in renal ammonium excretion resulting in an excess excretion of titratable acid, a lower urinary pH, and a loss of the normal alkaline tide. The reasons for this decreased ammonium excretion in this group of uric acid stone formers are not known. Suffice it to say that this excretion of a persistently acid urine places the patient at a great risk for uric acid stone formation.

Additional causes of a persistent acid urine excretion include various gastrointestinal diseases with diarrhea (due to dehydration and/or loss of bicarbonate), ileostomy (due to bicarbonate loss), and the use of acidifying medications.

Treatment of uric acid urolithiasis involves alkali administration to reduce urinary pH, adequate hydration, and use of allopurinol to reduce urinary uric acid saturation. Although allopurinol results in xanthinuria, xanthine urolithiasis is exremely rare.

D. Magnesium Ammonium Phosphate Urolithiasis

These are the so-called "infection stones" and essential to the pathogenesis of these stones is a prolonged urinary tract infection with urease-

(1) $H_2N-\overset{\overset{\displaystyle O}{\|}}{C}-NH_2 \xrightarrow[H_2O]{urease} 2NH_3 + CO_2$

urea

(2) $NH_3 + H_2O \rightleftarrows NH_4^+ + OH^-$

(3) $CO_2 + H_2O \rightleftarrows H_2CO_3 \rightleftarrows H + HCO_3^- \rightleftarrows CO_3^-$

Figure 16. Urease action on urea (1) and subsequent further hydrolysis (2 and 3).

producing organisms. The action of urease on urea and the subsequent further hydrolysis (Figure 16) results in an alkaline urine, supersaturated with respect to magnesium ammonium phosphate (struvite) and carbonate apatite $[Ca_{10}(PO_4)_6 \cdot CO_3]$. Subsequent crystallization yields the triple-phosphate stones (struvite plus variable amounts of carbonate apatites). For these stones to form, the urine must be alkaline as a result of the accumulation of ammonium hydroxide.

This type of stone accounts for about 5%–15% of urolithiasis in most series. Often it is difficult to ascertain the primacy of infection in the pathogenesis of a particular stone in a patient since infection can occur secondary to stone formation. Topographical analysis of the stone by optical crystallography (see page 526) will aid in the determination of whether the triple-phosphate component of the stone is primary or superimposed on an already existant stone of another etiology.

The aim of therapy in the treatment and prevention of triple-phosphate stones is acidification and maintained sterility of the urine. This is impossible in the presence of stone material. Since these stones, more than any other stone, tend to fill the renal pelvis (staghorn calculi), surgical extirpation is mandatory.

E. Cystine Urolithiasis

Cystinuria, an autosomal recessive inherited disorder, is a manifestation of a renal tubular transport disorder. This disorder affects the transport of the basic amino acids, lysine, arginine, ornithine, and cystine; and it is manifest in the small intestinal mucosa and the renal tubular epithelium. As depicted in Figure 17, the apparent reason for the cystinuria in this disorder is the inability of the tubular luminal membrane to reabsorb both the filtered and secreted cystine. Cystine, a metabolic product of dietary methionine, is the least soluble of the naturally occuring amino acids. The excess urinary excretion, as occurs in cystinuria, results in cystine urolithiasis and is a cause of 1%–2% of stone disease in the United States. The risk factors for the development of cystine stones include urinary oversaturation with respect to cystine as in cystinuria and an acid-concentrated urine. Treatment of this disorder is directed at reversal of the risk factors by forced hydration to minimize urine concentration, alkali administration to increase urinary pH, and the use of penicillamine to decrease cystine saturation in the urine.

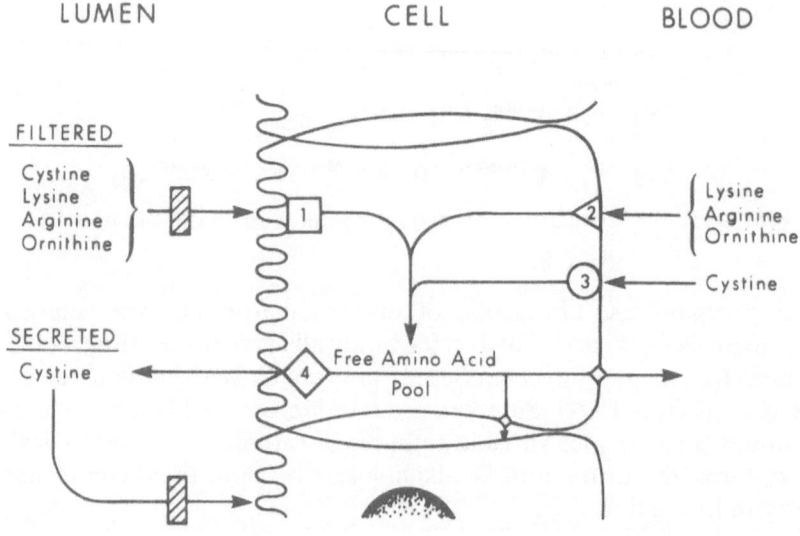

Figure 17. Schematic representation of the transport defect in cystinuria. Decreased uptake of both filtered cystine (1) and/or secreted cystine by the luminal membrane of renal tubular cells is proposed.

V. TREATMENT OF UROLITHIASIS

A. General Principles

1. Fluid intake

The most universal principle of urolithiasis therapy is to decrease concentration of the urinary solutes by increasing the urine volume. The volume required to sufficiently reduce solute concentration into the range of saturation may be quite large. Some patients find it intolerable to ingest the large amounts of water needed to sufficiently dilute the urinary solute concentrations, and this is the limiting factor in fluid therapy of urolithiasis. Therefore, high fluid intakes are rarely the sole treatment prescribed for urolithiasis, but attention to fluid intake is an important factor in the management of all patients. Most patients should be able to increase their fluid ingestion and thus the urinary volume to 2½–3 liters/day. This is a significant factor in successful treatment of a urolithiasis problem. Timing of fluid ingestion is important since it is necessary to break the normal cycle of urinary concentration. Normally, urine is most concentrated during sleep, and this is the most important time to add to the urine volume. A useful instruction is to have patients ingest 8–16 oz of fluid just before retiring. This is usually a sufficient volume to cause nocturia and prevent maximal urinary concentration. Additional fluid intake after awakening and voiding is also important.

The type of fluid used to increase urinary volume is important. Water is the most useful fluid. In most instances, fluids which will acidify the urine are not helpful since the acid load results in an increase in calcium excretion. Potassium-containing fluids may be helpful in patients who are taking diuretics as a primary treatment for urolithiasis. Finally, substitution of H_2O with carbohydrate-containing fluids should be avoided since carbohydrates have a calciuric effect.

2. Diet

Another obvious treatment for urolithiasis is the adjustment of the dietary intake of the substances related to the chemical composition of the renal stone. Historically, this has not been a particularly effective mode of therapy. However, with the advent of routine chemical analysis of the stones, and greater insight into the pathogenesis of certain stone types, important principles of dietary therapy have evolved. The role of the diet in each particular form of stone disease will be discussed below in the respective section for each stone type. Generally, unbalanced diets with excessive concentration on particular food types tend to be associated with urolithiasis. This is especially the case in the instance of purine intake and uric acid stones. Thus, a diet well balanced with each type of food is an important consideration for all patients with urolithiasis.

B. Specific Modalities of Therapy

1. Calcium Urolithiasis

a. General Principles

Increased rates of fluid intake are advisable for patients with calcium urolithiasis. Reduction of the urinary calcium concentration to normal, in a hypercalciuric subject with an excretion rate of 300–450 mg Ca/day, would require doubling or tripling of the normal fluid intake. This may not be feasible for many patients. However, all patients should be counseled as to the advisability of increasing their fluid intakes including ingestion of sufficient water before sleep to cause nocturia. Restriction of dietary calcium has long been advocated as a form of treatment for calcium urolithiasis. Its efficacy has been judged by controlled trials (Coe, 1977) and found to be ineffective. Its broad application over many centuries also leads one to the conclusion that it is not an especially effective mode of treatment. However, the ability to reduce urinary calcium excretion by decreasing dietary calcium intake in patients with idiopathic absorptive hypercalciuria is very clear. This reduction in calcium excretion should decrease the tendency for calcium salt precipitation and stone growth. Diets extremely low in calcium carry the risk of increasing oxalate absorption since much of the oxalate ingested in the diet is bound to calcium in the lumen of the gut. Also, a diet extremely low in calcium entails a long-term risk of aggravating or causing secondary hyperparathyroidism leading to the development of bone disease and dissolution of bone with release of calcium salts into the blood stream.

A reasonable dietary recommendation for patients with calcium urolithiasis which avoids the pitfalls of an extremely low-calcium diet is an intake of calcium in the range of 550–650 mg/day. This is easily provided with the simple instruction of providing one serving per day of a dairy product to an otherwise well-balanced low-calcium diet. This level of calcium intake will not contribute to dietary hypercalciuria, and yet it will be sufficient to prevent most of the side effects of a low-calcium diet.

b. Thiazide Diuretics

The thiazide diuretics have become the mainstay in the therapy for hypercalciuric calcium urolithiasis and may even be useful in normocalciuric individuals (Coe, 1977). Their ability to decrease calcium excretion chronically and to effectively prevent stone recurrence has been clearly demonstrated. This effect appears not to be limited to the cause of urolithiasis with the greatest rationale for thiazide usage, that of idiopathic renal hypercalciuria. Rather, thiazides appear to decrease calcium excretion in most individuals. For instance, they represent an effective mode of therapy for those patients with absorptive hypercalciuria. Their effectiveness is without decreasing the intestinal absorption of calcium or causing the development of hypercalcemia. Whether this represents actions of thiazides at sites other than the kidney or adjustments in calcium balance at the level of the bone or gut that have not yet been described remains unclear.

The side effects of thiazide therapy are generally not severe. They include hypersensitivity reactions including rashes, fever, and leukopenia, which are rare. They commonly cause hypokalemia, and if dietary adjustment of potassium intake is not sufficient to correct the hypokalemia, potassium supplementation is required. The initial sodium diuresis that accompanies initiation of thiazide therapy occasionally leads to extracellular fluid volume depletion and symptomatic hypotension. This side effect is usually overcome by temporarily stopping therapy and reinstituting it on a more gradual basis. Difficulties with impotence are also occasionally seen in male patients. Finally, the tendency toward hyperuricemia seen in patients on thiazide diuretics may present a problem in precipitating attacks of gout.

Use of thiazide diuretics as the major treatment for calcium urolithiasis requires several adjustments to be made in the diet. First, calcium restriction to 500–700 mg/day intake range may be employed as an adjuvant to therapy. Additionally, the diet should be enriched in sources of potassium. Sodium intake should be controlled in the range of 4–9 g/day. Higher intakes of sodium decreases the ability of thiazides to contract the plasma volume, and the hypocalciuric action of the drug is thereby decreased.

c. Orthophosphates

Inorganic phsophate salts have been employed for many years in an attempt to treat calcium urolithiasis, especially in hypercalciuric individuals. Currently, neutral phosphates (a mixture of sodium and potassium phosphates at a neutral pH) are usually used in doses of 1–2 g/day. The role of phosphates in preventing stone recurrence remains controversial. In the experience of Smith and Thomas, orthophosphate therapy has been effective. However, other investigators have failed to show a beneficial effect of orthophosphates especially in normocalciuric patients.

Orthophosphate therapy is accompanied by a reduction in urinary calcium excretion, but usually not to the same degree obtainable by thiazide therapy. The mechanisms whereby orthophosphates reduce urinary calcium excretion are not completely clear. First, as they cause a rise in plasma phosphorus and a reduction in serum calcium, parathyroid hormone may be stimulated and calcium reabsorption increased. Alternatively, in hypophosphatemic subjects, especially those with idiopathic hypercalciuria and hypophosphatemia, orthophosphate may increase the serum phosphorus toward normal and thus inhibit renal $1,25\text{-}(OH)_2\text{-}D$ synthesis and thereby reduce intestinal calcium absorption. The studies by Shen suggest that phosphate therapy works in part through this mechanism. In addition, orthophosphate therapy increases the urinary excretion of pyrophosphate, an effective inhibitor of calcium oxalate and calcium phosphate crystal growth.

Further studies need to be performed to clearly define the role of orthophosphates in the treatment of calcium urolithiasis. It should be noted that there are several theoretical risks to chronic phosphate administration. Most importantly, in patients with renal insufficiency, phosphate loading may contribute to the development of secondary hyperparathyroidism. Recent animal studies suggest that phosphate may accelerate progression of experimental renal disease. Finally, orthophosphate salts are cathartic in nature and may cause intolerable diarrhea in some patients. To the extent that accelerated loss of fluid through the intestine contributes to a reduction in urinary volume, the urinary calcium concentration may be increased and the tendency for calcium precipitation increased even though the total urinary calcium excretion is decreased.

d. Binding Agents

Cellulose phosphate, an ion exchange resin that complexes calcium, is the only calcium-binding agent that has been significantly tried in calcium urolithiasis. This agent is not generally available in the United States, but European experience with the drug is fairly extensive. Oral administration of cellulose phosphate enhances fecal calcium excretion by binding dietary calcium as well as calcium secreted into the intestine. Thus, urinary calcium excretion is decreased. The rationale of using cellulose phosphate therapy for absorptive hypercalciuria is obvious. However, the use of cellulose phosphate in instances where 1,25-$(OH)_2$-D synthesis is augmented by secondary hyperparathyroidism due to a renal calcium leak or other mechanisms may theoretically worsen the primary defect. In this setting, negative calcium balances and worsening bone disease would be possible complications of chronic cellulose phosphate therapy. Other studies have demonstrated that cellulose phosphate therapy is accompanied by increased urinary oxalate. This would offset the reduction in urinary calcium and lead to a change in cause but continuing calcium oxalate precipitation. The therapeutic role of cellulose phosphate thus remains unclear.

2. Oxalate Urolithiasis

Dietary oxalate is a ubiquitous food stuff. Diets very low in oxalate are usually unpalatable. However, it is fairly easy to avoid foods highest in oxalate content. A partial list of these include tea, rhubarb, chocolate, certain nuts, and certain green vegetables (such as broccoli, spinach, watercress, and beet root). Whether further reduction in dietary oxalate is indicated or not is open to question because of the normally low intestinal absorption of dietary oxalate which is in the range of 2%. However, in certain patients, oxalate absorption may be dramatically increased. These are patients on extremely low-calcium diets, those with inflammatory bowel disease, or those following intestinal bypass surgery. In these patients, dietary manipulation may be the mainstay of therapy.

Calcium salts have been used in an attempt to decrease oxalate absorption in patients with intestinal hyperabsorption of oxalate. However, its ability to bind oxalate is limited and its ability to reduce urinary oxalate excretion is not great. Additional modalities of therapy for hyperoxyluria in patients with intestinal hyperabsorption include control of steatorrhea by reduction of dietary fat. In patients with bile acid diarrhea, the use of cholestyramine or Taurine to decrease the glycine-conjugated bile salts have been utilized. The effectiveness of Taurine therapy has not been documented. In some patients, the presence of metabolic acidosis or hypocitric aciduria may be improved with alkali replacement in the form of bicarbonate of Shohl's solution. Some patients with intestinal hyperabsorption of oxalate and malabsorption also have magnesium deficiency. Replenishment of body magnesium stores increases urinary magnesium excretion, and magnesium oxalate is much more soluble than calcium oxalate.

3. Uric Acid Stones

In the population with gout, those with idiopathic hyperuricosuria and those with calcium urolithiasis and hyperuricosuria, a common finding in patients with uric acid stones, is a diet high in purines (Coe, 1976). Adjustment of dietary habits to a more balanced diet is usually very important in reducing uric acid excretion in these patients. However, since uric acid is a normal by-product of purine metabolism, endogenous production of uric acid may limit the usefulness of dietary purine restriction.

Inhibition of uric acid production by xanthine oxidase inhibitors, such as allopurinol, has become the mainstay of uric acid urolithiasis therapy. The drug is easy to administer since it requires only a single dose per day. However, it has frequent side effects which may be severe. These include exfoliative dermatitis, fever, and leukopenia. Finally, uricosuric agents should be avoided in patients with uric acid stone disease.

4. Magnesium Ammonium Phosphate Stones

High fluid intakes and urinary acidification may be helpful in patients with stones due to infection. However, the hallmark of therapy is successful treatment of the infection, which may require eradication of all precipitates. This is the case since urea-splitting bacteria may reside within the interstices of the stone, and thus may not be eradicated by otherwise appropriate antibiotic therapy. For this reason, antibiotics and surgery are intricately related in the successful treatment of infection stones.

The use of urease inhibitors to decrease the production of ammonia by urinary tract bacteria is a potentially important adjunct to therapy. Griffith *et al.* have reported considerable experience with the use of a urease inhibitor, acetohydroxamic acid, as an adjunct to antimicrobial therapy and in some instances for stone dissolution with long-term use. Urease inhibitors, in general, are not available for use independent of approved research protocols. There is also considerable interest in the use of irrigation with stone solvents for infection stones in the pyelocalyceal area. The most used stone solvent is a mixture of buffered citric acid and magnesium salts. One such solution, hemiacidrin, is marketed under the trade name Renacidin. Irrigation of renal stones with Renacidin via ureteral catheter or percutaneous nephrostomy tubes has been successful in dissolving struvite stones. However, frequent complications prompted the Food and Drug Administration to disapprove hemiacidrin as a renal irrigant. However, it remains available as a bladder irrigant. Considerable progress should be made in the near future regarding dissolution of various stone types by irrigation with stone solvents.

5. Cystinuria

Conservative management of cystinuria involves the general principles of increasing fluid intake, urinary alkalinization by bicarbonate therapy, and carbonic anhydrase inhibitors. In cases where conservative management is unsuccessful, penicillamine or α-mercaptopropionylglycine (Thiola) have been employed to form mixed disulfides with cysteine which are more soluble than cystine. The latter drug, α-mercaptopropionylglycine, is only an experimental agent in the United States. Penicillamine, although effective, has a high incidence of severe side effects. For this reason, the potential of a drug like Thiola, with fewer side effects, is very attractive for the future treatment of cystinuria. In addition, a recent report suggests that it may be used as a urinary stone solvent.

VI. CONCLUSION: SUMMARY OF PATHOGENESIS

No single pathogenetic factor can explain all the cases of urolithiasis. Rather, urolithiasis is a complex and multifactorial disease. The major risk factors for stone formation include hypercalciuria, hyperoxaluria, hyperuricosuria, inhibitor deficiency, and altered urinary pH. As discussed in the preceding sections, any one or a combination of these risk factors could predispose to stone formation.

SUGGESTED READINGS

General

Bordier, P., Ryckewart, A., Gueris, J., and Rasmussen, H.: On the pathogenesis of so-called idiopathic hypercalciuria. *Am. J. Med.* 63:398, 1977.
Coe, F. L. (ed.): *Nephrolithiasis*. Year Book Medical Publishers, Chicago, 1978.
Coe, F. L. (guest ed.): Nephrolithiasis, in Brenner, B. M., and Stein, J. H. (eds.): *Contemporary Issues in Nephrology 5*. Churchill Livingstone, New York, 1980.
Pak, C. Y. (ed.): Symposium on Urolithiasis, *Kidney Int.* 13:341, 1978.
Pak, C. Y. C., *et al.*: The hypercalciurias: causes, parathyroid functions, and diagnostic criteria. *J. Clin. Invest.* 54:387, 1974.
Robertson, W. G.: Physical chemical aspects of calcium stone-formation in the urinary tract, in Fleisch, H., Robertson, W. G., Smith, L. H., and Vahlensieck, W. (eds.): *Urolithiasis Research*. Plenum Press, New York, 1976.
Smith, L. H.: Urolithiasis, in Earley, L. E., and Gottschalk, C. W. (eds.): *Strauss and Welt's Diseases of the Kidney 3*. Little, Brown and Company, Boston, 1979.
Williams, H. E.: Nephrolithiasis. *N. Engl. J. Med.* 290:33, 1974.

Treatment

Coe, F. L.: Treated and untreated recurrent calcium nephrolithiasis in patients with idiopathic hypercalciuria, hyperuricosuria, or no metabolic disorder. *Ann. Intern. Med.* 87:404, 1977.
Coe, F. L.: Hyperuricosuric calcium oxalate nephrolithiasis. *Kidney Int.* 13:418, 1978.
Coe, F. L., Moran, E., and Kavalach, A. G.: The contribution of dietary purine overconsumption to hyperuricosuria in calcium oxalate stone formers. *J. Chronic Dis.* 29:793, 1976.
Griffith, D. P., Moskowitz, P. A., and Carlton, C. E.: Adjunctive chemotherapy of infection-induced staghorn calculi. *J. Urology* 121:711, 1979.
Griffith, D. P., Bruce, R. R., and Fishbein, W. N.: Infection (urease)-induced stones, in Coe, F. L., Brenner, B. M., and Stein, J. H. (eds.): *Contemporary Issues in Nephrology 5*. Churchill Livingstone, New York, 1980.
Halperin, E. C., and Thier, S. O.: Cystinuria, in Coe, F. L., Brenner, B. M., and Stein, J. H. (eds.): *Contemporary Issues in Nephrology 5*. Churchill Livingstone, New York, 1980.

Hayase, Y., Fukatusu, H., and Segawa, A.: The dissolution of cystine stones by irrigated tiopronin solution. *J. Urol.* 124:775, 1980.

Pak, C. Y. C.: *Calcium Urolithiasis: Pathogenesis, Diagnosis and Management,* Plenum Press, New York, 1978.

Smith, L. H.: Urolithiasis, in Earley, L. E., and Gottschalk, C. W. (eds.): *Strauss and Welt's Diseases of the Kidney 3.* Little, Brown and Company, Boston, 1979.

Smith, L. H.: Enteric hyperoxaluria and other hyperoxaluric states, in Coe, F. L., Brenner, B. M., and Stein, J. H. (eds.): *Contemporary Issues in Nephrology 5.* Churchill Livingstone, New York, 1980.

Shen, F. H., Baylink, D. J., Nielsen, R. L., Sherrad, D. J., Ivey, J. L., and Haussler, M. R.: Increased serum 1,25-dihydroxyvitamin D in idiopathic hypercalciuria. *J. Lab. Clin. Med.* 90:955, 1977.

Thomas, W. C., Jr.: Use of phosphates in patients with calcareous renal calculi. *Kidney Int.* 13:390, 1978.

Yendt, E. R., and Cohanim, M.: Prevention of calcium stones with thiazides. *Kidney Int.* 13:397, 1978.

VII

Renal Pharmacology

This last section contains a single chapter which deals with the role of the kidney in pharmacokinetics. The effects on the handling of drugs of renal insufficiency or heavy loss of protein by the kidney leading to hypoproteinemia are discussed. Another portion of this chapter describes the potential nephrotoxicity of drugs. In a separate section of the chapter the effects of drugs with a primary site of action on the kidney are considered. A special emphasis is given to the pharmacology of diuretic agents. This section should familiarize the reader both with the mechanism of action of drugs on the kidney and with the consequences of renal failure on the handling of drugs by the organism.

17

Renal Pharmacology

AUBREY R. MORRISON

I. THE KIDNEY AND PHARMACOKINETICS

The science of therapeutics of necessity requires a knowledge of the biochemical and physiological effects of drugs and their mechanisms of action. However, in the administration of a drug or drugs to man, consideration must be given not only to what the drug is doing to the body but also to what the body is doing to the drug. The dynamic nature of the events occurring subsequent to drug administration requires knowledge of the bioavailability, absorption, distribution, binding, metabolism, excretion, and elimination of the drug. Thus, the "drug of choice," its dosage, and its dosage interval can be profoundly influenced by concomitant administration of other drugs and disease states—factors which have significant effects on the absorption, distribution, and biotransformation (that is, the pharmacokinetics) of the drug.

A. Bioavailability

Chemically equivalent preparations which differ in their biological and therapeutic effects are said to differ in their bioavailability. This results from

AUBREY R. MORRISON • Departments of Medicine and Pharmacology, Washington University School of Medicine, St. Louis, Missouri 63110.

differences in crystal form, particle size, or some other physical characteristic of the drug preparation.

B. Route of Administration

The route of administration of a drug must be either enteral or parenteral (see Table I). Oral ingestion in the safest, most convenient, most economical, and most common method of administration. The major advantages of parenteral administration are as follows: (1) In emergency therapy the therapeutic levels can be attained rapidly and accurately; (2) in some situations parenteral administration is essential for the drug to be absorbed in active form.

C. Distribution

Most drugs are distributed throughout the body in the aqueous compartment. Unless the drug is one which acts topically, it must first permeate cellular plasma membranes and enter the blood where it will then reach the tissues at a rate determined by the physicochemical properties of the drug and by the local hemodynamics. The biochemical and physiological effects of most drugs are determined by the amount of drug reversibly bound to specific receptors in the tissue, and the concentration of drug in tissues is in turn directly proportional to the amount of the drug in plasma water. Figure 1 is a schematic representation of the fate of a drug in the body.

The apparent volume of distribution of a drug is the aqueous volume into which a drug is distributed. The calculation makes two assumptions: (1) that the body acts as a single compartment with respect to the drug and (2) that there is no metabolic degradation. Thus, the apparent volume of distribution is given by

$$V_D = \frac{\text{Total amount of drug in the body}}{\text{Concentration of drug in plasma}}$$

Table I. Possible Routes of Drug Entry into the Circulation

Enteral	Parenteral
1. Sublingual	1. Percutaneous
2. Oral	2. Subcutaneous
3. Rectal administration	3. Intradermal
	4. Intramuscular
	5. Intranasal
	6. Inhalation
	7. Intravenous
	8. Intraarterial

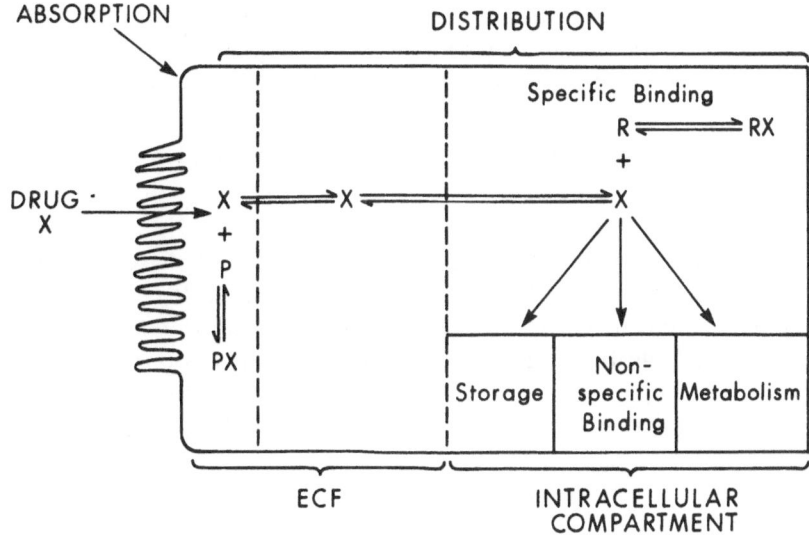

Figure 1. Absorption and distribution of drug X in body fluid compartments. P is a plasma protein and PX is a plasma protein–drug complex. R is a specific receptor, and RX is a receptor–drug complex. ECF is extracellular fluid. In the intracellular compartment the drug may be stored, it may undergo nonspecific binding, or it can be metabolized.

Weakly basic drugs actually accumulate in cells to slightly higher concentrations than in the extracellular fluid and thus have larger volumes of distribution. The converse is true for weak acids. This is due to the slightly lower pH intracellularly, pH 7.0, compared with that of the extracellular fluid, pH 7.4.

D. Protein Binding

1. Normal

Plasma consists of a heterogenous group of proteins in solution which have specific biological functions. These proteins interact with small molecules by ionic, hydrogen, van der Waals, and hydrophobic interactions. The metal-binding globulins, transferrin and ceruloplasmin, interact strongly with iron and copper, respectively, while the α- and β-lipoproteins bind the bulk of the lipid soluble molecules, e.g., vitamin D steroids and cholesterol. The major plasma protein contributing to drug binding is albumin. This protein has a molecular weight of about 69,000 and its isoelectric point occurs at pH 5. At concentrations of 4 g/100 ml and physiologic pH, 7.4, there are about 200 ionizable groups per molecule of albumin and it has a net negative charge. Nevertheless, it can interact with anions as well as cations. The binding of drugs by protein is reversible and often requires that the native configuration of the protein be intact.

If a drug is able to combine with n sites on each protein molecule with the same affinity in the absence of positive or negative cooperativity, then the kinetics of that interaction are defined by the law of mass action:

$$\underset{(D)}{\text{Drug}} + \underset{(nP)}{\text{protein}} \underset{K_2}{\overset{K_1}{\rightleftharpoons}} \underset{(DP)}{\text{Drug–protein complex}}$$

Since plasma proteins to a large extent remain in the vascular compartment, the intensity of the effect of any reversibly acting drug will be related to its concentration in plasma water, that is, free drug (D). Changes in nP, that is, the available binding sites on protein, will increase or decrease the drug protein complex (DP), thus decreasing or increasing the amount of free drug (D) available for specific binding to target receptors.

2. In Uremia

In patients with a marked reduction in renal function there is a decreased binding of many drugs to their plasma proteins. This is especially true for acidic or anionic drugs (low pK_a) (see Table II). Drugs of this type usually bind to one site on the albumin molecule. Drugs that are organic bases (high pK_a) may have normal or decreased binding (see Table III). Some of the basic drugs which have normal binding, such as quinidine, have more than one binding site on albumin, while drugs such as diazepam (basic), which have decreased binding in uremia, appear to bind primarily to one site on albumin. Two hypotheses have been advanced to explain the alterations of protein binding in uremia: (1) in uremia small molecules are retained which competitively displace drugs from normal binding sites and (2) there are changes in the albumin molecule itself which alter the binding sites qualita-

Table II. Binding of Acidic Drugs to Plasma Proteins in Uremic Patients

Drug	Binding
Sulfonamides	Decreased
Phenytoin	Decreased
Thyroxine	Decreased
Clofibrate	Decreased
Salicylate	Decreased
Benzylpenicillin	Decreased
Dicloxacillin	Decreased
Barbiturates	Decreased
Diazoxide	Decreased
Phenylbutazone	Decreased
Warfarin	Decreased
Furosemide	Decreased
Indomethacin	Normal

Table III. Binding of Basic Drugs to
Plasma Proteins in Uremic Patients

Drug	Binding
Desmethylimipramine	Normal
Quinidine	Normal
Dapsone	Normal
Triamterene	Decreased
Trimethoprim	Normal
Morphine	Slight decrease
Propranolol	Normal
Diazepam	Decreased
d-Tubocurarine	Normal

tively or quantitatively. There is good evidence supporting both mechanisms and in all probability both operate to differing degrees in different patients.

While the pharmacokinetic consequences of impaired plasma protein binding are readily discernible, the clinical consequences are more difficult to predict. On the one hand, the higher fraction of unbound drug, more intense effects and an increased incidence of adverse effects could be expected. On the other hand, impaired binding may also lead to enhanced clearance since some elimination processes follow first-order kinetics. Thus, elimination proceeds at rates proportional to unbound levels of drug. Of special interest to this chapter is the situation where the drug is eliminated via renal routes and there is impairment of renal function; this will be discussed later. Since the total available binding sites on plasma albumin will be reduced in the nephrotic syndrome, this becomes another clinical condition in which the steady state level of drug may be altered necessitating alterations in dosage interval or total drug administered.

E. Drug Elimination by the Kidney

The major routes of drug elimination are metabolism and excretion. Drugs are eliminated either unchanged or as metabolites. In general, more polar compounds are excreted unchanged while the less polar lipid soluble drugs are not readily eliminated until they are metabolized to more polar, less lipid soluble compounds.

Of the organs involved in excretion of drugs and their metabolites, the kidneys are the most important.

F. Clearance

The renal excretion mechanisms consist of glomerular filtration, tubular secretion, and any combination thereof. The concept of clearance is used to describe the elimination of a drug by the kidney. By definition the clearance of a drug is the volume of plasma perfusing the kidney that is cleared of the drug per unit time.

Thus, the renal clearance of drug (D) is given by the formula

$$C_D = \frac{U_D \times V}{P_D}$$

where U_D is urine concentration of drug, V is urine flow rate per min, and P_D is the concentration of the drug in plasma water.

It is also useful to consider the term *extraction ratio*, which is defined as the ratio of renal clearance to renal blood flow. When the extraction ratio is low, the drug is predominantly cleared by glomerular filtration and its renal clearance is sensitive to changes in binding by plasma proteins, whereas when the extraction ratio is high and approximates unity, the drug is cleared predominantly by tubular secretion and the clearance is very much affected by changes in renal blood flow and not by changes in binding to proteins. The renal excretory mechanisms which represent glomerular filtration, tubular secretion, and reabsorption may have the net effect of removing a constant fraction of drug presented to it. Stated in another way, the excretion rate is proportional to the plasma concentration (first-order kinetics). While the renal clearance of a drug gives information as to the amount of drug excreted in the urine per minute, the total clearance of the drug is obviously the sum of hepatic and renal clearances plus contributions from any other organs eliminating the drug(s), e.g., in sweat or milk.

For the clinician wishing to adjust drug dosages in patients with impaired renal function it becomes important to determine the extent to which the plasma concentration of the drug is altered by changes in the renal excretory process.

The relationship between renal clearance and overall elimination is thus of some importance.

Let K_E be the rate constant of elimination defined by the first-order equations $dc/cf = K_E C$, where C is concentration of drug in plasma water and V_D is the apparent volume of distribution. Then

$$K_E = \frac{\text{Clearance}}{V_D}$$

The half-life of an exponential process ($t_{1/2}$) is given by $0.693/K_E$. Therefore the elimination half-time for a drug excreted by the kidneys will be

$$t_{1/2} = 0.693 \, \frac{V_D}{\text{Clearance}}$$

From this relationship it can be seen that increases in volume of distribution or decreases in clearance can increase $t_{1/2}$, and conversely decreases in volume of distribution and increases in clearance will decrease $t_{1/2}$. Since V_D and clearance are potentially independent of each other, then the $t_{1/2}$ will depend on the ratio of these two parameters.

As indicated previously, the renal clearance of drugs depends on the net effects of glomerular filtration, tubular secretion, and tubular reabsorption.

Clearance of a drug by glomerular filtration is dependent on its concentration in plasma water and is very sensitive to changes in protein binding. On the other hand, for drugs excreted by tubular secretory processes, provided the binding to proteins is reversible, it makes no difference what fraction is bound to plasma proteins.

G. Tubular Secretion

Two types of renal secretory transport systems are present: (1) organic acid transport (e.g., penicillin, probenecid, hippurates, esters, glucuronides) and (2) organic base transport (e.g., procaine, mecamylamine). These transport systems are separate, energy dependent, and blocked by metabolic inhibitors (e.g., 2,4-dinitrophenol).

In newborn infants and especially premature infants there is underdevelopment of the renal tubular secretory mechanisms. In addition, there is low renal blood flow and glomerular filtration. Both of these conditions then can markedly reduce the renal clearance of drugs either excreted by glomerular filtration or by the transport systems. Such effects on drug metabolism in the neonatal and pediatric age groups are of great importance and concern to the clinician and underscore the importance of monitoring blood levels of drugs in these patients.

The pH of the urine is maintained within a range of 4.5–8.0. Marked acidification of the urine takes place in the distal tubule, which is a "tight" epithelium and can establish steep H^+ gradients between lumen and renal tubular cell ($\approx 1000:1$). The pH of the luminal fluid may, therefore, affect the ionic state of drugs in the lumen and thus have profound effects on the rate of drug excretion. Since the nonionized form of a weak acid or base can permeate biological membranes with much greater facility than charged ionic species, then an acid urine will increase the absorption of weak acids whose pK_a is in the neutral range and promote excretion of weak bases with pK_a values in the same range. By the same token, the urinary excretion of such drugs as phenobarbital (pK_a 7.2), acetyl salicylic acid (pK_a 3.5), and probenecid (pK_a 3.3) are markedly increased by procedures that increase urinary pH.

The ratio of ionized to nonionized species of a drug is dictated by the Henderson–Hasselbalch equation $pH = pK_a + \log (A)/(HA)$, where (A) is the concentration of ionized drug and (HA) the concentration of the nonionized species. Figure 2 shows the pK_a of some drugs.

H. Clearance by Dialysis

The same principles that govern elimination of drugs cleared predominantly by glomerular filtration govern the clearance of drugs by dialysis, that is, across artificial membranes (see Chapter 15). Thus, drugs that have

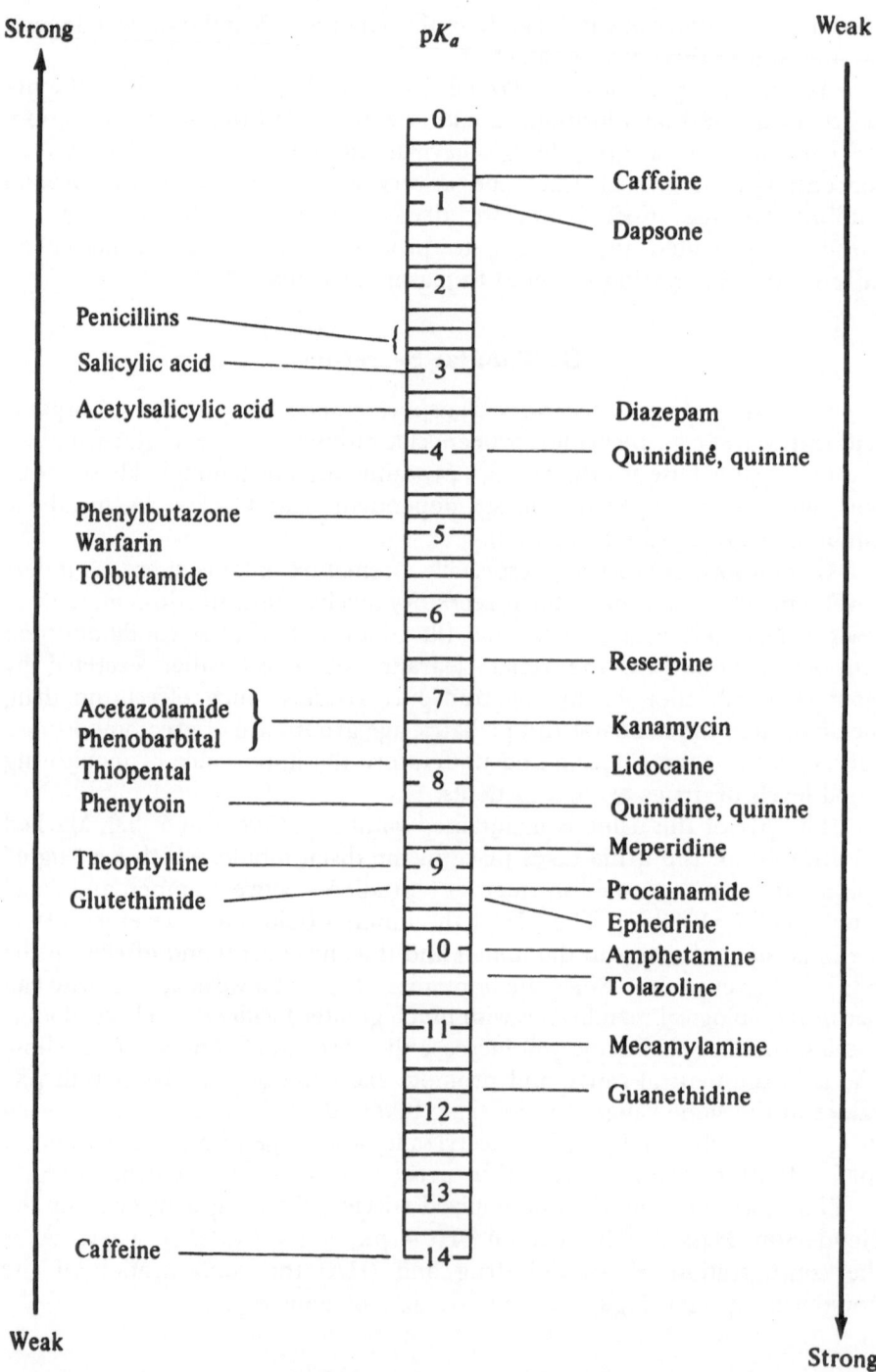

Figure 2. pK$_a$ values of a few acidic and basic drugs. Some of these drugs, like penicillin and acetylsalicylic acid (aspirin), are relatively strong acids. Others, like acetazolamide (diamox) or phenobarbital, are relatively weak acids at the pH of plasma (7.4). The same applies to some of the basic drugs.

Table IV. Drugs Usually Requiring Supplemental Dosage after
Dialysis

I. Antibiotics
  A. Aminoglycosides: streptomycin, kanamycin, gentamycin,
     tobramycin
  B. Cephalosporins: cephalothin, cephalexin, cephapirin, cephazolin
  C. Penicillins: penicillin, ampicillin, carbenicillin
  D. Other antibiotics: sulfonamides, chloramphenicol, trimethoprim,
     cycloserine, ethambutol, 5-fluorocytosine
II. Vasoactive drugs: aminophyline, methyldopa, procainamide
III. Immunosuppressive–chemotherapeutic agents: methotrexate, 5-
     fluorouracil, cyclophosphamide
IV. Miscellaneous: salicylates, phenobarbital

---

a large volume of distribution, e.g., propoxyhene, glutethemide, and digoxin, which have either high lipid partition coefficients or are significantly tissue bound, are not effectively cleared by dialysis. This would occur even through the dialyzer clearance may be high. The same observation obtains if a drug is very highly protein bound. Therefore, in considering dialysis for patients with drug overdoses several features must be taken into account in determining the efficiency of drug removal from the body: (1) volume of distribution, (2) degree of binding to plasma proteins, and (3) hematocrit (which influences the percentage of plasma water per volume of blood).

These same considerations must be borne in mind for patients undergoing chronic dialysis in whom a therapeutic regimen is instituted. Table IV shows a few drugs usually requiring supplemental drug dosage after dialysis.

I. Drug Metabolism

While an appropriate response to a drug in renal failure is most often a consequence of altered excretion, it must be borne in mind that the majority of drugs are not excreted unchanged. They are biotransformed to metabolites which are then excreted. Thus, renal failure may have significant effects on the rates of biotransformation of drugs. It has been observed that some drug oxidations that occur in the hepatic endoplasmic reticulum are accelerated in uremia, thus necessitating increased dosage of these drugs. While the mechanisms responsible for these pharmacokinetic observations are not known with certainty, they may in part be related to decreased plasma protein binding. On the other hand, other aspects of drug metabolism such as reductions and hydrolysis of ester linkages appear to be slowed. Thus, drug metabolism may be normal, accelerated, or slowed in uremic man, and the effects of uremia depend on the specific pathway of drug metabolism being studied.

J. Drug Regimen in Renal Disease

In uremia, therefore, the dosage of drug may need to be altered. The two basic mechanisms by which this is accomplished are (1) alteration in drug dosage and (2) alteration in dosage interval. In drugs which require a fairly constant plasma level the alteration of the drug dosage rather than the interval is to be recommended. Thus, if the clearance and site of elimination are known, it should be possible to predict and anticipate the influence of site of administration, protein and tissue binding, and hemodynamics in the disposition and kinetics of the drug. Unfortunately, there are no easy clinical tests which allow one to calculate the metabolic clearance of a drug; thus, it becomes very difficult to predict changes in the $t_{1/2}$ of a drug eliminated primarily by metabolism. However, in drugs eliminated predominantly by the kidney the $t_{1/2}$ of the drug determined under normal conditions may serve as a point from which to determine alterations in the $t_{1/2}$ when renal function is decreased. Bennett *et al.* have a useful table for drug modification in renal disease. Where the therapeutic level is critical and variability in metabolic clearance is expected, the plasma concentration of drug should be determined.

II. DRUG NEPHROTOXICITY

Drugs may influence renal function by directly or indirectly influencing renal hemodynamics, thus decreasing renal blood flow and glomerular filtration rate (GFR) per nephron. These effects can be considered prerenal when they have their effects on decreasing peripheral resistance and blood pressure or decreasing cardiac output. In addition, drugs like diuretics may decrease GFR by causing reduction of intravascular volume secondary to increased sodium and water excretion in the urine. Under these circumstances, there may be a decrease in GFR and renal function, without any intrinsic renal damage. On the other hand, certain drugs, like acetominophen, radiocontrast agents, cephalosporins and cephaloridine, aspirin, amphotericin B, and aminoglycosides, may cause direct toxic effects to renal tubular epithelium with consequent disorders of tubular function and decrease in GFR.

A. Direct Toxicities

The kidney contains an active microsomal system capable of metabolically activating drugs. In addition, the kidney receives 20%–25% of total cardiac output and contains elaborate transport processes for secretion and reabsorption. Thus, very high concentrations of certain drugs may be obtained in the renal parenchyma.

It has become evident that when the kidney oxidizes certain drugs, e.g., acetominophen, through the cytochrome P450 system (mixed-function oxidase), the reaction generates an alkylating or arylating intermediate which can then through nucleophilic attack on cell macromolecules eventually lead to cell death. Renal glutathione can be protective by combining with the nucleophilic metabolites and inactivating them. Thus, toxicity under these circumstances occurs when kidney glutathione is depleted or when the dose of acetominophen is large enough to exceed the glutathione available for detoxicification.

Cephaloridine also produces nephrotoxicity by a toxic intermediate again suggesting that oxidation is important for the toxicity. In contrast to acetominophen, however, renal glutathione does not seem to protect. The toxic reactant is presumably an electrophilic reactant since nucleophilic sulfydryl compounds decrease its toxicity. Salicylates also cause experimental necrosis of the renal proximal tubules. The lesion is markedly diminished by enzyme inhibitors of the cytochrome P450 system.

In contrast to the drugs which apparently require oxidation or activation to produce their effects, the toxicity of aminoglycosides is not influenced by enzyme inhibition of the cytochrome P450 system. Experiments with neomycin have shown profound effects on polyphosphoinositide metabolism by kidney *in vivo* and by renal homogenates *in vitro*. Because of the evidence for polyphosphoinositides in membrane function in secretory cells it is tempting to postulate an interaction of aminoglycosides with polyphosphoinositide components of the renal tubular cell thus influencing ion transport.

Table V shows drugs which produce toxicity by direct effects on renal tubular epithelium or glomerular structures leading to variable degrees of renal functional impairment.

Intrarenal obstruction may be produced as a secondary phenomenon by a variety of therapeutic agents. Uric acid precipitation in the lumen of renal tubules may occur as a complication of therapy for lymphoreticular malignancies leading to acute urate nephropathy. Methotrexate, an organic acid secreted into the distal tubule, may precipitate in the renal tubule either as the parent drug or a 7-hydroxylated metabolite under conditions of concentrated urine with low pH. This may lead to acute intratubular obstruction. Methoxyflurane anesthesia and ingestion of antifreeze (polyethylene glycol) may be associated with crystalluria and precipitation of oxalate within the renal tubule leading to acute renal failure. Other drugs, e.g., methylsergide, may be associated with retroperitoneal fibrosis and extrarenal obstruction.

Table V. Drugs Which Produce Nephrotoxicity by a Direct Effect on the Renal Parenchyma

1. Antibiotics: aminoglycosides, cephaloridine, polymixin B, colistimethate, demeclocycline
2. Metals: mercury, bismuth, uranium, arsenic, silver, iron, antimony, copper, and lithium
3. Solvents: carbon tetrachloride, glycols
4. Miscellaneous: acetominophen, sulfonamides, amphotericin B, chlorophenothane (DDT), snake venom, streptozotocin, radiological contrast agents, salicylates

B. Immunological

The penicillins, in particular methicillin, have been associated with an interstitial nephritis which is probably mediated via an immune mechanism. The immunopathogenesis of this syndrome is, in some cases, due to circulating antibodies to tubular basement membranes. In addition, there are a variety of glomerulonephritic lesions associated with penicillin G therapy in which an immune basis is suspected. Other drugs that cause similar syndromes are rifampin, sulfonamides, furosemide, cephalothin and phenindione.

III. DIURETICS

In the broadest sense, a diuretic is any agent capable of producing an increase in urine flow directly or indirectly. However, since it has become customary for most physiologists, pharmacologists, and clinicians to limit the definition of diuretics to drugs that act on the kidney to produce a net loss of sodium from body fluids, most of our discussion will be confined to such substances. Diuretics were discovered and used effectively by clinicians long before investigators in this century pondered their site and mechanism of action. Calomel (mercurous chloride) was combined with digitalis in the mid-nineteenth century (Guy's Hospital Pill). Earlier (1919) an astute medical student called the attention of a skeptical attending physician to the marked increase in urine flow recorded by a diligent nurse after administration of an organomercurial (merbaphen) for congenital syphilis. It was not until the 1950s after accidental discovery of the diuretic effect of sulfa derivatives that meaningful attempts were made to uncover the sites of action of diuretics.

A. Possible Renal Mechanisms of Action of Diuretics

Diuretics may exert their effects by (1) redistribution of renal blood flow, (2) altering membrane permeability, (3) directly inhibiting enzymes, e.g., Na–K-ATPase, or hypothetic carrier molecules involved in the translocation of sodium or chloride across cell membranes, or (4) inhibiting cellular metabolism or the supply of energy available for ion transport.

Diuretics generally act to inhibit the reabsorption of salt and water by the epithelial cells of the renal tubules, so that a greater proportion of the glomerular filtrate is excreted, i.e., the fractional excretion of sodium (FE_{Na}) is increased. These compounds for the most part have large effects on ion transport in kidney tubules and minimal effects on ion transport elsewhere in the body. Extensive studies have elucidated the sites of action of diuretics within the nephron and the transport systems affected. However, the molecular basis for their effects is still unclear.

While the primary effects of diuretics are on Na^+ balance, they may, in addition, directly or indirectly influence urinary excretion of other cations. The sites of action of diuretics along the nephron have been studied by (1) clearance techniques, (2) micropuncture, and (3) isolated perfused nephron segments.

The major sites along the nephron where diuretics act are the proximal tubule, the loop of Henle (thin), the thick ascending limb of Henle's loop, the cortical diluting segment, and the cortical collecting duct. Some diuretics have more than one site of action but generally each diuretic has a major site of action along the nephron with which it interacts and effects at this particular segment are responsible for the major portion of the diuresis (see Figure 3).

1. Sites of Action

a. Proximal Tubule Sites

The diuretics which have proximal tubular effects fall into the following classes: (1) carbonic anhydrase inhibitors, (2) osmotic diuretics, and (3) thiazides (weak carbonic anhydrase inhibitors).

i. Carbonic Anhydrase Inhibitors. Sulfanilamide was the first of these compounds and led to the development of the chemically similar acetazolamide, which is now the prototype for diuretics having carbonic anhydrase inhibition as their major mechanism of action. Other diuretics with the same mechanism of action are metazolamide and benzolamide.

Mechanism of action. Inhibition of carbonic anhydrase is noncompetitive and greater than 99% of enzyme in the kidney must be inhibited for effects to occur since the enzyme is in large excess. The concentration of the drug which causes 50% inhibition of the enzyme (IC_{50}) *in vitro* is 7.2×10^{-8} M and its effect on the proximal tubule is greater than its effect on the distal tubule.

Excretion. These drugs are readily absorbed from the gastrointestinal tract. Peak plasma concentrations occur in 2 hr. They are fairly well bound to plasma proteins and hence not readily excreted by filtration. However, they are excreted via the organic acid transport system and reach the tubular lumen via this route.

Effects. The major effects of the carbonic anhydrase inhibitors are to increase (1) HCO_3^- delivery out of the proximal tubule, (2) pH of urine, (3) K^+ excretion in urine, (4) Na^+ and H_2O excretion, and (5) inorganic phosphate excretion in the urine.

The diuretic effect is self-limited since as metabolic acidosis ensues there is a decrease in the filtered load of HCO_3^- presented to the proximal tubule. This causes the drug to lose its effectiveness although continued inhibition of carbonic anhydrase persists.

Uses. Principal uses of carbonic anhydrase inhibitors are the following: (1) Limited use as diuretic agents. (2) Main use in ophthalmology for the

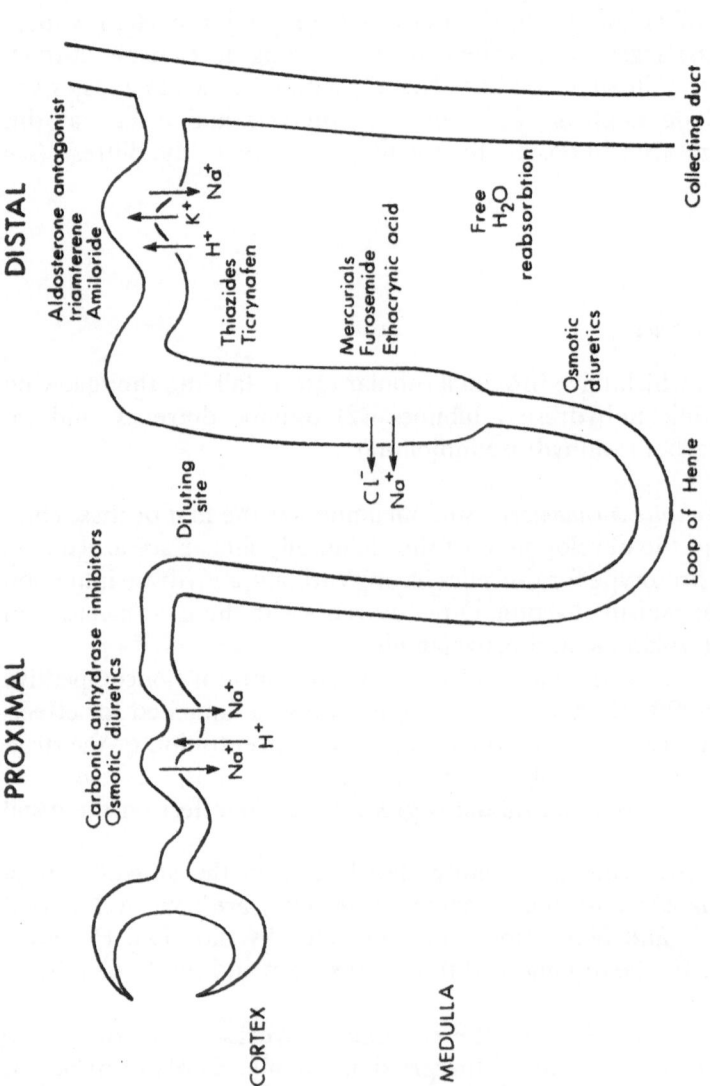

SITE OF DIURETIC ACTION

Figure 3. Sites of action of different diuretics along the nephron. Carbonic anhydrase inhibitors exhibit their major effect in the proximal tubules. Osmotic diuretics exert their effect on both the proximal tubule and the loop of Henle. Mercurials, furosemide, and ethacrynic acid have an effect on the thick ascending limb of Henle's loop. Thiazides and ticrynafen work on the diluting segment. Triamterene, aldosterone antagonists (aldactone), and amiloride exert their effect in the distal tubule and/or cortical collecting duct.

treatment of glaucoma since inhibition of carbonic anhydrase in the ciliary body decreases the production of aqueous humor. (3) Useful in certain conditions where alkalinization of the urine is required.

ii. Osmotic Diuretics. These are low-molecular-weight substances which are freely filtered by the glomerulus and remain in the tubular lumen in high concentrations because of a limitation in their reabsorption. The prototype, mannitol, has a molecular weight of 182. This simple sugar is not metabolized by the body and is not reabsorbed by renal tubules. Thus, it remains in the tubular lumen and exerts an osmotic effect on water movement. Glucose and urea, if present in final urine, may exert osmolar effects similar to mannitol and therefore promote salt and water losses.

Mechanism of action. The presence of an unreabsorbable solute in the proximal tubule reduces the quantity of water reabsorbed in association with active sodium transport by decreasing the osmotic driving force for outward water movement. As sodium is actively pumped out of the proximal tubule, the sodium concentration progressively falls. As this sodium concentration falls, the concentration gradient against which sodium must be transported increases, leading both to a decrease in outward sodium transport and an increase in passive backflux of sodium into the tubule (see Figure 12, Chapter 6). Typically, the urine lost during osmotic diuresis has a urine Na^+ concentration of 50–70 mEq/liter (hypotonic). In addition, recent evidence suggests that osmotic diuretics may cause redistribution to cortical nephrons with reduction of SNGFR in juxtamedullary nephrons.

iii. Thiazides. The thiazides are weak carbonic anhydrase inhibitors. This does not constitute the major mechanism of their diuretic action, which will be discussed fully later.

b. Thin Loops of Henle

At this site the only class of diuretics which have an effect are the osmotic diuretics. These drugs exert their effects by several mechanisms. They increase renal plasma flow and thus disrupt the countercurrent multiplier. This leads to dissipation of the hypertonic medullary interstitium. As a consequence of these alterations there is a decrease in the passive movement of Na^+ out of the thin ascending limb and a fall in the osmotic gradient favoring water movement out of the thin descending limb of Henle's loop (see Figure 13, Chapter 6).

c. Thick Ascending Limb of Henle's Loop

The diuretics which exert their major actions at this site are (1) mercurials, (2) furosemide, and (3) ethacrynic acid.

i. Mercurials. These drugs inhibit reabsorption of Cl^- from the thick ascending limb of Henle's Loop. Because of these effects, they inhibit the countercurrent multiplier and, therefore, decrease the osmolality of the medullary interstitium. These effects impair the ability of concentrate the urine, i.e., they decrease the negative free water clearance, $T^C_{H_2O}$. In addition, they impair the reabsorption of Cl^- and Na^+ out of the diluting segment and therefore impair the generation of free water, i.e., the free water clearance, C_{H_2O}. Thus, these diuretics increase urinary excretion of Cl^- and Na^+ and dramatically increase urine flow with the production of an isosthenuric urine. Mercurials are administered parenterally and are rapidly excreted by the kidney. Fifty percent of the administered dose can be recovered in the urine in 3 hr. They exert their effect from the luminal side of the tubular epithelium and are probably secreted into the tubular lumen via the organic acid transport system. Experimentally, the effects of the mercurial can be reversed by p-chloromercuribenzoate (a nondiuretic mercurial) and dimercaprol (a Hg^{2+} chelator), suggesting that these agents exert their action by interacting with sulfydryl groups on tubular epithelial cells.

In addition to their effects on the diluting segment, mercurial diuretics also act in the distal convoluted tubule and inhibit K^+ secretion, which explains why K^+ loss is less of a problem with mercurials than with other diuretics which do not have this effect. These effects on K^+ handling probably relate to the effect of mercurials on the membrane permeability of the cortical collecting duct epithelium.

Acidifying salts enhance the diuretic effect of mercurials while alkalinizing salts reduce their effectiveness. This was initially attributed to effects on urinary pH. However, *in vitro* experiments with isolated perfused tubules have failed to confirm that changes in luminal pH alter the effect of the diuretic on Cl^- transport. More recently the suggestion has been made that the levels of citrate whose excretion increases during alkalosis might inactivate the mercurials by chelation.

Preparations. Currently there are only two preparations: (1) Mercaptomerin sodium U.S.P. (Thiomerin) and (2) Meralluride N.F. (Mercurhydrin).

Mercurials are not used now because (1) they have to be administered parenterally, (2) more effective diuretics are available with less potential toxicity, and (3) they have considerable toxicity which includes arrythmias, flushing, gastrointestinal disturbances, and dermatitis.

ii. Furosemide (Lasix, Figure 4). Furosemide is a sulfamyl-benzene derivative of anthranilic acid and like the thiazides is a very weak carbonic anhydrase inhibitor. Its major effect and site of action, however, are unrelated to its modest inhibition of carbonic anhydrase. The drug is strongly bound to plasma proteins. Of an oral dose, two thirds are excreted by the kidney via filtration and tubular secretion and one third is excreted in the feces.

iii. Ethacrynic acid (Sodium Edecrin). Ethacrynic acid is one of a class of aryloxyacetic acids initially synthesized for their selective reactivity with functionally important sulfydryl groups, based on the belief that organic mercurials exert their effects by inhibition of sulfydryl-containing enzyme systems (Figure 4).

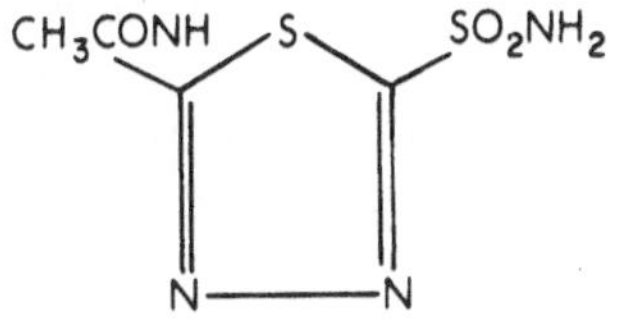

ACETAZOLAMIDE

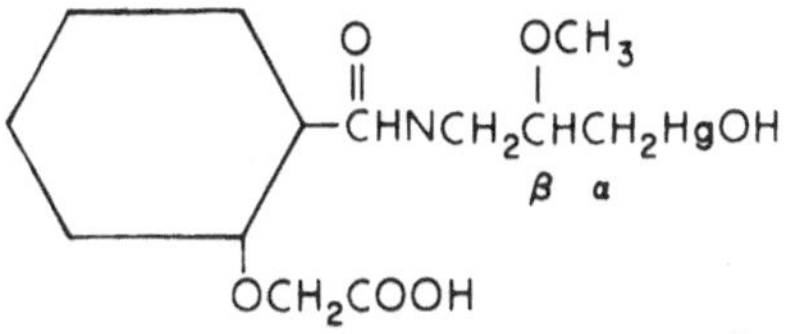

MERSALYL

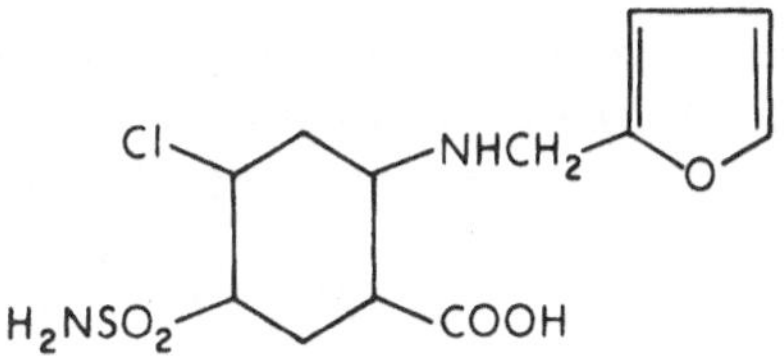

FUROSEMIDE

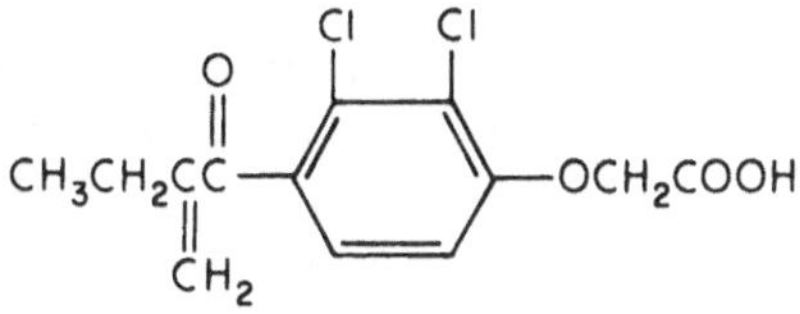

ETHACRYNIC ACID

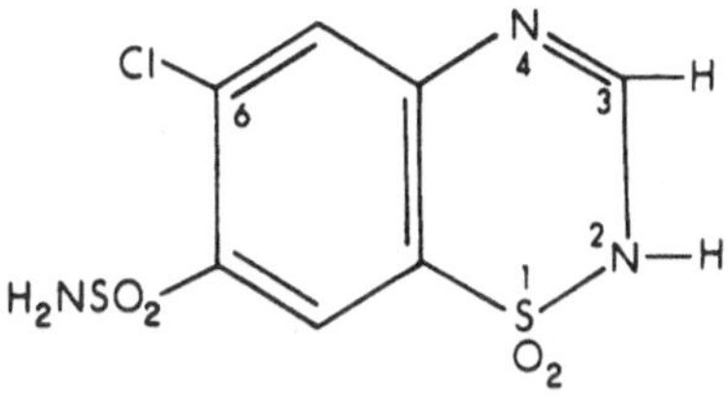

CHLOROTHIAZIDE

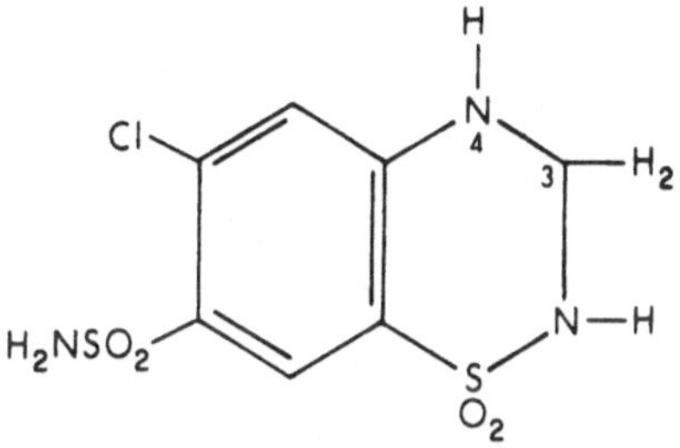

HYDROCHLOROTHIAZIDE

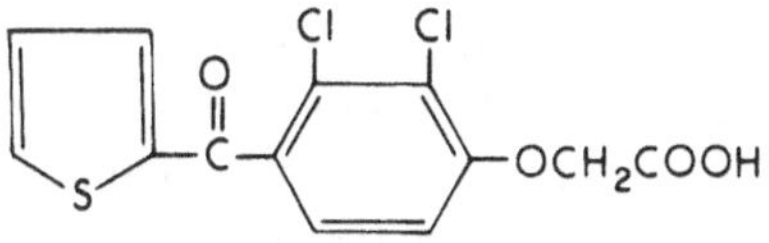

TICRYNAFEN

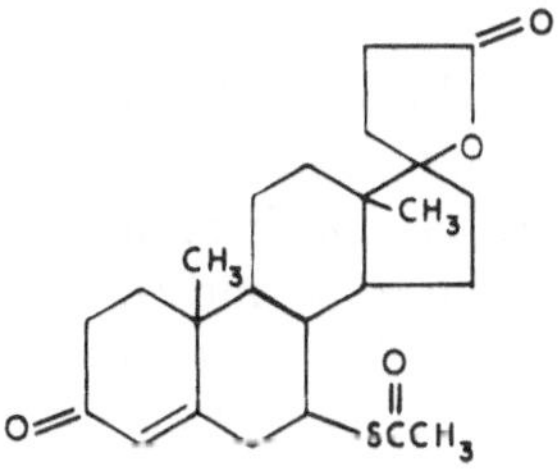

ALDACTONE

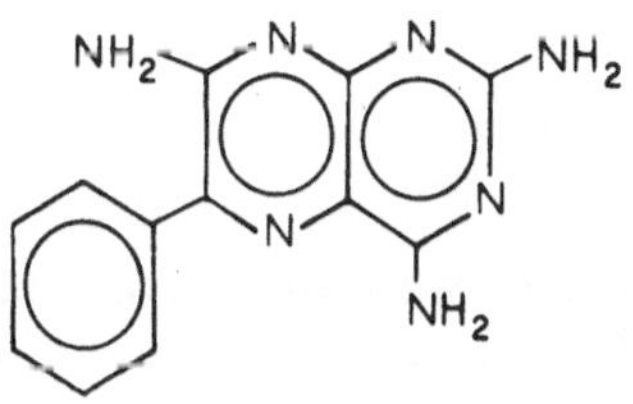

TRIAMTERENE

Figure 4. Structural formulas of commonly used diuretics.

This drug is highly bound to plasma proteins. An IV dose is excreted two thirds by the kidney and one third by the liver.

The drug is present in the urine in three forms: (1) parent compound, 30%; (2) cysteine adduct, 30%; (3) unstable metabolite of undetermined nature, 30%.

iv. Diuretic Characteristics of Furosemide and Ethacrynic Acid:

1. Prompt onset of action.
2. Rapid excretion (furosemide > ethacrynic acid).
3. Action independent of acid–base status.
4. Secreted by organic acid secretory mechanism of proximal tubule.
5. Inhibit active Cl^- transport and decreases transepithelial voltage in the ascending limb of Henle's loop, thus increasing U_{Na}, U_{Cl}, and urinary volume.
6. Decrease free-water clearance and decrease $T^C_{H_2O}$ (similar to mercurials).
7. Both exert their effects from the luminal side of the membrane, i.e., the urine side.
8. Inhibit membrane transport ATPase. However, at concentrations which cause diuresis *in vivo* there is very little evidence for inhibition of Na–K-ATPase *in vitro*.
9. Inhibit glycolysis.
10. Decrease mitochondrial O_2 consumption.
11. Cause marked increase in U_{Ca} and U_{Mg}.

In spite of these effects on metabolism, the mechanism of action of these drugs is not well defined. Most evidence suggests that they may act by decreasing the permeability of the luminal membrane of the thick ascending loop to chloride.

v. Special Effects. Ethacrynic acid. The active agent is probably an ethacrynic-cysteine adduct. Dimercaprol, an agent which antagonizes sulfydryl active reagents, poorly antagonizes the effects of ethacrynic acid. In addition, this drug is ototoxic and should be avoided in end stage renal disease.

Furosemide. In addition to its effects on thick ascending limb of Henle's loop, it is a weak carbonic anhydrase inhibitor. This drug is also a weak phosphaturic agent, thus indicating mild effects on proximal tubular function.

d. Cortical Diluting Segment

The two major classes of drugs acting at this site of the nephron are as follows:

i. Thiazides. The thiazides were discovered during testing for carbonic anhydrase inhibiting analogs of sulfanilamide. Although the renal activity of these drugs is in part related to carbonic anhydrase inhibition, this is not the major reason for the diuresis produced by these drugs because (1) the diuretic effect can be dissociated from the carbonic anhydrase inhibitory activity, (2) the diuresis is associated with minor alterations in urinary bicarbonate, and (3) increases in sodium excretion occur above the dose required for maximal carbonic anhydrase inhibition.

Structure–activity relationships. The simplest of the thiazides is chlorothiazide (Figure 4), which is referred to as a nonhydrogenated thiazide. Its potency can be increased by hydrogenation in positions 3 and 4 to form hydrochlorothiazide (Figure 4). Further increases in potency can be achieved by substituting benzyl or dichloromethane groups at position 3. The maximal diuretic effects of the thiazides are equivalent and their dose–response curves are parallel, suggesting similar modes of action (Figure 5). Thus, the same therapeutic effect can be attained by all the thiazides by using the appropriate dosage.

Site and mechanism of action. These drugs act at the cortical diluting segment of the loop of Henle inhibiting reabsorption of Cl^- and Na^+, thus increasing the osmolality of this segment of the nephron and impairing the ability to dilute the urine, thus impairing the generation of free water (C_{H_2O}).

In addition, by virtue of their carbonic anhydrase inhibitory properties thiazides decrease reabsorption of bicarbonate and sodium in the proximal tubule and increase bicarbonate excretion.

Absorption—fate and distribution. Thiazides are easily absorbed from the gastrointestinal tract. Their diuretic effect is seen within an hour of an oral dose. Chlorothiazide is distributed throughout the extracellular space and it passes the placental barrier to the fetus.

Thiazides are actively secreted by the organic acid transport system. Most compounds are excreted within 3–6 hr. In nephrectomized animals, chlorothiazide is excreted in the bile without metabolic alterations.

ii. Ticrynafen (Tienilic Acid). This drug is chemically a substituted phenoxyacetic acid and thus structurally related to ethacrynic acid (Figure 4). Its site of action is the cortical diluting segment of the distal nephron with effects similar to those of thiazides. However, it has a marked uricosuric effect due

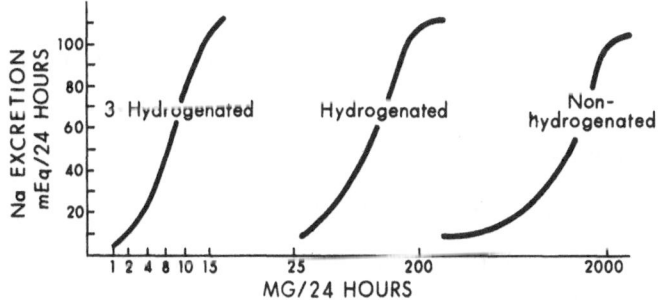

Figure 5. Parallel dose–response curves for various unsubstituted and substituted thiazides. The diuretic potency (Na excretion) increases with hydrogenation.

to inhibition of urate reabsorption, and may, therefore, be useful in treating hyperuricemia.

Ticrynafen is highly protein bound. Its diuretic effect is dependent on renal tubular secretion (by an organic acid pathway). Recently, this drug has been reported to cause hepatotoxicity, and has been removed from the market by the FDA.

e. Cortical Collecting Duct

i. Aldosterone Antagonist. Aldosterone acts on the cortical collecting duct to increase Na^+ reabsorption and promote K^+ excretion (see Chapter 7). Aldosterone (a mineralocorticoid) is first bound by a cytosolic protein which allows translocation of the compound to the nucleus of the responsive epithelial cells to cause transcription of messenger RNA which codes for the production of proteins which are involved in Na^+ transport. Thus, drugs with antagonize aldosterone would be natriuretic and kaliuretic. The prototype, spironolactone (Aldactone, Figure 4) is a competitive inhibitor of aldosterone. This drug (1) inhibits binding of aldosterone to cytosolic protein, (2) is effective only in the presence of aldosterone, (3) is a relatively weak diuretic, (4) decreases K^+ excretion (main attribute) in the urine, and (5) can cause gynecomastia in males, irregular menses, hirsutism, and deepening of the voice in females.

ii. Triamterene. This drug is a pteridine compound related to folic acid (Figure 4). It is rapidly absorbed when administered orally and excreted in the urine. The peak excretion in urine occurs one to two hours after ingestion. In plasma, about two thirds are protein bound and one third is free.

Its mechanism of action is independent of aldosterone. It decreases the transepithelial voltage in the distal convoluted tubule and decreases the electrochemical gradient for K^+ movement. It is effective on the luminal side of the membrane and inhibits the entry of Na^+ from lumen to cell. In addition, triamterene inhibits a H^+ ion pump on the luminal membrane, thus decreasing H^+ ion secretion in the distal tubule and increasing urine pH. As a diuretic, this drug is not very potent but is useful when used in combination with a thiazide to reduce the potassium losses in the urine.

iii. Amiloride. This drug is halopyrazine carboxamide, similar in site of action to triamterene. It is now available in the United States for human use.

2. Clinical Use of Diuretics

a. Na^+-Retaining States (Edema-Forming States)

These include (1) congestive heart failure, (2) nephrotic syndrome, and (3) hepatic failure with ascites. Although all of the above states have secondary hyperaldosteronism, aldosterone antagonists are not very useful as primary therapy because (1) the Na^+-retaining state is only in part related to increased mineralocorticoid-dependent Na^+ reabsorption, and (2) at best K^+-sparing diuretics and aldosterone antagonists can only result in the excretion of 1.5%–2% of the filtered load of Na^+. Therefore, diuretic agents like thiazides, furosemide, and ethacrynic acid are the drugs of choice.

b. Promotion of Negative Na^+ Balance

For promotion of negative Na^+ balance, e.g., in hypertensive patients, thiazides, either alone or in conjunction with antihypertensive agents, are useful. Aldosterone antagonists, e.g., spironolactone, may have specific effects when used in positive Na^+ balance states related to primary aldosteronism (Conn's syndrome). The major use of spironolactone and K^+-sparing diuretics is in conjunction with diuretics which induce K^+ loss in order to offset the K^+ losses generated by the more potent diuretics.

c. Nondiuretic Uses of Diuretic Agents

i. Nephrogenic Diabetes Insipidus. The thiazides are very useful since they produce volume contraction and decrease Na^+ and Cl^- delivery to the distal nephron segment. This results in a decrease in urine output.

ii. Treatment of Inappropriate Secretion of ADH. A drug like furosemide may be useful by increasing urinary water in excess of Na^+ while Na^+ losses are simultaneously replaced. This would tend to increase serum Na concentrations (see Chapter 6).

iii. Treatment of Hypercalcemia—Furosemide Plus Saline Diuresis. Furosemide inhibits reabsorption of Ca^{2+} in the renal tubule; thus it will produce a negative Ca^{2+} balance (see Chapter 9).

iv. Idiopathic Hypercalciuria—Thiazides. The thiazides decrease urinary calcium excretion by increasing proximal tubular reabsorption of calcium as a consequence of ECF volume contraction (see Chapters 9 and 16).

v. Glaucoma. Carbonic anhydrase inhibitors will decrease production of aqueous humor and decrease intraocular pressure.

3. Complications

The use of diuretics, like that of many other therapeutic agents, is associated with side effects and complications. Some of these are hypokalemia, hyperuricemia, and metabolic alkalosis.

a. Understanding Hypokalemia Induced by Diuretics

Increased K^+ excretion in the urine is produced by all diuretics which act at sites of the nephron proximal to the cortical collecting duct (site of K^+ secretion). Exceptions are mercurials because of their direct inhibitory action on K^+ transport.

The increased K^+ secretion may be related to increased distal tubular flow rate and the delivery of less permeant anions to these segments. Volume contraction, secondary to diuretics, and consequent hyperaldosteronism will also promote K^+ loss (for a detailed discussion of K^+ handling see Chapter 7).

Thus, hypokalemia is a very common complication of the most commonly used diuretics.

Some of the many abnormalities resulting from hypokalemia include the following:

1. Metabolic: Abnormal carbohydrate metabolism (deficient insulin release).
2. Cardiac effects: ECG changes, e.g., flattened T waves, and development of U waves; may accentuate digitalis toxicity and predispose to arrythmias.
3. Neuromuscular effects: Ileus, weakness, tetany, encephalopathy in patients with hepatic disease; rhabdomyolysis.
4. Renal effects: Polyuria and polydipsia; hypokalemic nephropathy.

b. Hyperuricemia

Plasma uric acid may rise as a consequence of the use of thiazides and/or furosemide. These drugs elevate plasma urate by increasing urate absorption from the proximal tubule due to ECF volume contraction and also decrease urate clearance by decreasing its tubular secretion. In patients with gout, the changes in uric acid handling produced by these diuretics may precipitate an acute attack of gout.

c. Metabolic Alkalosis

This is dealt with more extensively in Chapter 8. Suffice it to say that diuretic therapy will generate metabolic alkalosis by producing hypokalemia and maintain the alkalosis via volume contraction.

IV. MISCELLANEOUS DRUGS WITH RENAL ACTION

A. Probenecid

Probenecid is a benzoic acid derivative whose action is largely confined to the inhibition of the renal tubular transport of organic acids.

Probenecid has a high affinity for the organic acid carrier system and does not readily dissociate from it. Thus, it will interfere with transport of other organic acids without itself being significantly excreted. In addition, it has a high lipid solubility of its nonionized form which results in almost complete reabsorption by backdiffusion.

Uses of probenecid: (1) Probenecid increases the plasma levels and prolongs the action of penicillin by blocking the tubular secretion of the antibiotic. (2) Small doses inhibit tubular secretion of uric acid; however, larger doses inhibit reabsorption and thus are uricosuric. Because of its uricosuric action, probenecid is used in the treatment of hyperuricemia to enhance urinary excretion of uric acid. May be used by itself or in combination with colchicine.

B. Drugs Affecting Uric Acid Handling

i. Probenecid. See above.

ii. Diuretics. Thiazides, furosemide, and ethacrynic acid all may produce ECF volume contraction and all are transported by the organic acid pathway and effectively compete with uric acid for secretion by the tubule. Hence, hyperuricemia is a potential complication when using these diuretics.

iii. Ticrynaphen (tienelic acid). Ticrynaphen competes for tubular reabsorption of uric acid and thus is uricosuric.

iv. Other Drugs. Other drugs which may compete with uric acid for secretion via the organic acid carrier-mediated transport process are diodrast, PAH, salicylates, sulfinpyrazone, and pyrazinamide.

C. Drugs Affecting Prostaglandin Biosynthesis

Endogenous renal prostaglandin biosynthesis may, in part, be responsible for the distribution of regional blood flow within the kidney. Thus, inhibition of total prostaglandin biosynthesis by inhibition of the cyclooxygenase (the enzyme which is responsible for oxygenation of arachidonic acid) may cause redistribution of renal blood flow (see Chapter 3).

Drugs such as aspirin, indomethacin, and other nonsteroidal antiinflammatory agents have been shown to cause redistribution of blood flow from outer cortex to juxtamedullary areas. In addition, in situations in which dilator prostaglandins may be playing a role in maintaining renal blood flow (e.g., in cirrhosis of liver with ascites, low salt intake), therapy with indomethacin or ibuprofen may cause decreases in renal blood flow and GFR.

SUGGESTED READINGS

Bennett, W. M., Singer, I., Golper, T., Felig, P., and Coggins, C. J.: Guidelines for drug therapy in renal failure. *Ann. Intern. Med.* 86:754–783, 1977.

Bennett, W. M., Muther, R. S., Parker, R. A., Feig, P., Morrison, G., Golper, T. A., and Singer, I.: Drug therapy in renal failure: dosing guidelines for adults. I. *Ann. Intern. Med.* 93:62–89, 1980.

Bennett, W. M., Muther, R. S., Parker, R. A., Feig, P., Morrison, G., Golper, T. A., and Singer,

I.: Drug therapy in renal failure: dosing guidelines for adults. II. *Ann. Intern. Med.* 93:286–325, 1980.

Gennan, F. J., and Kassirer, J. P.: Osmotic diuresis. *N. Engl. J. Med.* 291:714–720, 1974.

Gilman, A. G., Goodman, L. S., and Gilman, A. (eds.): *The Pharmacological Basis of Therapeutics,* Sixth edition. Macmillan Publishing Co., New York, 1980.

Goldstein, A., Aronow, L., and Kalman, S. M.: *The Principles of Drug Action,* Second edition. John Wiley and Sons, New York, 1976.

Jacobson, H. R., and Kokko, J. P.: Diuretics: sites and mechanisms of action. *Annu. Rev. Pharmacol.* 16:201–214, 1976.

Koch-Weser, J., and Sellers, E. M.: Binding of drugs to serum albumin. *N. Engl. J. Med.* 294:311–326, 1976.

Melmon, K. L., and Morrelei, H. F. (eds.): *Clinical Pharmacology,* Second edition. Macmillan Publishing Co., New York, 1978.

Mudge, G. H., and Duggin, G. G. (eds.): Symposium on drug effects on the kidney. *Kidney Int.* 18:539, 1980.

Reineck, J., and Stein, J. H.: Mechanisms of action and clinical uses of diuretics, in Brenner, B. M., and Rector, F. C. (eds.): *The Kidney,* Second edition. W. B. Saunders, Philadelphia, 1981, Chap. 22, p. 1097–1134.

Symposium on drug action and metabolism in renal failure. *Am. J. Med.* 62:459–562, 1977.

Index

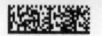